An Introduction to Practical Pharmacy: Designed As a Text-Book for the Student, & As a Guide for the Physician & Pharmaceutist. with Many Formulas & Prescriptions

Edward Parrish

W. G. Wayman
Feb 186.

INTRODUCTION

TO

PRACTICAL PHARMACY:

DESIGNED AS A

TEXT-BOOK FOR THE STUDENT,

AND AS A

GUIDE FOR THE PHYSICIAN AND PHARMACEUTIST.

WITH

MANY FORMULAS AND PRESCRIPTIONS.

BY

EDWARD PARRISH,

GRADUATE IN PHARMACY; MEMBER OF THE PHILADELPHIA COLLEGE OF PHARMACY, AND OF THE AMERICAN PHARMACEUTICAL ASSOCIATION; AND PRINCIPAL OF THE SCHOOL OF PRACTICAL PHARMACY, PHILADELPHIA.

SECOND EDITION, GREATLY ENLARGED AND IMPROVED.

WITH TWO HUNDRED AND FORTY-SIX ILLUSTRATIONS.

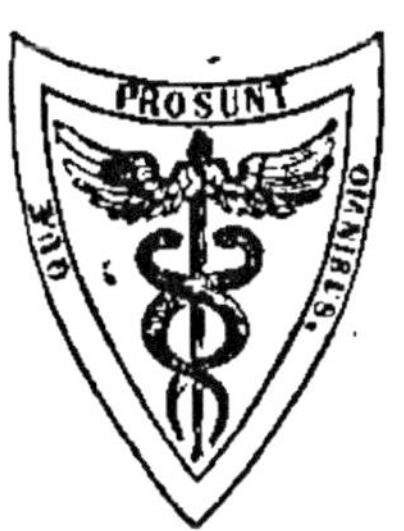

PHILADELPHIA:
BLANCHARD AND LEA.
1859.

PHILADELPHIA:
COLLINS, PRINTER, 705 JAYNE STREET.

TO

WILLIAM PROCTER, Jr.,

PROFESSOR OF THEORY AND PRACTICE OF PHARMACY IN THE PHILADELPHIA COLLEGE OF PHARMACY,
EDITOR OF THE AMERICAN JOURNAL OF PHARMACY, ETC.,

This Work is Inscribed

AS A TESTIMONIAL TO HIS ZEAL AND ABILITY

IN

PROSECUTING THE ART AND SCIENCE OF PHARMACY,

AND AS A

TRIBUTE OF THE ENDURING FRIENDSHIP AND ESTEEM

OF

THE AUTHOR.

PREFACE

TO THE

SECOND EDITION.

THE success of the first edition of this work has abundantly proved its adaptation to the wants of those for whom it was written, and has stimulated the effort, in its revision, to make it worthy of still more general acceptance.

To keep pace with the progress of pharmacy within the past few years has required the most persevering industry and zeal. Since the first publication of this work, numerous chemical, physiological, and therapeutical discoveries have added to the resources of the physician, with a corresponding enlargement of the domain of pharmacy, while the progress of scientific education and enterprise among pharmaceutists has multiplied the number and perfected the details of their processes.

Besides the increased size of the page, and the abundant use of smaller type in the least important parts, it has been found necessary to add nearly two hundred pages of new matter, and to provide a number of original drawings in addition to the very extensive series of illustrations contained in the first edition. In these additions I have kept steadily in view the elementary character of the work, which is appropriately styled, "An Introduction to Practical Pharmacy," and have kept the more strictly scientific facts distinct from those which are elementary and practical.

The extensive use of syllabi, which formed a conspicuous feature in the first edition, has been found so convenient as to be still further extended in the present. In this form we are enabled to present to the eye an immense number of facts in small space, and to display them effectively in their relations to each other. The syllabi in Part III. and Part IV. have been prepared with great labor, and are especially commended to careful study.

In the labor of the present revision, and especially in collating and extending the parts just named, I have been much assisted by my friend, John M. Maisch, of this city, to whose original investigations we owe many interesting facts in the history of the essential oils, and other valuable contributions to pharmaceutical knowledge.

In developing the important relations of pharmacy to organic chemistry, many recent foreign works have been consulted not generally accessible to students in this country, and it is confidently believed that the present issue will be found a fair exponent of the state of pharmaceutical science up to the time of its issue.

This volume is not the work of a secluded student in his closet, it has been composed by a practical pharmaceutist and druggist, in the midst of the daily routine of his shop, and surrounded by the difficulties incident to an active business career; it is, necessarily, imperfect in many of its details; but the first edition having been received with an appreciation of its scope and design, the second is commended to the favorable consideration of physicians and pharmaceutists.

Attention is called to the Instructions how to Study and Consult the Work, and to the Table of Contents, which follow.

INSTRUCTIONS

HOW TO

STUDY AND CONSULT THE WORK.

ERRATA.

P. 133, line 1 from bottom, for Cochineal ℥ss, read ʒss.

P. 372, line 15 from bottom, for "*bicarbonate of potassa*," read "*bichromate of potassa.*"

P. 472, the first paragraph, including formula, from "In presenting" to "Water —— 1 gallon," &c., should be inserted under head of "Liquor Magnesiæ Citratis."

P. 634, in Mixture of Acetone, &c., read Acetone fʒj instead of f℥j.

3. The Processes for preparing and dispensing medicines are fully detailed in Parts II. and V., especially those practicable with the ordinary facilities of the dispensing office and shop.

4. Of Chemical Compounds, organic and inorganic, the Composition is given in the syllabi; the Processes for their preparation, the Tests for their purity, and their Uses are given in the text.

5. In consulting the index, the most ready method of finding a preparation is to refer to the class to which it belongs. An inorganic salt is best found under the head of its metallic base, an organic compound by its most common name. Many of the organic compounds, as essential oils, mentioned only in the syllabi, are not placed in the index, as the arrangement of the syllabi facilitates a reference to them.

CONTENTS.

PART I.

PRELIMINARY.

CHAPTER I.

CHAPTER II.

CHAPTER III.

PART II.

GALENICAL PHARMACY.

CHAPTER I.

CHAPTER II.

CHAPTER III.

CHAPTER IV.

CHAPTER V.

CHAPTER VI.

CHAPTER VII.

CHAPTER VIII.

CHAPTER IX.

CHAPTER X.

CHAPTER XI.

CHAPTER XII.

CHAPTER XIII.

CHAPTER XIV.

CHAPTER XV.

PART III.

ON PHARMACY IN ITS RELATIONS TO ORGANIC CHEMISTRY.

CHAPTER I.

CHAPTER II.

CHAPTER III.

CHAPTER IV.

CHAPTER V.

CHAPTER VI.

CHAPTER VII.

CHAPTER VIII.

CHAPTER IX.

PART IV.

INORGANIC PHARMACEUTICAL PREPARATIONS.

CHAPTER I.

CHAPTER II.

CHAPTER III.

CHAPTER IV.

CHAPTER V.

CHAPTER VI.

CHAPTER VII.

CHAPTER VIII.

CHAPTER IX.

CHAPTER X.

CHAPTER XI.

PART V.

EXTEMPORANEOUS PHARMACY.

CHAPTER I.

CHAPTER II.

CHAPTER III.

CHAPTER IV.

CHAPTER V.

CHAPTER VI.

CHAPTER VII.

APPENDIX.

LIST OF ILLUSTRATIONS.

2

ALPHABETICAL INDEX

OF

CLASSES OF MEDICINES AND PREPARATIONS,

DISPLAYED IN THE FORM OF SYLLABI.

MISCELLANEOUS TABLES.

PRACTICAL PHARMACY.

PART I.

PRELIMINARY.

CHAPTER I.

ON THE FURNITURE AND IMPLEMENTS NECESSARY TO THE DISPENSING OFFICE OR SHOP.

THE various forms of apparatus required by the pharmaceutist in the preparation and dispensing of medicines, will be brought into view in connection with the pharmaceutical processes, successively described and illustrated throughout this work. In the present preliminary chapter, it will suffice to describe those most simple kinds of apparatus which are indispensable to the country practitioner in the performance of the manipulations coming within the range of his office practice, and are also useful as part of the necessary outfit of the apothecary.

Fig. 1.

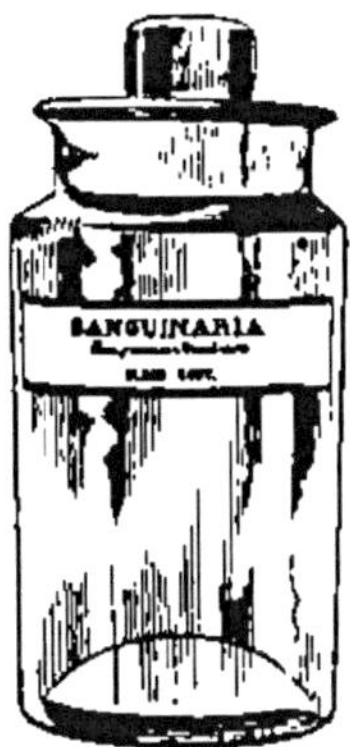

Broad German salt-mouth, adapted to materia medica specimens.

THE FURNITURE BOTTLES.—Much depends upon the selection of suitable bottles to contain a stock of medicines. They should be of flint glass, and fitted with well-ground glass stoppers. Recently our market has been supplied with a kind of German glassware, which possesses the advantage of cheapness and freedom from color. German bottles are generally of greater diameter in proportion to their height, and those designed for solids, possess wider mouths, and consequently larger stoppers than American bottles of the same capacity. Fig. 1 represents one of this description. They are well adapted for putting up specimens of the materia medica, for study and illustration, but are generally too thin and frail to serve a good purpose as furniture bottles. Besides these, there is a variety of German bottles known as mushroom stoppers, shown in Fig. 2, which are tall, and of small diameter. The stopper is less liable to be broken, and the shape is considered by many as in better taste.

Figs. 3, 4, and 5 are forms of German salt-mouth and tincture bottles, made extra heavy, adapted to containing chemical tests and re-

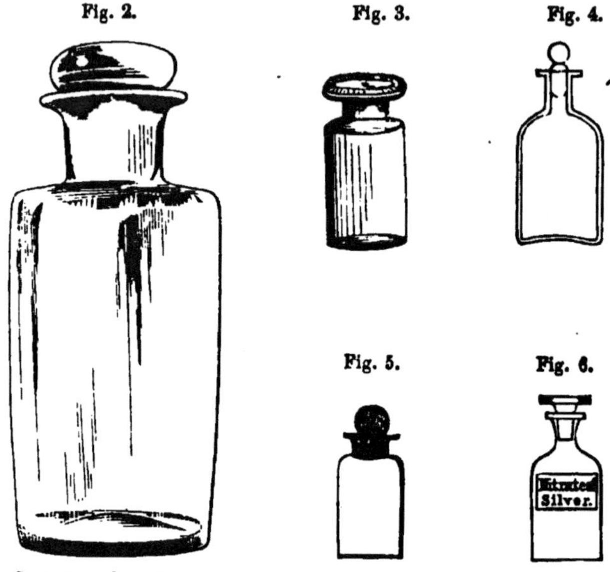

Fig. 2. German mushroom stopper. Fig. 3. Fig. 4. Fig. 5. Fig. 6.

agents, and much used in laboratories. Though of inelegant shapes, they are too expensive to be generally used by physicians and pharmaceutists.

Fig. 6 shows an imported bottle with enamelled label for solutions of nitrate of silver. This label being engraved in the glass is not liable to be corroded or washed off; though designed for chemical laboratories, this is a useful article of furniture in the dispensing office or shop.

The American made bottles are of two kinds, those blown and finished without a mould (Fig. 7), which are the most transparent and smoothest kind, and those blown in a mould (Figs. 8 and 9), to which I usually give preference in fitting up a physician's dispensing office from their greater uniformity of size and shape. The hollow stopper, shown in Fig. 8, is also moulded and afterwards ground; it has advantages over any other description of stopper.

The form of a bottle mould has much to do with the beauty and utility of the bottle. That used for my salt-mouth and tincture bottles is a solid iron cylinder so thick as to retain the heat imparted by the successive charges of fused glass blown into it, and thus to avoid the unpolished surface often produced on the glass by suddenly chilling it in contact with the sides of the mould. On the top of this solid iron cylinder is a pivot, near the outer edge, to which movable shoulder

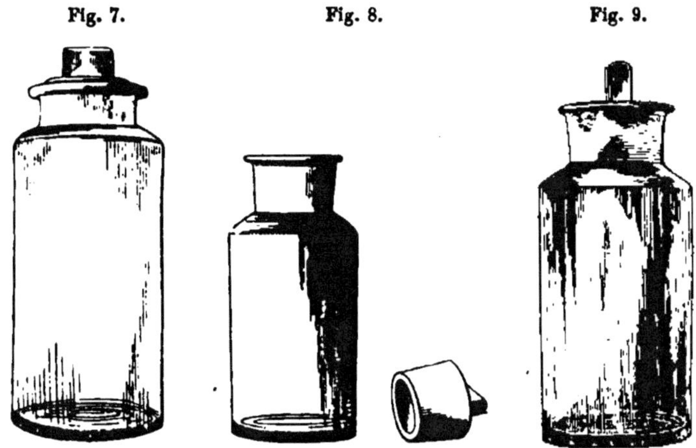

Fig. 7. American blown salt-mouth.

Fig. 8. Moulded salt-mouth, showing hollow stopper.

Fig. 9. Moulded salt-mouth.

moulds are attached; each of these is in two parts, opening and closing by a lever attached; when closed, they form the shoulder and neck of the bottle; the lip is finished in the usual way by a tool. As the bottle is to be drawn out of the mould with facility when blown, the cylinder is tapered slightly towards the bottom, but this is so slight as not to be observed in the bottle.

The advantages of this kind of mould over those which open through their whole length, are that there is no liability to a ridge down the side of the bottle, and that the same mould, by adapting to it different shoulder moulds, will furnish at pleasure salt-mouth or tincture bottles. Figs. 8 and 11 are made in the same mould with different shoulder attachments.

Bottles with wide mouths and ground glass stoppers, designed for solids, are called salt-mouths; those with narrow mouths and ground glass stoppers, for liquids, are called tinctures.

Tinctures with very long necks and narrow mouths, as shown in Fig. 10, though desirable sometimes for containing very volatile liquids, are inconvenient for syrups and the fixed oils, and very ill adapted to dropping. They are also less readily cleaned than the ordinary tincture bottles shown in Figs. 11 and 12, which have necks no longer than that of a salt-mouth; it is necessary, however, that the stoppers of these should be well fitted and ground.

Besides the foregoing, there are two kinds of bottles frequently employed in furnishing the physician's outfit, where cheapness is the chief consideration, viz:—

The *specia jar*, which consists of a wide mouth bottle without a lip e mouth of which is covered by a tin top. This is objectionable not excluding the air, and it is also less cleanly and neat than the lt-mouth. It is rather cheaper.

Fig. 10.

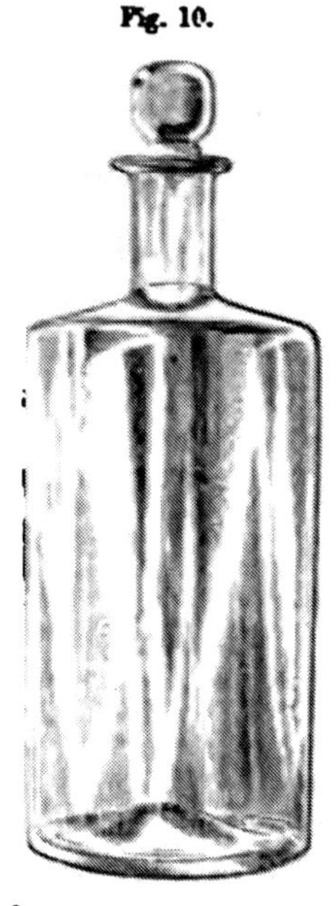

Long-neck German tincture.

Fig. 11.

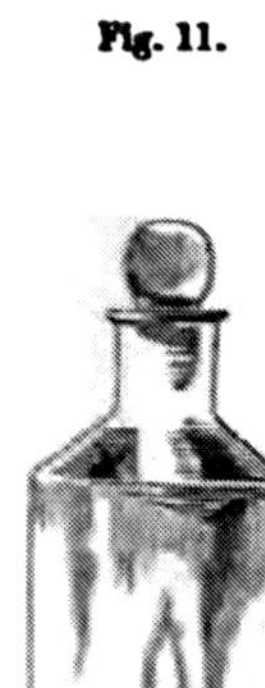

American moulded tincture.

Fig. 12.

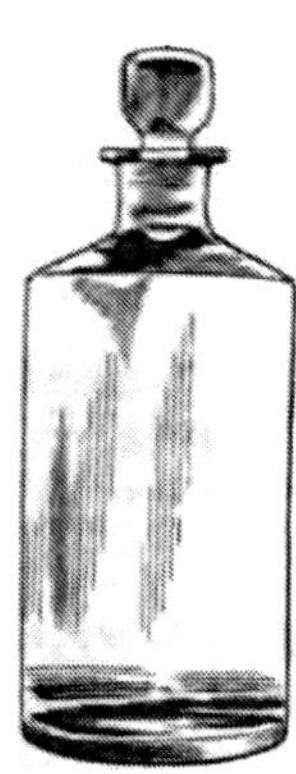

Ordinary American blown tincture.

Fig. 13 represents a bottle I have imported, which is admirably ntrived to keep fixed oils, for the purpose of dispensing. The lip of the bottle is furnished with a flange nearly at right angles to it, which is ground on the outer surface, so as to fit a cap shown separately in the right hand figure. Into the neck of the bottle is inserted a ground glass stopper, also shown separately in the drawing, which is perforated by a lipped tube, and has upon the side opposite the lip a groove for the admission of air in pouring out the oil.

Fig. 13.

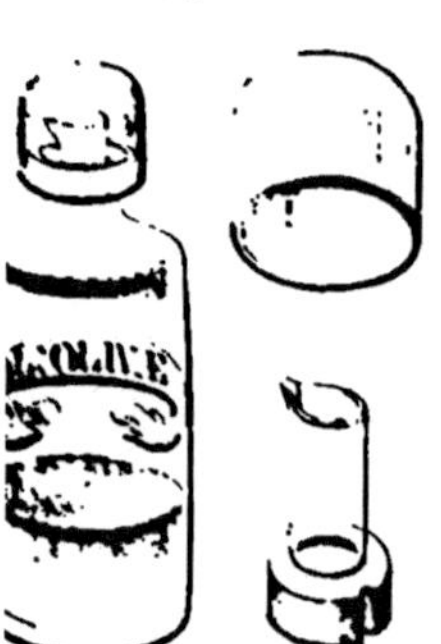

The object of this arrangement will be obvious. In drawing oil from the bottle it flows through the tubed stopper, running in a thin stream from the lip, and any portion which runs down the outside collects in the gutter formed by the outer lip and runs back into the bottle through the groove in e side of the stopper. The cap keeps this oily portion from becomg dusty, and protects the contents from the action of the air. A bottle of this description may be used for years without becoming greasy on the outside.

Fig. 14.

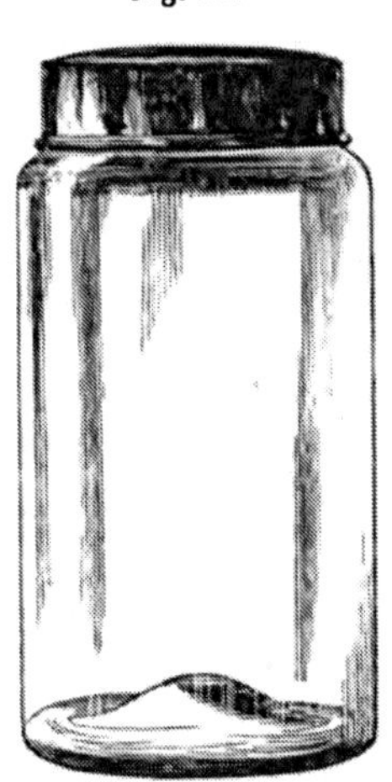

Specia jar.

Fig. 15.

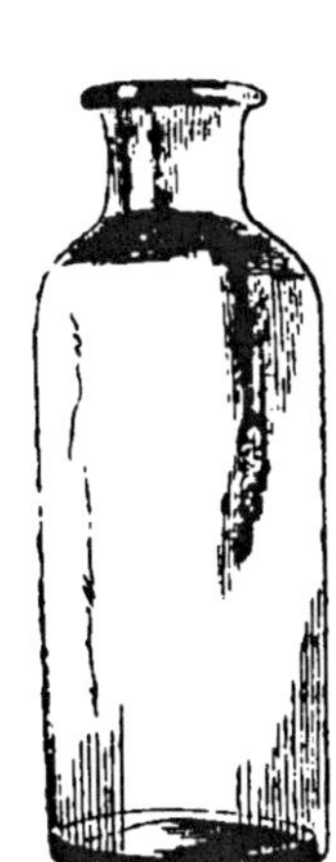

Common wide-mouth packer.

Packing bottles are made either with a wide mouth for solids, as in Figs. 15 and 16, or a narrow mouth for liquids, as in Figs. 17 and 18; these are stopped by corks, and are the least desirable kind of furni-

Fig. 16. Fig. 17. Fig. 18.

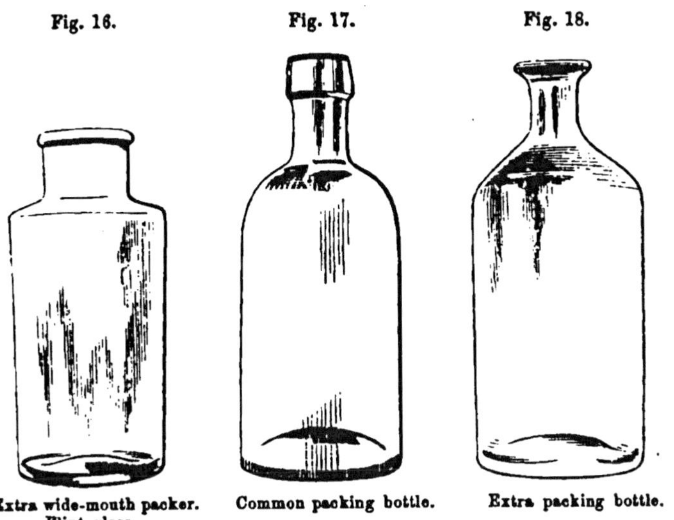

Extra wide-mouth packer. Flint glass. Common packing bottle. Extra packing bottle.

ture bottle, though very useful for transporting medicines, or for keeping extra supplies with which to replenish the regular furniture bottles. Packing bottles are comparatively cheap, and are generally stronger than salt-mouths or tinctures. They are usually made of green glass, and may be formed without a lip, called common (Fig 17), or with a lip called extra (Fig. 18). Those with the lip are the most approved, and hold somewhat more than their nominal capacity.

Neat round wooden boxes, some of which are imported and others manufactured in New England, have been recently introduced under the name, Arrow Root boxes. They are of different sizes, from about 4 ounces capacity to a quart, and serve a good purpose for preserving roots, barks, leaves and seeds in a dispensing office or shop. They are equally tight with a specia jar, and have the advantage of excluding the light.

The use of tin boxes of various patterns to suit the taste and of sizes reaching as high as several gallons is becoming more general in drug stores, and these have many advantages over glass bottles.

Uniformity in the size and shape of the furniture bottles adds much to the completeness of the physician's outfit. Care should be taken to apportion the different sizes, so that there will be enough of each to fill a shelf in the medicine case allotted to them. Thus, if there are twelve quart bottles, there should be fourteen pint, sixteen half pint, twenty four-ounce, or in about this proportion. In view of this fact, I have prepared catalogues which will be found in the appendix, embracing assortments more or less complete, of the most prominent articles of the Materia Medica, so apportioned as to quantity as that each shall constitute a uniform and well-arranged collection of medicines, and at a certain definite price, according to the extent and completeness of the outfit.

It is the practice of some druggists, in furnishing physicians' outfits, to label the furniture bottles with the common English labels used in ordinary dispensing operations; this is objectionable, for reasons which are sufficiently obvious. Others, though employing Latin labels, printed for the purpose, disfigure each bottle by a conspicuous card, announcing their name, occupation, and address.

In order to insure, as far as in their power, the use of correct nomenclature in labelling furniture bottles and drawers, the Philadelphia College of Pharmacy have published three sets of Latin labels, each containing an assortment, embracing several different sizes, according as the articles are kept in large or small quantities. These are sold by the druggists, and from their completeness, elegance, and cheapness, commend themselves to all who are about fitting up a shop or dispensing office. The yellow labels are sold at $1 and $2 50 per set; the bronze at $12 50. Specimen labels, such as shown in Fig. 1, are also published by the College.

After having pasted the label on to the bottle or drawer, by means of mucilage of tragacanth, or other convenient paste, and stretched it tightly over the part, it should be smoothed by laying a piece of thin paper upon it, and pressing it uniformly with the thumb. When it has become dry, it may be sized by painting over it a thin coating of clear mucilage of gum Arabic. This should extend a very little over the edges of the label. It should be then dried again, and varnished with spirit varnish; this not only improves the appearance of the label, but renders it durable and impervious to moisture.

JARS.—Ointments and extracts are usually kept in jars made of porcelain or queensware. These vary in quality, in color, and in shape. They should not be made of a very porous material, especially if designed for ointments, and should be well glazed, both on the inside and outside surfaces. The best are imported from England.

Fig. 19.

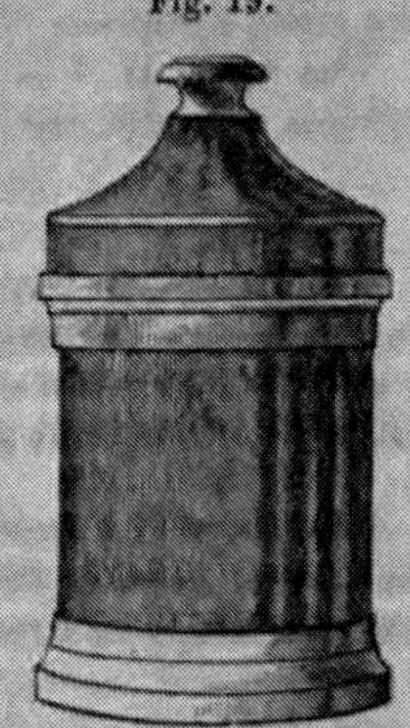

Canopy-top jar.

In regard to the shape of jars; the variety called canopy-top (Fig. 19) is generally preferred, as having a more finished appearance than the flat-top (Fig. 21).

Jars of this kind should never be labelled on the top, as the tops being about of the same size, are liable to be misplaced, and mistakes occasionally occur in this way.

Ointments and extracts are also frequently put into queensware jars without tops, called *gallipots* and *tie-overs* (Figs. 20 and 22). These are cheaper than covered jars, but are inconvenient and ill adapted to the preservation of the substances kept in them. They are usually tied over with kid, bladder, or parchment, the latter substance being the best. Extracts

Fig. 20. Fig. 21. Fig. 22.

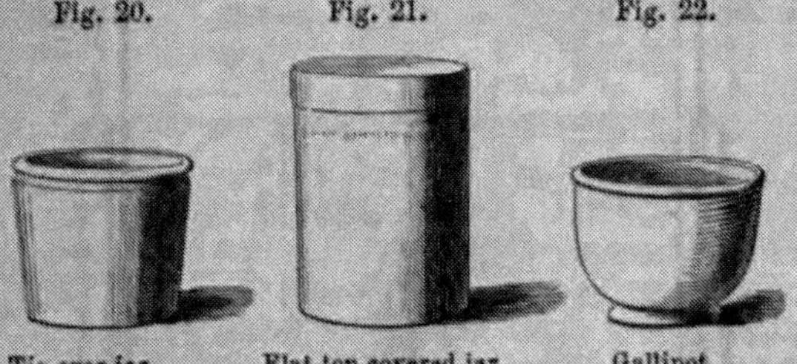

Tie-over jar. Flat-top covered jar. Gallipot.

rapidly lose their moisture when kept in tie-overs or gallipots, and those which contain volatile active principles, as extract of conium, soon become deteriorated. Ointments also undergo a change under these circumstances, frequently becoming rancid. When tie-over jars are used, it is well to cover the top with a piece of tin-foil, previous to securing the skin over it; this obviates in part the disadvantages to which they are liable.

PACKAGES.—Besides the medicines usually kept in bottles, jars, and boxes, there are many in the physician's outfit which are adapted to drawers, and are usually sent to him in paper packages, and as he is not always provided with a sufficient number of drawers to appropriate one to each article, they are frequently thrown together. Where this is the case, he should take care to have all those substances possessing a strong odor, as, for instance, valerian and serpentaria, kept separate from the others if not put into bottles. Packages of this description should be secured in two distinct papers, one of which should be thick and well glazed.

When drugs are to be preserved in packages, and have to be unwrapped every time a portion is taken out, they should be tied with good linen twine, passed at least twice around the package in the same direction, and connected by a bow knot.

The mode of folding, tying, and labelling paper packages will be spoken of under the head of dispensing medicines.

Implements.

The necessary implements for preparing and dispensing medicines in their more ordinary forms will be described in this place, leaving a reference to some of those not usually met with in the physician's office to subsequent parts of the work.

Scales.—The scales should be two in number. The pair for prescriptions, suitable for weighing one drachm and under, and the pair for weighing two drachms and upwards.

Fig. 23.

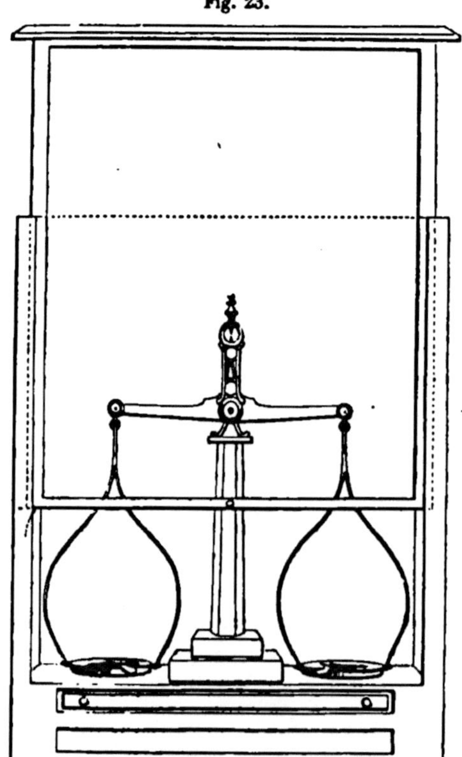

Prescription scales and case, with the sash raised to the proper height for use.

There are many different varieties of prescription scales in use; the most approved is that with an upright pillar, into the top of which is set a fulcrum, containing planes of hard steel, on which rest knife edges of the same material, placed at the centre of gravity of the beam; such scales are usually made of brass; the beam and scale dishes are frequently of silver. They vary in price according to their material and workmanship, from ten to twenty-five dollars. To preserve their delicacy, they should be kept in a suitable case, and in a position where they are not liable to a jarring motion, so prejudicial to the sharpness of the knife edges. In cleaning them, care should be taken to avoid bending in the slightest degree one or other arm of the lever. It is well to try the accuracy of the scales occasionally, as well by weighing exceedingly small quantities upon them when balanced by heavy weights as by weighing the same quantity successively on the opposite plates, by which means the least deflection in one or other arm of the lever may be ascertained.

Owing to the comparative expensiveness of these scales, another kind is more extensively purchased by physicians, in which the upright pillar is omitted. These are usually imported either from England, France, or Germany. They come in boxes of wood or tin, and have the advantage of being much more portable. The best are received from England, and have steel beams. The German variety is very inferior, and, indeed, frequently worthless. The physician who administers strychnia, veratria, or morphia in his practice may as well judge of the quantity by the eye as by the use of a pair of common German scales, which frequently fail to indicate it within half a grain or even a grain.

Fig. 24.

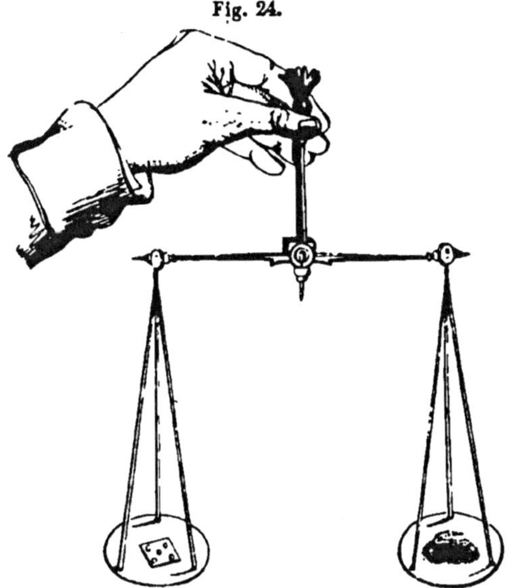

Prescription scales without upright.

Very good scales are imported from W. & T. Avery, Birmingham, and sold in this country at prices varying from $2 50 to $5 00 each; some have glass plates, adapting them to weighing corrosive substances. Fig. 24 exhibits this description of scales, with the manner of holding them.

A cheaper form has the ends of the beam open, and the cords attached to the plates secured to a little hook, which is slipped on to the curved ends, and readily movable; this arrangement is shown in Fig. 25. They are not generally so accurate as those with closed ends to the beams.

Fig. 25.

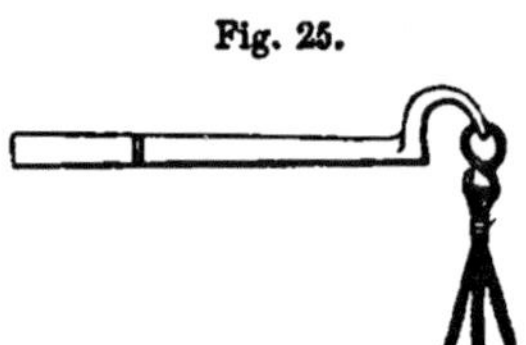

Fig. 26 represents a kind of scales for weighing ℥ss and upwards, which are less in use among medical practitioners than they ought to be; until recently it has been customary to guess at quantities which were too large for the prescription scales, the expense of the larger kind of scales being a great objection on the part of the young practitioner to purchasing them. A pair of large brass scales, made on the principle of those in Fig. 23, costs from twelve to thirty dollars. The kind here shown is selected on account of its cheapness; it is manufactured of iron, varnished, to protect it from rust, with a movable tin pan or scoop, and a platform arrangement of the beam. It is furnished the country physician or storekeeper for one dollar and twenty-five cents, and answers a good purpose.

Fig. 26.

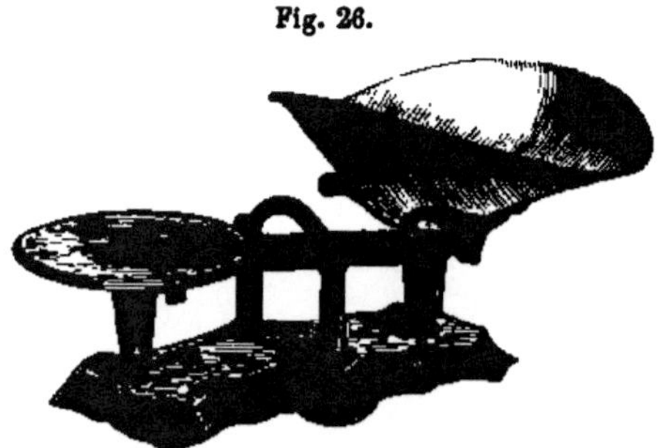

Cheap tea scales.

The best kind of platform balance for the dispensing counter is Beranger's pendulum scale, which is imported from France. The bearings, though complex, are protected from dust and corrosion, and insure great freedom of motion and consequent accuracy, combined with sufficient strength for considerable weights.

The best location for the scales is on a level counter by itself, away from the jarring occasioned by the ordinary manipulations of the shop. It should be adjacent to the paper drawers, and should have room on it for both sets of weights.

WEIGHTS, although sometimes made in this country, are usually imported, of the smaller kinds, with the box scales. Those for ten grains and upwards are made of brass cut into squares, and marked with the officinal signs for denoting the different denominations of weight. Those for six grains and under are of sheet brass cut into squares, and variously marked with the number of grains, as shown in Figs. 27, 28, 29, and 30.

Fig. 27. Fig. 28. Fig. 29. Fig. 30.

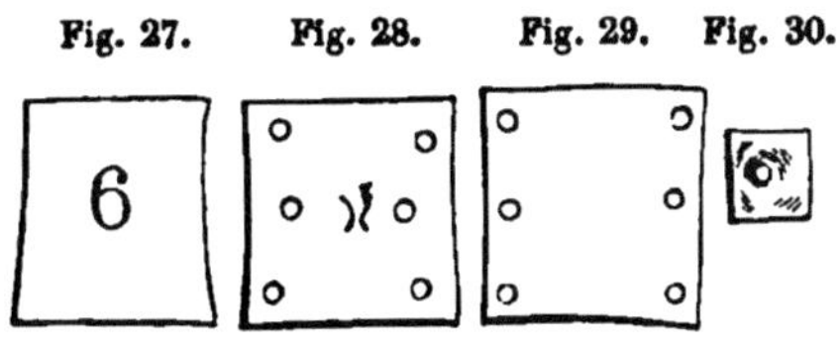

Weights of sheet brass.

The inexperienced operator is liable to error in using these small weights from the fact that they frequently have, besides the marks denoting the number of grains, a stamp placed on them by the manufacturer, which is the German sign corresponding with our gr. (grana). (See Fig. 28.) This is liable to be counted with the other indentations, and to add one to the actual number of grains; a two-grain weight is liable to be taken for a three-grain, a three-grain to be used instead of a four, and so on. Close observation, however, will exhibit a decided difference between the two kinds of indentations.

The mode of marking shown in fig. 27 is more liable to error than the others, especially when the weights become soiled and a little corroded by use.

In regard to accuracy, it must be admitted that most of the imported weights are very faulty; those made by W. and T. Avery, and by our own best scale-makers are to be preferred.

Within a few years past a description of weights from ʒij to ℈ss has become common in our market, quite preferable to the German square weights of the same denominations. These are round, or eight-sided, stamped out of brass plates, with very distinct inscriptions, as shown in Figs. 31 and 32. They are imported from England, being the manufacture of W. and T. Avery, of Birmingham, already referred to.

Fig. 31. Fig. 32.

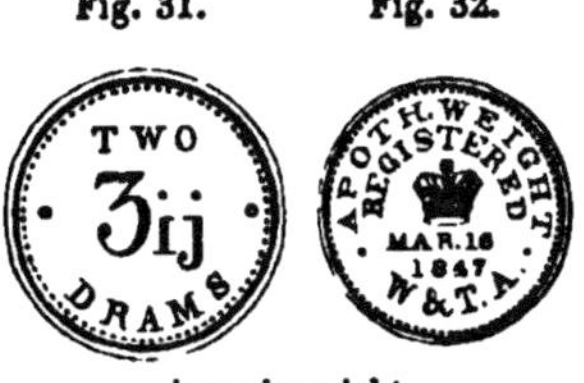

Avery's weight.

Some trials made with common German weights, convince me that few of those commonly met with are even reasonably accurate; a ʒj weight was found to weigh as high as 69.8 grains, and a gr. vj weight weighed 6.75 grains; others approximated more nearly; a ʒss weighed 30.25 grains, a ʒj 60.1 grains, a ℈ss 10.1 grains, a ʒij 120.5 grains, &c. None of Avery's that were tried, varied more than $\frac{1}{10}$ grain from their nominal weight.

The larger apothecaries' weights are almost invariably in the shape of cups, fitting into each other, the two inmost ones (Fig. 33) representing each two drachms; the next a half ounce, the next an ounce, and so on up to sixteen ounces in the larger nests. Now, as each cup represents a certain weight by itself, and as each is double that inside of it (excepting the two smallest, which are equal), the sum of any nest will be equal to that of any weight into which it fits; thus, the 16 oz. weight will balance the nest within it, which consists of an eight ounce, a four ounce, a two ounce, a one ounce, a half ounce, and two quarter ounces, and the entire nest will weigh thirty-two ounces.

Fig. 33.

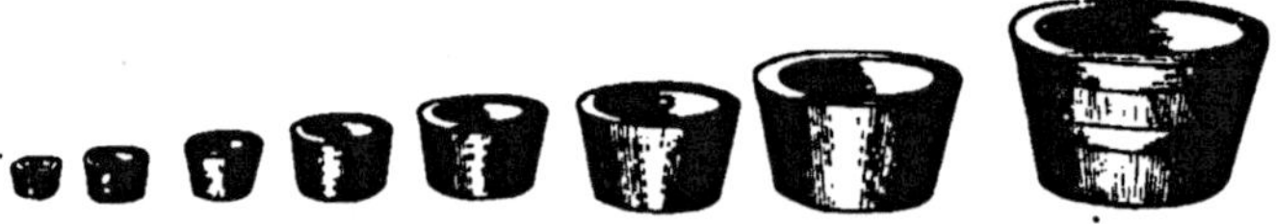

Series of apothecaries' or cup weights.

This arrangement of weights, though very compact and convenient, and furnishing a prominent distinction between the officinal and ordinary commercial weights, is more expensive than might be desired, considering the great utility to the apothecary and physician of having a good supply of such important implements of his art.

The physician about commencing practice in the country, and desirous of economizing in this department of his outfit, may procure sets of these weights ascending as high as four ounces, the nest weighing eight ounces. They will be found to answer his purposes in preparing tinctures, syrups, &c., in small quantities; in dispensing the vegetable medicines for infusions; and in his weighing operations generally, less disadvantage would flow from the exclusive use of apothecaries' than of avoirdupois weights. The subject of weights and measures is more fully presented in the next chapter, where drawings will also be found of the avoirdupois weights in use.

Measures.—As all liquid substances are generally dispensed by measure rather than by weight, and as our Pharmacopœia directs the use of the officinal standard of measurement in preparations containing liquids, with but few exceptions, one or more graduated measures are necessarily embraced in the physician's outfit. The most convenient for dispensing operations, is either a four or eight ounce conical measure, such as is shown in Fig. 34. These are of flint or of green glass, and are graduated down to one fluidrachm or half a drachm, which are the lowest denominations we generally wish to measure, and they can be filled several times in succession when it is desirable to measure a pint or quart.

Fig. 34.

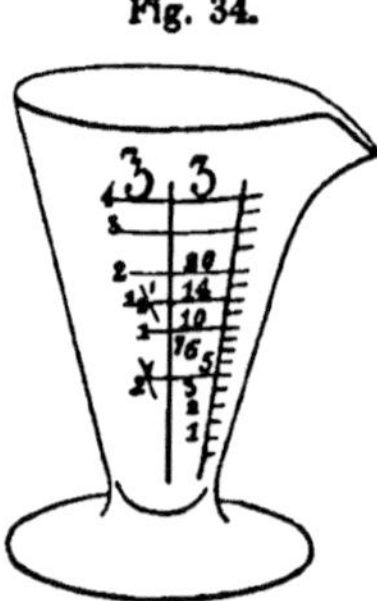

f℥iv graduated measure.

These measures are either made by our own glass manufacturers, and graduated here by persons following it as a business, or they are imported from Germany. The German measures are not to be relied on for accuracy, though from the quality of the glass, they are generally believed to be less liable than our own to break in measuring hot liquids.

Fig. 35.

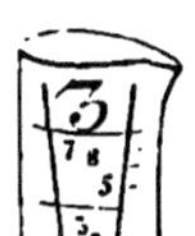

Medicine chest measure.

In selecting a measure, the chief points to be observed are, to have a good lip for pouring the liquids from, and clear and distinct marks both on the fluidrachm and fluidounce columns; the glass should not be very thick, as, by refracting the light, it interferes with accuracy in the measurement of small quantities. Large measures, which are not to be used for quantities under an ounce, may be made of the form shown in Fig. 35. These are less liable to be broken by careless handling. One ounce graduates of this description are sometimes made for medicine chests or saddle-bags where great economy of space is necessary.

Minim Measures.—For the divisions of a fluidrachm, the minim measure is employed. This is usually an upright cylinder of glass, with a lip at one extremity, and a glass pedestal at the other, and is graduated from sixty minims (one fluidrachm) to five minims. The kind used in fitting saddle-bags, and physicians' pocket cases, is made of glass tube with or without a foot, and does not occupy more space than an ordinary f℥ij tube vial. The inconvenience of employing a measure of this kind has led to the use of drops in prescription, instead of minims, and as essential oils and spirituous liquids drop so differently from aqueous liquids, and as the same liquid drops very differently from different vessels, discrepancies are likely to occur, unless the dispenser sufficiently understands and observes the distinction. (See tables of approximate measurement in next chapter.)

Fig. 36.

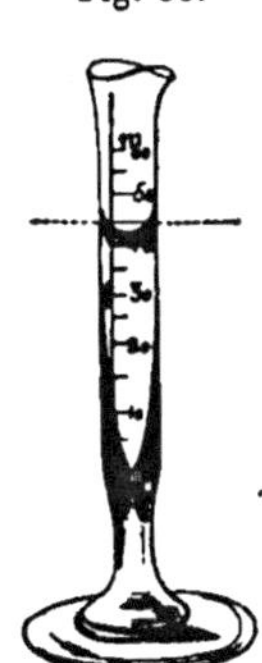

Minim measure.

Tin Measures.—Tin and copper measures of half pint, one pint, or two pints capacity, will be found very useful to the dispensing physician. They may be used for water, alcohol, syrups, and most tinctures, whenever the full quantity they will contain is prescribed.

MORTARS.—Mortars are necessary in so many processes of pharmacy, as to be among the most important items of an outfit. I shall describe the kinds usually sold, with their different uses, leaving to the physician the choice of one or more varieties, according to circumstances.

Wedgewood mortars are imported from England, and an inferior quality of similar ware is made in this country. They differ somewhat in their texture, though generally possessed of sufficient roughness to adapt them to the powdering of substances by trituration.

The best varieties are glazed enough to prevent their absorbing or becoming permanently stained by chemicals triturated in them, and yet are not so smooth as to allow substances to slip about instead of being retained under the pestle. At least one good wedgewood mortar is necessary. It should be of the shape indicated in Fig. 37,

Fig. 37. Fig. 38.

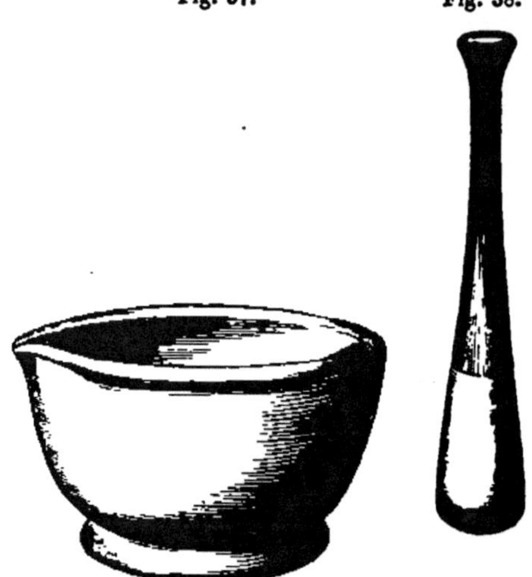

Wedgewood mortar and pestle.

perfectly flat on its base, so that it will stand firm during the process, and furnished with a good lip. The pestle should be, in shape, precisely adapted to the interior surface of the mortar; neither flattened nor pointed at its lower extremity, as is frequently the case. As the larger sized pestles always consist of two pieces, a wooden handle, and the rounded portion, which is of wedgewood ware, care should be taken to have the connection between them, which is made with cement, perfectly tight. When they become loosened, they may be secured by a cement made of resin, two parts; yellow wax, one part; and Spanish brown, three parts; melted together by heat.

For the purpose of solution, a *porcelain mortar* is convenient; such are frequently more shallow than the wedgewood variety. They are perfectly smooth, and highly glazed, and are not liable to be stained by chemical substances dissolved in them. They will also be found convenient in preparing such ointments and cerates as require to be introduced into a mortar, being more readily cleansed than wedgewood ware. The one shown in Fig. 39 has a pestle of the same material.

Fig. 39.

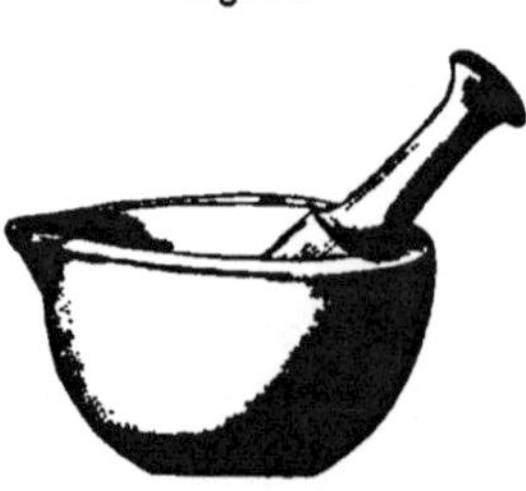

Porcelain mortar.

Glass mortars are frequently found in the office of the physician, and the shop of the apothecary. They are too soft for use in reducing hard substances to powder, but are adapted to forming solutions of readily soluble materials, and to use in making ointments. The small sizes are much employed in fitting up medicine-chests and medical saddle-bags.

The smoothness which occasions substances to slip about under the pestle in manipulating with glass mortars, may be overcome by grinding fine emery and oil of turpentine in them.

For large operations, as, for instance, in making syrup of bitter almonds, confection of roses, or mercurial ointment, a *marble mortar* is most convenient; a perfect block of hard and close grained marble of requisite size, is cut out into a shape corresponding with that of the perfect wedgewood mortar, represented in Fig. 37. The pestle is made of the same material, or of hard wood, fastened upon a long wooden handle, which may be projected into an iron ring above, secured properly over the centre of the mortar, so that while the operator gives the requisite grinding motion to the lower extremity of the pestle, the upper is held securely in its place.

Mortars of the kinds described are not adapted to contusing substances, either with a view to obtaining powders, or to employing them in a bruised condition. If used for this purpose, they are very apt to be broken on the first trial.

Fig. 40.

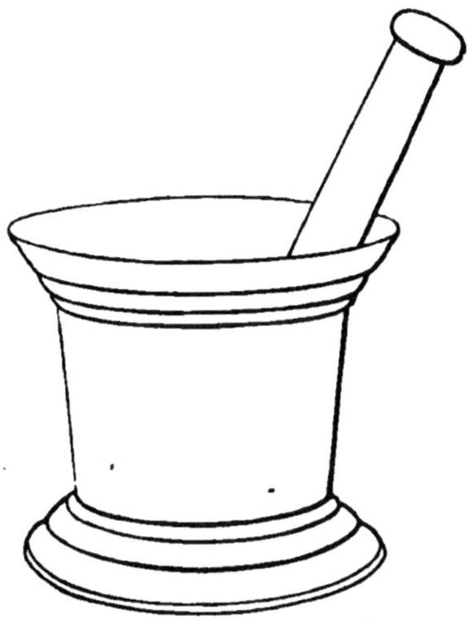

Mortar and pestle for contusion.

For contusion, an *iron, brass, or bell-metal mortar* of the shape here shown is best suited. Unlike mortars for trituration, these are flat at bottom, and the pestles terminate in a flattened ball; they are tall in proportion to their diameter, as seen in the drawing.

The laborious process of powdering drugs is greatly facilitated by the employment of mills; some of the varieties of coffee and spice-mills met with in iron or hardware stores are exceedingly useful in the comminution of vegetable substances, for the preparation of tinctures, infusions, &c., and even, assisted with suitable sieves, in their reduction to powder.

A very excellent mill, called Swift's drug-mill, is figured and described in the chapter on powdering.

Fig. 41 represents a spice-mill, which will be found convenient where the drug is not too large to be introduced into it, in which case I use a stout pair of shears, a tobacco knife, or a large iron mortar, for its previous reduction. This has the advantage of being secured to a table by a clamp, so as to be removable at pleasure.

Fig. 41.

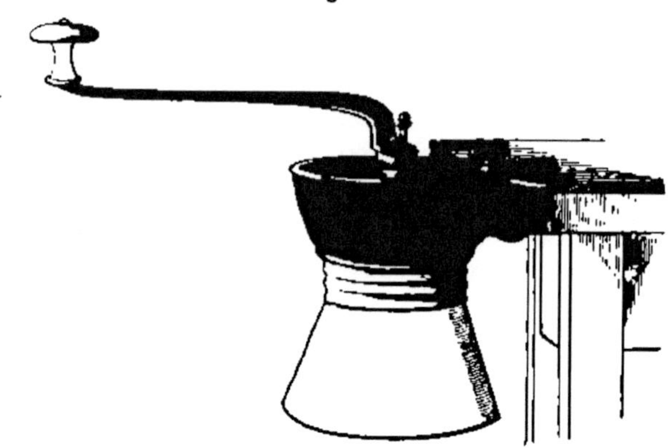

Spice-mill.

To the physician who prepares his own powders, one or more sieves will be found very useful. The most permanent and desirable kind is that made of wire gauze, though hair and bolting-cloth sieves are somewhat less costly. The latter answer very well if kept clear of moths; a sieve with a covering at top and bottom is preferable. These coverings should be made of leather, secured by hoops rather than of wood, which is liable to warp and crack.

I shall have occasion to speak of the employment of coarse sieves in the preparation of powders for percolation, and need only mention them in this place, to refer to the article on the displacement process.

SPATULAS.—Of these there are several kinds. The plain steel spatula, or palette knife, shown in Fig. 44, is, perhaps, best adapted to the general purposes of dispensing. In selecting them, care should be taken to have one very flexible, and another quite stiff, while, of course, they should be of two or more sizes. The balance handle spatula (Fig. 43) is also useful in dispensing operations, being gene-

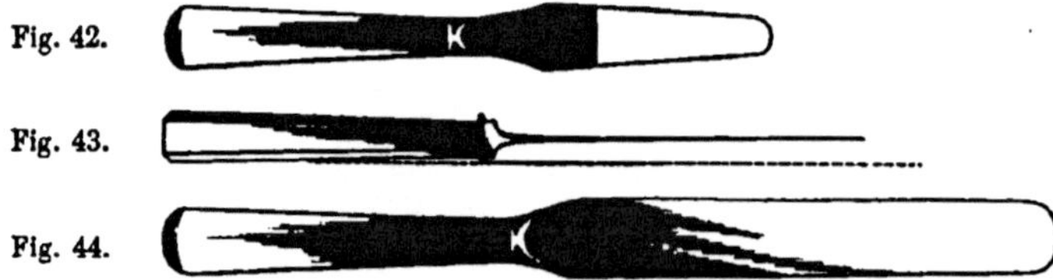

Fig. 42.

Fig. 43.

Fig. 44.

rally reserved for folding powders, and for other neat manipulations. It has the merit of lying on the table or counter without the blade coming in contact with it, a convenience when employed with pill masses or ointments. Three inch spatulas may be made with a tapering blade, as shown in Fig. 42, so as to allow of their being introduced into rather narrow-mouthed bottles, such as are usually put into saddle-bags and medicine chests.

Spatulas of glass, ivory, and bone are sometimes, though rarely, employed. They are useful in manipulating with corrosive substances which would act upon steel.

A *pill tile* (Fig. 45), made of porcelain or queensware, is a useful utensil in preparing certain ointments and pills. Tiles are made of various sizes, and are sometimes graduated, as seen in the drawing, to facilitate the division of masses into twelve or twenty-four pills.

The division of pill masses, however, is better accomplished by the aid of the machine, shown in the accompanying drawing. The mode

Fig. 45.

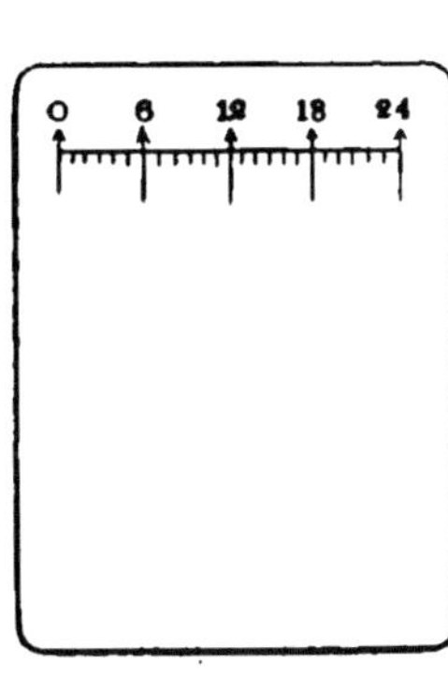

Graduated pill tile.

Fig. 46.

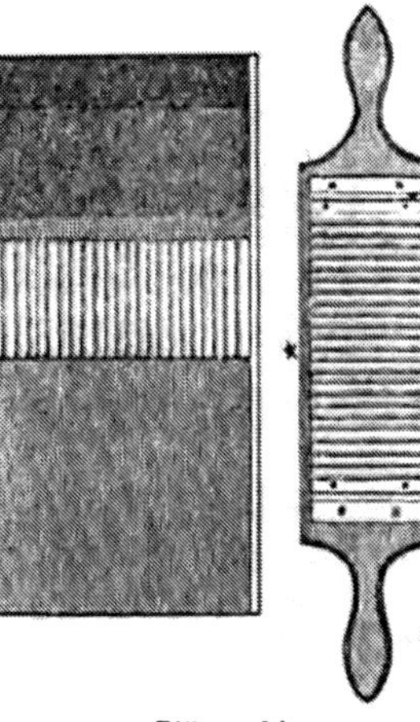

Pill machine.

of using this most useful instrument, is described in the chapter on dispensing medicines.

The *funnel*, sometimes called tunnel, is an article of every-day use in the dispensing shop or office. A porcelain or wedgewood funnel is represented in the plate. The sides should be straight, and at an angle of 60° to each other. The tube should be smallest at its lowest extremity, and should have one or more grooves upon its outer surface, to allow of the egress of air from a bottle, into the mouth of which it is fitted. Funnels which are grooved on their inner surface, are generally preferred for filtration, as allowing a more ready downward passage of the liquids, especially when the plain filter is employed. They may be made of glass, porcelain, Berlin or queensware, and tin; those of glass are generally furnished physicians in their outfits; but the porcelain variety is far less liable to breakage, and is equally cleanly.

Fig. 47.

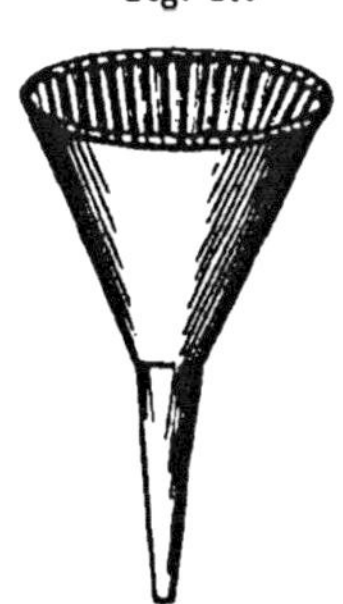

The porcelain funnel.

The *displacement apparatus* is now almost indispensable to the physician who prepares his tinctures, infusions, &c. The kind best adapted to a physician's outfit is a tin tube, of about 8 inches long, and $3\frac{1}{2}$ inches in diameter, terminated by a funnel, and containing one or two perforated diaphragms, fitting loosely into the tube, so as to be readily removed for cleaning (Figs. 48 and 49). There is also a kind made

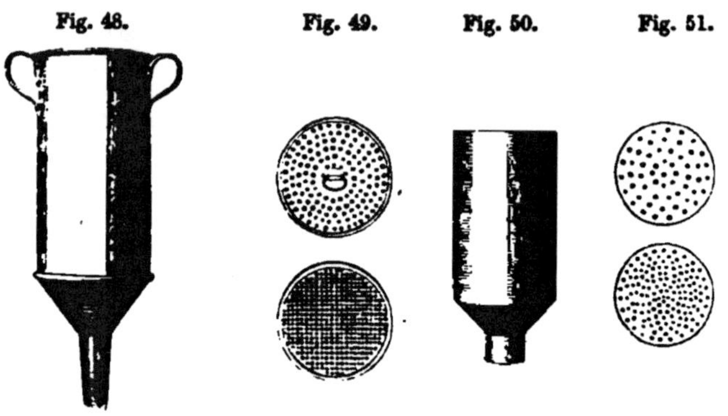

Fig. 48. Fig. 49. Fig. 50. Fig. 51.

Tin displacers, with upper and lower diaphragm.

Porcelain displacer, with two diaphragms.

of porcelain or earthenware resembling the preceding in shape, and containing diaphragms of the same material (Figs. 50 and 51). Under the head of the displacement process, the mode of preparing and using apparatus of this kind is more fully described.

One or more *evaporating dishes* of Berlin or fine porcelain ware, and a porcelain cup (Fig. 53), will be found convenient in the prepara-

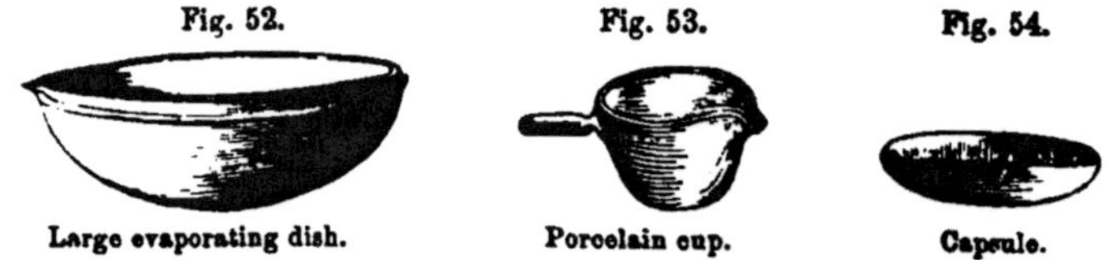

Fig. 52. Large evaporating dish.

Fig. 53. Porcelain cup.

Fig. 54. Capsule.

tion of many of the galenical and most of the chemical preparations appropriate to the office or shop. These dishes are of different prices according to quality, and range from the two gallon to the one fluid-ounce size. The smaller sizes from half pint down, adapted to experiments, are sold at 75 cents per nest.

The *flask* is a cheap and convenient mplement for small operations requiring heat, and especially for forming solutions of saline ingredients.

The *tripod* (Fig. 56), or a retort stand, should not be forgotten, as being necessary to the convenient use of the foregoing.

Vials.—The physician's outfit usually contains from a half gross to a gross of prescription vials, varying in size from f℥viij to f℥ss. As more of the smaller sizes are used than of the others, it is desirable to have about the following proportions in a gross: One doz. f℥viij, one doz. f℥vj, two doz. f℥iv, three doz. f℥ij, three doz. f℥j, two doz. f℥ss, though usually a larger number of the two smaller sizes are introduced at the expense of the three largest sizes. Several of the larger sizes should have wide mouths, for convenience in bottling solid substances, and also to adapt to the displacement apparatus. Vials in commerce are classified as flint, German flint, and green glass; as fluted and plain; and as long and short. Flint vials are considerably more expensive than the green, though they are far more elegant for prescription purposes. They are generally made in a mould. Of the fluted vials, the long (Fig. 57) are the most convenient for ordinary purposes; they admit of a larger label being pasted on them, which is sometimes desirable in case of prescriptions, and they are more convenient for medicines that are to be administered by drops.

Fig. 55. Fig. 56.

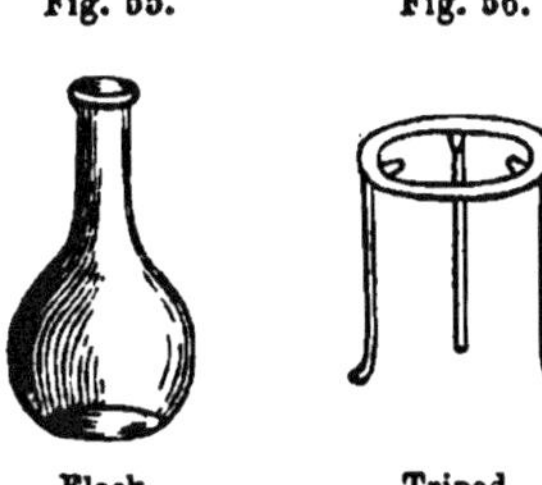

Flask. Tripod.

Fig. 58 represents a short fluted vial of the same size, and having a wide mouth, adapting it to solid substances. Fig. 59 is a flint vial,

Fig. 57.

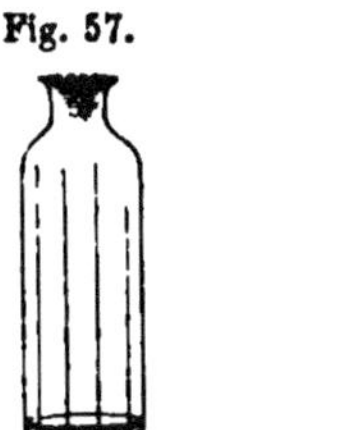

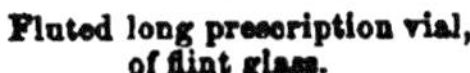

Fluted long prescription vial, of flint glass.

Fig. 58.

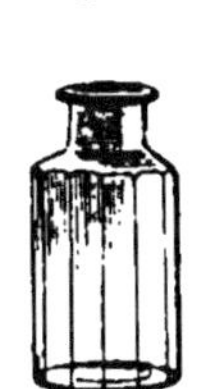

Wide-mouth flint fluted vial.

Fig. 59.

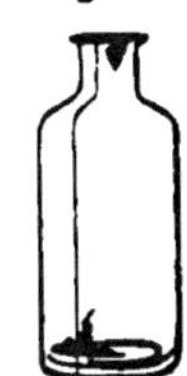

Plain prescription vial, of flint glass.

now very much in vogue, intermediate between the two preceding in height, and without the fluted surface; these are apt to show a crease down their whole length, at the point where the two halves of the mould in which they are made come together in shutting it, a common feature in all bottles made in moulds, which open and shut by what may be called a lateral suture. Figs. 60, 61, and 62 represent vials blown without a mould, or in an open clay mould, and finished by hand. These have a handsomer and smoother surface, though less regular and uniform in shape, as here the shape depends on the skill of the finisher, not the construction of his tools. German glass vials are intermediate in price between those of flint and common green glass. They are very well adapted to ordinary dispensing purposes, and, as made by our best manufacturers, leave little to desire.

The shape of the lip is one of the most important considerations in the selection of vials; if the lip is too narrow and rounded, a constant source of annoyance will occur from the liquid trickling down the

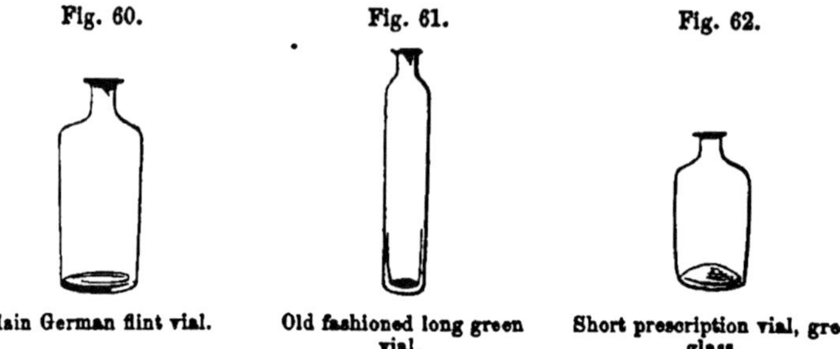

Fig. 60. Plain German flint vial.

Fig. 61. Old fashioned long green vial.

Fig. 62. Short prescription vial, green glass.

neck and sides of the vial after pouring from it, and it will be impossible to drop from it at all. Figs. 61 and 62 represent the old fashioned cheap green glass blown vials; that shown in Fig. 61 has the disadvantage of not standing up, and is usually suspended by a string.

Corks.—These are exceedingly variable in quality; the softest and most perfectly shaped varieties, though expensive, are so far preferable for use as to make them cheaper in the end. Tapering corks possess the advantage of being fitted to vials of various sized necks with great facility, and if sufficiently "velvety," will bear thrusting tightly and securely into their place. These remarks are equally true of the larger sizes, called bottle corks; of these we have pint corks, quart corks, demijohn corks, and flat or pot corks, the last being used chiefly for wide-mouth packing bottles and earthen jars. It is well to be supplied with a few of these, though vial corks constitute by far the largest proportion of the whole number required. There is a variety called "citrate corks," introduced since the invention of citrate of magnesia solution, very uniform in size and quality, and an improvement on the ordinary pint corks. "Homœopathic corks" are so called from their being adapted to small or tube vials; they are of elegant quality and tapering in shape.

Paper of different kinds should not be overlooked in making up an outfit. The most useful is druggist's white wrapping-paper, which should be fine without being heavy or spongy in its texture; it should not crack at the edges when turned over sharply. The sizes met with in commerce are medium, about 19 × 24 inches, and double medium, 24 × 38 inches. For directions in regard to dividing the sheets, for dispensing medicines in packages, see chapter on dispensing. The kind of paper called flat cap will be found very convenient in addition to the above for putting up powders, especially in very small doses.

Filtering paper should be without color, and of a porous texture, and yet sufficiently firm to sustain the weight of the liquid placed upon it.

The market is now freely supplied with a superior article in circular sheets, called French filters.

Fancy paper, employed for capping corks, or as a very nice outer wrapping to packages, is recommended to those who desire to practise neatness and elegance in dispensing. Tin-foil is also required for covering jars of ointment, deliquescent powders, &c.

Pill Boxes.—These are of three kinds: 1st. Paper pill boxes, adapted to dispensing pills. 2d. Wooden pill boxes, or chip boxes, made of shavings, and best suited for ointments, confections, &c.; of this article, a very beautiful style is imported from England, which commands nearly double the price of the American kind. 3d. Turned boxes. These have been recently introduced for dispensing pills, and are certainly more substantial than either paper or chip boxes. They do not, however, serve so good a purpose for ointments; the bottom, being cut across the grain of the wood, soon becomes saturated with the grease, and soils everything it is set upon. Pill boxes are usually sold by the dozen nests, wrapped in paper. Sometimes a nest contains three, and sometimes four boxes, ranging from about an ounce capacity to one-fourth that size.

The physician should provide himself with a tin case, in the shape of a closed cylinder, in which to carry his gum catheters and bougies, and another for adhesive plaster cloth, which otherwise is liable to become useless in our climate.

The other items to be mentioned are a few pieces of fine Turkey sponge for surgical use, and one for the inhalation of ether, if a friend to anæsthesia in surgery and obstetrics. A corkscrew, a ball of fine linen twine, a pair of scissors, a few coarse towels for wiping mortars, a tin cup for heating liquids, a sheepskin for spreading plasters, &c.

The apparatus and furniture here described, are such as may be regarded as necessary to the outfit of a country practitioner. I shall find occasion to refer to many implements in the subsequent parts of this work which it would be superfluous to describe in this place, though frequently included in the outfit.

CHAPTER II.

ON WEIGHTS AND MEASURES AND SPECIFIC GRAVITY.

METROLOGY embraces the science of determining the bulk, or extension of substances, called measurement, and their gravitating force, called weight, and the relation of these to each other, called specific gravity.

In the present essay, it is not designed to enter into the subject further than is necessary to the student of medicine and pharmacy. The reader is referred to an able essay on its historical bearings, compiled by the late Dr. Benjamin Ellis from the *Report on Weights and Measures*, made by Hon. J. Quincy Adams, when Secretary of State, to the U. S. Senate in 1821. (See *American Journal of Pharmacy*, vol. ii. pp. 111 and 188.)

WEIGHTS AND MEASURES.—So difficult has it been found to modify or materially alter the systems of measurement and weight handed down from the earliest antiquity, and tenaciously adhered to by the mass of the people, and so inadequate have been the efforts of the British Crown and Parliament to supply proper and invariable standards, that the present Troy and Avoirdupois weights are believed to be even less perfect and consistent with each other than the very ancient standards from which they were derived. The inconveniences attendant on the use of separate sets of weights and measures for different kinds of commodities, have probably always been felt, and are only partially remedied by adapting these to one common unit to which all can be reduced. This adaptation, in the case of our different standards, is through the grain or unit of weight; the systems of Troy, Apothecaries' and Avoirdupois weights, and of Wine measure, are all readily compared through this common standard—the *grain*.

Troy Weight is used by jewellers, and at the mints, in the exchange of the precious metals. Its denominations are the pound, ounce, pennyweight (= 24 grs.), and grain.

Apothecaries' Weight is used by apothecaries and physicians in mixing and prescribing medicines, and is officinal in the United States, London, and Edinburgh Pharmacopœias (not in that of Dublin). In buying and selling medicines, not ordered by prescription, the avoirdupois weight is used.

The denominations of the apothecaries' weight are pounds, ounces, drachms or drams, scruples, and grains. Its pound, ounce, and grain, correspond with the Troy weight.

Avoirdupois Weight is used in general commerce, and by apothecaries in their strictly commercial transactions, as in buying and selling medicines without the prescription of a physician, and also in compounding recipes for domestic purposes, and for use in the arts. Its higher denominations need not be named. As at present used, it has pounds, ounces, and fractions of the ounce.

Synonyms.—The names given above may be substituted, with advantage, by *officinal* for the apothecaries', and *commercial* for the avoirdupois, as more definite, and less likely to be confounded in the mind of the student.

A knowledge of these, and of their relations to each other, is of the highest degree of importance to the physician and apothecary, and, for want of giving due attention to them at the outset, many students are continually confused in the practice of pharmacy.

In the following table, I have endeavored to display, in the simplest and most comprehensive manner, the value of each denomination in the respective weights, and the relation of these to each other:—

Table of the Officinal Weights (Apothecaries').

20 grains = ℈j (one scruple)	= gr. xx.	
60 grains = ʒj (one drachm)	= ℈iij	(3 scruples).
480 grains = ℥j (one ounce)	= ʒviij	(8 drachms).
5,760 grains = ℔j (one pound, U. S. P.)	= ℥xij	(12 ounces).

Table of Commercial Weights (Avoirdupois).

437.5 grains = 1 oz. (one ounce).
7,000 grains = 1℔ (one pound, Com.) = 16 oz.

The *use of signs* is here seen to be of importance, as designating, when correctly used, to which system of weights the particular denomination refers; thus, ℥j means 480 grains—the officinal ounce; while 1 oz. means 437.5 grains—the commercial ounce. The sign for designating the pound is not so distinctive; ℔j is applied equally to the officinal pound, 5,760 grains, and to the commercial, 7,000 grains; so that, when a doubt may arise as to which is intended, the prefix *U. S. P.* would be well adapted to designate the officinal, and *Com.* or *Av.*, the commercial.

The *comparative value* of the different parallel denominations may be thus expressed:—

The officinal ounce contains 42½ grains more than the commercial.

The officinal pound contains 1,240 grains less than the commercial.

Or, thus:—

The officinal has the larger ounce, and the commercial has the larger pound, the former containing ℥xij (each 480 grains) in a pound, and the latter 16 ounces (each 437.5 grains) in a pound. Or thus:—

$$480 \times 12 = 5{,}760 \text{ (officinal).}$$
$$437.5 \times 16 = 7{,}000 \text{ (commercial).}$$

To the pharmaceutist who manipulates with large quantities of drugs, the use of apothecary's weights is very inconvenient, and a convenient rule for converting one system into the other is a desideratum. The following is the simplest rule for the purpose with which I am acquainted, and gives a pretty close approximation to the exact result.

To convert a given number of officinal ounces into avoirdupois ounces, add $\frac{1}{12}$ and $\frac{1}{200}$ to the number. For example, to find the value of 24 officinal ounces in commercial ounces—

$$24 + \frac{24}{12} + \frac{24}{200} = 26.12 \text{ or } 26\tfrac{1}{8}.$$

It must be remembered always that this rule is not accurate, only approximate. A table is inserted in the appendix for convenience in converting one system into the other.

Decimal Weights.—The attention of pharmaceutists and of commercial men has recently been directed to the subject of reforming the systems of weight and measurement in use in this country and in England, and the most prominent change now proposed is the entire substitution of the French decimal system for all those now in use. This system is now used in most analytical laboratories in this country, and throughout Europe, and although its general adoption for all the purposes of trade is considered rather chimerical, yet it is worthy the careful study of the scientific, and is so useful to all who pursue the study of chemistry and pharmacy, that the following table is inserted:—

Comparative Table of Decimal with Commercial and Officinal Weights.

NAMES.	Equivalent in Grammes.	Equivalent in Grains.	Equivalent in Commercial Weight.			Equivalent in Officinal Weight.			
			lb.	oz.	gr.	lb.	oz.	dr.	gr.
Milligramme . . .	.001	.0154							
Centigramme . .	.01	.1543							
Decigramme . . .	.1	1.5434							1.5
Gramme	1	15.4340							15.4
Decagramme . . .	10	154.3402		0¼	45			2	34.0
Hectogramme . .	100	1543.4023		3½	12.152		3	1	43.0
Kilogramme[1] . . .	1000	15434.0234	2	3¼	12 173	2	8	1	14
Myriagramme . .	10000	154340.2344	22	0¾	12	26	9	4	20

Scales and Weights.—The balance, or scales, is of course indispensable to the idea of metrology, and the possession of masses of previously ascertained gravitating force, called weights, is equally necessary. Scales are of various styles, although, for use in pharmacy, the simple kinds figured among the necessary implements for furnishing the physician's office, answer every purpose. In this place, it will be proper to call attention especially to the usual *forms* of *weights* of the different systems. The apothecaries' weights are invariably, for all denominations, made of brass or copper. The larger weights come in the *cup* form, as shown in Fig. 63. Each cup is equal to the sum of

Fig. 63.

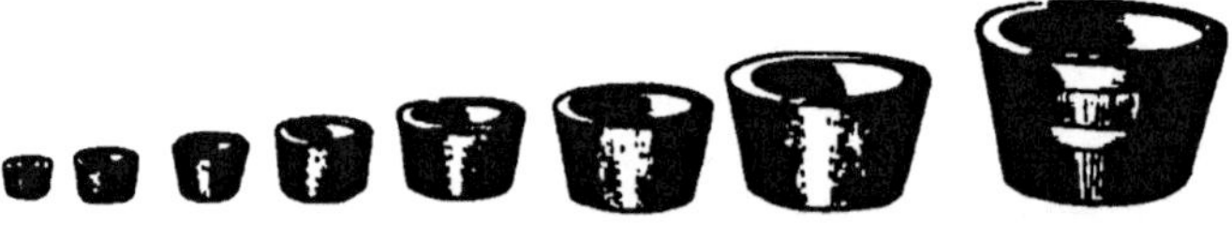

Series of apothecaries' or cup weights.

all those which fit in it, or is twice the sum of the next smaller. These weights are expensive, and, unfortunately, too little used by physicians, and even by some apothecaries. The small weights which accompany the box scales, and which are figured in the last chapter, are used for all denominations up to two drachms, and then the common commercial or avoirdupois weights, which are cheaper than the brass cup weights, are frequently brought into play.

Those are usually in *piles* of iron, brass, or zinc, of the form shown in the annexed figure, each weight being half that of the one below

[1] Abbreviated Kilo.

Fig. 64.

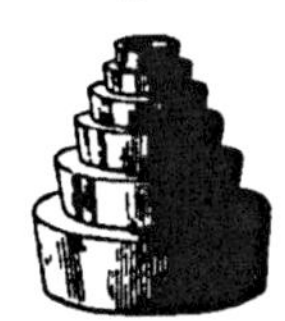

Commercial or avoirdupois weights.

it. In a large number of processes, one ounce, or two ounces, are ordered, and in these cases, if the commercial weight is used, a ℈ij, or ʒj and ʒss weight must be added from the small set. In the case of a pound being ordered, as there shown, 18 ounces from the pile, and a ʒj from the small set, will nearly approximate the required weight.

Measures of capacity are used for liquids, and, in the higher denominations, for corn and the cereal grains, but the only table of these we need present is that employed in medicine, called Wine Measure. The unit of this system is called a minim, and is equal to about .95 of a grain of pure water at 60° F.

Table of the Officinal, or Wine Measure.

Minims.						Grains of water.
60	=	fʒj	(one fluidrachm)	=	♏ lx =	56.9
480	=	f℥j	(one fluidounce)	=	fʒviij =	455.6
7,680	=	Oj	(one pint)	=	f℥xvj =	7,291.1
61,440	=	Cong. j	(one gallon)	=	Oviij =	58,328.8

Or thus:—

60 minims are one fluidrachm.
8 fluidrachms are one fluidounce.
16 fluidounces are one pint.
2 pints are one quart.
4 quarts are one gallon.

Besides the discrepancy occasioned by the minim not being equal to one grain of the natural liquid standard, it will be perceived at once that a wide variance exists in the denominations above an ounce. The fluidounce contains 480 minims, as the officinal ounce contains that number of grains; but in the pint are 16 fluidounces, while the corresponding pound contains only 12 ounces. From these causes, the adjustment of proportions of solids to liquids, when accuracy is required, is a matter of no little calculation. In England, this system of measures has been revised of latter years, so as to bring about a close relation between the solid commercial ounce and the fluidounce. In the Imperial measure, the minim is equal to .91 of a grain, and it is multiplied as follows:—

Imperial Measure.

Minims.						Grains of water.
60	=	fʒj	(one fluidrachm)	=	♏lx =	54.6
480	=	f℥j	(one fluidounce)	=	fʒviij =	437.5
9,600	=	Oj	(one pint)	=	f℥xx =	8,750[1]
76,800	=	Cong. j	(one gallon)	=	Oviij =	70,000

Graduated measures of glass of Oj, f℥viij, f℥vj, f℥iv, f℥ij, f℥j, fʒj capacity are manufactured, and sold by druggists; these are sometimes

[1] Equal to 1 lb. 4 oz. avoirdupois weight.

quite inaccurate, but may be readily verified by balancing them on the scales, and gradually adding pure water until the required weight in grains, as shown in the table, is attained. In the same way we may graduate our own measures, marking the denominations by the following ready process:—

Having coated one side of the glass with a thin coating of wax, balance it on the scales, adjust the weights, and add the required number of grains of pure water, observing to add it drop by drop toward the last; as soon as the weight is accurately counterpoised, remove it to a level table or counter, so high that it will be on a line with the eye, and carefully, with the point of a pin, mark the line formed by the surface of the liquid, and opposite this the appropriate sign; this may be rendered more clear and distinct afterwards. In the same way mark the various other denominations, having an eye to the temperature, which should not vary far from 60°. Now form a paste, by mixing a sufficient quantity of finely-powdered fluor-spar with sulphuric acid, and spread this over the marked surfaces, and set the measure aside for a day or two, after which wash it off and remove the wax; the graduated measure is now indelibly and distinctly marked, and, if we have used the proper care, more accurately than is usual with those sold. I have compared two, in which the one fluidrachm mark of one corresponded nearly with the two fluidrachm of the other, and in other respects they were almost as much at variance.

Fig. 65.

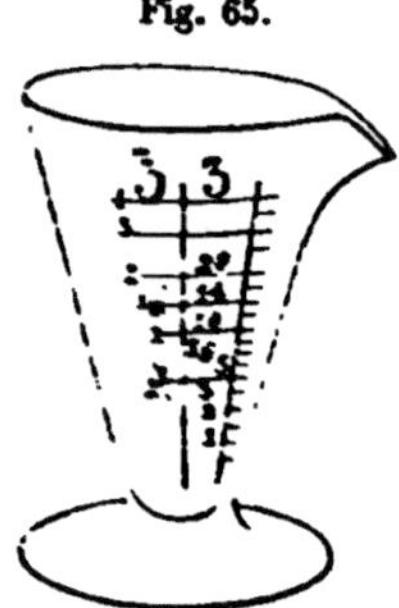

f℥iv grad. measure.

A precaution to be observed, whether in graduating or using a measure, particularly of small capacity, may be appropriately mentioned here.

Owing to the adhesion of the liquid to the sides of the measure, its surface is concave, and shows, from a side view, two lines; one where the edge of the liquid adheres to the glass, and the other, the line of the lower surface of the concavity. Now, in order to fix the true line in this case, it must be intermediate between the upper and lower edge of the liquid, and not at either surface. This is more obvious the smaller the diameter of the measure, and, in the accompanying drawing, the dotted line has been made at the proper point for measurement.

Fig. 66.

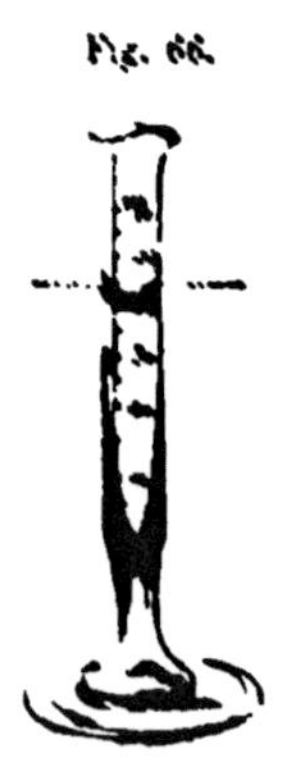

Minim measure.

Besides the common forms of glass graduated measures, a measure is used, especially by German pharmaceutists, made of block tin and graduated on the inside; each denomination is marked by a raised rim, and the quantity designated by an appropriate sign. These are especially convenient for measuring hot liquids, and if readily procurable would soon be generally introduced.

Approximate Measurement.—The approximate standards of measurement are very inaccurate, but they have no wider range than the doses of medicines, so that they are for the most part satisfactory. The following table exhibits those in common use:—

A gill mug, or teacupful	f℥iv.
A wineglassful	f℥ij.
A tablespoonful	f℥ss.
A dessertspoonful	fʒij.
A teaspoonful	fʒj.
A drop	from $\frac{1}{3}$ to $1\frac{1}{2}$ minims.

Of the above, it may be remarked that the wineglassful is frequently less than two fluidounces, although the champagne glass is nearer four fluidounces. I have observed that the modern teaspoons are larger than formerly, and that the more expensive silver spoons are larger than those of common metal of the same nominal size.

The size of drops varies from various causes, of which the nature of the liquid, the size and shape of the lip of the vessel from which dropped, and the extent to which the lip is moistened, are the most important. The following lists of liquids, with the number of drops in a fluidrachm, may be considered as furnishing good approximations to the relative size of their drops:—

Three lists are appended: 1st. That by Elias Durand, originally published in the *Journal of the Philadelphia College of Pharmacy*, vol. i. p. 169, and copied into most of our standard works; from this I have omitted several items, on account of their standard strength having been altered since the period of his experiments. 2d. That of Prof. Procter, published in the tenth edition of the *United States Dispensatory*, and confined to different essential oils. 3d and 4th. Lists I have prepared as the result of my own observations, chiefly confined to medicines not included in the foregoing.

1st. Durand's Table of the number of Drops of different Liquids equivalent to a fluidrachm.

	DROPS.		DROPS.
Acid, acetic, crystallizable . .	120	Tinctures of assafœtida, foxglove, guaiacum, and opium . . .	120
" hydrocyanic, medicinal . .	45	Tincture of chloride of iron . . .	132
" muriatic	54	Vinegar, distilled	78
" nitric	84	" of colchicum . . .	78
" sulphuric	90	" of squill	78
" " aromatic . .	120	Water, distilled	45
Alcohol	138	" of ammonia, strong . .	54
" diluted	120	" " weak . .	45
Arsenite of potassa, solution of .	57	Wine, Teneriffe	78
Ether, sulphuric	150	" antimonial	72
Oils of aniseed, cinnamon, cloves, peppermint, sweet almonds, and olives	120	" of colchicum	75
		" of opium	78

2d. Procter's Table of the number of Drops to a fluidrachm of Essential Oil, as dropped, A, *from the bottles from which they are commonly dispensed, and* B, *from a minim measure.*

	A.	B.		A.	B.
Oleum anisi	85	86	Oleum menthæ pip.	103	109
" cari	106	108	" " viridis	89	94
" caryophylli	103	103	" rosmarini	104	105
" chenopodii	97	100	" sabinæ	102	108
" cinnamomi	100	102	" sassafras	102	100
" cubebæ	86	96	" tanaceti	92	111
" fœniculi	103	103	" valerianæ	116	110
" gaultheriæ	102	101	Creasotum	95	91
" hedeomæ	91	91			

3d. Table of the number of Drops of different Liquids equivalent to f℥j, *as dropped from pint and half pint tincture bottles and from a minim measure. Thermometer* 80° F.—E. PARRISH.

Those marked *av.* are averages of several droppings.

	FROM ♏ MEASURE.	FROM Oj OR Oss TR.
Acetum opii	69	90
Acidum aceticum (commercial)	102	73
" " dilutum, *av.*	52.5	55
" nitricum dilutum	44	62
" sulphuricum dilutum	49	54
" " aromaticum	148	116
" hydrocyanicum dilutum, *av.*	52	[1]
Alcohol	143	118
" dilutum, *av.*	124.5	98
Aqua, *av.*	46	64.5
Chloroformum, *av.*	276.5	180
Extractum valerianæ, Fld.	126	115
Glycerina (first dropping)	135	53
" *av.*	84.7	55
Infusion digitalis, *av.*	60	62.5
Liquor ammoniæ	62	49
" iodinii compositus	75	75
" hydrarg. et arsen. iodid.	52	52
" potassæ arsenitis	63	60
Oleum menthæ viridis, *old*	103	110
" olivæ	99	76
" tiglii	92	80
Spiritus ætheris nitrici	148	90
" " compositus	140	90
Syrupus acaciæ	56	58
" scillæ	88	85
Tinctura aconiti radicis	130	118
" ferri chloridi	151	106
" iodinii	144	113
" opii	147	106
" " camphorata	110	95
" tolutani	138	120
Vinum antimonii, *av.*	84	62
" opii	92	78

4th. Number of Drops of Water equivalent to f℥j *dropped from* f℥j *vials.*

1st trial 34.	2d trial 48.	3d trial 32.	4th trial 48.
5th trial 60.	6th trial 50.	7th trial 65.	Average 48.1.

[1] From f℥j Tr. bot. 53.

The drop machines here figured are contrived to obviate, to a certain extent, the inequalities given in the above table; they are not

Fig. 67.

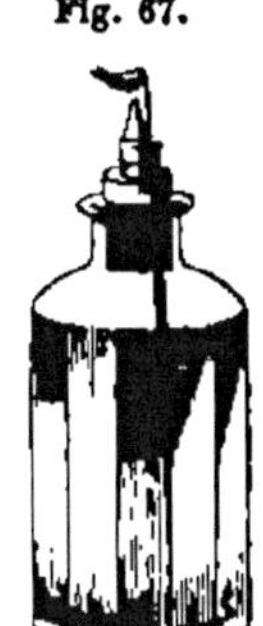

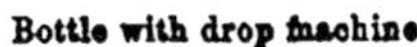

Bottle with drop machine.

Fig. 68.

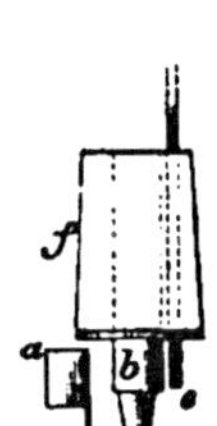

generally known, though quite useful to the physician and apothecary who has occasion to drop a large number of drops in succession. Their construction will be obvious from the drawing. A perforated cork with a tube, either of glass or metal, drawn out to a small orifice, and a capillary tube of metal passing above the surface of the liquid in the inverted bottle, so as to supply air to the vacuum created by the liquid as it drops out, constitutes all that is essential to the apparatus.

Specific Gravity.—In accordance with the general plan of this work, I shall endeavor to simplify this subject, and to divest it of unnecessary details, so as to leave no excuse to the student for neglecting to acquaint himself with it, so far as it is necessarily connected with his pursuits. In works on physics and chemistry, the subject of specific gravity is treated of as related to solids, liquids, and gases, but inasmuch as we are seldom under the necessity of trying the specific gravity of solids or gases except in experimental research, and as this text-book is designed merely to direct the practitioner of medicine and pharmacy in the necessary pursuits of his office or shop, I shall confine this essay to the specific gravity of liquids, which is the most important branch of the general subject.

It has been said at the commencement of this chapter that while extension and gravitation or weight, are each capable of a separate standard of measurement, it is impossible to bring them to a common standard—they are only capable of being *compared* with each other. To this comparison of the quantity of matter with its extension, we direct our attention under the head of specific gravity.

If we take a vial which will hold an ounce of water by weight, we find it will hold about an ounce and a half of nitric acid, and about three-quarters of an ounce of ether; hence we may say, approximately, that nitric acid is twice as heavy as ether, or that it is half as heavy again as water, while ether is only three-quarters as heavy. We thus compare these two liquids with a common standard, and one which, being universally diffused in a state of tolerable purity, furnishes the most ready means of comparing solid or liquid substances together. The relation which the weight of a substance bears to that of water is, therefore, called its specific gravity. Water being assumed as 1 in the illustration just given, nitric acid would be $1\frac{1}{2}$ or 1.5, and ether $\frac{3}{4}$ or .75. Upon this principle we may ascertain the specific gravity of all liquids by having a bottle, the capacity of which is well and accurately determined, filling it with these various liquids at a certain normal temperature, ascertaining their weight, and by a simple calculation bringing them to this common standard. The specific gravity of substances, when accurately ascertained, constitutes one of the most important items in their history. In pharmacy, it is much employed to indicate the strength and purity of medicines, particularly acids, alcohol, the ethers, and essential oils; and a physician is deficient in one of the most important aids to diagnosis who has not at hand the means of taking the specific gravity of *urine*.

The apparatus for ascertaining the specific gravity of liquids are of two kinds: first, specific gravity bottles; and second, hydrometers, or loaded tubes which mark the density of liquids by the depth to which they sink in them, according to known and purely artificial standards. The most convenient specific gravity bottles are graduated to hold 1,000 grains, or 100 grains of pure water at 60° F. Those made by Dr. W. H. Pile, of Philadelphia, are accurate and reliable; they are of two kinds, stoppered and unstoppered; the former are most approved; they are accompanied by a little counterpoise to be

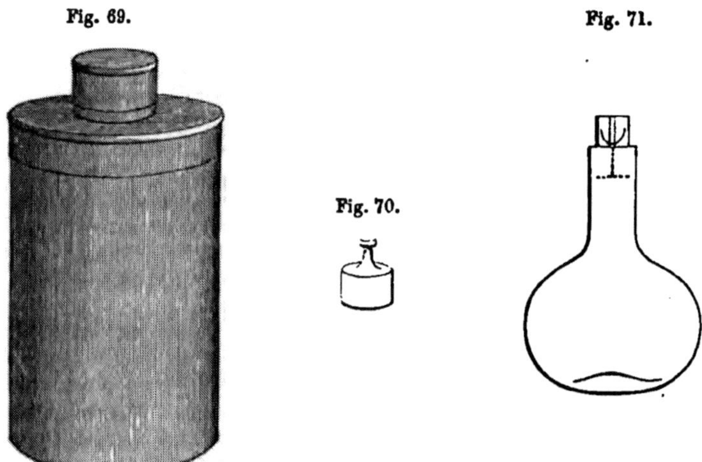

Fig. 69. Fig. 70. Fig. 71.

Stoppered specific gravity bottle, tin box, and counterpoise.

placed on the opposite scale plate, which exactly balances the empty bottle, so that the weights which balance it when filled and placed on the scale indicate the weight of its contents.

In filling the stoppered thousand grain bottle, it requires to be filled a little above the point in the neck to which the stopper will reach when replaced, so that this shall force out the air and a small portion of the liquid into the capillary tube drilled through it. The whole bottle is then wiped clean and dry, and weighed. The unstoppered thousand grain bottle is marked by the scratch of a file opposite the point in the neck to which the liquid must reach; this line should be intermediate between the upper and lower edge of the concave surface of the liquid in the neck when filled (see Fig. 66). The hundred grain bottles are of the same description, and used in the same way; they are convenient when only very small quantities can be obtained for testing, but are, of course, not quite so accurate. One particular merit of these bottles is, that the weight of a liquid, as obtained by filling and weighing them, expresses its specific gravity.

Fig. 72.

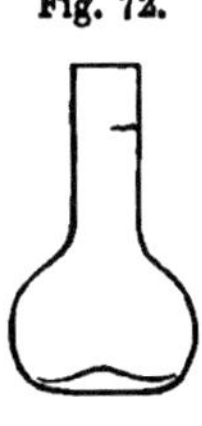

Specific gravity bottle, unstoppered.

The equation is this: as the weight of a certain bulk of water is to the weight of the same bulk of the liquid being tested, so is the specific gravity of water, which is unity, to the specific gravity of the liquid; or, as 1,000 is to the weight of the liquid, so is 1 to the specific gravity of the liquid. Having obtained the weight of this quantity of a liquid, we have its specific gravity; attention being required to the decimal mark merely. If, for instance, we fill the 1,000 grain bottle with alcohol, and find it weighs 835 grains, we write its specific gravity .835, placing the decimal mark before the figures, because the weight is less than the unit adopted. If we fill it with chloroform, and find the weight to be 1,490 grains, we state the specific gravity at 1.490, placing the decimal after the first figure; or, if we find it to hold 13,500 grains of mercury, we state the specific gravity 13.5, the decimal being varied for obvious reasons, but no calculation being necessary to ascertain their relation to water.

The specific gravity bottle I next proceed to describe does not exhibit the specific gravity of the liquid without a previous calculation, but possesses the advantage of being cheap and extemporaneous, and, if carefully made, is nearly as accurate.

Select a smooth and clean bottle, not too thick or clumsy, with a ground glass stopper; after first filing down the side of the stopper a small groove to subserve the purpose of the capillary orifice in the stopper of the 1,000 grain bottle, adjust it to one or more weights which counterpoise it, and put these aside for that use. Now find, by several trials, the exact weight of water it will hold at the proper temperature, and mark this on the bottle, or on a paper in which it is constantly wrapped; this is used in the same way as the 1,000 or 100 grain bottle, except that it is necessary to make a calculation after each weighing, to ascertain the specific gravity of the liquid. Suppose it to be a f℥ss bottle, and to contain, say 242.5 grains of pure water, and the liquids tested to have weighed 256 grains; now, to ascertain its specific gravity, a sum must be made as above stated: as the weight of a certain bulk of water is to the weight of the same bulk of this liquid so is the specific gravity of water to the specific gravity of this liquid:—

242.5 : 256 :: 1 : 1.055, or divide the weight of the liquid by the weight of the same bulk of water, thus $\frac{256}{242.5} = 1.055$.

I have, though rarely, been able to select f℥ss bottles, which, by modifying their size by filing the stopper, would hold exactly 250 grains, or $\frac{1000}{4}$, so that it was only necessary to divide the ascertained weight by 4 to get the specific gravity. This plan of taking the specific gravity is more accurate than that by hydrometers, that these extemporaneous or home-made bottles, when well made, and used with good scales, are to be preferred to the best hydrometers. These rarely mark with precision more than the second decimal, which is reached without difficulty with a bottle, even when the scales do not indicate the fractions of a grain: unstoppered specific gravity bottles are still more readily made.

The greatest practical difficulty in accurately adjusting a specific gravity bottle, and in taking the specific gravity of liquids, has relation to the temperature. The proper temperature for liquids to be measured by the specific gravity bottle is 60° Fahrenheit's scale, which at certain seasons of the year, in our climate, is readily attainable, but in hot weather the temperature of water will reach 90° or more; the dew-point then rises above 60°, so that if the water be brought to that temperature artificially and put into the bottle, the moisture deposited upon the outside of the bottle while weighing it will sensibly increase its weight. In order to obviate this difficulty, it is more convenient to have tables giving the variations of specific gravity by elevation or depression of temperature. The tables of this description formerly in use are unsatisfactory and conflicting, and have led Dr. Pile to prepare an original table, founded upon many hundred trials at all temperatures from 50° to 93°. This he has kindly furnished me for publication. The utility of this table in verifying the accuracy of the specific gravity bottle at any temperature will be apparent.

It may be remarked that as the glass bottle itself expands and contracts, experiment has shown it will contain about .013 grains more for every degree above 60°, and as much less below it. In weighing liquids above or below that temperature, we do not obtain directly the true specific gravity, but the conjoined result of the expansion or contraction of the water and the glass bottle. If the actual specific gravity is sought, it will be necessary to make the proper corrections both for the liquid on trial and for the glass bottle. This has been done in the following table.[1]

[1] For tables showing the variation in specific gravity of alcohol by changes of temperature, see Booth's *Encyclopædia of Chemistry*, Art. Alcoholometry, Tab. III. and IV.

Table of Apparent Specific Gravity of Water as observed in a Glass Bottle at different temperatures; also its true Specific Gravity. By W H. PILE, M. D.

Temp. Fahr.	Sp. gr. in Glass Bottles.	True Sp. Gr.	Temp. Fahr.	Sp. Gr. in Glass Bottles.	True Sp Gr.
50°	1000.54	1000.67	72	998.94	998.78
51	1000.50	1000.62	73	998.83	998.66
52	1000.46	1000.56	74	998.72	998.53
53	1000.41	1000.50	75	998.60	998.40
54	1000.36	1000.44	76	998.48	998.27
55	1000.30	1000.37	77	998.35	998.13
56	1000.25	1000.30	78	998.22	997.99
57	1000.20	1000.23	79	998.08	997.84
58	1000.14	1000.16	80	997.94	997.68
59	1000.07	1000.08	81	997.79	997.52
60	1000.00	1000.00	82	997.64	997.36
61	999.92	999.91	83	997.49	997.20
62	999.84	999.82	84	997.35	997.04
63	999.72	999.72	85	997.20	996.87
64	999.68	999.63	86	996.94	996.60
65	999.60	999.53	87	996.78	996.43
66	999.51	999.43	88	996.62	996.26
67	999.42	999.33	89	996.46	996.08
68	999.33	999.23	90	996.29	995.90
69	999.24	999.12	91	996.12	995.72
70	999.14	999.01	92	995.96	995.54
71	999.04	998.90	93	995.79	995.36

Schiff has proposed a very simple arrangement for the determination of the specific gravity of solid and liquid bodies. It consists merely of a test glass of even width graduated into cubic centimeters from the bottom and resting in a wooden or cork foot. It is used by pouring a convenient quantity of any liquid into the tube, noting its height and weighing the apparatus in grammes; the solid body is then introduced in a coarse powder, the apparatus weighed again and the height of the liquid noted. The difference of weight indicates the weight of the body, the difference of measure gives in cubic centimeters the amount of liquid displaced, and (as one cubic centimeter of water weighs one gramme) also the weight of distilled water in grammes displaced by the above body; consequently the weight of the body divided by the difference of measure in cubic centimeters gives the specific gravity.

To find the specific gravity of any given liquid, this is introduced into the tube previously weighed, the difference of weight in grammes after and before filling it, is simply divided by the number of cubic centimeters occupied by the liquid, to furnish the specific gravity.

The greatest density of water is at 39° F., and as the specific gravity is usually taken at 60° F., there is a slight discrepancy in the weight of water, which is exactly one gramme for each cubic centimeter at 39°; but the expansion of water between 32° and 212° is not more than .012, and the difference of its weight at 39° and 60° so slight that for ordinary purposes it may be overlooked.

HYDROMETERS.—These are instruments designed to be plunged into liquids to ascertain their comparative density or specific gravity although not capable of the same accuracy as the specific gravity bottles above described, they have the advantage of great convenience, and answer well for approximate results.

The application of this instrument depends upon the well ascertained law that a body immersed in any liquid sustains a pressure from below upwards equal to the weight of the volume of the liquid displaced by such body, and the use of the hydrometer dates back to the discovery of that principle, a period about three hundred years before the Christian era.

Hydrometers are now named with reference to the class of liquids for which they are designed, and to the scale upon which graduated. The kinds most sold in this country are imported; they are called, Baumé's hydrometers or areometers, and are also called saccharometers, when adapted to the measurement of syrups; acidometers, to acids; elæometers for oils, and urinometers for urine.

Cartier's hydrometer, which is somewhat used in France, is only applicable for light liquids; it is a modification of Baumé's Pése Esprit, and, having some points in the scale which correspond, is generally confounded with it. Without intending to confuse the student with unnecessary details, I shall give in a few words the method of obtaining the standards on the respective scales, and the mode of converting them into specific gravity and the reverse rule, omitting the tables, which will be found in the *Dispensatory* and chemical works.

Baumé had two instruments, one for liquids heavier than water, and one for liquids lighter than water; the former called *Pése Acide*, or *Pése Sirop*, and the latter *Pése Esprit*.

The zero for heavy liquids was water, and the point to which the instrument would sink in a solution containing fifteen per cent. of salt was marked 15°. The interval doubled gave 30°, the next 45°, and so on. The zero for lighter liquids, or *pése esprit*, was obtained by immersing the tube in water containing 10 per cent. of salt in solution, and the point to which it would sink in pure water he made 10°; dividing the stem into like intervals, he obtained 20°, 30°, &c., the intermediate degrees by subdivision.

Now it will be at once perceived that the slightest error made in obtaining the first interval by this process becomes increased in every extension, so that with all care and precaution to insure accuracy, scarcely any two instruments could be made to correspond precisely.

This mode of graduating hydrometers has long since been superseded by the equally practicable and more accurate method of obtaining the specific gravity of two known liquids at a certain fixed temperature. These are placed at the extremes of the scale, and the intermediate space is accurately subdivided into the requisite number of degrees.

The liquids ordinarily used for this purpose are, for liquids heavier than water, sulphuric acid and water; for those lighter than water, ether (highly rectified) and water. The specific gravity of these being of course ascertained before each trial by a standard hydrometer, or by the use of the 1000 grain bottle, but authorities are not agreed precisely in fixing their specific gravities, so that even the most accurate manipulators are liable to error from this fact, unless by having a common definite rule accuracy is ascertained. Another difficulty in regard to Baumé's hydrometers as usually imported, is, that they are marked by arbitrary numbers, which have no necessary connection with the specific gravity, and they can only be used with facility when access can be had to the tables published in chemical works, in which the degrees of Baumé, with their corresponding specific gravity numbers are represented.

The following simple formula has been contrived for the purpose of finding the specific gravity of any liquid, the degree of Baumé being known, or the reverse.

For Liquids heavier than Water.

1. To reduce Baumé to sp. gr. Subtract the degree of Baumé from 145, and divide into 145; the quotient is the specific gravity.

2. To reduce specific gravity into Baumé. Divide the specific gravity into 145, and subtract from 145; the remainder is the degree of Baumé.

For Liquids lighter than Water.

1. To reduce Baumé to sp. gr. Add the number of the degree to 130, and divide into 140; the quotient is the sp. gr.

2. To reduce sp. gr. to Baumé. Divide the sp. gr. into 140, and subtract 130 from the quotient; the remainder will be the degree of Baumé. In this manner, the tables at the end of this article were calculated.

The *rationale* of this formula is more difficult to understand than its application. The modulus or constant number here used, is the proportion which the space of one degree (or the bulk which one degree occupies) bears to the space or bulk of the whole hydrometer below the water line.

Or, it may be stated to be the proportion, which the weight of water displaced by the hydrometer when floating in water, bears to the weight of water equal in bulk to one degree.

For example, suppose the weight of a hydrometer to be 200 grs., it is floated in water and marks the water line (10° B. in pése esprit, or 0° B. in pése acide); now to sink it one degree in the first case, $\frac{1}{140}$ of its weight must be added, or 1.428 grs.; 140 is therefore the modulus of the scale for light liquids; in the other case, we must withdraw $\frac{1}{145}$ of its weight, or 1.38 grs., to enable the hydrometer to rise one degree; 145 is therefore the modulus of the pése acide: from this it will appear that the modulus determines the size of the degrees. That here presented was selected (as most consistent with the practice of manufacturing chemists, and according with the tables published in the *United States Dispensatory*) by Henry Pemberton, Practical Chemist, of this city, to whose able article showing the inconsistency of the standards in use, published in the *American Journal of Pharmacy*, vol. xxiv. p. 1, the reader is referred.

The inconvenience of an arbitrary scale, as that of Baumé, has long been felt, and has led to the manufacture of the new style of hydro-

Fig. 73.

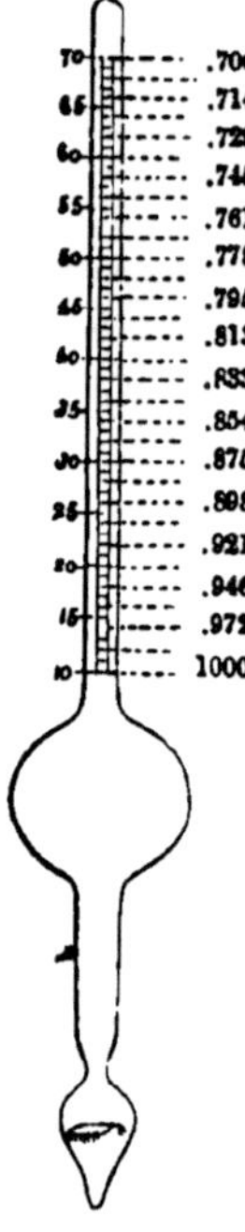

Hydrometer for liquids lighter than water.

meter, which is here figured; these have the scale of Baumé, with the actual specific gravity corresponding to it written opposite each other on the tube.

This article, as manufactured by Dr. W. H. Pile, before referred to, is unexceptionable. He makes a large size containing two in a series, one for liquids heavier, and the other for liquids lighter than water, each having an extensive range, and also a small size, consisting of two for light, and three for heavy liquids. The advantage of the series of five small instruments is, that the scales having a much less range, are capable of exhibiting more accurately slight differences in sp. gr. than in the other case. In the drawing, one of the large instruments is exhibited, considerably reduced in size; and as the scales with the two sets of figures could not be represented in a single view of the tube, the printer has appended on either side the figures representing the degree of Baumé, and a part of those representing the sp. gr.

Besides these hydrometers, Dr. Pile makes others for special applications, and graduated to suit particular objects; one of the most curious of these is the Lactometer, for the measurement of milk, which, as we get it in large cities, is liable to adulteration, and especially to dilution with water. (*See* Lac Vaccinum, Part III.)

Of all the practical applications of the art of determining specific gravity, none is more important and interesting than its use in ascertaining the qualities of urine. The urinometer is the most delicate of this class of instruments; it is a hydrometer tube with a very small range, only going from 1.000 to 1.060 specific gravity; within these limits, all the variations of urine from its normal standard may be ascertained. So delicate are these determinations, that the variations of temperature, important in all cases, here require special attention; and accordingly many of the urinometers are accompanied by a little thermometer to be plunged into the urine simultaneously with the tube; sometimes the thermometer is inclosed in the tube, and at others, as in the apparatus, Fig. 74, accompanies it in a neat box containing also a graduated glass for containing the urine.

The thousand grain bottle, with proper observance of the thermometer, is, however, in this as in all other cases, the surest test of specific gravity.

Fig. 75 represents the urinometer removed from the box and floated in the vessel accompanying it (in which the graduation marks are not seen). The graduation of the urinometer is such, that each degree represents 1·1000, thus giving the actual specific gravity by simply adding the number of degrees on the scale corresponding with the surface of the liquid, to 1000. Thus, supposing the number cut by the surface of the fluid to be 30, as shown in the figure, the specific

Fig. 74.

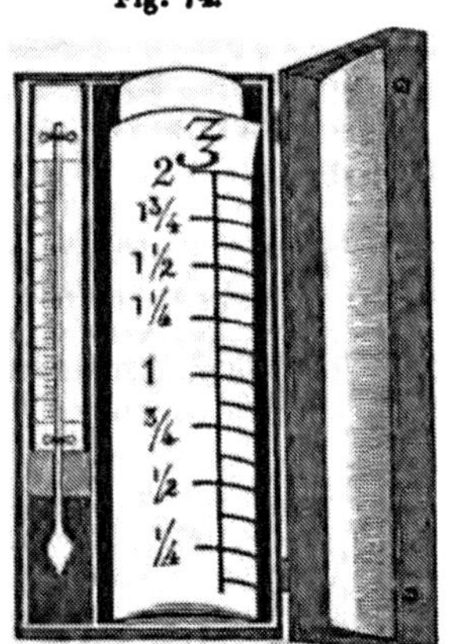

Urinometer box containing thermometer, graduated glass vessel, &c.

Fig. 75.

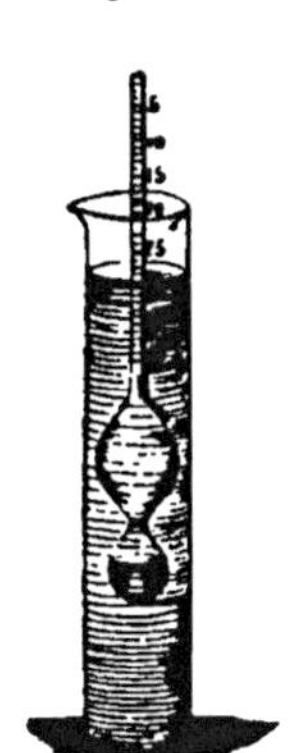

Urinometer in use.

gravity would then be 1.030. The average density of healthy urine is about from 10° to 25° of this scale, at 60° F., or sp. gr. 1.010 to 1.025. That of diabetic urine ranges from 30° to 60°, or sp. gr. 1.030 to 1.060.

Figs. 76 and 77 represent a hydrometer and glass jar adapted to containing the liquid to be tested; unless this vessel has considerable depth, the hydrometer is liable to touch the bottom, which would prevent its measuring. These vessels are sold by the principal dealers in chemical apparatus.

Fig. 76. Fig. 77. Fig. 78.

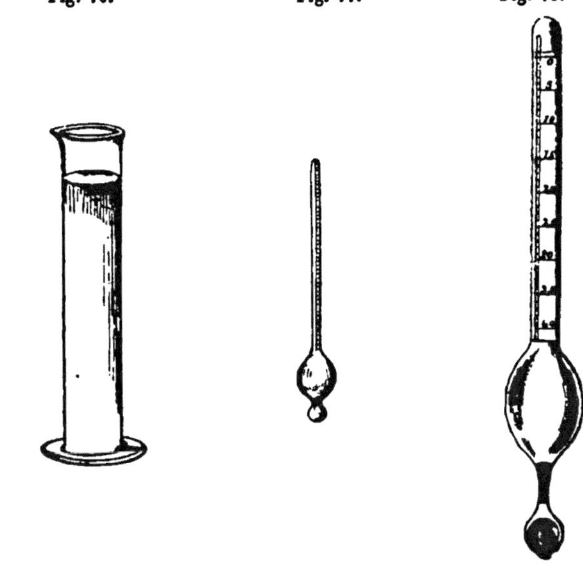

Hydrometer, with vessel for floating it.

Saccharometer.

Sometimes hydrometers for liquids heavier than water are manufactured of small size, for the special purpose of measuring the strength of syrups. Fig. 78 represents one of these, which is graduated to Baumé's scale. It floats at 30° in a solution of the sp. gr. 1.26, the density of saturated simple syrup when boiling.

BAUMÉ'S DEGREES, WITH THEIR CORRESPONDING SPECIFIC GRAVITY.

Table for Liquids lighter than Water. Temp. 60° Fahr.

Degrees of Hydrom.	Specific Gravity.	Degrees of Hydrom.	Specific Gravity.	Degrees of Hydrom.	Specific Gravity.
10	1.000	31	0.870	51	0.773
11	0.993	32	0.864	52	0.769
12	0.986	33	0.859	53	0.765
13	0.979	34	0.854	54	0.761
14	0.972	35	0.848	55	0.757
15	0.966	36	0.843	56	0.753
16	0.959	37	0.838	57	0.749
17	0.952	38	0.833	58	0.745
18	0.946	39	0.828	59	0.641
19	0.940	40	0.824	60	0.737
20	0.933	41	0.819	61	0.733
21	0.927	42	0.813	62	0.729
22	0.921	43	0.809	63	0.725
23	0.915	44	0.805	64	0.722
24	0.909	45	0.800	65	0.718
25	0.903	46	0.795	66	0.714
26	0.898	47	0.791	67	0.711
27	0.892	48	0.787	68	0.707
28	0.886	49	0.782	69	0.704
29	0.881	50	0.778	70	0.700
30	0.875				

Table for Liquids heavier than Water. Temp. 60° Fahr.[1]

Degrees of Hydrom.	Specific Gravity.	Degrees of Hydrom.	Specific Gravity	Degrees of Hydrom.	Specific Gravity.
1	1.007	26	1.218	51	1.543
2	1.014	27	1.229	52	1.559
3	1.021	28	1.239	53	1.576
4	1.028	29	1.250	54	1.593
5	1.036	30	1.261	55	1.611
6	1.043	31	1.272	56	1.629
7	1.051	32	1.283	57	1.648
8	1.058	33	1.295	58	1.667
9	1.066	34	1.306	59	1.686
10	1.074	35	1.318	60	1.706
11	1.082	36	1.330	61	1.726
12	1.090	37	1.343	62	1.747
13	1.098	38	1.355	63	1.768
14	1.107	39	1.368	64	1.790
15	1.115	40	1.381	65	1.813
16	1.124	41	1.394	66	1.835
17	1.133	42	1.408	67	1.859
18	1.142	43	1.422	68	1.883
19	1.151	44	1.436	69	1.908
20	1.160	45	1.450	70	1.933
21	1.169	46	1.465	71	1.959
22	1.179	47	1.480	72	1.966
23	1.188	48	1.495	73	2.014
24	1.198	49	1.510	74	2.042
25	1.208	50	1.526		

[1] These tables accompany Dr. Pile's hydrometers on the label.

CHAPTER III.

ON THE UNITED STATES PHARMACOPŒIA.

The necessity of accurate standards for the regulation of the strength and purity of medicines has been felt ever since medicine has been cultivated as a liberal profession, and in modern times has led to the adoption of authoritative works, called Pharmacopœias. Those published in Great Britain and on the continent of Europe were generally used in America during the last and the early part of the present century; though much confusion grew out of their different and sometimes conflicting directions.

The want of a national standard for the preparation of medicines having thus been felt for some time by practitioners of medicine and pharmacy, in 1818 a practicable plan for originating such a work was proposed at the suggestion of Dr. Lyman Spalding, by the New York State Medical Society. This was so generally acceptable to physicians, that in accordance with it, on the first day of the year 1820, a convention of medical delegates met in the city of Washington, over which Dr. Samuel L. Mitchell, of New York, presided, and Dr. Thomas T. Hewson, of Philadelphia, acted as secretary, in which essays prepared by the district conventions previously held in the Eastern and Middle States were duly considered, and the first edition of the *Pharmacopœia of the United States* was adopted, its publication being intrusted to a committee, who issued it before the close of the same year. This work, from the respectable authority which issued it, and from its general adaptation to the wants of physicians and apothecaries, was calculated to supersede the standards previously in use, although its general adoption was not rapidly brought about.

With a wise forethought to correct the imperfections of their work, and to adapt it to the future progress of pharmaceutical knowledge, the convention of 1820 provided for the choice of delegates to meet in convention after the lapse of ten years for revising the *Pharmacopœia*. The convention of 1830 elected Dr. Lewis Condict,[1] of New Jersey, its president, and after discussing the proposals submitted to them, referred the work of revision to a committee, of which the late Dr. Thomas T. Hewson was chairman, which met in Philadelphia, and by general correspondence and comparison of views with those residing in other localities, were enabled to add much to the value of the work. No small share of the labor of this committee was borne by Drs. Wood and Bache, who, by the publication, in 1831, of the *U. S. Dispensatory*,

[1] Dr. Condict, who, at the period of issuing this edition, is still an active and capable physician, participating with zeal in all the progressive movements of the profession, is perhaps the oldest living graduate of the University of Pennsylvania, having taken his degree in 1794, and been a practitioner of medicine for 65 years.

a work of great utility, in which the pharmacopœia was fully explained, commented on, and compared with similar foreign works, aided greatly in giving it the character it has ever since enjoyed, of a national standard for the preparation of medicine. The decennial revisions, in 1840 and 1850, were accomplished under similar auspices. The conventions which assembled at the capital in those years were presided over by Drs. Lewis Condict and George B. Wood, respectively, and the committees charged with carrying out the views of the body met in Philadelphia.

In the three decennial revisions, the Colleges of Pharmacy of Philadelphia and New York have borne an active, though not a conspicuous part; only in the last convention were they officially represented. There can be little doubt that the excellence of most of the formulæ of the *Pharmacopœia* is due in great measure to the valuable practical suggestions of the committees of pharmaceutists appointed by those organizations. Previous to the conventions of 1840 and 1850, large and efficient committees of practical pharmaceutists subjected all the proposed changes to the most rigid experimental scrutiny before submitting them to the convention, and through Professor Procter, their representative in the committee of revision and publication, their influence was made available in the final arrangement and completion of the work.

Upon the object and scope of the *Pharmacopœia* little need be said; its influence in producing uniformity in nomenclature, and in the strength and efficiency of medicinal preparations, has been widely and increasingly felt, although it is to be regretted that it is less in the hands of physicians and apothecaries than its importance demands. In this connection it may be proper to speak of the comparative utility of the *Pharmacopœia* and *Dispensatory*, especially as so many students of medicine and pharmacy confound the two works with each other. Every physician who practises pharmacy, as most country practitioners do, and every apothecary, should possess a copy of each of these works. The *Pharmacopœia* for use as a guide book in making preparations, and the *Dispensatory* for reference as an encyclopêdia of materia medica, therapeutics, and pharmacy.

While the *Dispensatory* is justly regarded as indispensable, and has certainly contributed more than any other work to the general diffusion of pharmaceutical knowledge, those very qualities which give it its true value unfit it to substitute the *Pharmacopœia* as a Recipe-book. The conciseness and brevity of the latter work, the clear and conspicuous type, and the absence of unnecessary detail, adapt it especially to the purpose named, that of indicating the ingredients, the proportions, and the mode of preparation of the officinal preparations. Liability to mistakes is greatly lessened by the clearness and accuracy of a recipe, which should always be open before the operator, and should be continually consulted in the course of his manipulations.

It will be in place to explain, in this connection, the use of the term *Officinal* in this work. While by some, this word is meant to apply to all permanent preparations; by others, it has an application to those only which are generally known and recognized by physicians and pharmaceutists in the particular locality referred to, and spoken of in the *Dispensatory*, or in foreign *Pharmacopœias*. I have preferred to restrict the use of the term to drugs and preparations mentioned in the *U. S. Pharmacopœia;* and I have carefully distinguished these throughout the work, from such as are either new remedies since the *Pharmacopœia* was last revised, or were omitted from the work from any other cause. It appears to me that this is the only limit of the term *officinal* which renders it definite and precise, and with this meaning it certainly is most useful in a work like the present.

To lay before the student the whole plan of the *Pharmacopœia*, and especially the principles which have regulated its nomenclature, the following extracts from the preface to the last edition are inserted here:—

"The contents of the work are arranged in the two divisions of Materia Medica and Preparations; the former enumerating and defining medicines as they are derived from nature, or furnished by the manufacturer, the latter containing formulæ, or rules, by which they are prepared for use.

"The subdivision of the Materia Medica into a primary and secondary list, is a peculiarity of our national standard. It has the advantage of permitting a discrimination between medicines of acknowledged value, and others of less estimation, which, however, may still have claims to notice. Many substances, at one time much employed, are passing out of use, without having been wholly discarded; while others are brought to the notice of the profession, and are undergoing trial, without having been generally adopted. It is very convenient to have a section into which such doubtful medicines may be thrown, to await the decision of experience for or against them. Without being entirely lost sight of, they are thus kept in a subordinate position, which may prevent misapprehension as to their real or estimated value. It is necessary to be understood, that the primary list contains not only all substances of recognized efficacy, but others of little or no apparent importance as medicines, which, however, are employed in some one or more of the 'preparations,' and are therefore essential. Without this explanation, the propriety of introducing such bodies as *Animal Charcoal*, *Bone*, *Cochineal*, *Marble*, and *Red Saunders*, into the primary list might be disputed.

"Both in the Materia Medica and the Preparations, the alphabetical arrangement has been adopted. In a work intended not for regular perusal but for occasional reference, it has the great merit of convenience. It has, moreover, the advantage that, making no claim to scientific classification, it is not liable to the charge of failure, so often and so justly urged against more ambitious systems. In relation to the preparations, it will be noticed that they are arranged in groups, the titles of which are placed in the alphabetical order. The pharmaceutical processes naturally throw themselves into such groups, which could not be divided and otherwise distributed without great inconvenience. Their affinity consists either in closely analogous modes of treatment, as in the decoctions, extracts, infusions, &c.; in having some common base, as in the preparations of the different metals; or in a certain resemblance of character, as in the acids and ethers. It happens, fortunately, that the several individuals in these groups are so named, that they fall into the general alphabetical order, with but very few and insignificant exceptions. It is proper to observe that the order of succession is based on the Latin names throughout the work.

"The Pharmacopœia was originally published both in the Latin and English languages. This was, at the time, an innovation upon general usage; as codes of this kind had been almost always issued by the dignified bodies from which they emanated exclusively in the Latin, which was considered as the language of science. In the revision of 1840, the Latin was dropped; as it did not offer advantages equivalent to the trouble of adapting a dead language to facts and processes for which it had no terms, and to the double cost of the work which it occasioned. The Latin names, however, of the medicines and preparations, have been retained, as they are still generally, and often very conveniently, used in prescription; and it is desirable that medicines should have designations by which they may be recognized in all civilized countries.

"The system of nomenclature of the Pharmacopœia of the United States is one of its chief merits. Adopted at a period when it was without example in other works of the kind, and improved with each successive revision, it now prevails to a considerable extent in all the Pharmaceutical codes recognized where our vernacular tongue is spoken. Its aim is to be simple, expressive, distinctive, and convenient. In relation to medicines of vegetable origin, it adopts for those which have been long and well known, the names by which they have at all times been recognized, and which have withstood, and will no doubt continue to withstand all the mutations of science. In this category are such titles as *Ammoniacum*, *Camphora*, *Galla*, *Opium*, *Senna*, *&c.* For medicines of more recent origin, which had received no distinctive officinal designation, it takes either the generic or specific title of the plant or animal from which the medicine is derived. Thus, we have the generic names *Anthemis* from Anthemis nobilis, *Chimaphila* from Chimaphila umbellata, *Eupatorium* from Eupatorium perfoliatum, *Gillenia* from Gillenia trifoliata, *Lobelia* from Lobelia inflata, &c.; and the specific names, *Senega* from Polygala Senega, *Serpentaria* from Aristolochia Serpentaria, *Taraxacum* from Leontodon Taraxacum, &c. A very large proportion of the names have been formed in this way; and, as the generic or specific title of the plant had its origin, in many instances, in the vernacular name, the original designation is thus fixed and perpetuated.

"When it happens that two different medicines are obtained from different species of the same genus, it becomes necessary to adopt either for both, the whole botanical title of the plants, or for one of them the generic or specific name, and for the other the whole name. Thus we have *Cassia Fistula* and *Cassia Marilandica*, *Quercus alba* and *Quercus tinctoria*, as titles both for the plants and their medicinal products; and, in the case of the different species of Gentiana, the generic name *Gentiana* for the product of G. lutea, and the whole name, *Gentiana*

Catesbæi, for that of the species so designated in scientific arrangements. When different parts of the same plant are recognized as distinct medicines, they are designated by attaching to the generic or specific title, the name of the part employed. Thus are formed the names *Colchici Radix* and *Colchici Semen* from Colchicum autumnale, and *Stramonii Folia*, *Stramonii Radix*, and *Stramonii Semen* from Datura Stramonium. When these names become established in pharmacy, it does not follow that they are to be changed with the changing scientific titles. On the contrary, it is generally best to retain them, unless, by doing so, injurious confusion may be occasioned. Thus we have *Prunus Virginiana* as the name of wild-cherry bark, though the plant from which it is derived is now usually designated by botanists as Cerasus serotina. It will be noticed that the Latin names are generally used in the singular number, even though the idea of plurality may be essentially connected with the medicine. Thus, *Cantharis*, *Caryophyllus*, *Ficus*, *Galla*, *Limon*, &c., are used instead of the plural of these terms respectively; and, in reference to the names derived from the part of the plant employed, the same plan is mostly followed, as in the case of *Stramonii Semen*, *Colchici Semen*, &c. In this the example of the Roman medical writers, particularly of Celsus, has been followed. The leaves, however, are expressed in the plural, as *Stramonii Folia*, &c., which is also in accordance with the practice of the same classical author.

"In the use of English names, it is not deemed necessary that they should be literal translations of the Latin terms; but that title is preferred which custom and the genius of the language seem to sanction. Thus, the English name corresponding to *Linum* is not *flax*, but *Flaxseed*; and, on the same principle, *Fœniculum* is called *Fennel-seed*; *Ulmus*, *Slippery Elm Bark*; *Glycyrrhiza*, *Liquorice Root*, &c. Nor are the English names always in the same number as the Latin. We may correctly say, *Caryophyllus*, *Galla*, *Prunum*, and *Rosa*; but the genius of our language requires that we should translate these terms *Cloves*, *Galls*, *Prunes*, and *Roses*.

"The plan of nomenclature in relation to medicines of mineral origin is to give the proper scientific name, when convenience, or some higher principle does not call for a deviation from that rule. Hence, the names of most mineral medicines are in strict accordance with existing scientific usage. But, in some instances, short and old established names are preferred to the scientific, especially when these happen to be somewhat unwieldy. Thus, *Alumen*, *Calamina*, and *Creta* have been preferred to the chemical names *Aluminæ et Potassæ Sulphas*, *Zinci Carbonas Impurus*, and *Calcis Carbonas Mollis*. In other instances, the chemical designation is more or less unsettled, or the composition of the substance has not been decisively determined. In such cases, either an old name is retained, as *Acidum Muriaticum* instead of either *Acidum Hydrochloricum* or *Acidum Chlorohydricum*; or some name is preferred generally expressive of the composition without aiming at chemical accuracy, as *Calx Chlorinata*, taken from the London Pharmacopœia, and *Ferrum Ammoniatum*.

"In other cases, it is considered safest to designate very active medicines which, if their strict chemical titles were used, might be dangerously confounded, by names which, though upon the chemical basis, have some epithet attached expressive of their distinctive character, as *mild chloride of mercury* and *corrosive chloride of mercury*, instead of *protochloride of mercury* and *bichloride of mercury*. Sometimes, for convenience sake, when no risk of confusion can possibly arise, names are adopted sufficiently expressive of the nature of the substance, though not precisely so; as *sulphate of iron* instead of *sulphate of protoxide of iron, hydrated oxide of iron* instead of *hydrated sesquioxide of iron*, &c. If any part of the nomenclature of mineral bodies should seem at first sight somewhat incongruous, it will be found to have been adopted in accordance with some one of the principles here stated, or in some other way to have the advantage of convenience or utility. Not a single name has been given or retained without careful consideration.

"When the officinal names of particular medicines may be supposed not to have yet become universally known, and the old names are still extensively used, the latter are given as synonymes in a subordinate type and position; and those officinal titles which have been superseded by others adopted at the present revision, are inserted beneath, with a reference to the Pharmacopœia of 1840.

"In the MATERIA MEDICA, the Latin and English officinal names are first given, and immediately afterwards, in a distinct paragraph, a definition fixing the precise character of the substance referred to; designating, for example, the plant or animal from which it is derived, and the part employed, if it be of vegetable or animal origin; and defining it by the precise chemical name, if mineral. When the officinal name sufficiently explains itself, as in the case of *Magnesiæ Sulphas, Potassæ Nitras*, and *Sodæ Carbonas*, no definition is given. To most of the mineral substances brief notes are appended, containing, in short and precise terms, an enumeration of those properties by which their identity can be determined, and of the tests by which their freedom from adulterations or accidental impurities may be ascertained. The same plan has been extended to many of the chemicals among the preparations. In relation to most of the medicines of organic origin, it has not been thought advisable to offer similar tests of genuineness and purity; as the means of judging are much less precise, and could not be readily expressed in a few brief rules.

"Among the PREPARATIONS will be noticed several substances which are now seldom made by the apothecary, being obtained almost exclusively from the manufacturing chemist. They have been retained in their present position, because, in our widely-extended country, circumstances may not unfrequently render it desirable that the apothecary should be able to prepare them in the absence of a due supply; and, though the processes might not have been introduced if now claiming admission for the first time, yet, having a place already in the Pharmacopœia, it has not been deemed advisable to omit them, and transfer their products to the Materia Medica. The circumstance that these substances are placed among the preparations does not preclude their purchase from the manufacturer when they can be procured of the proper quality.

"To one familiar with the British Pharmacopœias, it will be obvious that, in the preparation of our own, many of the processes have been taken from them with little alteration. This has been done advisedly. It is of the highest importance that medicines having the same names should have the same composition; and, as British works on medicine are much read in this country, it would lead to never-ending confusion if the substances they refer to by name should differ materially from those known by similar names with us. It has, therefore, been a general aim to bring our pharmacy into as near a correspondence as possible with that of Great Britain; but in all cases in which greater purity or efficiency in the medicine, or greater convenience and economy in the process, or any peculiarity in the relation of the preparation to our own circumstances and wants, called for deviation from the British standards, modified or wholly original processes have been adopted."

PART II.

GALENICAL PHARMACY.

CHAPTER I.

ON THE COLLECTION AND DESICCATION OF PLANTS.

THE plant may be conveniently divided into the root, stem, bark, buds, leaves, flowers, fruits and seed, and these different parts require the observance of different rules in regard to their collection, desiccation and preservation for use in medicine.

ROOTS of annual plants should be dug immediately before the time of flowering; of biennials, or perennials, late in the fall, or very early in the spring. If the latter, it should be immediately after the first appearance of the plant above the ground. Perennial roots should not be gathered till after two or three years' growth. Rhubarb is allowed to mature for four or five years—asparagus till three years old.

Fleshy, or succulent roots, require to be cut previous to drying, so as to expose a large surface to the air; the mode in which they are sliced, whether longitudinally or transversely, is of interest in judging of certain foreign drugs, but is little regarded by herbalists in preparing the indigenous roots for market.

In all cases, it is important that the root, or other part of the plant, should be thoroughly dried. In the case of taraxacum, parsley, and other succulent roots, it is necessary to apply a heat of about 150° F., in order to destroy the eggs deposited by insects, which, through neglect of this precaution, may occasion the speedy deterioration of the root by worms.

The smaller and more fibrous roots, and especially those contai n ing essential oils, require to be less thoroughly dried, and, as soon as their condition will admit of it, should be carefully put away into tight drawers, bottles, or tin cans. The stems of herbaceous plants should be gathered after foliation, but before flowering, unless the flowers are to be used with the stem.

BARKS of trees are best gathered in the spring, of shrubs in the autumn, at which seasons they can be most easily separated from the wood. They should be generally deprived of their epidermis, and dried spontaneously, their porous texture and comparative tenuity facilitating the process. Wild-cherry bark is often deficient in quality, from being gathered at the wrong season, and from the wrong part of the plant. It should be taken from the root in the eighth month—August. I have known it to become mouldy and lose its aroma by being put away too damp; when of fine quality, it has a strong and characteristic odor. The bark of wild cherry is preferred to be taken from the root of the tree, and that of sassafras is always derived from the root.

LEAVES should be gathered when fully developed, and before they have commenced to wither and fall; those of biennial plants, as the solanaceæ and digitalis, during the second season. After the appearance of the flowers, the leaves begin to lose their activity, the juices going to develop the fruit. In labiate plants the leaves are more aromatic as they approach the flowering tops, and the upper ones are frequently gathered with the tops.

HERBS, in which term are included whole plants, and such parts of the same plant as are collected and sold together, should be gathered when in flower. Plants which have thick and branching stalks or stems, should be deprived of these before being put up for sale.

FLOWERS may be gathered just before they are perfectly developed. The scent is less lively, and the color paler in fully expanded flowers, in consequence of the ovary growing at the expense of the accessory organs. The French or red rose is always gathered in bud, the astringent principle and beautiful red color being then best developed. A clear, dry morning, after the dew is dissipated, is to be preferred in either of these cases. They are dried in the shade, without artificial heat; the floor of a garret, through which is a draft of dry air, is well adapted to this purpose. Fleshy fruits, when designed for preservation are generally plucked before they are quite ripe. It is found that raspberries, strawberries, blackberries and mulberries yield a less glutinous and more agreeable juice when not perfectly ripe—"dead ripe;" the vegetable acids are then not so completely converted into sugar, and the aroma is fresher and stronger. The fruit of persimmon (*Diospyros*, U. S.) is directed to be collected before ripening, owing to its abounding in tannic acid, which, as it ripens, seems to be converted into sugar and apotheme.

SEEDS, which are the least perishable of vegetable productions, should be perfectly ripe when collected; they require very little drying.

The "United Brethren," called Shakers, at their settlement in New Lebanon, New York, have very extensive and convenient arrangements for drying these vegetable materials. Series of shelves of wire network are disposed in layers at suitable distances from each other, in large and well ventilated apartments; upon these the herbs are carefully placed, and allowed to remain subject to the desiccating action of the air, circulating below as well as above, until completely dried. They are then removed to capacious bins, of which many are arranged along the sides of the room, and preserved until nearly ready for pressing—an operation which, in common with some other herbalists, the Shakers practise upon every article of the vegetable Materia Medica which they collect for sale.

This practice, while it has its advantages, is liable to some objections. It has been said that, owing to the moist condition to which the plants require to be brought before pressing, the packages are liable to become mouldy in the middle. I have never met with an instance of this kind, however, and believe that the excellent reputation the Shaker herbs have attained is well founded. Another objection to these herbs, of a very different character, is, that they are not adapted to the examination of the physical characteristics of the plants; a pharmaceutical student, placed in an establishment where they are sold to the exclusion of the dried plants in bulk, enjoys no opportunity of familiarizing himself with the physical and botanical characters of this extensive class of medicines; to this may be added the difficulty in noticing any deficiency in quality, any intentional or accidental adulteration, or error in labelling the articles.

Very large quantities of several of the American medicinal plants enter into our commerce; spigelia and serpentaria are collected chiefly in the southern and southwestern States; sassafras and wild cherry bark, the root of asarum Canadense, and the leaves of hyoscyamus, belladonna, and conium, are naturalized in the New England States and in Canada, while taraxacum, eupatoreum, lobelia, geranium, lappa, inula, dulcamara hydrastis, and many others are gathered almost all over the country. The sources of the vast supplies of many of the leading American plants which enter into commerce are studiously concealed by the principal manufacturers and dealers, and the prices of the more important are subject to considerable fluctuations.

The business of collecting and drying medicinal plants is pursued in the vicinity of many of our large cities by herbalists, who realize a living from it. These have it in their power, by taking students of medicine and pharmacy with them on their excursions into the woods and fields, to extend a knowledge of medical plants among a class to whom it cannot fail to be in the highest degree useful and interesting.

There are few pursuits better calculated to relieve the monotony of a student's life, or to impart healthfulness and variety to the sedentary occupations of the apothecary, than a systematic out-door pursuit of the useful and ennobling science of botany; and the pharmaceutist or physician, by giving it a practical application to his business, may, in many instances, combine pecuniary with mental and physical advantage. For the benefit of students residing or sojourning in Philadelphia, a catalogue is inserted in the appendix, containing the name, time of flowering, and precise habitat of the wild plants growing within a few miles of the city.

The *cultivation* of medicinal plants in this country, for sale as such, is mainly confined to the beautiful valley in Columbia County, N. Y., already referred to, where it is pursued by the Shakers, and by Tilden

& Co. This district seems especially adapted to the purpose, and, like the celebrated "Physic Gardens" of Mitcham, in England, furnishes a great variety, and in large quantity.

Immense plantations of peppermint for the production of the oil exist in St. Joseph's County, in the southern part of Michigan, and in Ohio and Western New York. These are estimated to comprise an area exceeding 3,000 acres, and to yield in oil of peppermint over $63,000 per annum.

For an interesting account of the "Physic Gardens of Mitcham," see *American Journal of Pharmacy*, vol. xxiii. p. 25; for some details in regard to the N. Lebanon Gardens, see the same *Journal*, vol. xxiii. p. 386; and for an account, by F. Stearns, of the peppermint plantations of Michigan, see *Proceedings of Am. Pharm. Association*, 1858.

The question of how far the cultivation of plants diminishes or modifies their medicinal activity, is at present an undecided point; it is, however, universally admitted, that climate and soil exercise an important influence on their virtues.

The opinion is adopted by many that most plants are more fully developed in the country in which they are indigenous, than in any to which they may be transplanted; but that there are many exceptions to this rule, if it be a general rule, must be quite apparent.

In the present state of our knowledge upon this subject, we cannot go further than to say that of plants indigenous to the temperate zones, some flourish equally on either continent, while others, owing to some want of congeniality in climate and soil, will only develop their peculiar properties fully in the localities to which they are indigenous.

At the gardens in New Lebanon, the narcotic herbs indigenous to Europe are cultivated with apparent success, and the extracts prepared from them are among the best manufactured.

The classification of the vegetable materia medica best adapted to the purposes of the druggist is that which groups the different parts of plants together, as indicated at the commencement of this chapter. This is the arrangement adopted in the course of instruction in the Philadelphia College of Pharmacy; without any claim to a scientific basis, it is convenient, and affords especial advantages to the student who applies himself to the study of the physical peculiarities of the drugs. In examining students with the special object of teaching them to distinguish different drugs, I am accustomed to take up those most resembling each other in succession, relying chiefly upon the exhibition of characteristic specimens, and the application of the ready tests supplied by the senses. If every physician, druggist, and pharmaceutist were to make full use of this method, there would be very few instances of mistaking aconite root for taraxacum or briony for colombo.

CHAPTER II.

ON THE POWDERING OF DRUGS AND ON POWDERS.

According to the plan adopted in this work, the first class of preparations to be treated of is that of powders.

The preparation of the material for powdering, consists of garbling or sorting, and drying it. The former process pertains to the druggist, and the latter mainly to the drug grinder.

The object of *garbling* is to separate any impurities or adulterations, and any decayed or deteriorated portions of the drug. In nearly all foreign drugs imported into this country, especially those of vegetable origin, there are great variations in quality, and even in the same lot there are frequently very good and quite worthless specimens. As an illustration of this, Chinese rhubarb may be instanced: the roots, when broken, are found to vary exceedingly in quality, even in the same case; some are heavy and compact in their structure, breaking with a very uneven fracture, presenting a red and yellow marbled appearance, giving a gritty impression between the teeth, and the peculiar bitter, astringent taste, characteristic of the drug, while other roots are comparatively light, spongy in their internal structure, and almost destitute of the peculiar color and taste; some are worm-eaten, others which have the requisite specific gravity and the external appearance of a good article, are dark colored within and quite inferior. The custom of some, when about to send a lot of rhubarb to the drug-mill to be ground, is, either to send it in the mixed condition in which it is imported, or to select from it the finest pieces for separate sale, and for a sample, and send all the inferior roots, with perhaps only a small portion of the best, to be powdered.

A druggist who exhibits the best roots, selected in this way, as a sample of the kind powdered, cannot be acquitted of a gross and unpardonable fraud upon his customers. If he sends the whole case, containing good, bad, and indifferent, as originally imported, he may at least claim that, though he has not improved the quality of the medicine in reducing it to powder, he has not rendered it worse. But, with a view to furnishing a good and reliable medicinal agent, without regard to price, he would garble his rhubarb, by cracking each root, rejecting the decayed and otherwise defective pieces, and preserving in the form of powder only that which is of value. This is done by some druggists and pharmaceutists, who are more desirous of a reputation for the quality of their drugs than for cheapness.

Notwithstanding the difficulty of distinguishing the quality of medicines in powder by their sensible properties, we have in the case of rhubarb, general indications of excellence in a bright yellow color, a heavy and compact character in which the particles are not dustlike and mobile on the surface, and a well-marked and unmixed rhubarb odor. By a careful study of the characteristics of powders, their colors, compactness or mobility of particles, and, above all, their resemblance in odor and taste to good specimens of the drug, the physician and pharmaceutist may reach considerable skill in judging of their quality, and even in detecting adulterations.

In a subsequent chapter, I shall have occasion to refer to the variable quality of powdered gum Arabic; this is mainly owing to the neglect of garbling, or to the use of the rejected portion, after garbling, for reduction to powder. It is desirable to have the whole gum free from dusty and gritty particles; in this condition, it is more elegant and convenient for chewing, and for making the nutritive mucilaginous drinks, so much used by invalids, and it commands a better price. It is therefore customary to sift gum, as taken from the case, and the inferior kinds of powder are made from these siftings, which contain the dust, particles of sand, and other impurities.

A good powdered drug must invariably command an advance on the price of the drug in its crude state, the loss by drying, waste, cost of powdering, from 6 to 12 cents per pound, and other incidental expenses, to say nothing of the loss by garbling, furnishes a sufficient answer to those who complain of the high price of choice powders.

The chief reason for the deficiency in the quality of medicinal powders, is found in the reluctance manifested by the public, and retail apothecaries and physicians, to pay a liberal price for them. Powders are not unfrequently sold at a less price than the whole drug, especially when the article is costly, and of variable quality in commerce. This is true, especially of rhubarb, jalap, gum Arabic, and the spices, which, as a general thing, cannot be recommended in powder with the same confidence as in the unpowdered condition, or in the form of Galenical preparations, prepared from the whole or contused drug.

In garbling digitalis, hyoscyamus, and some other leaves, whether for powdering, or for use in making tinctures, as before stated, care should be taken to remove the midribs and petioles, which are comparatively inactive.

Drying and Powdering.—When a drug is sent to be ground in its ordinary condition, it generally requires drying, previously to being submitted to the action of the mill.

Moist and tenacious substances, such as the gum resins, opium, aloes, squill, and jalap, colocynth, and all fresh roots and herbs, require this treatment to a certain extent, and the drug-mills are supplied with apartments, or steam baths, adapted to it. These are heated to a temperature of about 120° F., and the drug is allowed to remain in them as long as is deemed necessary to deprive it entirely of water.

Some drugs are injured by this process; the volatile ingredient, so often the active principle, suffers great loss, and the resulting powder is comparatively inefficient. Myrrh and assafœtida furnish good illustrations of this.

On the other hand, substances possessed of no active volatile ingredient, but containing a large amount of water, as opium, are enhanced in value by drying and powdering. Some specimens of opium diminish in drying and powdering, to the extent of 20 per cent., which, if the process is properly conducted, increases the efficiency and value of the drug in that proportion. Experiments under my own supervision show about an average loss of 9 per cent., in reducing tolerably hard opium to the pulverulent condition. It is on this account, and from the fact that the powder, when unadulterated, is more nearly uniform in its composition than the drug in mass, that the U. S. Pharmacopœia directs the use of powdered opium in making all the Galenical preparations of that drug.

Elecampane root is said to lose seven-eighths of its weight in drying; stramonium leaves, nine-tenths; hyoscyamus and belladonna leaves, nearly as much. If these plants lose nothing but moisture in the process, and retain all their active medicinal properties unimpaired, it is obvious that they are seven or eight times stronger when in powder, or in a dry condition, than when recent. It is moreover a generally received opinion that vegetables yield their virtues by infusion more readily when dried than when they are fresh.

A difficulty, liable to occur in powdering drugs at the mills, is due to the accidental admixture of foreign substances with them. The extensive grinding surface employed becomes so completely covered with the fine powder, that it is cleaned with great difficulty; so that the next substance introduced becomes contaminated with it, sometimes to its great disadvantage. I have repeatedly observed this in the cases of certain articles of delicate flavor, as orris root and vanilla.

The plan of *dusting* powders, which insures their extreme fineness, and the separation of any earthy impurity, has gained in favor of recent time. The apparatus now used is constructed so that the powdered drug, when it has passed between the grinding surfaces, is thrown by a draught, artificially created below, to a height of about five feet, and is then allowed to settle upon the adjacent parts, from which, after it has collected in sufficient quantity, it is removed.

It will be appropriate, in this place, to give some observations upon powdering, as practised, on a small scale, in the shop and laboratory. This is accomplished by means of mortars, suited to the different processes of contusion and trituration, and by mills.

Mortars for contusion are usually made of iron, brass, or bell-metal, of the shape shown in Fig. 79. Contusion is employed for powdering and bruising ligneous substances generally, being adapted to breaking apart their fibres, and, by the violent attrition of the coarser particles with each other, reducing the whole to a more or less fine powder.

Care must be taken to avoid treating any corrosive substance in the iron mortar, thus allowing it to become rusty; or, if this should occur, it should be carefully washed out with diluted muriatic acid, and scoured with clean sand, to fit it for use. Any adhering material should be cleaned away immediately after the mortar is out of use, as

Fig. 79.

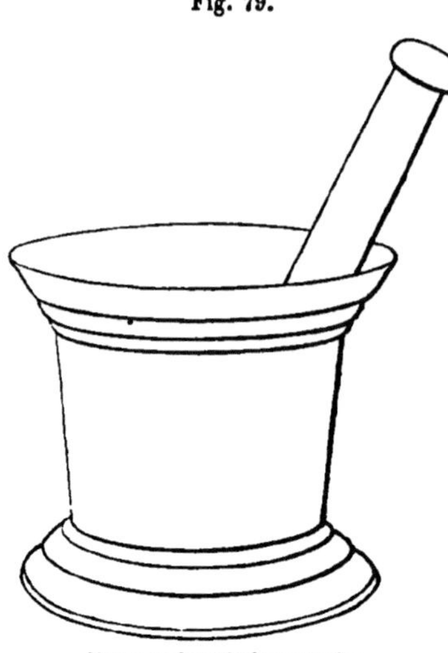

Mortar and pestle for contusion.

it is then more easily removed than if allowed to remain and harden. The mortar is then always ready for use.

In powdering substances by contusion too large a quantity should not be introduced into the mortar at one time; if the mortar is small, sufficient to cover the bottom for the depth of an inch or two; the flattened extremity of the pestle is then to be brought into direct and violent contact with it, each successive stroke being aimed at the same spot in the centre of the circle formed by the sides and bottom of the mortar. When part of the contents under treatment assumes the condition of a fine powder, which is exhibited by the air becoming charged with the dust, it is well to sift it, and thus separate the fine from the coarser particles, these last being returned to the mortar, and further contused until a second sifting becomes necessary, and so on till it is finished. A small portion of the drug is usually left in powdering, which it seems impossible to reduce sufficiently; this is part of the ligneous portion, which is frequently inert; the drug-grinder who obtains a considerable quantity of this *gruff*, as it is called, usually retains it for admixture with the next lot of the same drug he is called upon to grind, in this way reducing somewhat the loss upon it: he is usually allowed a small percentage for this necessary deficiency in the powdered product.

The mortar and pestle adapted for trituration are shown in Figs. 80 and 81. Such a mortar requires to be more carefully handled than one for contusion. It is adapted to the reduction of saline substances and chemicals generally to powder, by the friction of their particles with each other, between the hard and rough surfaces of the mortar and pestle. The ware being brittle, should not be subjected to blows with the pestle; it should be carefully wiped out and laid away, after using, so as to be dry and clean whenever needed.

The mode of manipulating with the wedgewood mortar and pestle, after placing in it the material to be ground to powder, is to grasp the pestle firmly with the right hand, holding the mortar with the left if necessary, and gradually to traverse the mortar with the pestle from the centre outwards, reaching the circumference gradually, by a series of rotary motions; and then, by reversing the direction of these motions, to bring the pestle again to the centre; in this way all parts are brought fully and equally under the action of the pestle. When the contents of the mortar become caked, and cease to fall towards the centre, when agitated, which often happens when the powder becomes very fine, a spatula should be occasionally run around the sides and bottom, to loosen and mix together the different portions.

Fig. 80. Fig. 81.

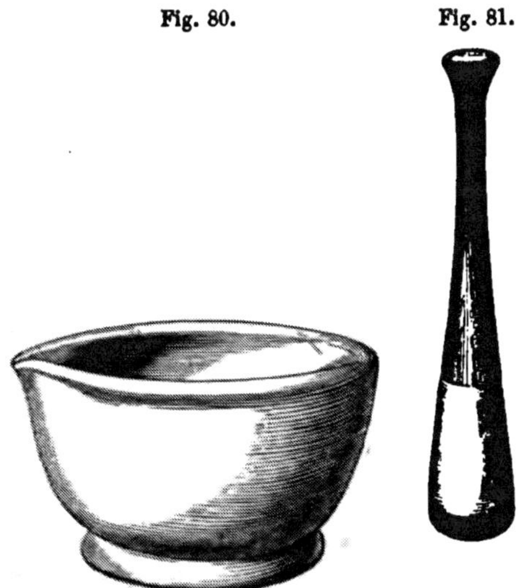

Wedgewood mortar and pestle.

A loose and careless way of triturating substances is productive of no saving of labor; the conditions most favorable to pulverization by trituration are a constant, uniform, and hard grinding motion communicated to the pestle, the layer of powder intervening between it and the mortar being thin, and the mortar so shaped as to present all parts of it equally to the action of the pestle.

Many substances can neither be reduced to powder by the process of contusion nor by that of trituration; of these, nutmeg may be instanced as one which is most conveniently grated, or scraped off with

Fig. 82.

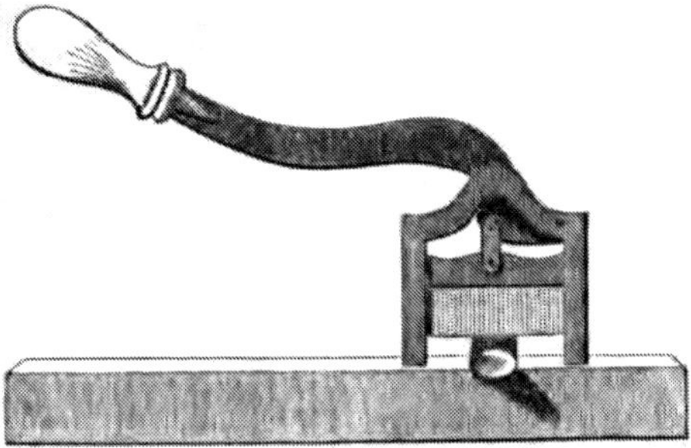

Tobacco knife.

the blade of a knife; vanilla is another instance, this may be cut into short pieces with shears and afterwards triturated with a third substance; if reduced with a view to infusion or displacement with alcohol, sand may be conveniently employed; if water is to be used, or if it is to be dispensed in a dry condition, hard lumps of sugar may be advantageously substituted. Many oily substances such as nutmeg and cardamoms and other aromatic seeds, can be made into convenient powders with dry and ligneous substances, although themselves unsuited to this form of preparation. Orange-peel, slippery elm, mezereon bark, liquorice root, are best comminuted by cutting them with a pair of shears, or a knife fastened on a lever, such as tobacconists use for cutting tobacco into plugs, and then drying them and introducing them into a suitable mill. The mode of cutting a piece of liquorice root into convenient pieces for chewing, is shown in the drawing.

Quassia, guaiacum, logwood, and red saunders are chipped by machinery, the two latter especially, for use in arts.

Camphor is easily reduced to powder by adding to it a small portion of some liquid in which it is soluble, as, for instance, alcohol, and triturating to dryness; the proportion of alcohol proper to be added to camphor for this purpose is about one minim to three grains. As camphor will not retain its impalpable condition alone, it is desirable to incorporate with it immediately, any dry powder with which it is designed to be mixed, as, for instance, precipitated carbonate of lime, where it is to be used as a dentifrice.

Figs. 83 and 84 represent very convenient forms of labor-saving apparatus for the physician and pharmaceutist. Swift's drug-mill is in very common use, both for fine and coarse powders; and the spice-mill represented on the next page will often do to substitute it, being more portable, and readily removed and replaced again upon the edge of the counter or office table. The grinding surfaces in both are of cast iron, in the one case toothed, and in the other grooved, so as to tear apart the substances with facility. In each case, the coarseness of the product may be varied by the use of a screw, which is so arranged as, by tightening it, to approximate the grinding surfaces, and effect a finer division, or, by loosening, to furnish a coarser powder by removing the comminuting surfaces further apart. The article to be powdered should be well dried, and, for grinding in the small mill, should not be in pieces larger than a hickory-nut.

Fig. 83.

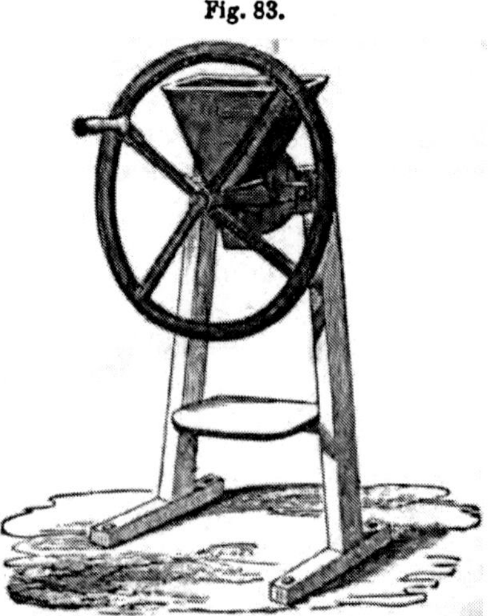

Swift's drug-mill.

Muriate of ammonia, and carbonate and nitrate of potassa, and other saline substances, are conveniently reduced by the process of *granu-*

Fig. 84.

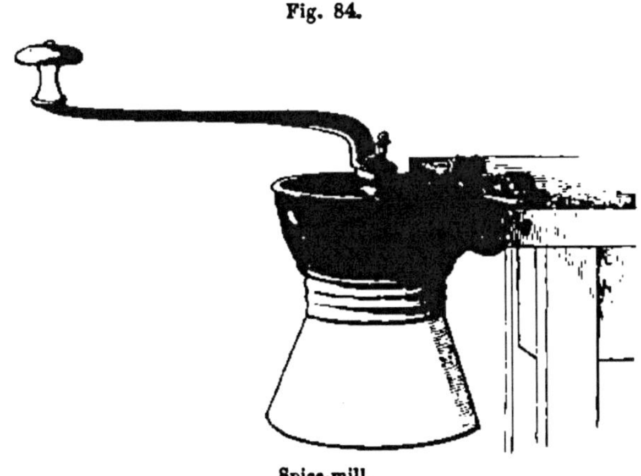

Spice-mill.

lation, which consists in dissolving the salt in water, and evaporating to dryness, constantly stirring. The process is only applicable to a few articles which are freely soluble, and not readily decomposed or volatilized by heat; the granulated powders thus produced are generally quite different from those made by mechanical means; they are neither so fine nor so free from water.

Many of the insoluble powders are obtained by precipitation; as, for example, precipitated sulphur, prepared by dropping muriatic acid into a solution of bisulphuret of calcium and hyposulphite of lime; the calcium and chlorine present, uniting with the acid, form chloride of calcium and water; the former being extremely soluble, the sulphur, which is insoluble, is thus precipitated as a fine powder. (See *Sulphur.*)

On the same principle the precipitated carbonate of lime is prepared by adding a solution of carbonate of soda to a solution of chloride of calcium. As a result of the reaction, the soluble carbonate of lime is produced and is thrown down in the form of a powder. (See *Alkaline Earths.*)

It is worthy of remark, in regard to these powders generally, that they are composed of very small crystals. Their fineness is dependent upon the temperature and degree of concentration of the liquids when mixed. When the solutions are hot and concentrated, the reaction takes place suddenly, and the powder is very fine; when they are cold and more dilute, the precipitate is gradually deposited, and more perfectly assumes the crystalline form.

Tartar emetic is obtained in a very fine powder, suitable for preparing the ointment, by dissolving it in water, so as to form a strong solution, and then adding alcohol to this. The strong affinity of water for alcohol causes it to unite with it, and the tartar emetic being less soluble in the alcoholic liquid is thrown down in an impalpable powder.

Sifting.—The fineness of powders may be regulated by the use of sieves which will separate particles of different degrees of division; the finest bolting cloth will only pass those which are almost impalpable, while sieves of from 40 to 60 meshes to the linear inch are adapted to the preparation of coarser powders for displacement. In all cases when the powder is to be used in divided portions, care should be taken to mix the different siftings thoroughly together, as the more ligneous and least active portions usually resist the operation of the pestle longest and are in the last siftings.

Fig. 85 represents a sifting machine, patented by Samuel Harris, of Springfield, Mass., which is well adapted to facilitate the process. It consists of a wooden box, with a flange, upon which an oblong sieve is made to move by a wheel and crank, the construction of which is shown in the drawing; by closing the lid the dust is prevented from rising in the air, and one of the most common causes of waste and annoyance is thus obviated. The sieve is movable, so as to be emptied without inconvenience, and by having sieves of different degrees of fineness, it will be obvious that the apparatus may be adapted to all the purposes of the pharmaceutist. The sizes of this apparatus are so varied as to suit numerous purposes, not only in pharmacy, but in the arts and in agriculture.

Fig. 85.

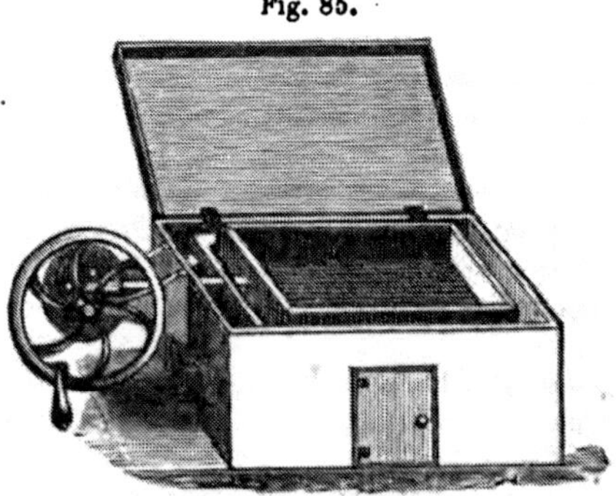

Harris' sifting machine.

The operation of *sifting* may also be varied according to the degree of fineness required in the powder. To pass the finest particles only the sieve should be gently agitated, the powder being laid lightly upon it, and the operation being suspended as soon as it has ceased to pass through readily; the plan of rubbing the powder over the sieve with the hand, thus using more or less pressure to force it through the meshes, may be pursued when the fineness of the powder is not so much desired as the rapidity of the process.

Powders, as a class of medicinal remedies, possess the advantage, when skilfully prepared, of uniting all the proximate principles of the plant, in their natural condition, and may be administered without the intervention of any menstruum. They may be used in bulk, taken into the mouth with water or some viscid liquid; or may be made into pills; or suspended in liquids in the form of mixtures. See Part V. *Extemporaneous Pharmacy.*

The disadvantages' attendant upon their use, are these: they are frequently too bulky for convenience, the dose being so large as to be repulsive to the patient; generally vegetable powders contain a considerable proportion of inert ligneous matter, many of them are liable to undergo an unfavorable change by exposure to the influence of the atmosphere, especially when it is charged with moisture; and they are liable to be injured by light. Vegetable powders are also subject to adulteration, the detection of which is difficult.

Except in the few cases, such as opium and cinchona bark, where we may isolate the active principle, and ascertain the proportion contained in a given sample, it is difficult to judge with certainty of the quality of a powdered drug; the best safeguard of the physician against fraud or the effects of carelessness, where the vegetable powders are concerned, is to buy them of careful and conscientious druggists, who either powder them, or exercise a strict supervision over the process as conducted by the drug-grinder.

Extreme fineness is very much sought after in powders, especially of latter times; and we are not without evidence of its conferring great superiority in some cases. Ferri pulvis of the U. S. Pharmacopœia is an instance of the advantage of minute division.

The fineness of powders affects their color, as is manifest in the case of white saline substances, which become whiter by long trituration.

There is no separate class of *simple* powders in the Pharmacopœia; they are understood to be included in the Materia Medica list. The *compound* powders which are officinal, are included in this work under the general head of extemporaneous powders and pills, and designated by U. S. P. A table of them will, however, be useful to the student in this connection.

Pulveres, U. S. P.

Name.	Proportions.	Med. Prop.	Dose.
Pulvis Aromaticus . . .	Cinnamon 2 p. Ginger 2 p. Cardamoms 1 p. Nutmeg 1 p.	Carminative	
" Aloes et Canellæ . . (Hiera Picra)	Aloes 4 p. Canella 1 p.	Stomachic Laxative	20 grains.
" Ipecac et Opii . . . (Dover's Powder)	P. Ipecac 1 p. P. Opium 1 p. Sulph. Potass 8 p.	Sedative Diaphoretic	10 grains.
" Jalapæ compositum .	P. Jalap 1 p. Bitart. Potass 2 p.	Cathartic	20 grains.

The necessary practical hints in regard to the mode of preparing and dispensing these, are given under the appropriate head in the chapter on *Dispensing.*

CHAPTER III.

ON SOLUTION, FILTRATION, AND THE MEDICATED WATERS.

THERE are two objects in view in this process, and the principal feature in the classification of solutions is founded on this fact.

The simplest kind is that in which, by the use of an appropriate liquid, we overcome the attraction of aggregation in a solid body, rendering its particles more susceptible to chemical action, and more readily assimilated when taken into the stomach. The liquid used for this purpose is called a solvent; and water, the great neutral solvent, is most used in preparing this class, which may be designated *simple solutions*, whenever on evaporation the solid ingredient may be recovered unaltered.

When we speak of the solubility of any solid substance, we have reference to its relation to water, the term being an approximate one. Very few substances exist in nature wholly insoluble; and as there is no line between the least soluble, and those which are freely dissolved under ordinary circumstances, the term is not adapted to use where accuracy or precision of language is required.

Solution is accomplished by bringing the material under treatment, into contact with the solvent under favorable circumstances; these relate, 1st, to temperature; 2d, to the state of aggregation of the solid; 3d, to its position in relation to the solvent.

Hot liquids dissolve substances with greater facility than do cold; with exceptions, among which are lime, magnesia, and chloride of sodium. Though heat favors solution, there are no liquids wholly insoluble in the cold, which dissolve by the aid of increased temperature. In addition to the greater solvent power of hot liquids, the currents produced by the process of heating them, favor the more rapid solution of the contained solids, as shaking up the vessel favors the same result.

To facilitate solution in a small way, mortars are much employed; they serve the double purpose of reducing the solid to powder, and of promoting its intimate mixture throughout the liquid. Mortars of porcelain ware (Fig. 86) are most suitable for this purpose; they are used as follows. The substance to be dissolved, is first placed in the mortar and rubbed into a powder more or less fine. The process of solution proceeds more slowly as the liquid becomes more nearly saturated, hence a small portion of the solvent is first added

Fig. 86.

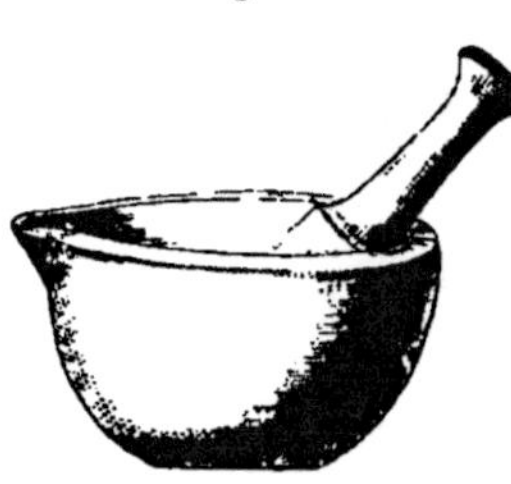

Porcelain mortar.

and triturated with the powder; as soon as this portion seems to be nearly saturated, it is poured into another vessel, and an additional portion of the solvent added, triturated, and poured off in the same way; a fresh portion again being added, the process is repeated, and so continued till the powder has disappeared. The liquids thus obtained, being mixed, furnish a stronger solution than could be prepared in the same length of time under the ordinary circumstances of contact.

When a weak solution is to be made, especially of a delicate chemical substance, like nitrate of silver, a good way is to drop the crystals or powder into the liquid previously placed in a clean vial of suitable size, to which a cork has been fitted, and to shake it up until dissolved. This should only be done in the case of very soluble substances, and the shaking should be continued as long as any portion remains undissolved.

A good arrangement for effecting solution is to place the solid on a perforated diaphragm resting beneath the surface of the liquid, or to inclose it in a bag of some porous material, and suspend it by a thread in the vessel near its top. By this contrivance, that portion of the liquid having the greatest solvent power, because the least saturated, is always in contact with the solid; the solution, as it becomes saturated, sinks to the bottom, and displaces the portion less charged with the solid ingredient, which, in consequence of its less specific gravity, tends to the top, thus keeping up a continual circulation in the fluid favorable to the object in view. In large operations in the arts where it is impossible to shake or to stir the liquid conveniently, an arrangement based upon this principle is adopted, and in smaller pharmaceutical operations Squire's infusion mug, figured in the next chapter, will be found to answer a good purpose.

The term *saturated*, besides its application as above, is employed to signify that an acid is neutralized by an alkali, or *vice versa;* or, in other words, that an equivalent proportion of one substance has combined with an equivalent proportion of another, for which it has an affinity; they are then said to have saturated each other. The term, when used for this purpose, may be said to be a strictly chemical one, but when employed as above, to designate the point at which a liquid ceases to dissolve a solid body, it is used in a pharmaceutical sense. It is worthy of remark that the saturated solution of one salt is frequently a solvent for other salts, a quality of great value in the preparation and purification of salts in the arts.

Rapid solution, even when not accompanied by chemical reaction, generally causes a reduction of temperature, and thus retards the process to a certain extent, so that, in arrangements for solution on a large scale, it is important to counteract this effect by contrivances for keeping up the temperature of the liquid.

A large number of the solutions used in medicine are effected by inducing chemical changes among the ingredients introduced into them, sometimes yielding soluble compounds, where one or more of the original ingredients were insoluble.

The solutions officinal in the U. S. Pharmacopœia, are not arranged as a separate class of preparations, but being generally composed of the metallic salts dissolved in water, they are dispersed throughout the work under the heads of the salts themselves, and will be noticed in detail either in the consideration of the extemporaneous combinations, or under separate and appropriate heads, being designated by the initials U. S. P. The following syllabus embraces them at a single view:—

Solutions officinal in the U. S. Pharmacopœia.[1]

OFFICINAL NAME.	REMARKS.	USES AND DOSES.
Liquor Ammoniæ	Solution of the gas, sp. gr., .960	Externally
" " Fortior	" " .882	"
" " Acetatis	From the Carbonate and Dil. Acet. Acid	fʒj, f℥ss
" Barii Chloridi	From Carb. of Baryta and Muriatic Acid	5 drops
" Calcii Chloridi	From Carb. of Lime and Muriatic Acid	30 drops
" Calcis	Saturated Solution of Hydrate of Lime	f℥j
" Potassæ	From Carbonate by Hydrate of Lime	10 dps in milk
" " Arsenitis	64 grs. Arsen. Acid and Carb. Potas. to Oj	10 drops
" " Carbonatis	℔j to f℥xij water	"
" " Citratis	See Extemporaneous Preparations	f℥ss
" Sodæ Chlorinata	From Chlorinated Lime and Carb. Soda	Antiseptic
" Magnesiæ Citratis	By direct combination, flavoring, &c.	f℥xij
" Plumbi Subacetatis	From Acetate of Lead and Litharge	Externally
" " " dilutus	fʒij to Oj water (Lead Water)	"
" Ferri Iodidi	By direct combination and sugar	15 drops
" " Nitratis	" "	10 drops
" Iodinii Comp.	Iod. 22½ grs., Pot. Iod. 45 grs. to f℥j	5 drops
" Hydr. et Arsenici Iod.	Gr. xxxv of each to Oss	5 drops
" Morphiæ Sulphatis	1 gr. to f℥j	fʒj

FILTRATION.—In this place it is appropriate to introduce an account of the process of filtration. The object of this is to separate any un-

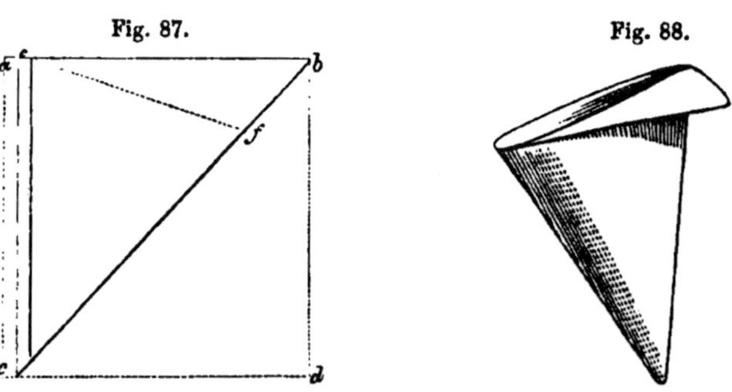

Fig. 87. Fig. 88.

Flannel strainer.

dissolved or precipitated substance suspended in a liquid from the liquid itself. When the liquid is viscid, and contains only motes of an appreciable size, as, for instance, when a syrup has been prepared from sugar contaminated with insoluble impurities, a sufficient filter

[1] Solutions in alcohol are called tinctures or spirits, as Tinct. Ferri Chloridi, Tinct. Iodinii, and Spiritus Ammoniæ.

may be constructed of flannel or Canton flannel by folding over a square piece in the manner indicated in the figure, the line *c d* being laid over the line *c a*, and united by a seam; the bag thus formed is pointed at *c*, and open from *a* to *b*, the line *a c* being lapped over to form the seam. In using this strainer, the long end projecting toward the point *b*, beyond the dotted line *e f*, may be turned over the side of the vessel, by which the strainer will be kept in its place while the liquid is poured into the opening at the top.

This process is called *straining*, though a kind of filtration. In pharmacy, infusions, decoctions, syrups, fixed oils, and melted ointments are subjected to it in order to separate foreign ingredients. They pass through the strainer with much greater facility when quite hot, though in the case of the fixed oils and syrups, clearer products are obtained by conducting the operation in the cold, and by using several thicknesses of the flannel, or by employing Canton flannel with the nap on the inside. Coarse linen is sometimes better than flannel, especially when considerable pressure is to be employed, as in extracting the juice from the pulp in making fruit syrups.

Fig. 89.

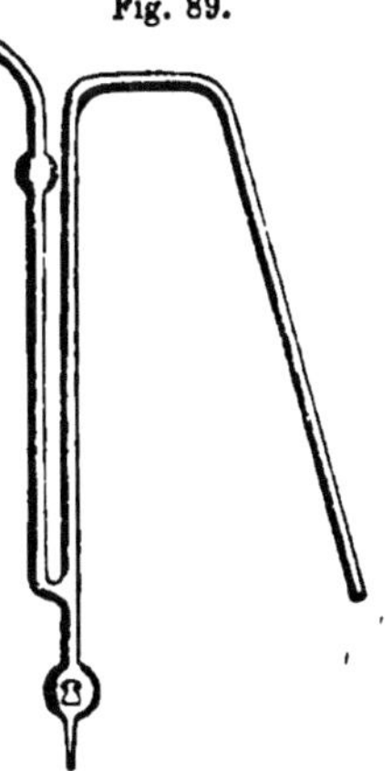

Siphon.

Filtration differs from clarification in its mechanical action. The latter term is applied where the impurities to be separated are deposited on account of their greater specific gravity, or by being rendered heavier by the application of heat, or where, by the addition of a foreign substance, they are aggregated together and separated as a coagulum. In separating a clear supernatant liquid from a deposited precipitate, or for drawing off liquids from vessels ill adapted to decantation, a siphon (Fig. 89) may be advantageously used.

The mode of using this instrument is to insert the shorter leg in the liquid, to apply the finger to the open end of the longer leg, and then draw the whole tube full of the liquid by sucking at the mouth-piece; when this is done, the finger is withdrawn, and the liquid will commence to flow, and continue till it reaches the same level in the receiving vessel that it has in the other.

Figs. 90 and 91 represent an apparatus I have been using for some time past for straining syrups. Fig. 90 is a tin bucket, into which a funnel-shaped wire support, Fig. 91, is suspended, resting on the bucket by a projecting rim at the top; a jelly bag is here unnecessary, as a sufficiently large square or round piece of flannel laid upon the wires will assume a convenient position for use.

Fig. 92 represents in section a contrivance for straining jellies attributed to the late Dr. Physick, and made by Isaac S. Williams, of Philadelphia; a wire support fits into a funnel, which is soldered into a vessel designed to be kept full of hot water so as to prevent the cooling and thickening of the jelly during straining.

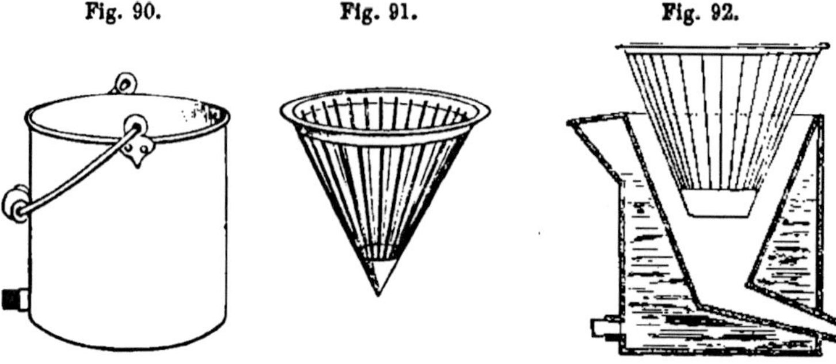

Fig. 90. Fig. 91. Fig. 92.

Apparatus for straining syrups, &c. Physick's jelly strainer.

For ordinary aqueous, alcoholic, and ethereal liquids, the process of *filtration*, employing the term in its more limited sense, is used, the filtering medium being paper. The best filtering paper is porous and free from any kind of glazing; that made from cotton or linen rags is the best for ordinary purposes; the kind made from woollen materials seems better adapted to viscid liquids, being thicker and more porous, but seldom free from coloring matter. It is, also, more soluble in alkaline solutions, and unfit for filtering such. Good filtering paper for delicate analytical processes should contain no soluble matter and should not give more than $\frac{1}{250}$ to $\frac{1}{280}$ of its weight of ashes; the soluble matter may be removed by washing it, first with very dilute hydrochloric acid, and secondly with distilled water.

The construction of paper filters is an extremely simple thing when once learned, and is easily taught the student by a practical demonstration; it is, nevertheless, a difficult thing to describe clearly without giving to it more space than may appear at first sight due to so small a matter.

There are two kinds of paper filters, the *plain* and the *plaited;* the use of the plain filter is in cases where we desire to collect the solid

Fig. 93. Fig. 94.

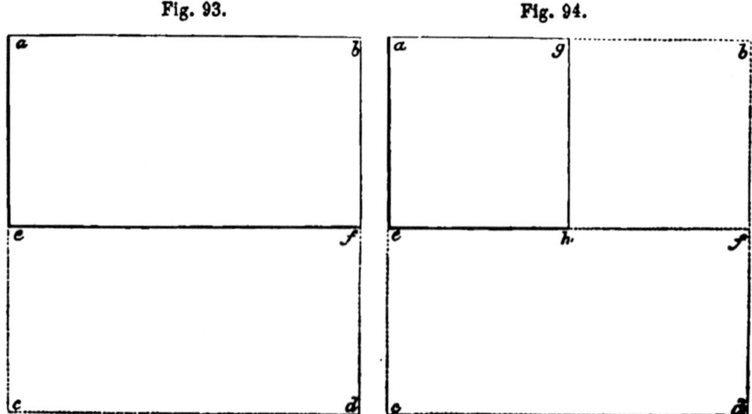

ingredient present in the liquid, and to remove it afterwards from the paper. It allows the passage of the liquid through it with less rapidity, and yet, owing to its being so readily folded, it is in very common use. The method of folding the plain filter is similar to the first steps to be taken in folding the plaited filter.

In the following description I have endeavored to convey an idea of this process.

A square piece of filtering paper, *a b c d* (Fig. 93), is folded over in the middle so as to form a crease at the line *e f*; the edge *c d* being laid directly over *a b*. The parallelogram, *a b e f*, represents the paper thus folded; the line *b f* being now laid upon the line *a e*, a crease is formed as represented by the line *g h* (Fig. 94); the folded paper, if opened, makes a cone, having the point *h* at its base, and by cutting off the projecting angle *a*, by a curved line from *e* to *g*, a plain filter will be the result, as shown in Fig. 95.

Fig. 95.

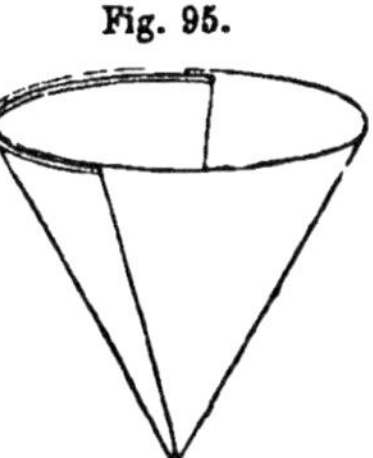

The *plaited filter* is made as follows: Take the paper before being cut, as above, and having opened it again so as to expose the parallelogram, the line *e h* (Fig. 96) is laid upon the line *c h*, forming a crease at *a h*. This being opened again the line *e h* is laid upon the line *a h*, pro-

Fig. 96. Fig. 97.

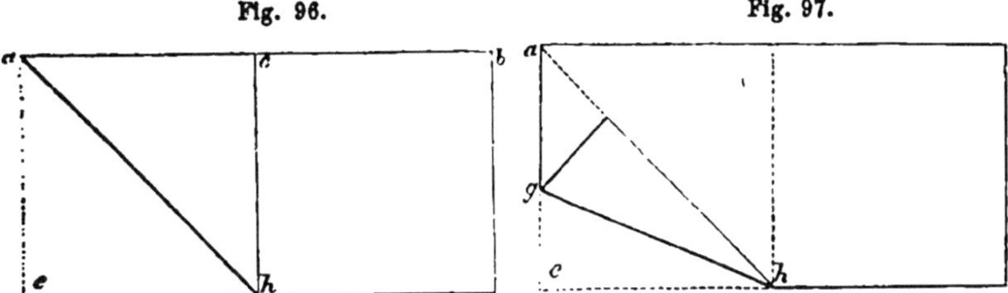

ducing an additional crease at *g h* (Fig. 97). The crease *j h* (Fig. 98) is next to be formed by folding *a h* upon the middle dotted line (Fig. 98), as shown in Fig. 99.

Fig. 98. Fig. 99.

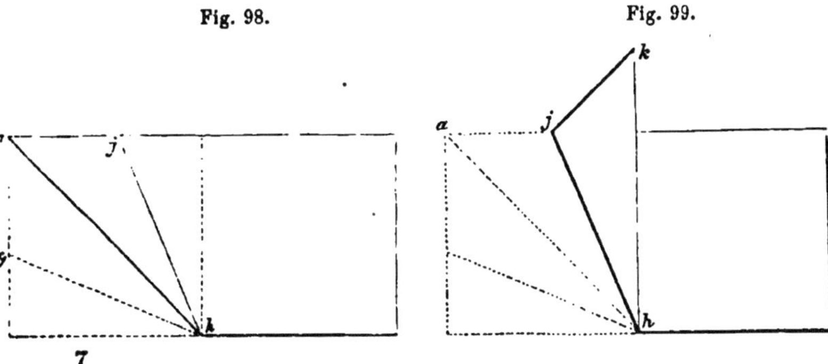

One-half of the parallelogram having thus been creased, we proceed to form on the other the corresponding creases *m h*, *b h*, and *k h* (Fig. 100), all of which are in one direction, forming receding angles. The next thing to be done is to divide the eight sections thus formed by a

Fig. 100. Fig. 101.

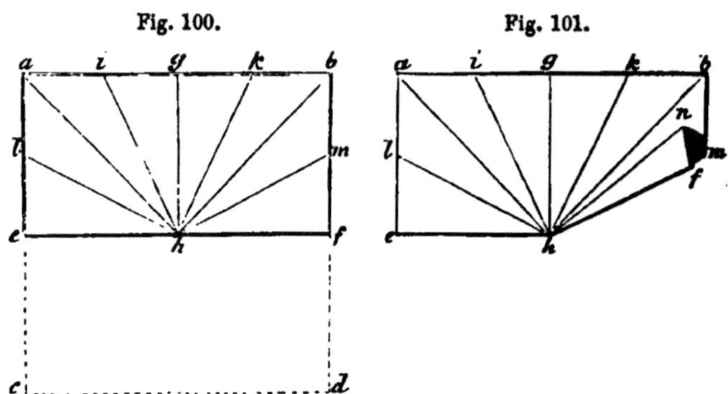

crease through each in the opposite direction. To do this, the edge *f h* is laid in the crease *b h*, and then turned back, as shown in Fig. 101, producing the crease *n h*. In the same way an intermediate crease is formed in each of the spaces. This is better accomplished by turning the paper over, so that each of the receding angles shall project upward, and in this way be more readily brought together, as shown in Fig. 102, producing a receding angle in forming the intermediate creases.

Fig. 102.

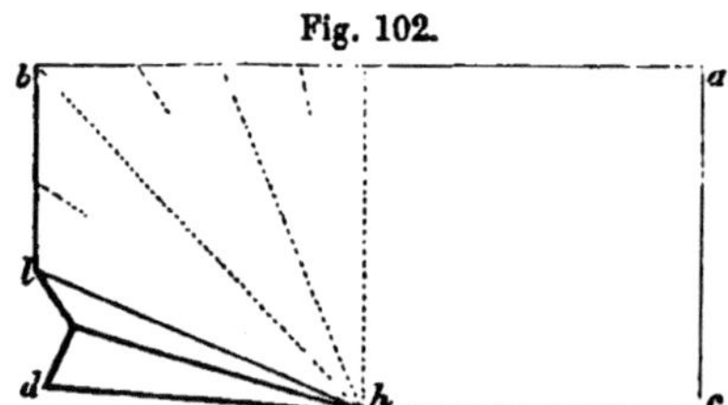

The paper will now have the appearance of a fan, represented by Fig. 103, folding it up in each of its creases like a shut fan (Fig. 104). The projecting points, *a* and *b*, may be clipped off with a pair of scissors at the dotted line, and upon opening the originally doubled halves made by the first fold at *e f* (Fig. 93), it will be found to present the appearance indicated in Fig. 105.

In the filter, as thus constructed, the creases occur alternately, except near the line *e f*, where the two creases occurring next each other are in the same direction. Sometimes, to obviate this, the space intervening between these is folded backwards, as shown in the figure, so as to make a narrow crease in the opposite direction.

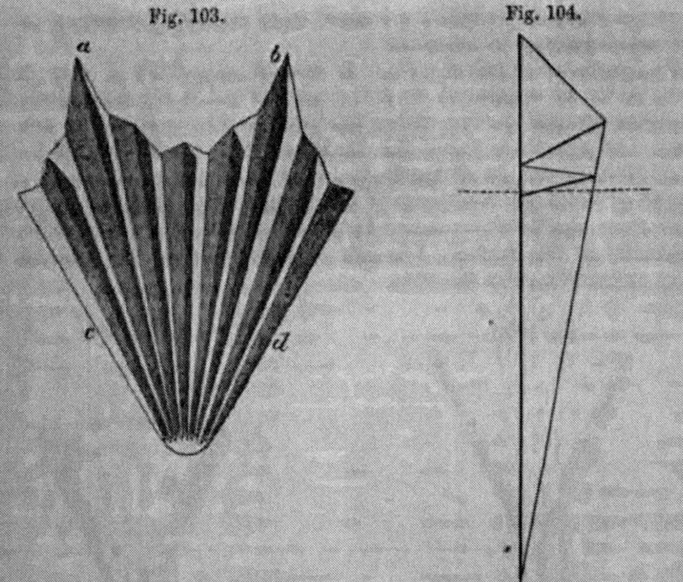

Fig. 103. Fig. 104.

The plaited filter, as thus formed, is exceedingly useful for general purposes, exposing the entire surface of the paper to the action of the liquid, and allowing the process to proceed more rapidly than in the case of the plain filter, first described.

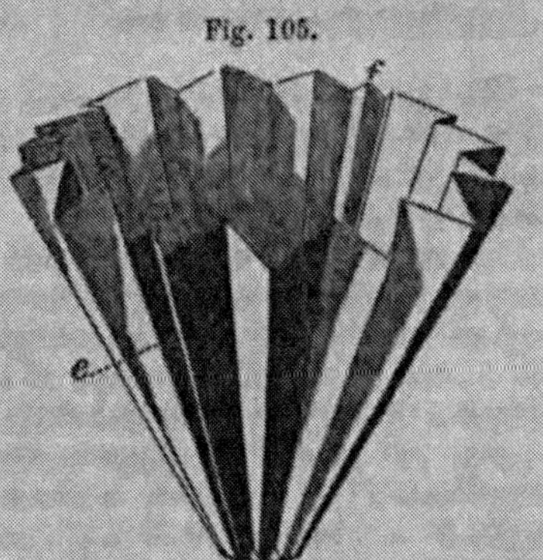

Fig. 105.

A funnel, such as described and figured on page 49, is employed for supporting a filter of either kind, and is, as there stated, better adapted to ordinary use when grooved on its inner surface, so as to allow the free downward passage of the liquid, after it has permeated the paper, and a groove on the outside of the tube, so that, when inserted tightly into the neck of a bottle, the air within may find ready egress.

If the tube of the funnel is smooth and ungrooved, a small plugget of folded paper, a piece of thick twine, or a small wedge shaped splinter of wood, should be inserted in the neck of the bottle, along with the tube of the funnel; this will obviate one of the most common annoyances connected with filtration.

In filtering into an open vessel, it is well to place the lower extremity of the funnel in contact with the side of the vessel, thus preventing any inconvenience from the liquid splashing on the sides or over the top, and by creating a downward stream, promoting the free and rapid passage of the filtrate.

The paper of which the filter is formed, especially if very porous, is liable to be weakened by being plaited as above described; it is therefore advised not to make the creases firmly down to the very point, but rather to leave the terminus of an undefined shape; and when there is danger of breakage, either from the great weight of the liquid or from the weakness of the paper at its point, a very small plain filter may be advantageously placed under the point at the lowest extremity of the funnel; this acts as a support to the weakest and most exposed part of the filter.

Fig. 106. Fig. 107.

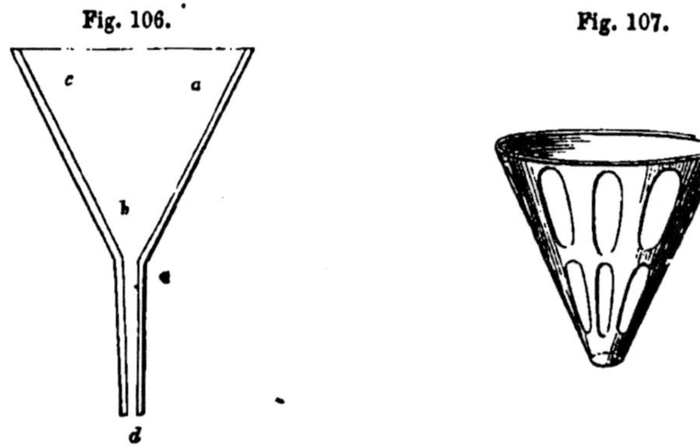

Section of a well-formed funnel. Filter support.

The proper shape of a funnel for filtration is shown in section at Fig. 106. The lines *a b* and *c b* are straight, and *a b c* and *a c b* are angles of 60°, making an equilateral triangle, into which the filter just described will fit perfectly.

In consequence of the unequal degree of firmness of the different creases, some of these are liable to float up from the sides of the funnel, to obviate which a filter weight has been invented, which consists of a wire frame of the shape of the funnel, and with a wire for each crease; this is laid upon the filter, and keeps it perfectly in its place.

Fig. 107 is a filter support adapted to the rapid passage of liquids in filtration; it, however, requires to be used in connection with an open or wide-mouth receiving vessel or a funnel, otherwise the liquid might not be perfectly collected as it passes downwards.

The filtration of small quantities of liquid, as in chemical experiments, may be performed without a funnel or filter support by inserting a plain filter directly into the open top of beaker glass or other open vessel, or into a ring of glass or earthenware laid on top of an open vessel; a filter of this kind, that will hold one fluidounce, will filter many ounces of certain liquids in an hour.

When paper filters are of large dimensions, or used for fluids which soften the texture of the paper, or for collecting heavy powders or metallic precipitates, they may be supported on linen or cotton filters of similar shape. This is best done by folding the cloth with the paper, and in the same way as would be done with doubled paper, observing to place them in the funnel so as to be in perfect contact toward the bottom.

A newly-invented filter of E. Waters, Troy, New York, consists of a circular sheet of paper of double thickness, composed of loose cotton and woollen fibre, and contains a piece of lace about four inches square covering the point of the filter; this is introduced between the sheets when they are "couched," so that the pulp unites through the meshes of the lace, and thus effectually overcomes the difficulty of breaking.

A process discovered by the inventor obviates the liability to break at the point by being folded, a difficulty which is increased in proportion to the thickness of the paper. From the limited trial I have as yet given them, I believe the invention to be an improvement.

Oils are filtered on a small scale in the way already described for other liquids, but in large quantities may be passed through felt hat bodies, which are to be had in the large cities generally, or through bags of Canton flannel, which are usually made about twelve or fifteen inches in diameter and from four to eight feet long. These may be inclosed in bottomless casings or bags of coarse canvas, about five to eight inches in diameter, for the purpose of condensing a great extent of filtering surface into the smallest possible space. Several of these bags secured on the inside to the bottom of a tinned cistern are inclosed in a closet with suitable arrangements for maintaining a slightly elevated temperature, though this is not always desirable, and the oil is introduced from above, and collected as it passes from the filter. For further particulars on the filtration of oils, &c., see *Cooley's Cyclopædia of Practical Receipts*, London, 1856.

In filtering very volatile liquids, particularly in hot weather, some contrivance must be resorted to to prevent evaporation from the wide surface exposed, while, at the same time, the escape of air from the receiving vessel must be provided for. The drawing here given (Fig. 108), from Mohr & Redwood, represents an arrangement of the kind. The glass funnel is fitted by a cork into the receiving vessel; its top is ground to a smooth surface, on which is laid a plate of glass, *c;* a little simple cerate will furnish a good luting; *b* is a very small glass tube laid down the inside of the funnel between it and the filter, and so twisted at its lower end as to be supported in its place; this forms a connection between the air below and that above the liquid, without allowing any evaporation.

The use of a guiding rod in pouring a liquid upon a filter is found a great convenience; a glass rod is well suited to this purpose. The lower extremity is directed against the side of the filter near the apex, while the middle portion is placed against the mouth of the vessel, as shown in the drawing; by this means the stream is made to fall steadily, and not with too great force, and against the strongest part of the filter; the liquid being poured, is also prevented from running back upon the containing vessel, and thus wasting, a very annoying circumstance, which is especially liable to occur when the vessel,

Fig. 108. Fig. 109.

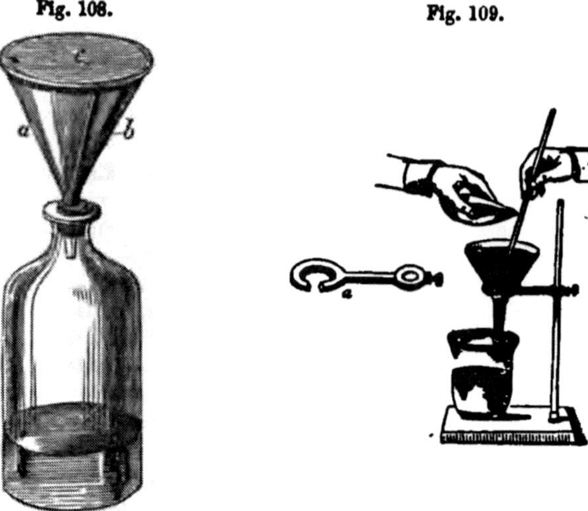

Filter for volatile liquids. Pouring with a guiding rod.

whether a flask, a vial, or an evaporating dish, is furnished with no lip, or a very poor one, for pouring.

A useful precaution in pouring liquids from bottles may be mentioned in this connection. It nearly always happens that the last drop or two of the liquid being poured remains on the lip of the bottle, and is liable, if the lip is ill formed, to run down the outside; this may be obviated by touching the stopper to the edge where the liquid is collected, thus transferring this drop to the end of the stopper previous to inserting it in the neck of the bottle.

Much of the filtration in pharmacy has for its object the separation of the insoluble ligneous portions of vegetable medicines, after they have been sufficiently macerated. A practical difficulty in this case is deserving of mention here. If a measured portion, say one pint of liquid, has been macerated with two, four, or six ounces of a vegetable substance for the purpose of making a tincture or infusion, and, after the proper lapse of time, the whole is thrown upon a filter, the clear liquid that will pass will measure as much less than a pint as the vegetable substance holds by its capillary attraction. In order to obtain the whole quantity desired, some have diluted the filtered liquid till it reached precisely the required measure; but by the discovery of the principle of displacement (see Chapter V.), it is found that an additional portion of liquid, if presented to the saturated powder, under favorable circumstances, will displace the portion of the original menstruum remaining in its pores. To secure this is more important from the fact that it is usually most highly impregnated with the active principles of the plant; and, therefore, in transferring the macerated preparation to a filter, the swollen mass of powder should be carefully compacted into the filter, and after the liquid has drained off, a fresh portion of a similar liquid should be added till the preparation measures the quantity originally intended.

THE MEDICATED WATERS.

Closely resembling the solutions proper, are the medicated waters. —*Aquæ Medicatæ, U. S. P.*

These are generally solutions in water of the essential oils, made by triturating the latter with a third substance (carbonate of magnesia, usually), which, either by dividing them mechanically, and thus presenting them to the water under favorable circumstances, or by a chemical union with them, renders them soluble to a limited extent, and imparts their sensible properties to the medicated waters thus formed.

The same result is obtained by mixing the fresh herb with a quantity of water in an apparatus for distillation, and allowing them to remain in contact until the water has, to a certain extent, dissolved out the essential oil, extractive matter, coloring principle, &c.; and then, by the application of heat, volatilizing the water and the essential oil, and collecting them in a refrigerated receiver. If the oil is in excess, it will be found on standing to collect on the surface of the liquid in the receiver, but a certain amount is retained in solution by the water, imparting to it the fragrance peculiar to the herb employed. (See Chapter on *Distillation.*)

A third method of preparing medicated waters is to impregnate pure water, generally refrigerated, with gases, either by the aid of pressure or by simple absorption. Some of those prepared in this way are usually classified as *chemical preparations.*

In the tabular view appended, the officinal medicated waters are classified according to the methods of preparing them:—

AQUÆ MEDICATÆ.

(Unofficinal in Italics.)

FIRST CLASS.—*By trituration with an insoluble substance which is afterwards separated by filtration.*

Officinal name.	Proportions.		Comp.		Dose.
Aqua camphoræ,	Camphor ʒj,	Carb. magnes.	ʒij to Oj=3 grains to f℥j		f℥ss.
" amygdalæ amaræ,	Oil ♏xvj,	do.	ʒj to Oij=1 drop to f℥j		f℥j.
" cinnamomi,	Oil ♏xvj,	do.	ʒj to Oj=2 drops to f℥j		f℥ij.
" fœniculi,	do.	do.	do.	do.	do.
" menthæ pip.,	do.	do.	do.	do.	do.
" " virid.,	do.	do.	do.	do.	do.
Aqua anisi,	do.	do.	do.	do.	do.

SECOND CLASS.—*By distillation.*

Aqua rosæ,	Rose petals ℔j to Oj	Vehicle for collyria, &c.	
Aqua sambuci,	Elder flowers,	do.	do.
" *flor. aurantii,*	Orange flowers,	Sedative adjuvant.	
" *mali Persicæ,*	Peach leaves,	do.	do.
" *lauro-cerasi,*	Cherry-laurel leaves,	do.	do.

THIRD CLASS.[1]—*By charging water with gas.*

Aqua acidi carbonici,	5 parts of CO_2 to 1 of water.
Liquor chlorinii,	Contains twice its bulk of the gas.

REMARKS ON FIRST CLASS.

The manipulation in preparing those of the first class is quite simple, and, except in the case of camphor water, is precisely uniform. The carbonate of magnesia is removed by filtration, and only serves the purpose of dividing the oil and rendering it more soluble in the water. It may be substituted by prepared chalk, powdered silica, or some other insoluble substance in very fine powder.

In making *camphor water*, the chief point to be observed is to secure the complete division of the camphor; this is accomplished by triturating it with alcohol, which brings it into a pasty mass; this mass must now be brought completely between the triturating surfaces of the pestle and mortar, for if any portion escapes it will be lumpy and granular, and not in a favorable condition for solution. The carbonate of magnesia may be triturated with the moist camphor before it has passed into the condition of a powder, and after thorough incorporation the whole may be passed through a fine sieve; the water is then gradually added. The undissolved carbonate and camphor should be thrown on the filter with the first portion of the liquid, so that it may be percolated by the liquid during its filtration.

In the preparation of extemporaneous solutions or mixtures, the medicated waters of the first class are very convenient; but where the one required is not at hand, it may be substituted by dropping the essential oil on a small piece of sugar, or, if in a mixture containing gum, upon the powdered gum, and triturating with a sufficient quantity of water. The proportion of the oil used, as shown in the table, is in all cases, excepting that of the bitter almond water, one minim (which is frequently substituted by two drops) of the oil to one fluidounce of the liquid.

REMARKS ON SECOND CLASS.

ROSE-WATER is the only medicated water directed by the *Pharmacopœia* to be made by distillation. This is very much employed in prescription for the preparation of solutions of nitrate of silver, as a substitute for distilled water. It is liable to undergo a change, depositing a sediment, and becoming quite sour if long kept, especially in warm weather. On this account, and in consequence of the greater facility and cheapness of the process, some pharmaceutists make rosewater in the same way as the other medicated waters, by triturating the oil or attar of rose with magnesia, and then with water, and afterwards filtering. The proportions usually employed are four drops of the oil to a pint of water; when made in this way, however, it is not

[1] For liquor ammonia, and other medicated waters not classified under this head, see Part IV.

so well adapted to the uses above mentioned, though suitable for flavoring pastry, &c.

THE DISTILLED WATER OF ELDER FLOWERS is a very delicate vehicle for saline substances in solution for *collyria*. It is much used in Europe, but is seldom kept by our pharmaceutists, rose-water being used for the same purpose to its exclusion.

ORANGE-FLOWER WATER.—A well known and delightful perfume, imported from France and Italy, and obtained by distillation from the flowers of the bitter orange tree. It is one of the most agreeable of flavors for medicinal preparations, though, until recently, confined almost entirely to the purposes of the perfumer. Its sedative effects, which are not generally known in this country, and not noticed in our works on materia medica, adapt it especially to use in nervous affections. In doses of a tablespoonful it is found to allay nervous irritability and produce refreshing sleep.

PEACH WATER, which is chiefly used as a flavor in cooking, is made by a similar process from the leaves of the *mali Persica*, peach-tree. It is generally substituted by the officinal *aqua amygdalæ amaræ*.

CHERRY-LAUREL WATER, officinal in the *Edinburgh and Dublin Pharmacopœia*, is directed to be made by distilling one pound of fresh bruised leaves of cherry-laurel with water till one pint (Imperial measure) of the distilled water is obtained. To this the Edinburgh College directs the addition of an ounce of comp. spt. of lavender, to distinguish it in color from common water. This preparation is recently much prescribed, especially by German practitioners, in doses of thirty minims to a fluidrachm, as a sedative narcotic. It contains a varying proportion of hydrocyanic acid, and deteriorates very much by keeping. In view of this fact, I have recently adopted the following recipe for its artificial preparation, suggested by Dr. W. H. Pile:—

Take of Diluted hydrocyanic acid, *U. S. P.*, f℥j;
Ess. oil of bitter almonds, . . ♏iij;
Alcohol, ... f℥iij;
Water, ... f℥iiss.—M.

The distilled water of wild-cherry tree leaves has been recommended as a substitute for cherry-laurel water.

REMARKS ON THIRD CLASS.

The medicated waters of this class seem to belong properly to the chemical preparations, with liquor ammoniæ, &c.; but, in the *Pharmacopœias*, carbonic-acid water and chlorine water are exceptions, and placed among aquæ medicatæ.

CARBONIC-ACID WATER is frequently, though incorrectly, called soda water; its proper synonym is mineral water. In most large cities, the manufacture of this is a separate branch of business, and it is purchased by the apothecary in copper fountains lined with tin holding about fifteen gallons. The chief impurities to which it is liable are the carbonates of copper and lead, derived from the fountain and pipe from which it is drawn. These, particularly the former, render carbonic-acid water not only worthless, but absolutely injurious; they may be detected by the metallic taste they impart to it, by the addition of ammonia, which gives a blue tint to the salts of copper, and by the ferrocyanide of potassium, which gives a garnet-colored precipitate, if copper is present. Iodide of potassium indicates the presence of lead by a yellow precipitate.

The chief use of carbonic-acid water in prescription is for dissolving saline substances in making aperient and antacid draughts, for suspending magnesia, for making solutions of citrate of potassa, and occasionally by itself as a grateful drink to allay thirst and lessen nausea. As a vehicle for magnesia or saline cathartics, eight fluidounces are usually prescribed, to be taken at once, or in divided portions frequently repeated. It parts with the gas upon exposure, and should, therefore, be used as soon as possible after the cork has been drawn. Sometimes, when prescribed in small doses, it is dispensed in one-ounce or two-ounce vials, the contents of each being taken separately, while cold and in a state of effervescence, preferably, directly from the mouth of the vial.

Many pharmaceutists use expensive apparatus for the preparation of this article as a beverage, and the number of those in use has greatly increased during several years past. In the first edition of this work two of these were figured, but as they are generally described in the circulars of the makers, which are accessible to all who wish to acquaint themselves with their relative advantages and price, I omit them here and insert the following convenient form of apparatus.

Fig. 110 represents a French *gasogene*, such as are imported of various sizes, from one quart to five gallons capacity.

This is a strong glass vessel consisting of two bulbs joined together at their point of union by a tube of about half an inch bore extending into the upper one to near the top. The upper bulb is surmounted by a metallic cap, on to which is screwed a draught pipe with a valve, opened by pressing with the thumb upon the button at the upper extremity of a rod; attached to this draught pipe is a long glass tube of small diameter, passing through the larger tube, occupying the central space, to near the bottom of the apparatus. The object of this mode of construction is to permit the charging of water placed in the lower bulb, with gas, generated from carbonated alkali and acid placed in the upper bulb, without contaminating the water with the salts.

Fig. 111 shows the mode of filling the lower bulb with water by a long funnel, *e*, extending through the cap and neck of the apparatus, *d*, into the large tube, *f*; this obviously prevents any portion of water escaping into the upper bulb; the lower bulb is designed to be filled in this way about three-fourths full of cold water.

Fig. 112 illustrates the ingenious arrangement for introducing the bicarb. soda and tartaric acid (one of which should be in crystals partially powdered) into the upper bulb; *a* is a rod with a metallic

Fig. 110.

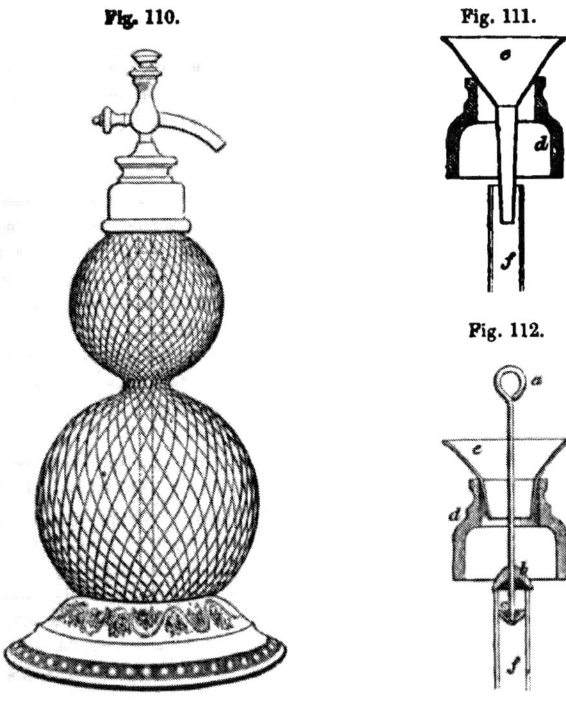

Gasogene.

Fig. 111.

Fig. 112.

cone, *b*, of a diameter greater than the glass tube, *f*, and a leather washer, *c*, which is thrust into the tube and completely closes it. The wide-mouth funnel, *e*, is introduced into the cap and neck of the apparatus, and the dry salts, mixed, thrown into it; these, falling over the cone, *b*, lodge in the upper bulb; the rod and funnel are now removed and the draught pipe screwed on.

By tilting the apparatus, some of the water runs through the larger tube into the upper bulb, and starts the mixed powders to combining; a brisk evolution of carbonic acid ensues, and, by shaking, its absorption by the water is facilitated. By opening the valve in the draught pipe, the charged water, by its own elasticity and the pressure of the excess of gas, is driven up the narrow tube and through the valve, and escapes. The object of the wire coating is to protect from injury in case of explosion, a purpose it out imperfectly fills.

The water introduced may be flavored with syrup, or it may be drawn into a glass containing the flavoring ingredient. The absorption of the gas is greatly facilitated by the refrigeration of the water, and by frequently shaking it up.

This apparatus may serve the purpose of pharmaceutists who do not desire to dispense carbonic-acid water as a beverage. It is a luxury for family use, and should be more generally introduced. They are sold for six dollars and upwards.

Mineral water *coolers* and *syrup holders* are necessary to all who dispense this beverage. One of the best forms of cooler consists of a coil of half inch pipe disposed around the inside of a circular cedar tub placed under the counter; the pipe is terminated by a small air-chamber, in which any excess of the gas is allowed to collect, so as to be drawn off by a screw; this appendage may be omitted where the bore of the pipe exceeds ½ of an inch, and where it is not very long. The size of the tub and length of the pipe may be regulated by circumstances; where the demand for the water is constant in hot weather, the tub should hold half a bushel of ice, and the pipe be at least fifty feet in length. An objection to this arrangement is found in the fact that the portion of the pipe between the top of the tub and the end of the draught pipe is not kept cold, and the water it contains and the first which passes through it are invariably drawn off first into the glass. This is obviated by the construction of a cooler upon the counter, which may or may not supersede the necessity of the cooler just described.

The cooler for the counter may combine an ornamental vase and draught pipe with the advantage of a coil surrounded by ice, an arrangement now very generally adopted. Connected with this, the cooling of the syrups, also, is a desideratum, and I have recently contrived a vase, which consists of a central, oval cylinder of galvanized iron, closed at the lower end, and containing a coil of block-tin pipe thirty feet long, which is coupled on to a lead pipe communicating with the copper fountain underneath, and is terminated by a draught pipe in the side of the vase; this central cylinder holds about half a peck of broken ice; outside of this, and fitting closely against it, are eight syrup cans with a plated faucet at the base of each, arranged as closely as possible to admit of their being conveniently used, and all proceeding from the part of the vase facing behind the counter. This ice cylinder and series of cans form a perfect circle with straight sides, and over the whole a tin casing fits accurately, having the proper external contour to form a graceful vase, and the intervening space between this and the inside cylinders being occupied by an air-chamber, which furnishes a non-conducting medium between the ice and the external warmth. In order to have the syrup cans movable for the purpose of repairs, the faucets are all on a line corresponding with the floor of the vase, and the external casing has scollops cut out at its base corresponding with these and the draught pipe, so that the whole fits accurately together, and may be taken apart at pleasure.

This apparatus is well adapted to an establishment where the sale is limited or the supply of ice small. The number of syrups it contains being limited, a further assortment requires to be kept in bottles, or in a separate syrup cooler.

The principle of this cooler is carried out on a much larger scale by O. S. Hubbell, of Philadelphia, in a cooler of 2½ feet in diameter on top of his counter, which, being so well protected by a layer of two inches of non-conducting material, and holding so large a quantity of ice, requires replenishing only once in several days, except in the hottest weather; this has 12 syrup cans of one gallon each, enough for a full assortment of syrups, and, except for its inconvenient size, leaves nothing to desire.

The inconvenience in drawing syrups from a faucet, of a drop collecting at the tip of the pipe after it has been shut off is obviated by an invention of Isaac S. Williams, of Philadelphia, by which a flat disk of metal moves with the lever and closes the end of the pipe as soon as the flow is stopped; by this contrivance the intrusion of flies and ants into the faucet is guarded against.

ARTIFICIAL SARATOGA WATER may be made as follows:—

Mix	Chloride of sodium	℥j.
	" magnesia, solution[1]	f℥ij.
	Bicarbonate of soda	ʒj.
	Solution of iodine (Lugol's)	fʒss.
	Tincture of chloride of iron	fʒss.
	Carbonic-acid water	Oiss.

Filter. Into a Oj tumbler introduce f℥j of the mixture, fill it up with carbonic-acid water, and drink immediately.

CHLORINE WATER, which is officinal in the Dublin and Edinburgh *Pharmacopœias*, and in the appendix to the London, is made by connecting a retort adapted to generating chlorine gas to a vessel containing half a pint of pure water, and mixing in the retort—

Hydrochloric acid	A fluidounce.
Binoxide of manganese	Two drachms.

The chlorine which is evolved is absorbed by the water. This preparation should be made fresh when needed; it is used chiefly as an antiseptic, and resembles our officinal *liquor sodæ chlorinatæ*, though stronger. It is also employed in testing quinia and morphia.

CHAPTER IV.

ON MACERATION AND THE INFUSIONS.

THE kind of solution spoken of heretofore is quite simple, and in most cases easily accomplished; but substances which are soluble only to a limited extent, or are composed of proximate principles associated mechanically, some of which are much more soluble than others, as the bark, leaves, wood, &c., of plants, require different and less ready modes of treatment.

The first thing to be done is to reduce the drug to a more or less fine powder, or to bruise it, after which the liquid, which in this case is called the menstruum, is brought into contact with it.

[1] Commercial muriatic acid saturated with magnesia.

When the quantity of the medicinal agent is small in comparison with the menstruum, as in most of the infusions, and where rapidity is not an object, the process of *maceration* is chiefly resorted to.

This is accomplished in a covered queensware vessel, a common pitcher or bowl, for instance, or sometimes in a tin cup or measure, care being taken in the case of astringent infusions to avoid the use of a defective tin or an iron vessel. Maceration consists in pouring the liquid upon the medicinal substance previously bruised or coarsely powdered, and allowing it to stand for a greater or less period of time, according to circumstances. The longest period directed in the *Pharmacopœia* for infusions is twenty-four hours, as in the case of infusion of wild cherry; the shortest, ten minutes, as in the case of infusion of chamomile. In preparing tinctures, wines, vinegars, &c., seven or fourteen days are generally prescribed.

Fig. 113.

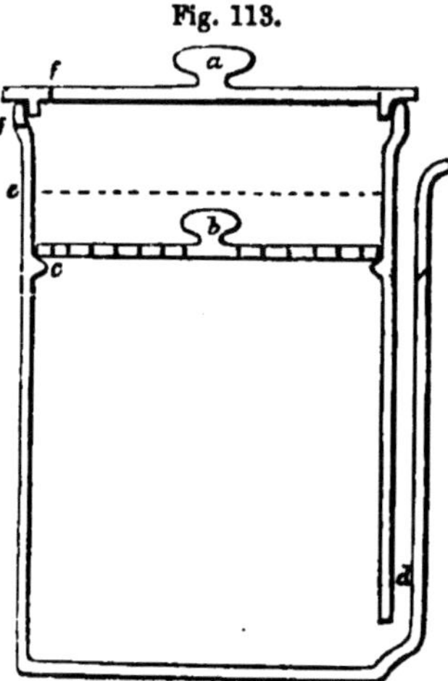

Section of Alsop's infusion mug.

Infusions are conveniently prepared in a vessel made for the purpose, here figured, called Alsop's infusion mug, which contains a perforated diaphragm, *b*, near the top, on which the substance to be macerated is placed; the liquid is introduced so as barely to cover this, reaching, perhaps, to the line *e*; a circulation is thus induced and continued in the liquid by which the least impregnated portions are brought constantly in contact with the drug, and the most completely saturated portion, by its greater specific gravity, sinks to the bottom.

Squire's Infusion Pot is an improvement on Alsop's; it is a very neat pharmaceutical implement adapted to making the galenical liquid preparations generally. In Fig. 114, we have a section, *B* and *D*, being two cup-shaped perforated diaphragms, either of which may be

Fig. 114.

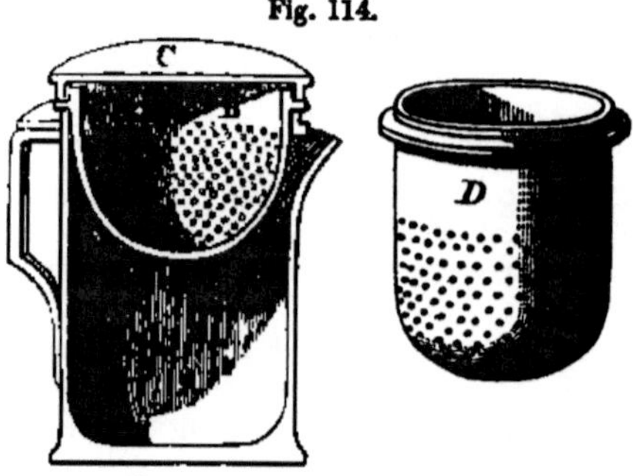

Section of Squire's infusion pot.

used at pleasure. The vessel must be of such capacity that the substance placed on the diaphragm shall be under the surface of the liquid when properly filled. N. Spencer Thomas, of Philadelphia, manufactures a good stoneware imitation of this apparatus. A modification of this is used in some large establishments for the preparation of tinctures; it has many advantages over ordinary apparatus for maceration, and is not unlike displacement in the beauty and efficiency of the preparations made in it.

In preparing large quantities of tinctures or infusions by maceration, there is considerable loss of the saturated liquid, unless a suitable press is used to obtain the last portions. The pattern here figured, which is sold by Bullock & Crenshaw, of Philadelphia, price $10, is among the best in the market.

Fig. 115.

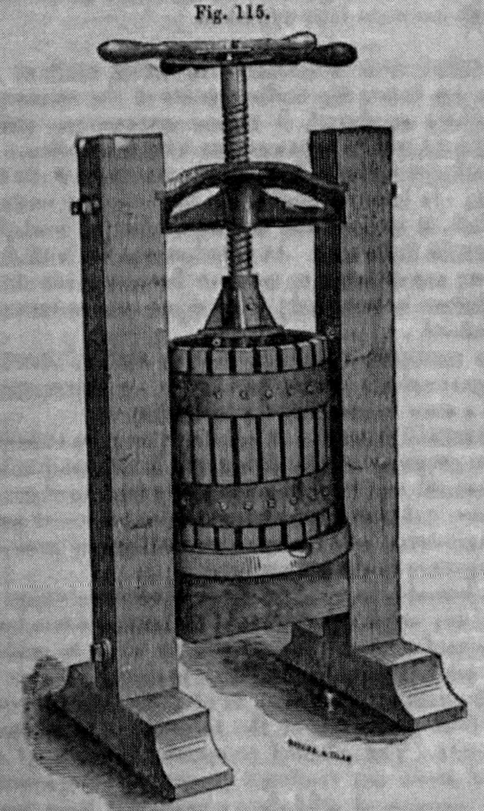

It is substantial, and permits the application of considerable force. The frame is oak, 3½ inches square. The hopper is made of strong oak pieces separated ⅛ inch from each other—the pieces are firmly held together by two broad iron bands, through which a screw passes into each piece, securing it in its place. The hopper is 11 inches high, and 8 inches in diameter, having a capacity of 3 gallons—it stands upon a circular base of oak, which is grooved to receive and collect the expressed liquid, and has a lip to discharge it. The screw is iron, with square thread, 1½ inch diameter, and passes through a heavy iron casting. Both the iron head-piece and the support for the hopper are let into the oak uprights, and secured by heavy iron bolts.

In using the Press, a press bag, having about the diameter of the hopper, should be used—the bag should be made of strong canvas of an open texture; or the hopper may be lined with clean straw, after the manner of the Cider Press. The hopper being open at both ends, and movable, is readily cleared of its contents and cleansed. Jenk's Kitchen Press is a smaller and cheaper kind sold by the dealers in housekeeping articles, at prices varying from $1 75 for five inch cylinders to $3 for eight inch cylinders.

Digestion differs from maceration in being confined to elevated temperatures, yet below the boiling point of the menstruum; as the term is generally employed, it means maceration, with continued application of heat, and is synonymous with simmering.

The term *infusion* includes both maceration in its more limited sense and digestion. It is often applied to the ordinary mode of making infusions, which is to pour the hot liquid on the bruised drug, and allow it to remain until cool. In a recipe worded with due regard to accuracy, if we are directed to *macerate* for any given time, we know that *cold* infusion is intended; if to *digest*, we understand that *hot* infusion is desired.

In making tinctures, digestion, though seldom directed, is often very useful, particularly where rapidity is an object, and where we wish to form a very concentrated preparation.

Of the proximate principles of plants, it may be remarked that hot water has the property of dissolving the starch, and cold water the vegetable albumen, and both dissolve the gum, sugar, extractive, and other principles liable to fermentation; the absence of any antiseptic in infusions and decoctions renders them extremely prone to undergo change on exposure to the atmosphere.

When it is desirable to preserve these aqueous solutions for a longer period than a day or two, they should be bottled while hot, the bottle being filled completely and corked tightly, so as to exclude the air, and then set aside in a cold place in an inverted position. The addition of ⅓ to ¼ quantity of alcohol, or of some tincture not interfering with the medical properties of the infusion, is recommended where not objectionable. The officinal compound infusion of gentian and infusion of digitalis are rendered permanent preparations by this means. The infusion of wild-cherry bark will keep for some days without any addition to it, owing to the antiseptic influence of hydrocyanic acid it contains.

The following substances should not be prescribed mixed with or dissolved in infusions, being incompatible with one or more of the proximate principles usually present in them: Tartrate of antimony and potassa, corrosive chloride of mercury, nitrate of silver, acetate and subacetate of lead; in some cases, the alkalies, lime-water, and tincture of galls, and, in the instance of astringent infusions, the salts of iron.

When mixed with either of the tinctures made with strong alcohol, a resinous precipitate is deposited, and the mixture if strained loses much of its activity; the same is the fact, to a less extent, with many of the tinctures made with diluted alcohol.

Many of the infusions which are clear when freshly prepared, become turbid soon after by the deposition of vegetable albumen, apotheme, and other insoluble principles; these precipitates are likely to carry down with them a portion of the active ingredients. The infusions of cinchona prepared by maceration with hot water do not become clear, even by filtration through paper.

Infusions made by maceration may frequently be poured off clear from the vessel in which they were prepared, leaving the dregs in the bottom; this, however, is always attended with the loss of the last portion of the liquid; they may be strained through a muslin or flannel strainer, and, by using a little force in expressing the dregs, very nearly the whole portion of liquid may be obtained, or this may be done more satisfactorily, by displacement, in filtering them.

This class of medicinal preparations is one of the least elegant in use, and is mainly confined, in this country, to domestic practice. Even when prescribed by physicians, the infusions are generally made by the nurse or attendant upon the sick, rather than by the apothecary. The infusions of cinchona bark, infusion of digitalis, and compound infusion of gentian, form the chief exceptions to this.

The process of displacement, treated of in the next chapter, is applied with great advantage to some of these preparations, and I believe, in a majority of cases, the substitution of cold water for hot, and of displacement for maceration or digestion, would be found to produce a more elegant and equally efficient infusion, and one which, from containing less coloring matter, fecula, resinous, and other inert principles, would keep better, and be more acceptable to the stomach. Some experiments, recently reported, tend to show the superiority of cold infusion of senna over that made by the officinal process.

When an infusion is intended as an emetic draught, or to promote the operation of emetics, or as a diaphoretic, it is usually given while hot, and, of course, to all such cases the above remark does not apply. Nor is it equally applicable to the demulcent infusions of flaxseed, buchu, and slippery elm, although the former may be made very well with cold water, and is then less oily in its character.

The following syllabus is offered as presenting the whole officinal class of infusions, so that the student may conveniently study their composition, proportions, mode of preparation, and uses.

8

SYLLABUS OF INFUSIONS.

INFUSA, *U. S. P.*

FIRST CLASS.—*Made with boiling water by maceration.*

GROUP I.—℥j to Oj.

Infusum cinchonæ flavæ,	Tonic.—Better made with cold water.
" " rubræ,	Tonic. do.
" cascarillæ,	Stimulant; tonic.
" eupatorii,	Tonic.—Given hot as a diaphoretic and emetic.
" krameriæ,	Astringent.
" sarsaparillæ,	Alterative; diaphoretic.
" ulmi,	Demulcent.
" buchu,	Demulcent; diuretic.
" armoraciæ (with mustard-seed, ℥j),	Stimulant; diuretic.
" sennæ (with coriander, ʒj),	Cathartic.

GROUP II.—℥ss to Oj.

Infusum angusturæ,	Stimulant; tonic.
" anthemidis,	Tonic; emetic, when hot.
" colombæ,	Tonic.
" serpentariæ,	Tonic.
" valerianæ,	Stimulant; antispasmodic.
" capsici,	Arterial stimulant. Dose, f℥ss.
" zingiberis,	Carminative.
" humuli,	Tonic; mild narcotic.
" spigeliæ,	Anthelmintic.
" catechu comp. (with cinnamon, ʒj),	Astringent.
" lini comp. (with liquorice-root, ʒij),	Demulcent.

GROUP III.—Proportions varied.

Infusum caryophylli,	ʒij to Oj.	Stimulant.
" rhei,	do.	Cathartic.
" tabaci,	ʒj to Oj.	Sedative injection in hernia.
" digitalis,	ʒj to Oss,	+ Tr. cinnam., f℥j.—Narcotic. Dose, fʒij. (Withering's.)
" rosæ compositum,	℥ss to Oiiss,	+ Sugar, and diluted sulphuric acid.—Adjuvant to astringent gargles, &c.
" taraxaci,	℥ij to Oj.	Diuretic.

SECOND CLASS.—*Made with cold water by maceration or percolation.*

Infusum cinchonæ comp.,	℥j to Oj,	+ Aromat. sulph. acid, fʒj.—Tonic.
" pruni Virginianæ,	℥ss to Oj.	Sedative; tonic.
" quassiæ,	ʒij to Oj.	Tonic.
" gentianæ comp.,	℥ss to Oj.	+ Bitter orange-peel, coriander, dil. alcohol.—Tonic.
" sassafras medullæ,	ʒj to Oj.	Demulcent.

The general dose of infusions is f℥ij, or a wineglassful, frequently repeated. This is to be varied in the case of infusion of senna, compound infusion of flaxseed, and others, in which a much larger quantity may be taken at a draught.

There are two infusions which it would be improper to give in the above general dose; these are *infusion of digitalis* and *infusion of cap-*

sicum; both are given in doses of a tablespoonful or less. The chief use of *infusion of sassafras pith* is as an external application to inflamed eyes.

Compound infusion of rose is said to be an excellent addition to Epsom salts in solution for overcoming its bitterness.

UNOFFICINAL INFUSIONS.

An immense number of substances are frequently prescribed in the form of infusion, which it would be unnecessary to introduce here; in fact, it is a common way of prescribing most of the vegetable tonics and alteratives. The following recipes for compound infusions seem to belong in this place:—

Dr. Mettauer's Aperient.

Take of		
	Aloes (soc.)	ʒv.
	Bicarb. soda	ʒxj.
	Valerian (contused)[1]	℥j.
	Water	Oj.
	Comp. spirit of lavender	fʒvj.

Make an infusion.

DOSE.—A tablespoonful containing about 9 grs. aloes, 20 of bicarb. of soda, and 14 of valerian. As a laxative for constipation, &c.

Dr. Gerhard's Tonic Tea.

Take of		
	Contused gentian	℥ss.
	" rhubarb	ʒj.
	" ginger	ʒij.
	Bicarbonate of soda	ʒj.
	Boiling water	Oj.

Make an infusion.

When designed to be preserved for some time, I usually add half a fluidounce of compound tincture of cardamon.

DOSE.—A wineglassful three times a day.

Black Draught.

Take of		
	Senna	℥ss.
	Sulphate of magnesia	℥j.
	Manna	℥j.
	Fennel-seed	ʒj.
	Boiling water	f℥viij.

Macerate in a covered vessel till the liquid cools.

DOSE.—One-third, to be repeated every four or five hours till it operates.

Physick's Medicated Lye, or Alkaline Solution.

Take of		
	Hickory ashes	℥viij.
	Soot	℥j.
	Water	Cong. j.

Digest for twenty-four hours and strain.

DOSE.—A wineglassful. In dyspepsia.

[1] Some recipes omit the valerian.

Parrish's Cider Mixture.

Take of Juniper berries,	
Mustard-seed,	
Ginger, ...	each 2 ounces.
Horseradish,	
Parsley-root, ...	each 4 ounces.
Cider	1 gallon.

Macerate for a week and strain, or make by displacement, adding a little alcohol if designed to be kept long.

DOSE.—A wineglassful three times a day, increased at discretion. In dropsy.

Mistura Aloes Composita.—I. J. GRAHAME.

Recommended as a substitute for compound decoction of aloes of the British *Pharmacopœias.*

Take of Extract of liquorice	½ ounce.
Liquorice-root in moderately fine powder	1½ ounces.
Carbonate of potassa	1 drachm.
Aloes, myrrh, and saffron in moderately fine powder, each	1½ drachms.
Compound tincture of cardamon . .	6½ fluidounces.
Distilled water	18 fluidounces.

Rub well together the aloes, myrrh, and carbonate of potassa; add the remaining powder, and mix all intimately. Having mixed the water and compound tincture of cardamon, pour off this liquid on the compound powder, sufficient to dampen it; pack moderately in a suitable displacer, and, having placed over the surface a piece of perforated filtering paper, pour on the remainder of the liquid, and when it has ceased to pass, add water sufficient to make the filtrate measure in all twenty-four fluidounces. A clear, rich, reddish-brown liquid.—*Transactions Md. Col. Phar.*, 1858.

Elixir Clauderi.

℞.—Carbonate of potassa	℥j.
Aloes	ʒij.
Guaiacum	ʒij.
Myrrh	ʒij.
Saffron	ʒij.
Rhubarb (contused)	ʒij.
Water	f℥xviij.

Macerate a few days and decant.

DOSE.—A tablespoonful.

The concentrated infusions, of which several are in common use in England, properly belong to the class of fluid extracts, and under that head a recipe will be found for infusum cinchonæ spissatum, of the *London Pharmacopœia.*

CHAPTER V.

PERCOLATION, OR THE DISPLACEMENT PROCESS.

THE displacement process is the neatest, most rapid, and productive method for extracting the soluble principles from vegetable substances. It is directed in the *United States Pharmacopœia* for preparing a large number of the officinal tinctures, wines, vinegars, syrups, fluid extracts, extracts, and some of the infusions. It is frequently coupled, however, with directions for the employment of maceration, so that a physician or pharmaceutist, who may not have acquired a practical knowledge of its details, may choose the older and more familiar process for their preparation.

As a number of the most concentrated officinal preparations cannot be made by any other process, and as this possesses advantages in nearly every case, a knowledge of it is justly regarded as indispensable to the pharmaceutist, and the physician who may be called upon to practise pharmacy.

History.—The process of displacement has been employed from time immemorial in the preparation of coffee in the celebrated *Cafetière de Doubelloy*, an instrument much used in France, and occasionally in this country at the present time. It consists of an ordinary tin coffee-pot, surmounted by a movable cylinder, usually varying from three to five or six inches in diameter, and from eight to ten inches in length, and which contains two perforated diaphragms, one permanent and soldered on to the lower extremity of the cylinder, and the other movable, so as to be supported either upon the top of the mass of coffee in using the apparatus, or upon a projection in a movable upright tube, open at both ends, and so situated as to allow the free passage of the air from the lower to the upper part of the vessel.

The French coffee pot is a displacement apparatus of convenient construction, and had been long celebrated for the production of a clear and strong coffee, possessing a finer aroma than that made by decoction, but, until the year 1833, the idea seems not to have occurred of applying it to the production of pharmaceutical preparations. This application is due to M. Boullay & Son, French pharmaciens, who, by their admirable and well-conducted experiments, first demonstrated the adaptation of percolation to the general purposes of the shop and laboratory, drew the attention of the profession to its merits, and pointed out the best forms of apparatus, and the best modes for using them.

In 1836, an article by M. A. Guillermond, translated from the *Journal de Pharmacie*, was published in the *American Journal of Pharmacy*, vol. vii. p. 308, and in 1838, the late Augustine Duhamel, a scientific pharmaceutist of Philadelphia, published in the *American Journal of Pharmacy*, vol. x. p. 1, his first communication upon the new process. In the following year, in connection with William Procter, Jr., now Professor of Pharmacy in the Philadelphia College of Pharmacy, he engaged further attention to the subject in an able article of the same journal, vol. xi. p. 189, in which a series of careful experiments in the preparation of extracts, tinctures, infusions, and syrups were detailed, which so conclusively proved the superiority of this over the ordinary processes in use that intelligent pharmaceutists generally were induced to try, and eventually to adopt it.

The process of percolation so far found favor with the committee having under care the decennial revision of the *Pharmacopœia* in 1840 that it was sanctioned to a considerable extent in the edition of our national standard of that year. At the present time, it is so extensively employed in the preparation of the Galenical solutions as to a great extent to supersede the process of maceration.

THE APPARATUS.—In describing the common forms of displacement apparatus or percolators, I shall confine myself chiefly to the more simple and extemporaneous kinds adapted to the physician's office.

The common *tin displacer* consists of a cylinder varying in size, but at least twice as long as its diameter, terminated at one end by a funnel, the neck of which is made small enough to insert conveniently into a common tincture or narrow-mouth packing bottle; two perforated diaphragms of the size of the cylinder, and loosely fitting into it; each of these has a small ring of wire soldered on to it to facilitate its removal. Sometimes these cylinders are made larger at the top, tapering toward the lower end, and there is an advantage in this shape over straight sides, as shown in the drawing. The lower diaphragm should be of finely perforated tin plate; the finest sold is not objectionable, while the upper may be made of ordinary tinned iron, pierced with comparatively large holes. Occasionally the lower diaphragm is soldered to a very small tin tube, open at both ends, of nearly the length of the cylinder, near the top of which is a ledge on

Fig. 116. Fig. 117.

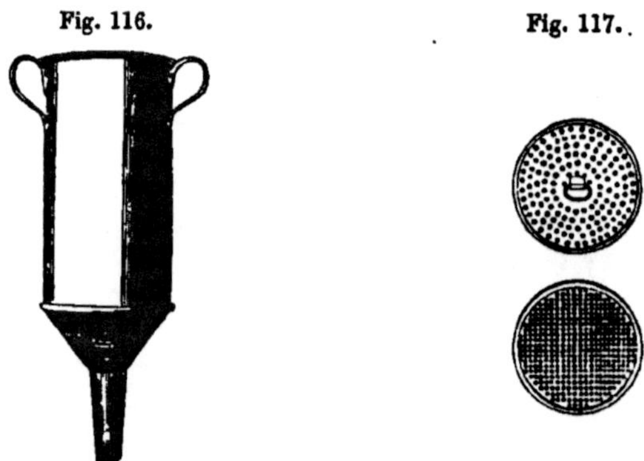

The displacer, with upper and lower diaphragm.

which the upper diaphragm is made to rest, as in the French coffee-pot and in the air-tight displacer (Fig. 123); the object of this is to allow the passage of air from the lower or receiving vessel into the top of the cylinder.

The Queensware Displacer.—This is the same as the above in shape; the material is considered more cleanly; it is not liable to corrosion with acid liquids, nor to impart a black color and metallic taste to solutions of the vegetable astringents.

Fig. 118. Fig. 119.

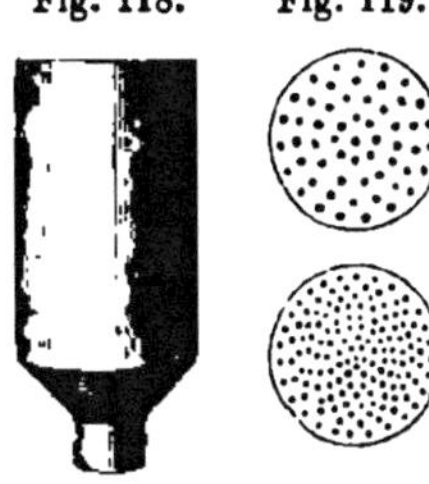

Porcelain displacer, with two diaphragms.

The Common Funnel.—This may be employed for displacement, by inserting a plug of carded cotton or of fine sponge into the neck, and by using a piece of perforated paper, or some thin cotton cloth, or other fabric for the upper diaphragm.

Since the first edition of this work was written, I have had occasion to try numerous experiments in displacement, and have found unexpected advantages from the use of the common funnel. The swelling of the solid contents of the displacer during the progress of its saturation with the menstruum frequently almost arrests the passage of the liquid when the common form of cylinder is used; but in an ordinary funnel the lateral pressure is forced into an upward direction, owing to the tapering direction of the sides of the funnel, and while the mass is rendered sufficiently compact, it is not so compressed as to interfere with the regular operation of capillary attraction and the displacement resulting from the pressure of the superincumbent liquid.

Lamp-chimney Displacers.—No form of apparatus is cheaper for small operations than ordinary lamp-chimneys, either plain (Fig. 120) or with bulb (Fig. 121). The smaller end of the chimney is filled with a cork cut so as to allow the free passage of the liquid, at the same time that it affords a mechanical support to the mass, or covered with a piece of gauze, book-muslin, or other coarse fabric, tied securely by a string round the chimney near its lower edge, and a little carded cotton being placed on it, the under diaphragm is rendered complete; the upper one may be made of paper, when necessary, as before described, or, where the diameter is small, may be omitted.

These, having no funnel-shaped terminations, require to be inserted in a wide-mouth bottle; one which answers the purpose should be selected and always kept at hand; a piece of thick pasteboard, or other firm substance, may be used as a support for an apparatus of this description by cutting a hole in it of the required size, so as to suspend it over a dish, or by the aid of a retort stand into a suitable jar or measure, as shown in Figs. 120 and 121. Lamp-chimneys with bulbs are still more convenient in this respect.

Fig. 123 represents a tin displacer with a water-joint near the top for covering and preventing evaporation in making ethereal or other very volatile preparations; the little tube *e* serves for the escape of

Fig. 120. Fig. 121.

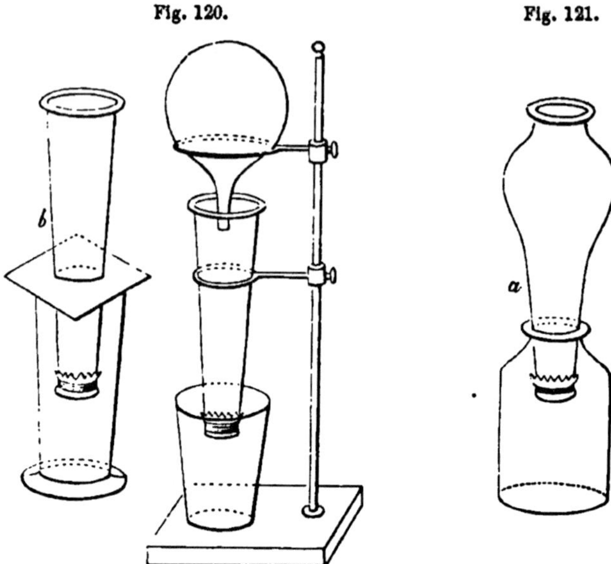

Lamp-chimney displacer with supports.

the air from the lower vessel *B*, so as to equalize the atmospheric pressure between the top of the air-tight displacer and the receiving

Fig. 122. Fig. 123.

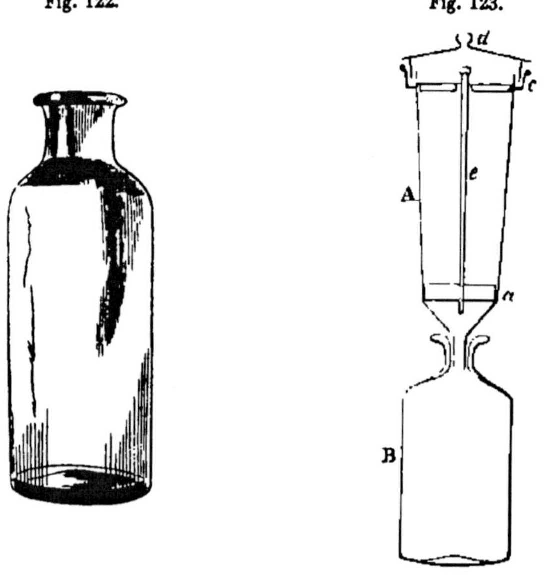

Receiving bottle for displacement. Tin displacer for volatile liquids.

bottle; the lower diaphragm *a* is soldered on to the top of this tube, and the upper diaphragm rests on it; *c* represents the gutter into which the top *d* fits, and which, being filled with water, constitutes an air-tight connection. The displacer fits into the narrow-mouth bottle either by the aid of a cork or not, as the case may require.

Broken Bottles.—A portion of the broken bottles in a shop have the bottom cracked uniformly off, which is likely to occur when hot liquids are poured into them; they furnish a cylinder-shaped vessel not unlike the tin displacement apparatus above described; a plug of cotton is used for a diaphragm, as in the case of the funnel. The bottoms of bottles may be cracked off for this purpose by passing gradually round them a red-hot rod of iron in contact with the glass, and, when fractured, removing the sharp edge by a file, or by inserting the bottle in a shallow vessel of cold water, so as to be immersed just up to the line to be fractured, and filling it nearly to the same line with water, then pouring in a sufficient quantity of oil of vitriol suddenly to raise the temperature on the inside, the bottom will generally drop out.

I have recently had made the very convenient and economical glass displacement funnel (Fig. 124). These are made of three sizes, the larger three and a half inches in diameter, and eight inches in length, exclusive of the neck; it is in shape like a broken bottle, but thicker and more uniform, and with a smooth edge at both ends; the neck is drawn out with the view to inserting it into a bottle, and it may be conveniently covered with a suitable piece of glass when desirable. No diaphragms accompany the apparatus; sponge, cotton, or broken glass is invariably used.

Fig. 124. Fig. 125.

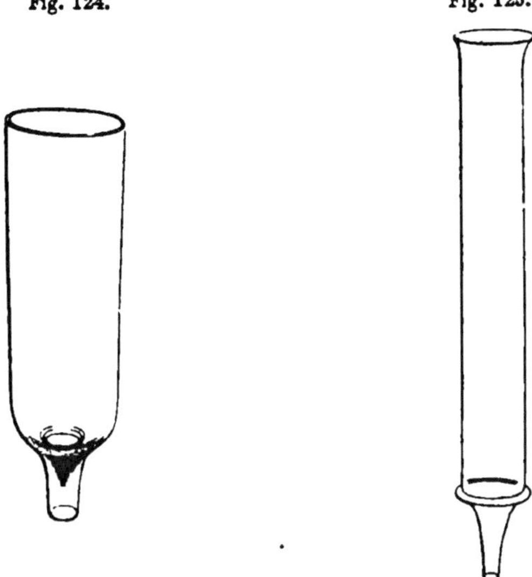

Glass displacer. Small syringe pattern displacer.

Availing ourselves of the very cheap and common production of syringes from glass tubes, which extend to one and a quarter inch in diameter, and can be furnished at a very low price, we have procured the apparatus represented in Fig. 125. It is a glass syringe of the largest size, without the piston or cap. It can only be used for small operations, for which, however, it is well adapted. In treating Spanish flies and other substances with ether, we have found it convenient from the facility with which the top can be corked up, preventing evaporation; a variety of preparations may be conveniently made with the syringe pattern displacer.

For reasons that will more fully appear when speaking of the process, it is necessary that the receiving vessel should be of such size as to hold precisely the quantity it is proposed to make, or be suitably graduated to this quantity. A convenient plan adopted in the school of practical pharmacy, where a variety of preparations are going on at the same time, is to mark upon a narrow slip of paper the name and quantity of the preparation about being made, and paste this upon the receiving vessel before commencing the process, in such a position that when the required quantity has passed it will just reach the top of the slip of paper; if a graduated measure of sufficient capacity is used, the necessity of this is obviated. It is convenient to a physician for his office purposes to keep one or more graduated bottles, made by pasting a slip of paper longitudinally on the bottles marked with a pen to the f℥viij, f℥x, f℥xij, Oj, and f℥xx denominations, as shown in this cut; the paper may be rendered impervious to moisture by collodion or other varnish.

Fig. 126.

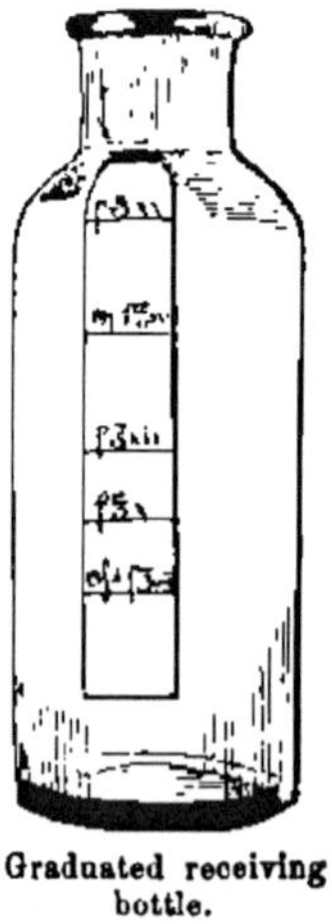

Graduated receiving bottle.

THE PROCESS.—The following is the usual direction for the treatment of substances by displacement:—

Saturate the substance in the form of powder with the appropriate menstruum, and after maceration (if necessary), transfer it to the apparatus; pack it more or less tightly in the cylinder, and gradually add sufficient of the menstruum to make, when it has passed, the required quantity of the preparation, care being taken to return the first portions of the liquid till it passes clear, and not faster than drop by drop.

Notwithstanding the apparent simplicity of this manipulation, skill in managing it is only attainable by experience, and hence the care observable throughout the *U. S. Pharmacopœia* of 1840, and even in that of 1850, to present directions for maceration with those for displacement, thus giving to the operator a choice of either process, and also enjoining a more or less protracted maceration previous to displacement.

With a view to imparting a preliminary knowledge of this process, which will facilitate the attainment of a practical familiarity with its details, I proceed to state the principal facts and circumstances which experience has suggested as important to be observed.

The *fineness of the powder* must be regarded by the nature of the substance and the menstruum; very porous and mucilaginous substances, as rhubarb, squill and gentian roots, senna, conium, and buchu leaves, colocynth pulp, &c., are treated most conveniently, where an ordinary displacer with straight sides is used, in powder, such as will pass through a sieve of six meshes to the square inch, or even coarser. Hard and close-grained drugs, such as stramonium, nux vomica, and most other seeds, quassia wood, ginger, serpentaria, valerian, and black snakeroots, and aconite and matico leaves, should be in comparatively fine powder. Water and diluted acetic acid, as a general rule, require coarser powders than diluted alcohol, and the latter menstruum coarser than alcohol and ether. This circumstance is among the most important to be learned in connection with displacement. In no case is it desirable to employ a coarse powder in treating drugs with strong alcohol or ether, and in scarcely any where diluted alcohol is the menstruum. A sieve of fifty meshes to the linear inch answers the best purpose in preparing powders for alcoholic preparations, though no sieve need be employed by those familiar with the degree of fineness by observation.

Previous maceration, though directed in nearly every instance in the *Pharmacopœia*, is not necessary, except in a few cases; the direction is there given for the purpose of guarding against the effects of careless manipulation, and it is an excellent precaution to insure the material being thoroughly permeated by the fluid, which may otherwise fail of taking place, owing to careless packing, or to a too partial division of it.

Porous materials, such as swell very much on the addition of a liquid, and some ligneous powders, which part with their active principles with difficulty, may be previously moistened, and allowed to macerate as designated in the *Pharmacopœia*, while many barks, roots, and leaves may be introduced in the state of dry powders, and small portions of the menstruum being successively added with judgment and care, the preparation may be quite as thoroughly made as by previous maceration.

One of the best criterions by which to measure the completeness of the process is its *rapidity;* if the addition of a portion of the menstruum is accompanied by a brisk stream running from the lower end of the apparatus into the receiving vessel, the process of displacement is going on but partially or not at all; it will then be necessary either to repack it again or to cork it up below, and allow the material to macerate until it has fully swelled up, and the fine particles have settled more completely into the interstices of the mass.

If, on the contrary, the addition of the fresh fluid fails to displace any portion of that with which the mass has been saturated, the whole may require to be removed from the apparatus and more loosely packed; or, as is sometimes done, the addition of a considerable column of the liquid, by its greater hydrostatic pressure, may be made to overcome the difficulty; and after it has once commenced to pass slowly, it will often increase in rapidity until the whole of the preparation is obtained.

The *packing of the powder* in the cylinder, whether it be dry or previously moistened, is an important point in conducting percolation; in this, as in regulating the fineness of the powder, reference must be had to the nature of the substance treated, and of the menstruum. Drugs of a porous structure, when dry, require to be rather loosely packed to allow for the swelling produced on the addition of the liquid, though, if previously saturated with the liquid, they may be somewhat compressed; hard, ligneous seeds or roots should be tightly packed. It may be said to be a rule in this case that the firmness of the packing should be inversely as the solvent and softening power of the liquid upon the solid under treatment. The packing should be accomplished at intervals during the filling in of the powder, so as to be uniform throughout the cylinder.

Repassing the first portions of the Liquid.—In a majority of cases the liquid first passes clouded, portions of powder sometimes being found in the receiving vessel, or the soluble principles, partially dissolved, having escaped through the diaphragm. In these instances, the liquid should be returned into the cylinder until it passes perfectly clear; it is, also, a good precaution in almost every case where maceration has been omitted to return the first portions of the liquid until they appear nearly saturated, reserving a portion to be added after the strength of the mass is nearly extracted. In making the saturated preparations, such as tincture of aconite root and wine of colchicum root, this preparation is especially important, and the necessity for its observance is increased in proportion to the rapidity with which the process is conducted, and to the quantity of material to be exhausted.

When a substance in sufficiently fine powder has been macerated (if necessary), and then properly packed in an apparatus, so that, on the addition of the liquid above, it will pass drop by drop, and, the first portions being returned, give a clear and very strong preparation, *the last portions of liquid will pass almost destitute of the soluble principles* contained in the drug. This is the clearest indication of the success of the experiment; it also proves that, by displacement, we may entirely obviate the necessity of any means of expressing the last portions of liquid from a porous mass.

In making preparations by displacement, we should aim by skilful manipulation to extract nearly all from the drug that is soluble before adding the last few ounces of the menstruum, which may be used to displace the last portion held by the dregs, and to dilute the liquid to the proper point.

After maceration, the dregs are almost always saturated with the strongest portion of the liquid, which is wasted unless some means of expression are resorted to; but, if the dregs be thrown upon a filter, and a portion of water or other convenient liquid be poured upon it, the last drop may sometimes be displaced without a resort to the troublesome process of expression.

If the liquid thus added to the dregs is different from the menstruum originally employed, and especially if it is a heavier liquid, it is liable to mix with it, and sometimes results in injury to the preparation. By adding about one-third less of the displacing liquid than the supposed quantity of menstruum remaining in the dregs, this inconvenience is generally obviated.

In the preparation of a tincture it will sometimes happen that the last portion cannot be recovered by adding water. In making large quantities of alcoholic extracts or tinctures made with strong alcohol, this is a great loss, and requires the use of a press. Convenient screw-presses are made in the cities, and sold at moderate prices; that shown on page 111 is well adapted to the object in view; it is a useful instrument to the pharmaceutist in several processes.

Grahame's Process.—Professor Grahame, of the Maryland College of Pharmacy, has proposed a modification of the displacement process, which experience has convinced me is an improvement on the foregoing. It may be thus stated:—

Reduce the substance by contusion to a powder which will pass though a sieve of forty meshes to the linear inch (if of close texture a sieve of sixty meshes is to be preferred); now add just sufficient of the menstruum to dampen the powder without wholly destroying its mobility; this usually requires about one-fourth as much menstruum as of the powder. Now transfer to *a glass funnel* with a plug of cotton in the neck, and pack it with little or much pressure, according to its tenacity or disposition to adhere (more firmly when alcohol or ether is the menstruum than when water is to be used); if the particles of the moistened powder move freely on each other, the packing should be with as much force as a glass vessel will bear, the whole of the powder being introduced at once, and packed with a pestle or packing-stick. The whole quantity of the menstruum may now be poured on, or to the capacity of the funnel, and the process allowed to proceed to completion, without in any case repassing the first portions of the liquid. By this process, if carefully followed, very concentrated solutions are obtained; indeed, most of the fluid extracts may be completed with little or no evaporation.[1]

Of the Solution of Gum Resins, &c., in Displacement Apparatus.—Vegetable products of this class are usually so soluble in the menstrua employed for their extraction as to render it a matter of little importance whether they are treated by maceration or displacement. They should be thoroughly divided in order to expose an extended surface to the action of the liquid, and, if displaced, should be mixed with an equal bulk of sand to facilitate the process; when made by maceration, they require to be filtered to free them from impurities suspended in them, the necessity of which is obviated when they are treated by displacement. It has been stated that tincture of kino made by the displacement process is less disposed to gelatinize than that made by maceration, and there seems little doubt of this, when the macerated article is allowed to stand in its dregs.

The management of this process sometimes requires the frequent attention of the manipulator to add fresh portions of the menstruum

[1] See paper by the author, Am. Journ. Pharm., vol. xxxi.

from time to time; but, if percolation is fairly commenced, the first portions having been returned if necessary, and coming through slowly and clear as above described, the following arrangement for *continuous displacement* may be adopted:—

A bottle or globe, capable of containing the quantity of menstruum necessary to complete the preparation, is fitted with a perforated cork, in which is inserted a glass tube of such length as that, being inverted over the displacement cylinder, the tube will descend below the surface of the liquid contained in it. The lower end of the tube should have a short curve turned on it; the bottle or globe being filled and arranged in this manner will not discharge any of its contents into the displacer until the surface of the liquid contained in it falls below the extremity of the tube; a bubble of air will then pass up into the bottle, and a corresponding portion of the liquid will descend. In this way, the supply in the displacer will be kept up until the bottle has emptied itself; and, if the quantity of the liquid has been accurately estimated, the preparation will be finished without further attention.

Instead of having merely a straight piece of tube inserted in the mouth of the bottle from which the liquid is supplied, two tubes may be used, as shown in Fig. 127. In this case, the afflux tube *a* is turned up at the end, as recommended above, and as the liquid runs out here air enters at *b*. The surface of the liquid into which *a* is immersed must, however, be so far below the lowest point of *b* as to enable the air to depress the liquid in the external ascending part of *b*, and thus to enter the bottle.

Fig. 127.

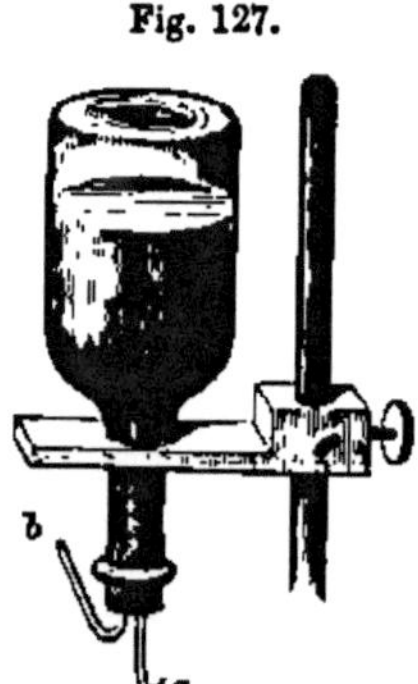

Bottle for continuous filtration and displacement.

The size of the tubes must be also so arranged that the liquid will not run from *a* unless the orifice of the tube be in contact with the contents of the filter, so that the cohesive attraction of the liquid may overcome the capillary attraction.

The process of percolation is very similar in its *modus operandi* to that of filtration; both are due to capillary attraction. In ordinary filtration, the capillarity of the paper causes the absorption of a certain quantity of liquid, but, on more than enough to wet it being added, the pressure of this drives out the first, taking its place, and so on. Precisely the same thing occurs in percolation; a porous substance being saturated with any liquid for which it has an affinity will yield this up, if a portion of liquid be poured on above, from the force of gravitation merely; and hence, in proportion to the height of the column of liquid, other things being equal, will be the rapidity of the process.

The fact that alcohol and ether pass through most plants so much more rapidly than water is due, perhaps, in part to these liquids being less forcibly held by this species of attraction, but mainly to their dissolving less freely the organic proximate principles most abounding in plants, and which render aqueous liquids so thick and viscid as to pass with difficulty.

Rhubarb, senna, squill, and a few other porous substances, containing a large proportion of mucilaginous and extractive matters, cannot be conveniently treated by displacement with aqueous liquids owing to this cause; in treating these, either by water, diluted alcohol, diluted acetic acid, or any other menstruum containing a considerable proportion of water, the following points are to be observed:—

a. The powder must not be too fine, though uniform.

b. The coarse powder must be thoroughly saturated with the menstruum before being introduced into the displacer; or, when it is introduced dry or only moistened, it must be at first loosely packed, otherwise, being swelled very much on the absorption of the liquid, it may become too tight. The common funnel is to be preferred under these circumstances, as directed by Prof. Grahame.

c. When the process proceeds with difficulty, from the causes above described, or from otherwise defective manipulation, it may be partly obviated by adding a considerable column of the menstruum above the mass; this, as already stated, acting by hydrostatic pressure, forces the liquid through with increased facility.

d. Time and patience will, to a certain extent, correct the same difficulty; after the first portions of the liquid, which pass so slowly from being highly charged with the soluble principles, and from the continued swelling of the powder, the remaining volume will come through more readily, increasing in rapidity to the end.

e. The admixture of sand serves a good purpose in this case, as in that of the gum resins.

f. Alcohol, diluted in various proportions with water, is used instead of water alone, in making by displacement fluid extract of senna, fluid extract of pink-root and senna, syrup of rhubarb, syrup of seneka, compound syrup of squill, and perhaps some other preparations, mainly on account of the difficulty of conducting the process.

Displacement, applied to hot liquids, requires some modification, both as regards the apparatus and the manipulations which next claim attention.

The deterioration to which vegetable infusions are liable by boiling is adverted to under that head; the chief use of displacement with steam or hot liquids is to obviate this, at the same time that the advantages of high temperature are secured.

The steam displacement apparatus, invented by C. Augustus Smith, of Cincinnati, Ohio, figured on the next page, consists of two distinct parts, *B*, the displacer, and *C*, the boiler, connected by a tube of tin or lead, *D*. *A* is a tin cap luted on to the top of a common displacement tube terminating in the funnel-shaped appendage below. This is surrounded by a tin jacket, into the bottom of which the conical tube *G* conducts cold water, while the spout *H* discharges the warmed water from the top. The substance to be treated being placed in the displacer, and the liquid designed to be applied to it put into the boiler, the connections are luted on, and heat applied by the lamp *E*, or preferably by a gas furnace. The vapor which is generated passes through the tube *D*, and penetrates the whole mass in the displacer, the jacket being now filled with cold water, the steam is condensed and passes out below, where it is collected in the receiver *F*. The advantage is thus gained of penetrating the powder thoroughly by the aid of heat, while the deteriorating influence of decoction is avoided.

Fig. 128.

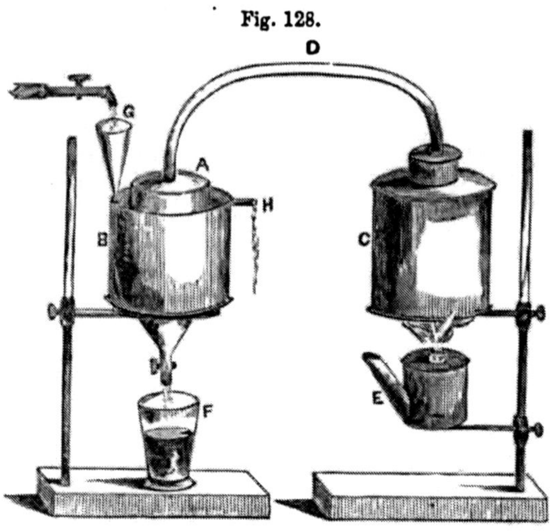

Smith's steam displacer.

Repeated experiments with this instrument have convinced me that it possesses advantages over the ordinary means for extraction with hot liquids which should recommend it to general favor; it is not only useful as a substitute for decoction, but obviates the difficulty above adverted to of extracting certain porous and largely soluble vegetables with water. The steam, whether of water or alcohol, being generated in the boiler and passed into the displacer before the addition of cold water to the cooler, is maintained at an elevated temperature until it has thoroughly permeated the mass; it is then, by refrigeration, converted into liquid, which finds ready egress through the lower orifice of the displacer, and is highly charged with the soluble vegetable principles present. The removal of these, added to the pressure of the steam, continually kept up from the boiler as fast as it is condensed, renders the flow rapid and the preparation concentrated.

Fluid extract of senna can be prepared in the steam displacer in less than twelve hours, without the use of alcohol as a menstruum; so concentrated is the decoction obtained in the first instance as to require comparatively little evaporation to bring it to the officinal standard.

The apparatus, as above described, is imperfectly adapted to treating substances with diluted alcohol; if that liquid be placed in the boiler, the effect of the heat applied is to drive over the alcohol first and then the water, so that the first portion being stronger of the resinous principles, and the latter of the starch and extractive, the mixture of the two would be turbid, and the extract not freely soluble. To obviate this, two boilers are sometimes adapted to one cylinder, one for alcohol and the other for water, and, by a proper regulation of the heat to each, the vapors may be brought over in nearly equal proportions at the same time. The cylinder should not be made of too great diameter nor length; but I am informed by the inventor that he uses cylinders of the capacity of a barrel; this is perhaps the largest size that would answer well in practice; where larger quantities of the same substance are to be treated at once than will fill such a cylinder, or where several different operations requiring the same menstruum are to be conducted simultaneously, two or more cylinders may be attached to the same boiler, and placed in the same cooler.

Substances heretofore digested in hot alcohol, a very inconvenient process, may be treated with that menstruum with great facility by using this apparatus as above described.

For *percolation with ether*, an ingenious apparatus, invented by Prof. Mohr, is figured in his work. It combines the advantages of a good air-tight displacer with that of a still for recovering the ether; it is, however, a complex apparatus, and rather troublesome to use. I omit a drawing of it, as being accessible in that work.

For percolation at ordinary temperatures, especially where a small amount of the medicinal substance is to be treated with ether, common displacer may be used, care being taken to cover it and the receiving vessel, to prevent evaporation; a narrow lamp-chimney, fitting below into a wide-mouth bottle, will be found to serve a good purpose, or, if large enough, a syringe pattern displacer. An adapter, such as is used in retort operations (Fig. 129, *A*), may be inserted through a perforated cork into a convenient bottle, the top being covered with a piece of bladder pierced with pin-holes, or fitted rather loosely with a cork to prevent evaporation.

Fig. 129.

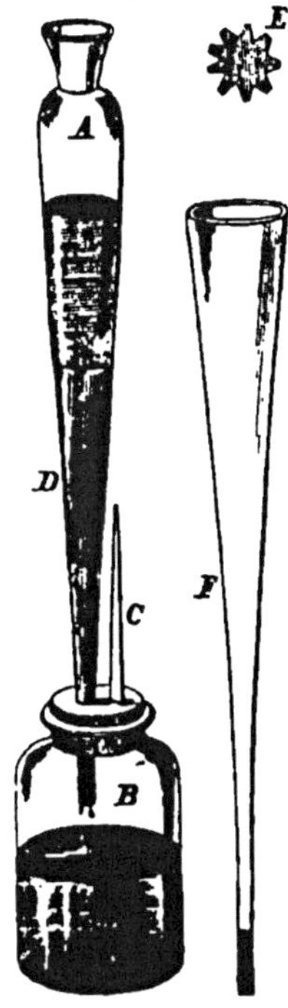

Extemporaneous glass displacers.

Fig. 129 represents two forms of displacers for ether and other volatile liquids; *A* is an adapter. The tube *C* is drawn out into a fine point, so as to admit the passage of the air without favoring evaporation. *E* represents a notched cork diaphragm, *F* a broken retort beak, suited to similar operations.

The application of a vacuum to promote the rapidity of the displacement process, is an important improvement in certain cases, and several very ingenious forms of apparatus have been contrived by the French with this end in view; perhaps the best of these are the coffee-pots, in which the pressure of steam is first brought to bear in penetrating the mass with the hot liquid, and then, by the withdrawal of the source of heat, the steam is immediately condensed, creating a vacuum which hastens the downward passage of the liquid. In using Smith's steam displacer, though at no time a very complete vacuum is formed, yet this principle comes into play, and undoubtedly facilitates the percolation of the mass under treatment, in the same way that it operates in a vacuum displacer.

CHAPTER VI.

TINCTURES.

The consideration of the process of displacement has prepared the student to enter upon those Galenical solutions in the preparation of which it is employed. Prominent among these, as the most numerous and most varied, is the class of tinctures.

The study of these and other Galenical solutions is less attended to by students than their importance demands; in some respects, a knowledge of pharmaceutical preparations is more important than a familiarity with the drugs themselves. It is the preparations that enter into the prescriptions of the physician almost exclusively; he should be acquainted not only with their doses, but with their proper therapeutical and pharmaceutical adaptations, as modified by the menstrua employed in their preparation, by their degree of concentration, their miscibility with other liquids, &c.

With a view to conveying this knowledge, as far as practicable, I shall devote the present chapter to the consideration of the tinctures officinal in the *U. S. Pharmacopœia*, and those unofficinal tinctures which are commonly used in this country.

Tinctures invariably contain alcohol, more or less diluted, as the vehicle for their active ingredients.

Alcohol, as officinal in the *U. S. Pharmacopœia*, is a colorless, limpid, very volatile liquid, of a peculiar penetrating odor, and burning taste, having a specific gravity of .835. Its chief impurities, as found in commerce, are as follows: Water, which increases its specific gravity in the ratio of its proportion; fusel oil, a constituent of whiskey, which being volatile, though less so than alcohol, is generally imperfectly separated in the distillation; this may be detected, by its imparting the peculiar odor of whiskey to the alcohol, and particularly by the odor left on the hand, after the alcohol has evaporated from it: and coloring matter, which is generally derived from the casks in which it is kept.

For a description of the mode of manufacture and chemical characters of alcohol the reader is referred to Part III., where it is treated of as a product of Fermentation.

Alcohol, of .835 sp. gr., called druggist's alcohol, contains 85 per cent. of pure or absolute alcohol; it is an excellent solvent for a large number of vegetable substances, as resins, camphor, benzoic acid, tannic acid, the balsams, grape sugar, the vegetable alkalies, castor oil; also for some inorganic substances, as iodine, carbonate and muriate of ammonia, caustic potassa and soda, nearly all deliquescent, and a few other salts. It mixes freely in all proportions with water, ether, acetic acid, and most of the essential oils, and reacts with several acids, forming ethers.

Besides its extensive solvent powers, qualifying it for so many uses in pharmacy, it is a most convenient antiseptic, effectually preventing fermentation in organic solutions to which it is added.

By the low temperature at which it evaporates, it is well suited to the preparation of concentrated medicines, requiring long evaporation.

In connection with these valuable physical properties, its therapeutical relations should not be overlooked. Alcohol is a very powerful arterial stimulant; even in small quantities it produces fulness of pulse, and a general excitant influence on the system; and hence the tinctures, especially those given in large doses, should not be used in the treatment of inflammatory diseases, and should be employed with prudence in all chronic cases, lest the continual stimulus derived from the alcohol they contain, should lead to the habitual use of intoxicating drinks.

The use of this strong alcohol in the preparation of tinctures, is confined to a comparatively small number, chiefly such as contain a considerable proportion of essential oil, of resin, or of resinoid principles. These constitute the second class in the syllabi which follow.

Diluted Alcohol—Alcohol Dilutum, U. S. P.—This is more extensively employed as a menstruum for tinctures; it consists of equal parts by measure of alcohol and water; its specific gravity is .935. Containing water, the great natural solvent, in so large proportion, this liquid is capable of extracting from plants, gum, extractive matter, vegetable albumen, and most coloring matters which are soluble in that menstruum, and to a certain extent, resinous matters, essential oils, and vegetable alkalies, soluble in alcohol; also sugar and tannic acid, soluble in both.

It has been supposed that the affinity for each other of the two ingredients in this liquid, interferes somewhat with the solvent powers of each; so that substances wholly insoluble in water would not be so thoroughly extracted by a given quantity of diluted alcohol, as by half the quantity of strong alcohol; and so in the case of substances insoluble in alcohol, they would not be so thoroughly extracted by the mixture as by water alone; but, according to the experiments of M. Jaques Personne, published in the *American Journal of Pharmacy*, vol. xviii. pp. 21, 103, the reverse of this is the fact, and a mixture of alcohol and water is stated to be a better solvent of the resinous and extractive principles of plants, than the same quantity of these two liquids separately employed.

Whatever may be the truth in theory, diluted alcohol is found in practice to answer a good purpose; furnishing tinctures which are reasonably permanent, at the same time that they are less stimulating than those made with strong alcohol, and are generally miscible with aqueous solutions without any portion of their active principles precipitating.

Several observers have, however, lately directed attention to the deposits universally occurring in tinctures after long standing, and the conclusion has been reached, in several instances, by experiment, that these contain appreciable quantities of the active ingredients of the preparations.

There are, no doubt, advantages gained by varying the proportions of water and alcohol to suit particular drugs.

There are several preparations officinal in our own *Pharmacopœia*, which are exceptions in the proportion of alcohol contained in them. The infusion of digitalis, and compound infusion of gentian, as before stated, are rendered permanent by small quantities of alcohol added to them, or by being made with very weak diluted alcohol.

Numerous fluid extracts are also made with varied proportions of alcohol and water in extracting the drugs, and also with a small proportion of alcohol, added for its antiseptic properties.

Tincture of aloes, which, for convenience, is noticed here, is an exception to the usual proportions of alcohol and water used as the menstruum for its preparation.

	Composition.		Dose.	Medical Properties.
Tinctura Aloes—	Powd. aloes, ℥ss Ext. liquorice, ℥iss	Alcohol, f℥iv Water, f℥xii	f℥ss	Mild cathartic.

With the object of presenting to view the composition, doses, and medical properties of the officinal tinctures, I have prepared the following series of Tables.

SYLLABUS OF TINCTURES.

Officinal in the *U. S. P.*[1]

Class I.—*Made with Diluted Alcohol.*

Group 1.—These are all made in the proportion of two ounces of the active ingredient to one pint of diluted alcohol. They may be nearly all classed as *narcotics*, though with properties modified in each case. Doses vary from 10 drops to f℥j.

Officinal Name.	Med. Properties.	Dose.	Remarks.
Tinctura aconiti foliorum	Nervous sedative	20 to 30 drops	See tinct. aconiti radicis.
" belladonnæ	Narcotic	do.	
" stramonii	do.	do.	Made from the seeds.
" conii	Alterative, narcotic	30 to 60 drops	Misnamed tinct. cicutæ.
" hyoscyami	Narcotic, laxative	do.	
" digitalis	Diuretic, sedative	10 drops	From English leaves of 2d year.
" lobeliæ	Emetic, narcotic	f℥ss to f℥j	Emetic dose, f℥ss.
" sanguinariæ	do.	do.	do.
" scillæ	Emetic, diuret., expect.	10 to 30 drops	See Acet. scillæ.
" colchici seminis	Diuretic, &c.	20 drops to f℥j	See Vin. & Acet.

[1] See Galenical Preparations of Opium.

GROUP 2.—These are made in varying proportions. They are generally quite incompatible with salts of iron, forming inky solutions. They are all astringents or tonics, or both. Doses, from fʒj to f℥ss.

Officinal Name.	Proportions.	Dose.	Med. Properties.
Tinctura gallæ	℥ij to Oj	fʒij	Astringent.
" catechu	℥iss to Oj with ʒj cinnam.	do.	do.
" kino	℥iss to Oj	fʒj	do.
" krameriæ	℥iij to Oj	do.	do.
" cinchonæ	do. (yellow bark)	f℥ss	Tonic
" " comp.	{ red bark ℥ij B. orange peel ℥iss serpentaria ʒiij saffron ʒj saunders ʒj } to f℥xx	do.	do. aromatic. (Huxham's.)
" colombæ	℥ij to Oj	do.	Tonic
" gentianæ comp.	{ gentian ℥j B. orange peel ℥ss cardamom ʒij } to Oj	do.	do. aromatic.
" quassiæ	℥j to Oj	fʒij	do.
" humuli	℥iiss to Oj	do.	do. sedative.

GROUP 3.—Of varying proportions, chiefly stimulants and aromatics. Doses, generally from fʒj to fʒij.

Officinal Name.	Proportions.	Dose.	Med. Properties, etc.
Tinctura valerianæ	℥ij to Oj	fʒij	Tonic, antispasm.[1]
" serpentariæ	℥iss do.	do.	Stimulant, tonic.
" cubebæ	℥ij do.	do.	Stimulant (added to copaiba mixt.) &c.
" cantharidis	℥ss do.	gtt. xx	Stimulant, diluted largely.
" capsici	do. do.	fʒj	do. do.
" cinnamomi	℥iss do.	f℥ss	Carmin., adjuvant.
" cardamomi	℥ij do.	fʒj	do. do.
" cinnamomi comp.	{ cinnamon ℥ss cardamom ʒij ginger ʒjss } to Oj	f℥ss	do. do.
" cardamomi comp.	{ cardamom ʒiij cinnamon ʒiiss caraway ʒj raisins ℥iiss cochineal ℥ss } to f℥xx	f℥ss	do. do.

[1] See Fluid Extract of Valerian.

GROUP 4.—Of varying proportions. Cathartics with modified properties. Chiefly compound. Doses generally, f℥ss.

Officinal Name.	Proportions.	Dose.	Med. Properties, etc.
Tinct. hellebori	℥ij to Oj	fʒj	Emmenagogue, cath.
" jalapæ	℥iij to Oj	do.	Cath., always used in combination.
" rhei	rhubarb ℥iss, cardamom ʒij } to Oj	f℥ss	Tonic, cathartic.
" " et aloes	rhubarb ʒv, aloes ʒiij, cardamom ʒij } to Oj	do.	Mild cathartic. (Elixir sacrum.)
" " et gentianæ	rhubarb ℥j, gentian ʒij } to Oj	do.	Laxative, tonic.
" " et sennæ	rhubarb ℥ss, senna ʒj, coriander ʒss, fennel ʒss, saunders ʒj, saffron gr. xv, liquorice gr. xv, raisins ℥iij } to Oiss	do.	Carminative, laxative. (Warner's Cordial.)
" sennæ et jalapæ	senna ℥iss, jalap ℥ss, coriander ʒij, cardamom ʒj, caraway ʒij, sugar ℥ij } to Oiss	do.	Carminative, laxative (Elixir salutis.)

REMARKS ON TINCTURES OF THE FIRST CLASS.—The tinctures made with diluted alcohol, are here found to be susceptible of division into four groups, arranged chiefly with a view to their medical properties, but generally having other features in common.

The first Group are easy of preparation by percolation, the herbs usually yielding their active principles and coloring matter before the whole amount of menstruum has passed. Stramonium and Colchicum tinctures should be made out of the finely powdered seeds: the former is remarkable for having a peculiar green or fluorescent appearance when seen by reflected light, though very clear and of a decided brown color by transmitted light.

The majority of them are narcotics, and are given in the dose of from 20 to 60 drops: they are all made in the proportion of two ounces of the drug to one pint of the menstruum. Considered therapeutically the six first named in the table form a very natural group; the remaining four have fewer points of resemblance, and several cannot be classed with narcotics without doing some violence to their true position. The tincture of digitalis is not only peculiar in its therapeutical action, but forms an exception in the dose, which should not exceed ten drops.

The second Group may be conveniently made by displacement. Tinctures of kino and catechu when made by maceration, should be filtered off from the dregs before standing away for use in dispensing; they are even then liable to gelatinize, particularly the first named;

it was thought that this might be obviated by the employment of displacement in their preparation, but this is doubtful. When made by displacement they require the use of sand or some other inert substance to separate their particles. In the preparation of compound tincture of cinchona the omission of the saunders prescribed, would be a great improvement.

The tonic and astringent preparations are appropriately associated, though differing among themselves. Tincture of quassia is *sui generis* in containing no astringent principle. The dose of these will be observed to be much larger than of the first group, ranging from two fluidrachms to half a fluidounce.

The third Group has less points of resemblance among its members than either of the others. The last four of this group are, however, all used for the same purposes, as adjuvants to other medicines, in extemporaneous solutions and mixtures. The compound tincture of cardamom is a very rich and elegant one for this purpose. When made by displacement the raisins, which are directed to be deprived of their seeds, should be placed in the receiving vessel and allowed to macerate in the tincture, though I have observed that when allowed to stand on them for a long time it loses, to a great extent, its rich color.

The fourth Group, with the exception of tinctures of hellebore and jalap, is a very natural one; these are what are called stomachics, and are much used in debilitated states of the stomach and bowels, following protracted illness. They should be used with caution, for fear of inducing intemperate habits.

The tincture of rhubarb and senna is directed in the *Pharmacopœia* to be made by maceration, but, with the exception of the raisins, which should be separated and macerated in the tincture, the ingredients if properly powdered and mixed, are well adapted to displacement.

The doses named in the tables may be considered as average adult doses; it is impossible to state their variations in a table.[1]

Class II.—*Made with Officinal Alcohol, sp. gr.* .835.

Group 1.—Saturated tinctures, or nearly so.

Officinal Name.	Proportions.	Dose.	Medical Properties.
Tinctura aconiti radicis	℥vj to Oj	gtt. v to x	Nervous, sedative.
" nucis vomicæ	℥iv to Oj	gtt. v to xv	Nervous, stimulant.
" *veratrum viride*	℥viij to Oj	gtt. v to xv	Narcotic (unofficinal).

[1] See Unofficinal Tinctures.

GROUP 2.—Resinous tinctures.

Officinal Name.	Proportions.	Dose.	Medical Properties.
Tinctura myrrhæ	℥ij to Oiss	fʒj	Astringent, emmenagogue.
" aloes et myrrhæ	aloes ℥iss saffron ℥ss tr. myrrh Oj	fʒj	Laxative, emmenagogue. (Elixir proprietatis.)
" guaiaci	℥iij to Oj	fʒij	Alterative, diaphoretic.
" assafœtida	℥ij to Oj	fʒj	Antispasmodic.
" castorei	℥j to Oj	fʒss	Antispasmodic.
" lupulinæ	℥ij to Oj	fʒj	Tonic, narcotic.
" tolutani	℥iss to Oj	fʒss	Stimulant, expectorant.
" benzoini comp.	benzoin ℥iss storax ℥j bals. tolu ℥ss aloes ʒij to Oj	fʒss	Stimulant, expectorant. (See Turlington's balsam.)
" zingiberis	℥iv to Oj	fʒj	Carminative.

GROUP 3.—Simple solutions in alcohol.

Officinal Name.	Proportions.	Dose.	Medical Properties.
Tinct. camphoræ	℥ij to Oj	gtt. xx	Stimulant.
" ol. menth. pip.	f℥ij to Oj	gtt. xx	Carminative.
" ol. menth. viridis	f℥ij to Oj	gtt. xxx	Carminative.
" iodinii	℥j to Oj	gtt. xv	Alterative.
" iodinii comp.	iodine ℥ss iod. potas. ℥j to Oj	gtt. xv	Alterative.
" saponis camphorata	soap ℥ij camphor ℥j oil rosem'y fʒij to Oj		Used externally. (Liquid opodeldoc.)

REMARKS ON TINCTURES OF SECOND CLASS.—It will be observed that tinctures of this class are generally given in smaller doses than those of the first class.

They are, as a class, more active preparations.

The first group, and tincture of ginger of the second, require great care in the management of the displacement to insure the complete extraction of the soluble active principles from so large a proportion of the respective drugs.

Each of the drugs should be powdered and passed through a sieve of at least 60 meshes to the linear inch, then the process should be conducted as recommended by Prof. Grahame, the powder being dampened with alcohol in an open dish or bowl, without losing its mobile or pulverulent condition, and then packed tightly into a funnel, to which the menstruum is to be added till the requisite quantity of tincture has passed. Should it happen that the whole strength has not been extracted up to the time or near the time of the full quantity having passed, it is better to set aside the tincture which has been collected and pass the remainder into an evaporating dish, in which it may be concentrated at a very low temperature and added to the first portion.

This class, especially the 2d group, and tinctures of camphor and iodine of 3d group, are all incompatible with aqueous liquids, which, by rendering the basis insoluble, precipitate it. Notwithstanding this apparent disadvantage, these tinctures are sometimes added to mixtures containing a large proportion of water, and answer a very good purpose, where sugar or gum are added as ingredients. Some of the resinous tinctures are much given on sugar, which being allowed to dissolve slowly in the mouth, is well calculated to develop their taste and odor.

The tinctures of essential oils, of which those of peppermint and spearmint are officinal, are commonly known as essences; but most of the essences sold are much below the officinal standard, as might be inferred from their price. (See chapters on *Distillation* and on *Essential Oils.*)

Tinctures of tolu and ginger are used in the preparation of the officinal tolu and ginger syrups. The latter is extensively known as essence of ginger, and is one of the most popular of carminatives.

I do not see the propriety of the use of strong alcohol in all the tinctures of this class; in several of those of the 2d group, diluted alcohol would seem to be the proper menstruum. In myrrh, there are 44 parts of gum to 40 of resin, and 2 of essential oil, so that one would suppose the proportion of diluted alcohol would be exactly suited to its solution.

In assafœtida there are about 65 parts of resin and 31 of gum, which would seem to indicate the use of about 2 parts of alcohol to 1 of water.

CLASS III.—*Ammoniated Tinctures.*

Made with Aromatic Spirit of Ammonia.[1]

Tinct. guaiaci ammoniata	℥iv to Oiss	Stimulating diaphoretic,	Dose, f℥j.
" valerianæ "	℥ij to Oj	Antispasmodic,	do.

Aromatic spirit of ammonia, itself an admirable stimulant and antacid, and extensively used as a remedy for sick headache, is used as a menstruum in this class of tinctures; it has the advantage, from the quantity of carbonate of ammonia it contains, of increasing the solubility of resinous bodies, and also adding to their stimulating effects and comparative medicinal efficiency in certain cases.

The "officinal volatile tinctures," as they are called, are both often prescribed; that of guaiac in gouty affections with an acid diathesis, that of valerian in hysteria, &c. It is very much superseded of late by the unofficinal Pieclot's solution of valerianate of ammonia.

TINCTURES NOT OFFICINAL IN *U. S. P.*

Under this head only a few of the more important will be introduced. The reader is referred to Medical Formularies for such as are not selected for insertion here.

[1] See chapter on Alkalies and their Salts.

Tinctura Cinchonæ et Quassiæ Composita.—Tonic Tincture.

Take of Cinchona,
Quassia,
Colombo,
Gentian,
Serpentaria,
Chamomile, of each . . ℥ss.
French brandy . . . Oij.

Powder suitably, mix and macerate 14 days, or extract by displacement.

A very valuable combination of bitters, which, by the absence of the disagreeable resinous coloring matter of Saunders, and by the employment of an acceptable form of alcohol as the menstruum, is adapted to supersede Huxham's tincture of bark. Dose, fʒj to f℥ss.

Bitter Tincture of Iron. (Dr. Physick.)

Take of Iron filings . . . . . . ℥iij.
Bruised ginger,
" gentian, of each . . ℥j.
" orange-peel . . . ℥ss.

Infuse in one pint of old cider for two weeks, in a bottle without a stopper, and filter.

Although not an elegant preparation, this is an efficient and popular chalybeate tonic. Dose, 30 drops, three times a day.

The following modified recipe is that I now employ with great success, forming one of the most approved remedies of its class:—

Take of Iron filings . . . . . . ℥iij.
Old cider . . . . . . Oj.
Acetic acid . . . . . . f℥j.
Citric acid . . . . . . ʒss.
Ginger . . . . ℥iv.
Gentian . . . . . . ℥iv.
Orange-peel . . . . . . ℥ij.
Alcohol . . . . . . Oij.
Water . . . . Oj.

To the iron filings in a wide mouth bottle add the cider and acetic acid; digest for several hours by the aid of a very moderate heat. Displace the aromatics with the mixed alcohol and water. Now add the citric acid to the cider preparation, mix the liquids, and after a few hours pour off the clear liquor, filter the remainder into this, and bottle for use. As thus made, this preparation has a rich wine color, becoming darker by age, but not black and grumous like the foregoing.

Tinctura Cinchonæ Ferrata.

On account of the large number of cases in which the tonic effects of cinchona and aromatics are indicated with ferruginous preparations, it is desirable to contrive a method of combining these without producing the inky and grumous appearance resulting from the diffusion of tannate of iron in the preparation. A tincture, with the above title, was announced some time since by Samuel Simes, of this city, as combining the advantages of cinchona and iron. A specimen of this being examined by Alfred B. Taylor, was pronounced to contain less than half a grain of the iron salt to an ounce; this occasioned the publication of a recipe by S. Simes, directing the precipitation of the cinchotannin, from the compound tincture made with brandy, by adding an excess of hydrated sesquioxide of iron; after filtration, and washing the precipitate with alcohol to recover any alkaloid which might otherwise be lost, sixteen grains of ammonio-citrate of iron were directed to be dissolved in each fluidounce, which, according to the statement, would produce no precipitation of the inky tannate.

Experiments carefully performed by myself and others, show that this precipitation may be avoided by the presence in the tincture of a considerable excess of citric acid, previous to the addition of the iron salt, even without the previous treatment prescribed in the recipe of Simes. This preparation, then, is conveniently prepared extemporaneously by the proper admixture of compound tincture of cinchona, or preferably tinctura cinchonæ et quassiæ composita, with citrate of iron, and an excess of citric acid (gr. vj to f℥j). (See *Extemporaneous Prescriptions.*)

The citric acid is to be first dissolved in the tincture, and the citrate of iron added afterwards. A bulky precipitate of a brownish color is apt to be thrown down, but a specimen of this, derived from ten ounces of the tincture, yielded on analysis only three grains of iron, though the full proportion, one hundred and sixty grains of the citrate, had been added.

Tinctura Arnicæ.

Take of Arnica flowers . . . . ℥iv.
Alcohol . . . . Oj.

Digest together, express and filter, or displace.

This is a very useful and popular external application to bruises; it is also used internally as a diffusible stimulant. Some pharmaceutists make it with diluted alcohol, obtaining a dark-colored, but less stimulating tincture. We have no authoritative formula to use in its preparation. (See *Arnica Liniment.*)

Tinctura Matico. (Dublin Ph.)

Take of Matico leaves, in coarse powder, . 8 ounces (commercial).
Proof spirit . . . . . . 2 pints (imp'l measure).

Macerate fourteen days, strain, express, and filter.

Dose, from f℥j to f℥iij. Used as an alterative stimulant and hæmostatic.

The solution of the alkaloids in alcohol constitutes a class of tinctures which are convenient and very readily prepared, though none of them are officinal in the *U. S. Pharmacopœia.*

Tinctura Quiniæ Composita. (Dublin Ph.)

Take of sulphate of quinia . . . . ℨv, ℈j.
Tincture of orange-peel . . . Oij (imperial measure).
Digest for seven days, or till dissolved.
Dose, fℨj, containing a grain of the quinia salt.

The tincture of orange-peel, which is not officinal here, may be substituted by tinct. gentianæ comp., *U. S.*

Tinctura Strychniæ.

Take of Strychnia . . . . . . gr. iij.
Alcohol . . . . . . fℨj.

Make a tincture.
Dose, ♏v to xvj.

This is perhaps about the strength of tincture of nux vomica (as shown below), for which it is sometimes substituted.

Name.	Proportions.	Dose.
Tinctura nucis vomicæ, *U. S.*,	℥iv to Oj alc.,	5 to 15 minims.
" strychniæ,	gr. iij to fℨj (16 minims = $\frac{1}{10}$ grain),	do.

Tinctura Cannabis Indicæ. (Dublin Ph.)

[1]Take of Purified extract of Indian hemp . . ℥ss.
Alcohol (Oss, imperial measure) . . f℥ixss.

Dissolve the extract in the alcohol.

The dose, as stated elsewhere, is forty drops; but when made of Squire's extract this is too much; in several instances of which I have been cognizant, it has produced alarming symptoms; so that I should prefer to begin with ten drops, to be repeated if necessary.

Flemming's Tincture of Aconite.

Take of Aconite root (dried and finely powdered) ℥xvi (Troy).
Rectified spirits . . . . . . Sufficient.

Macerate for four days with sixteen ounces of the spirits, then pack into a percolator, add more until twenty-four ounces of tincture are obtained.

This is the strongest of the tinctures of aconite, and is compared with the others in the following syllabus:—

Name.	Proportions.	Dose.
Tinctura aconiti foliorum, *U. S.*,	℥ij leaves to Oj dil. alc.,	20 to 30 drops.
" " radicis, *U. S.*,	℥vj root to Oj alcohol,	5 drops.
" " (Flemming's),	℥viij root to f℥xij do.,	3 to 5 drops.

There is not perhaps so great a difference between the last two as their relative proportions would indicate, both being nearly saturated. Great care should be taken to distinguish these by their full name in prescribing.

[1] See Extracts.

Dewees' Tincture of Guaiac.

Take of	Guaiacum resin	℥iv.
	Carbonate of potassa	ʒiss.
	Pulv. pimento	℥j.
	Diluted alcohol	Oij.[1]

Digest for two weeks. DOSE, from f℥j to f℥ij.

Tinctura Rhei Aromaticus.

Take of	Rhubarb,	
	Caraway,	
	Orange-peel, of each	℥ij.
	Brandy	Oij.

Macerate for two weeks or displace. DOSE, f℥j to f℥ss.

[For Ethereal Tinctures see next chapter.]

CHAPTER VII.

MEDICATED WINES, VINEGARS, ETHEREAL TINCTURES, ELIXIRS, AND CORDIALS.[2]

VINA MEDICATA, *U. S. P.*

THIS class of Galenical solutions is less numerous than the tinctures, to which it is closely allied.

There are two kinds of wine officinal in the *U. S. Pharmacopœia:* vinum album (vinum of the older Pharmacopœias), which is sherry wine (Teneriffe and Madeira are sometimes used in its stead), and vinum rubrum, which is port wine. The former contains about 20 per cent. of alcohol, sp. gr. .825, and the latter near 26 per cent.

In all the medicated wines which are officinal, white wine is directed as the menstruum. This is a clear, amber-colored liquid, having an agreeable pungent taste, and destitute of acidity. It possesses the advantage over either alcohol or diluted alcohol, of being less stimulating, and more agreeable in its taste and in its effects on the system. It is chiefly objectionable as a substitute for diluted alcohol, from its liability to decompose when impregnated with the soluble principles of plants. To meet this objection, it is customary with some to add from one to two fluidounces of alcohol to a pint of the wine, and this course is directed in the Pharmacopœia in the case of vinum rhei.

[1] The original recipe of Dr. Dewees directed diluted alcohol, one pound, but as the custom of weighing liquids has become obsolete, and as the preparation is nearly saturated, it has been changed as above.

[2] See chapter on Fermentation, Alcohol, and Ethers.

SYLLABUS OF OFFICINAL MEDICATED WINES.

White or Sherry Wine, used in making them.

Officinal Name.	Proportions.		Dose.	Med. Properties.
Vinum aloes	℥j + cardamom, ginger, āā ʒj	to Oj	fʒij to f℥ij	Carminative, aperient.
" rhei	℥ij + canella ʒj dil. alc. f℥ij	do.	fʒj to f℥ss	do.
" colchici rad.	℥vj (English root)	do.	gtt. x to fʒj	Diuretic, nerv. sedat.
" " seminis	℥ij (Powdered seed)	do.	fʒj to fʒij	do.
" ergotæ	℥ij	do.	fʒj	Excito-motor stimulant.
" ipecacuanhæ	℥j	do.	fʒj to f℥ss	Expectorant.
" tabaci	℥j	do	gtt. xx.	Diuretic.
" veratri albi	℥iv	do.		
" antimonii	2 grs. tart. emet. to f℥j		fʒj to f℥ss	Expect., emet.

REMARKS ON THE MEDICATED WINES.

The two *wines of colchicum* are much prescribed in rheumatic and gouty affections; that of the root, as seen in the Syllabus, is much the stronger. Prepared by displacement according to Grahame's method, a fine powder, dampened with the menstruum, pretty well packed in a common funnel, and subjected to the action of successive portions of the liquid, furnishes a very efficient preparation. The wine of the seed should be made of the finely-powdered, fresh, and well-preserved seeds; it is preferred by many as a more uniform preparation. Large quantities of wine of fresh colchicum root are imported from England, and it is said to be more efficient than that prepared of the dried root. Some of the best pharmaceutists in England, however, prefer to use the dried root as furnishing uniform and satisfactory results.

Wine of white veratrum, improperly called white hellebore, seems to have been overlooked by practitioners; it much resembles Norwood's tincture, though made from the English species of the plant, not our own.

Antimonial wine should be made by trituration in a mortar, though, owing to the comparative insolubility of the tartrate of antimony and potassa in alcoholic liquids, I usually prefer to dissolve it in one-half or one-third the quantity of water, and add this to wine to make the quantity ordered. The dilution of the wine in this case, though not directed in the Pharmacopœia, is an advantage in all respects.

Wine of ipecac. is an elegant and very popular preparation, being much used by itself, and along with other expectorant and diaphoretic remedies; it is not as depressing in its effects as wine of antimony, and yet about equally efficacious as an emetic and nauseant. It has just double the strength of the syrup of ipecac.

Wine of ergot is perhaps more used than any other preparation of that drug; it has no other fault than its proneness to decompose in hot weather, which makes it necessary to add a little strong alcohol, or to keep it in a cool place, and in well-stopped bottles.

WINES NOT OFFICINAL IN *U. S. P.*

Aromatic Wine.

Take of Wormwood,
Peppermint,
Rosemary,
Thyme,
Hyssop,
Sage,
Lavender,
Sweet marjoram, of each . . ℥ij.
Port wine . . . . . Oij.

Macerate seven days and displace.

The principal use of aromatic wine is as an astringent and stimulating wash, applied particularly to buboes.

Wines of Iron.

Under this name a variety of preparations have long been sold in the shops. The old recipe prescribed iron filings, one ounce, to sherry wine, one quart. The solution of the iron was here quite dependent on the presence of acid in the menstruum, and even when most successfully made, it seldom contained more than one grain of iron to the fluidounce. An improvement on this, proposed some years ago, consisted in the solution in sherry wine of tartrate of iron and potassa nearly to saturation; a common recipe called for one ounce to a pint.

Several new preparations of iron salts in wine have recently originated and obtained considerable popularity in this city. The following recipes were originated by my friend and former pupil, Thomas Weaver:—

Wine of Iron.

Take of Citrate of iron . . . . . 128 grains.
Sherry wine,
Water,
Sugar, and
Tincture of orange-peel, to make 1 pint.

Dissolve the citrate in hot water and add to it the other ingredients in proportion to suit the taste.

DOSE, a teaspoonful.

Modified Wine of Iron.

Take of Citrate of iron . . . . . 128 grains.
Ammonio-citrate of zinc . . 32 grains.
Water,
Sugar,
Tincture of orange-peel,
Sherry wine, to make a pint.

Dissolve as in the other case.

DOSE, a teaspoonful.

Bitter Wine of Iron.

Take of Citrate of iron . . . . 128 grains.
Extract of calisaya (Ellis) . 16 grains.
Sherry wine,
Water,
Sugar, and
Tincture of orange-peel, to make 1 pint.

DOSE, a teaspoonful.

Dissolve the citrate of iron and extract cinchona separately in hot water, adding a small excess of citric acid; then add the sugar and tincture of orange-peel, and lastly the wine. The chief secret in preserving the bouquet of the wine in contact with the iron salt is to add it after the utmost dilution.[1]

Wine of Pepsin.

I have recently experimented with a view to the preparation of a permanent solution of pepsin from the glandular skin of the pig's stomach, and have made a preparation containing aromatic tonics, and this peculiar digestive principle in solution in a weak, vinous menstruum. At the period of going to press, with this edition, however, I am unable to say with certainty how far it is a permanent and efficient representative of the starchy powder of Boudault, and therefore omit the recipe. The following, which has been recently published from *L'Union Médicale*, may be inserted in its place.

Take of Starchy pepsin, de Boudault . . . ʒiss.
Distilled water . . . . . ʒvj.
White wine . . . . . . ʒxv.
White sugar . . . . . . ℥j.
Spirit of wine . . . . . ʒiij.

Mix until the sugar is quite dissolved, and filter. One tablespoonful, equal to the ordinary dose of pepsin de Boudault. Taken after every meal, for indigestion.

Wine of Wild Cherry Bark.

Take of Alcoholic extract (from 24 ounces of
wild cherry bark) about . . . ℥vss.
Sweet almonds . . . . . . ℥iij.
Water . . . . 1 pint.
Sherry wine . . . . . . 2 pints.

Beat the almonds with the water to a paste, rub down the extract with half a pint of the wine, and mix the two liquids in a bottle of the capacity of three pints, stop it closely, and permit it to stand for three days, with occasional agitation; then add the remainder of the wine, allow it to stand a week, and filter. By this mode of proceeding, opportunity is afforded for the development of the hydrocyanic acid before the menstruum is made so alcoholic as to retard the reaction which favors its formation.

[1] See Preparations of Iron.

Thus made, wine of wild cherry bark is a transparent, wine-red liquid, having an astringent, bitter almond taste and odor, much less agreeable than the syrup, and of about the same strength.

The dose of this preparation is a teaspoonful.

Wine of Cinchona and Cocoa.

Take of	Red bark	℥j.
	Calisaya bark	℥iij.
	Ceylon cinnamon	℥ss.
	Cloves	ʒij.
	Caracas cocoa (the nuts)	℥viij.
	Boiling water	Oij.
	Water	Oss.
	Alcohol	Oij.
	Sugar	℔ij.

Powder the cinchona bark, cinnamon and cloves, and extract them with the alcohol; powder the cocoa, including the hulls, and place it in a separate funnel and pour the boiling water upon it; then mix the dregs, and treat them by percolation with the mixed percolates, adding the half-pint of water to the contents of the funnel at the close of the operation; then add the sugar.

This preparation has been recently introduced in this country from France; its utility consists in the bitterness of cinchona being more or less completely covered by the peculiar properties of cocoa.

DOSE, a teaspoonful to a tablespoonful.

Wine of Tar—Tar Beer—Jews' Beer.

A formula for this preparation was published in the 14th volume of the *American Journal of Pharmacy* (p. 281) by the late Augustine Duhamel, in which a quart of bran, a pint of tar, half a pint of honey, and three quarts of water, are mixed together in an earthen pipkin, allowed to simmer over a slow fire for three hours, then suffered to cool, half a pint of yeast added, and, after it has stood thirty-six hours, strained for use.

If these directions are followed to the letter, the product is exceedingly unsatisfactory, will not keep well, and is impregnated with but a small amount of the medical virtues of the tar. The addition of the tar at the first part of the process is the chief objection to this formula, as, by its antiseptic properties, it checks the fermentation, and thus diminishes the production of alcohol, and consequently the amount of tar dissolved.

The office of the bran is to disintegrate the tar so that the water may act on a largely exposed surface. Ground malt answers this mechanical purpose equally well, and as it is acted on by ferment when placed in water, this is an additional reason why it should be preferred to the bran. When, therefore, malt is substituted for bran, and the mixture of malt, honey, water, and yeast is suffered to react for thirty-six hours before adding the tar, so much alcohol is generated that it enables the fluid to dissolve a much larger proportion of that substance, and to keep perfectly well. The following is the formula proposed by Professor Procter:—

> Take of Ground malt, honey, and tar, of each one pound.
> Yeast, half a pint.
> Water, a sufficient quantity.

Mix the malt, honey, and three quarts of the water in an earthen vessel, keep them at the temperature of 150° F. (about), with occasional stirring for three hours, then suffer the whole to cool to about 80° F., and add the yeast.

Fermentation soon sets in, and should be promoted by maintaining the temperature between 70° and 80° F. during thirty-six hours. The supernatant fluid should then be decanted from the dregs of the malt, and the tar added gradually to these in a small stream, stirring constantly so as to distribute it uniformly among them, and prevent its conglomerating in masses. The decanted fluid is then returned to the vessel, and the whole well stirred up from time to time for several days or a week, observing to add water occasionally to keep the original measure. The whole is then thrown on a piece of Canton flannel or other close strainer, the fluid allowed to pass, and the dregs expressed strongly to remove as much as possible of the fluid inclosed. The expressed liquid is then filtered for use; there is an advantage in allowing it to stand until it gets nearly clear by subsidence, before filtering it. When first made, before filtering, wine of tar has but little color, but soon acquires a reddish-brown hue by exposure. It smells and tastes strongly of tar, is slightly acid, is not unpleasant to most persons, and, when prepared as above, is undoubtedly a valuable auxiliary to the physician in pulmonary diseases.

The dose of wine of tar is a tablespoonful.

Aceta, *U. S. P.*

In the list of the Pharmacopœia, Acetum (vinegar) is described as impure diluted acetic acid, prepared by fermentation. One fluidounce of it is said to be saturated by about 35 grains of crystallized bicarbonate of potassa. From this is prepared—

Acetum destillatum, officinal among the preparations, prepared by distilling vinegar, rejecting from each gallon the last pint, which contains the impurities. This liquid, which is nearly pure *weak* acetic acid, is about the same strength as the crude vinegar from which it is obtained, and possesses the same saturating power.

Distilled vinegar was directed in the Pharmacopœia of 1840, as the menstruum for the preparation of the officinal *aceta*, but in the last edition, it has been substituted by *acidum aceticum dilutum.*

The chief reason for this change has been that the latter liquid is cheaper and much more easily obtained. The immense production of *acetic acid* for use in the arts as well as in medicine, has reduced its price to a much lower point than formerly. The small bulk of the strong acid recommends it for transportation, and it may be readily and immediately diluted to the point desired. It is free from organic impurities, while the ordinary product of the distillation of vinegar is not, as shown by the fact that, while the latter is apt to turn brown on the addition of an alkali, the former remains clear and colorless.

The chief impurities likely to be present in acetic acid of commerce, are sulphuric, nitric, and muriatic acids, and traces of acetates of lead and copper.

Sulphuric acid is detected by the addition to a quite dilute solution of a small portion of a solution of chloride of barium, or nitrate of baryta, which will form a white precipitate of sulphate of baryta, if sulphuric acid be present. *Muriatic acid*, by the addition to another portion of a very dilute solution of nitrate of silver, will throw down white chloride of silver. *Nitric acid* is known to be present when, upon the addition of a small piece of metallic silver, a portion of the latter is dissolved, and may be precipitated as a white chloride upon adding a drop of muriatic acid. *Acetate of lead*, if present, may be detected by adding to a small quantity of the diluted acid, saturated with ammonia, a solution of iodide of potassium, which will give the bright yellow iodide of lead; it being insoluble, will separate as a precipitate. *Acetate of copper*, if suspected, may be proved to be present when a precipitate falls after the addition of a solution of ferrocyanide of potassium to a portion of the dilute acid, saturated with ammonia.

Acetic acid of commerce, sometimes designated as "No. 8," has, or should have, the sp. gr. of 1.041. The best method, however, of ascertaining its strength, is to saturate a given portion of it with bicarbonate of potassa in crystals: if of standard strength, 100 grains by weight of the acid will be accurately saturated by 60 grains of the crystals. The point of saturation is ascertained by the use of litmus paper, which should not change to a decided red color on immersing it in the liquid, after the addition of the bicarbonate. This experiment requires care, in order to secure a satisfactory result; if it should be found that the solution is decidedly acid, when tried by the test-paper, a further addition of bicarbonate should be made, noting the quantity. If considerably more than 60 grains are required to make it neutral, it is too strong, and generally the presence of some foreign acid may be suspected. If the proportion of bicarbonate is more than sufficient to make the solution neutral, the acid is then deficient in strength. Owing to the delicacy of the test by litmus paper, a specimen of acetic acid will seldom be found which will be *accurately saturated* by the required quantity of this or any other salt, and in estimating the value of the sample, the experimenter must be satisfied if the result is approximately correct, especially as carbonic acid, being liberated by the bicarbonate, is present in the solution, and is liable to influence slightly the behavior of the test-paper. Practically, no material disadvantage results, in the preparation of medicated vinegars, if the acetic acid happens to vary somewhat from the standard strength, provided it be free from foreign substances.

Acidum Aceticum Dilutum.—This liquid is made by adding to one part of acetic acid seven parts of water (making eight parts), so that the proportions may be stated as one part of strong acid in every eight parts of diluted. As 60 grains of bicarbonate of potassa saturate 100 grains of the strong acid, 7½ grains (one-eighth of sixty) will saturate the same quantity of the diluted acid; or, observing very nearly the same proportion, 35 grains will saturate one fluidounce.

Syllabus of Officinal Vinegars.

Aceta, *U. S. P.*

Officinal Name.	Proportions.	Dose.	Med. Properties, &c.
Acetum colchici	℥j to Oj: Alc. f℥ss	gtt. xxx to f℥ij	Diuretic, sedative, &c.
" scillæ	℥ij to Oj	do.	" "
" opii	℥viij to Oiij f℥iv	gtt. v to x	See Preparations of Opium.

The use of diluted acetic acid as a menstruum is confined by the *U. S. Pharmacopœia* to colchicum, squill, and opium.

In the case of colchicum, it is used with a view to furnish the active principle colchicia in the form of acetate; it is milder in its action than wine, and is suitable for combining with magnesia and sulphate of magnesia.

It forms an admirable menstruum for squill, its acid taste recommending it over both water and alcohol, and its medical action promoting that of squill in most cases to which that medicine is adapted.

In the case of opium, the object in employing this acid is to assist in dissolving and extracting the morphia, with which it combines, furnishing a soluble salt, and one which is considered more agreeable in its action than the meconate, as it exists in laudanum and other solutions prepared with neutral menstrua.

The antiseptic properties of diluted acetic acid are inferior to those of diluted alcohol, and on that account these preparations are more liable to change than the tinctures. A small addition of alcohol is sometimes made to obviate this. I have never known either of the officinal "aceta" to ferment by keeping. A syllabus of this class is appended.

The addition of acetic acid as an antiseptic to several of the syrups most liable to ferment has recently been recommended, and it is found to fill a useful place as a menstruum.

In the preparation of emplastrum ammoniaci, it is employed to dissolve the gum, and afterwards evaporated so as to leave it in a pure and softened condition suitable for spreading on kid. (See *Emplastra.*)

Acetic acid is further treated of among the derivatives of Wood (which see), and

The acetates are described under the heads of the several bases they contain.

Unofficinal Ethereal Tinctures.

The use of ether in its several forms as a menstruum in tinctures which is not directed in the *Pharmacopœia*, is somewhat objectionable, owing to the variations in strength to which these are liable from the rapid evaporation of the ether, even at ordinary temperatures, and in the transfer of the liquid from the bottles.

Several preparations, used by Dr. Mettauer, of Virginia, containing spt. ætheris nitrici, and spt. ætheris compositus, have been made public, from which the following are selected:—

Mettauer's Ethereal Tincture of Cantharides.

℞.—Cantharid. . . . . ℥iij.
Spt. æther. nit. . . . . . . Oiiss.

Macerate for eight days, and filter.

The ethereous menstruum seems to promote the tendency of the flies to the genito-urinary organs without producing strangury. It is also used as a blister for the scalp of infants.

Mettauer's Ethereal Tincture of Cubebs.

℞.—Cubebæ pulv. . . . . . . ℥iv.
Spt. ætheris nit. . . . . . . Oij.

Macerate for eight days, and filter.

Used for subacute inflammation of the bladder, urethra, &c., and of the mucous lining of the stomach and bowels. Dr. M. also uses spirit of nitric ether as a menstruum for colchicum, guaiac, squill, ergot, ipecac, &c. (See *Virginia Med. and Surgical Journal*, Nov., 1853.)

Asiatic Tincture for Cholera.

This is a most valuable application of the Ethereal Liquor of Hoffman, the diffusible character of which is admirably adapted to heighten the effect of the powerful stimulants prescribed. It has attained considerable celebrity within several years past.

Take of Opium . . . . ℥j.
Camphor . . . . . . ℥j.
Oil of cloves . . . . . . f℥j.
Capsicum . . . . . . ℥j.
Hoffmann's anodyne . . . Oj.

Macerate ten to twenty days, or prepare by displacement.

Adult dose, 20 to 60 drops every second, third, or fourth hour, according to circumstances, in a little sweetened water.

Ethereal Tincture of Guaiacum.

Take of Resin guaiacum . . . 3 oz.
Spirit of nitric ether (Squibb's) 1 pint, or q. s.

Treat by displacement or maceration, till one pint of the tincture is obtained.

DOSE, a teaspoonful.

Ethereal Tincture of Colchicum.

Take of Colchicum . . . . 6 oz.
Spirit of nitric ether . . 1 pint, or q. s.

Treat by displacement or maceration, till one pint of the tincture is obtained.

DOSE, 20 to 30 drops.

Ethereal Tincture of Cannabis Indicæ.

Take of	Squire's extract of cannabis .	Half an ounce.
	Spirit of nitric ether . .	Half a pint.

Triturate together in a mortar, till the extract is dissolved.
DOSE, 5 to 15 drops.

The foregoing preparations are used jointly for rheumatic and neuralgic symptoms. (See *Extemporaneous Prescriptions.*) They are also well adapted to substitute the alcoholic tinctures of the same drugs.

ELIXIRS AND CORDIALS.

Under these names a variety of unofficinal preparations are sold, most of which are mixtures of aromatic wines and tinctures with sugar, the latter predominating. Two preparations of this description are appended by way of illustration:—

Elixir of Calisaya.

Take of	Calisaya bark . .	One ounce.
	Recent orange-peel .	Half ounce.
	Ceylon cinnamon,	
	Coriander,	
	Angelica seeds, of each	Three drachms.
	Caraway,	
	Aniseed,	
	Cochineal, of each .	One drachm.
	French brandy . .	A sufficient quantity.
	Simple syrup . .	Ten fluidounces.

Displace the cinchona and aromatics with the brandy, until ten fluidounces are obtained. Continue the displacement with equal parts of brandy and water, till twenty-two fluidounces are obtained, then add the syrup.

Curaçao Cordial. (Imitation.)

Take of	Curaçao bark (bitter orange) .	℥j.
	Peel of sweet oranges . .	℥ss.
	Cloves,	
	Canella, of each	gr. xv.
	Brandy	Oss.
	Neutral sweet spirits . . .	Oij.
	Distilled orange-flower water .	f℥iij.
	Sugar	℔j.

Prepare a tincture by percolation with the aromatics, brandy and sweet spirits, then add the distilled orange-flower water and the sugar.
The genuine Curaçao cordial is imported from Rotterdam and is highly esteemed. This recipe, furnished me by L. M. Emanuel, of Philadelphia, forms a good imitation of it. Its chief use in medicine is as a remedy for nausea, especially when a symptom of pregnancy.

CHAPTER VIII.

GALENICAL PREPARATIONS OF OPIUM.

These preparations assume an importance to the student not belonging to others, from the extensive use made of opium in almost every form of disease, and from the unusual number and variety of Galenical solutions made from it.

No student should neglect to study these especially and carefully, so as to be familiar with their relative degrees of activity, and their effects as modified by the menstrua employed. On this account I have devoted a separate chapter to their consideration.

The following syllabus embraces the officinal Galenical solutions of opium, and also the solution of sulphate of morphia.

	Composition and relative strength.	Dose
Tinct. opii camphorata, (Paregoric),	Opium ʒss, Camphor ℈j, Benzoic acid ʒss, Oil of aniseed fʒss, Honey ℥j } to Oj dil. alc. — 1 gr. in 256 ♏	fʒj to f℥ss.
Tinct. opii (Laudanum),	Opium ℥j, ʒij to Oj = 1 gr. in 13 ♏	gtt. xxv.
Tinct. opii acetata,	Opium ℥j, Alcohol f℥iv, Vinegar f℥vj — 1 gr. in 10 ♏	gtt. xx.
Vinum opii, (Sydenham's Laud.),	Opium ℥ij, Cinnamon, Cloves, āā ʒj } to sherry, Oj. — 1 gr. in 8 ♏	gtt. xx.
Acetum opii, (Black Drop),	Opium ℥viij, Nutmeg ℥iss, Saffron ℥ss, Sugar ℥xij } to Oiij f℥iv when fin'd. — 1 gr. in 6½ ♏	gtt. v to x.
Liquor Morphiæ sulphatis,	⅛ gr. morphia = ¾ gr. opium to fʒj	fʒj.

The mode of preparation and uses of each of these will require separate mention.

All the preparations of opium are directed to be made from the powdered drug; this is designed to prevent variations in strength, resulting from the different degrees of dryness of different specimens, as found in commerce. In most instances, however, the apothecary or physician prefers to select the drug in its crude condition, and in the absence of conveniences for drying and powdering it in large quantities, uses it in lump. I shall, therefore, describe the processes with reference to both the powdered and the crude opium, premising that the manipulator should always make the preparation with the Pharmacopœia before him, in this as in all other cases.

Camphorated tincture of opium is made by dropping the opium as finely divided as its condition will admit of, the benzoic acid, camphor, and oil of aniseed, into a suitable bottle, and pouring the diluted alcohol upon them; after standing for two weeks, with occasional agitation, the tincture is filtered and the honey is added to complete it. The chief use of paregoric is for children, to whom it is given in doses varying according to the age of the child from ten drops to a teaspoonful. The adult dose is as stated in the table. It is used in mistura glycyrrhizæ comp., and in other expectorant medicines.

This tincture, in the Pharmacopœia of 1830, was directed to be made with a portion of extract of liquorice, which, as it gave it a dark color, resembling that of laudanum, was substituted in the two last editions by honey. It has a rich brown color, and a rather agreeable aromatic taste.

Tincture of opium is directed to be made by macerating powdered opium in diluted alcohol for fourteen days, expressing and filtering through paper. It may be prepared in a few hours by mixing the powdered opium with near its own bulk of sand, packing it in a funnel and pouring on the menstruum, in divided portions, as directed under the general head of the displacement process. If the drug in powder is not at hand, the following formula may be used: Take of opium, sliced, one ounce and two drachms, add to it two fluidounces of hot water, and by the aid of a pestle and mortar, work it into a uniform pasty mass; to this add six fluidounces of water, and eight fluidounces of alcohol, making in all one pint of diluted alcohol; allow it to macerate for two weeks, occasionally shaking it, and throw the whole upon a filter—to the pulp, remaining after the liquid has drained off, add about two fluidounces of water, which will displace the last portion so as to make the whole of the tincture measure exactly the pint.

Laudanum is more used than any other preparation of opium. It is employed internally in small doses, combined with stimulants, and frequently repeated, to excite the nervous and arterial systems, as in the typhoid forms of disease. (See *Prescriptions.*) It is also used by itself or in combination to allay nervous irritation, and to promote sleep and relieve pain; for these purposes, it generally requires to be given in full doses, especially when the case is urgent. It is sometimes employed in cancerous and other very painful diseases, and in mania a-potu, in doses of half a fluidrachm to one fluidrachm (60 to 120 drops), and repeated. Camphor water and compound spirit of ether are much used with it in its more strictly anodyne and sedative applications. In nervous and spasmodic affections, it is given with other antispasmodic medicines, or by itself. To expectorant mixtures it is a very frequent addition, though the camphorated tincture is generally preferable in this instance. Combined with astringents and chalk, it is much used in the treatment of diarrhœa, dysentery, and cholera morbus, and is a frequent addition to mistura cretæ. For its diaphoretic effects, the best combinations contain an emetic, as wine of ipecac or of antimony, or frequently spirit of nitric ether. It is often added to castor oil, to correct griping or excessive purging from its use.

Laudanum is much used in enemata, collyria, and in lotions of various kinds. In an enema it may be used in three times the quantity employed by the mouth, with a view to the same effect. In an eye wash, wine of opium, or a solution of the aqueous extract, is preferred, as obviating the stimulant effects of the alcohol. It is frequently added to cataplasms or poultices.

Laudanum is made of deficient strength by some druggists, in order to sell it cheap; the usual wholesale price for a good article is from sixty-two to seventy-five cents per pint, or by retail, twelve to eighteen cents an ounce. If it has become turbid from the evaporation of a portion of alcohol, it is above standard strength, and should be filtered to free it from the precipitate.

Acetated tincture of opium is not commonly designated by any synonym, and must be carefully distinguished from black drop, to be noticed presently. It may be prepared by macerating the opium in powder with the vinegar and alcohol for two weeks, or displacing as in the case of laudanum. If the opium is in mass, it may be worked into a paste with a small portion of the vinegar, after which the remainder of that liquid and the alcohol may be added, macerating for two weeks as in the other case.

This tincture is sometimes recommended in preference to laudanum, as less liable to produce those nervous symptoms, which often follow the use of opium. As shown in the table, it is stronger than laudanum, but much weaker than black drop.

Wine of Opium.—This officinal substitute for Sydenham's laudanum may be made by a similar process to the foregoing. It is made with a much larger proportion of opium to the quantity of menstruum employed, than laudanum, and yet the dose directed in the books is the same; this must be owing to a supposed inferior solubility of the active principles in wine, than in diluted alcohol. A great many extemporaneous prescriptions for collyria contain this ingredient.

Vinegar of Opium, or Black Drop.—The strongest of the preparations of opium is made by a series of processes, not quite so simple as those last detailed. The opium, either in coarse powder or worked into a paste as before described, is mixed with saffron and grated nutmeg, and digested with a given quantity of diluted acetic acid, for forty-eight hours. This may be conveniently accomplished in an ordinary beaker glass, or, if the heat is carefully regulated, in a wide-mouth packing bottle or bowl, placed on top of a stove in a bed of sand, care being taken to avoid a heat which would boil the preparation; after straining off this first portion of the liquid, the residue is again digested, with a fresh portion of the menstruum, for twenty-four hours, and this drained off. In order to displace the portion of menstruum which would otherwise remain in the mass, to insure the more thorough extraction of its soluble principles, and to obtain the liquid clear, the mass is now transferred to a displacement funnel, and the whole of the liquid passed through it, returning the first portion till it passes clear, and continuing the process by the addition toward the last of fresh portions of the same menstruum, till exactly the required measure is obtained. The clear solution is now transferred to the vessel first employed, the sugar added to it and dissolved, and finally, should it not make exactly the required quantity of the preparation, it is further evaporated to the right point.

Black drop is deservedly esteemed as a most valuable preparation. The morphia it contains is in the condition of acetate; which is considered by many to be more agreeable in its mode of action than the native meconate existing in the drug. One grain of opium being represented by 6½ minims, the dose will be only from five to ten drops, because, although in the case of laudanum, two drops are frequently required to make a minim, in this case, sugar being used instead of alcohol, the drops are larger, and frequently reach a minim in bulk.

The popularity of black drop with persons who use opium habitually, is one of the strongest evidences of its superiority over laudanum. I was informed by one lady, who is a victim to this vice, and who procures her black drop by the gallon, that in comparing her own condition with that of others within the range of her acquaintance, who have used laudanum to no greater excess than she uses black drop, that while they soon exhibited in their persons the evidences of its poisonous effects, she was enabled to preserve to a great extent the natural freshness and fulness of her features; this she attributed to the form in which she took the drug. Her statement cannot of course be received as evidence of the difference referred to, though it accords with the testimony of others, and also corresponds with the observation of some physicians of large experience.

Solution of sulphate of morphia (U. S), though its strength is usually estimated as stated in the syllabus, is weaker in proportion to the other preparations than is there stated. The dose is frequently f℥ij.

Magendie's solution, much used in New York and Boston, is made in the proportion of sixteen grains to the fluidounce. Care should be taken in prescribing and vending this, to distinguish between it and the officinal solution.

Unofficinal Solutions of Opium.

Elixirs of Opium.—There are several preparations vended under this name, of which the most popular is McMunn's Elixir. This is a weaker preparation than laudanum, the common dose being varied from twenty to forty or even sixty drops; being an aqueous solution, with probably the smallest proportion of a spirituous ingredient that is sufficient to preserve it, the drops are large and the quantity named approaches f℥j. McMunn's Elixir borders on the confines of quackery, though much used by regular practitioners. Its composition is concealed, although the fact of its being a nearly pure aqueous solution of opium seems generally understood. Several pharmaceutists have from time to time called attention to the superiority of water as a menstruum for opium. The late Augustine Duhamel was in the habit of making laudanum by digesting the opium with water alone, and adding the alcohol after filtering, believing that in this way he avoided the extraction of the resinous ingredient supposed to occasion the unpleasant after-effects. The separation of the narcotine from opium by digestion with ether previous to making laudanum from it, was at one time recommended, but is now little resorted to.

Eugene Dupuy, pharmaceutist of New York, published in 1851 the following recipe for a substitute for McMunn's Elixir, which he stated had been used for some six years with satisfaction, being found to possess the sedative property peculiar to it without any of the unpleasant effects attributed to laudanum. The proportion of opium is the same as in the officinal tinctura opii.

Take of		
	Opium	℥x.
	Water	q. s.
	Alcohol (95 per ct.)	f℥iv.

The opium is to be made into a thin pulp with water; the mixture allowed to stand in a cool place 48 hours, then transferred into an elongated glass funnel, containing filtering paper. A superstratum of water, equivalent to the bulk of the whole mass, is added. When the filtered liquid reached f℥xij, the alcohol is added to the filtered liquid, making Oj—about two thirds of the substance of the opium is contained in the solution; the resin, narcotina, &c., being chiefly contained in the residue. The dose by minims would be the same as that of laudanum.

Professor Procter's recipe for a similar preparation is as follows. It is more difficult of execution and more expensive, but makes a fine preparation, and one which has been found to answer a very good purpose:—

Take of		
	Opium, in powder	℥x.
	Ether,	
	Alcohol, of each	f℥iv.
	Water	q. s.

Macerate the opium in half a pint of water for two days, and express; subject the dregs to two successive macerations, using six fluidounces of water each time, with expression; mix and strain the liquors, evaporate them to two fluidounces, and agitate the liquid with the ether several times during half an hour. Then separate the ether by means of a funnel, evaporate the solution of opium to dryness, dissolve the extract in half a pint of cold water, pour the solution on a filter, and after it has passed, wash the filter with sufficient water to make the filtrate measure 12 fluidounces, to which add the alcohol and mix, making a pint.

This has the same strength as laudanum.

By the ether in this process, the odorous principle and resin dissolved to a certain extent by the water are extracted and dissipated; any portions of thebania, meconin, codeia and meconate of narcotine, contained in the aqueous solution, are also removed; the evaporation to dryness and re-solution in water, remove the ethereal odor, and separate a portion of acid resin and extractive.

Incompatibles.—All the preparations of opium are pharmaceutically incompatible with the alkalies, and their mono-carbonates generally, on account of their precipitating the morphia in an insoluble condition from its meconate. With acetate of lead, they give a precipitate, chiefly of meconate of lead, the morphia remaining in solution as acetate. Astringent infusions and tinctures generally throw down tannates or gallates of morphia, which are quite insoluble. Some of the metallic salts may be considered as incompatible, but in practice there is no difficulty in mixing small quantities of laudanum with diluted solutions of these. In fact, the chief point to be observed, in the mixing of these preparations in prescription, is to add them after the full degree of dilution is obtained; in this manner they may be mixed without disturbance, in the great majority of instances, especially where, as is mostly the case, the quantity added is small.

Treatment of Poisoning by Opium.—When opium is taken in quantities sufficient to produce death, the first and invariable remedy is to evacuate the stomach, by administering an active emetic dose, as for instance, five grains of tartar emetic or sulphate of zinc, or, as is frequently more convenient and equally efficacious, large doses of mustard suspended in warm water. The patient should also be kept in motion, if possible, the face and head being splashed with cold water, when a disposition to sleep seems to be gaining the mastery; in this way, patients may very frequently be restored, even after taking large doses of laudanum. Instances of the kind have been of frequent occurrence within the last few years in this city.

Two cases have come under my own notice, in which the galvanic battery has been employed as a last resort, with the effect of restoring one patient permanently, and the other temporarily, the reaction not being sufficient in the latter instance to establish convalescence, though life was prolonged for several weeks. Artificial respiration has occasionally been resorted to, when the prostrating influence of the poison had arrested the natural process, life being prolonged by this means, until the impression of the narcotic had passed off: recovery has been effected in this way.

The Abuse of Opium.—The habitual use of the preparations of opium as a means of intoxication, is an evil, the extent of which is scarcely appreciated by the profession, or by the community at large. There are shops in the outskirts of our large cities in which the sale of laudanum forms one of the principal items of business. These peddle it out to every poor victim, who can produce a few pennies to purchase a temporary relief from imaginary pains. So common is this article of trade that even little children are furnished with it, on application, as if it were the most harmless drug. It is sold in these shops at half the price maintained by respectable establishments, and there can be no doubt that its intoxicating effects are sought by many, who use it as a substitute for alcoholic drinks. Individuals who would shrink from the habitual use of spirituous liquors, employ this *medicine*, under a false persuasion that it is useful or necessary to allay some symptom of a chronic disease, until they become victims to one of the worst of habits. There is scarcely an apothecary in our large cities who cannot relate instances of opium intoxication that have come under his own notice, and been served at his own counter. Females afflicted with chronic disease; widows bereft of their earthly support; inebriates who have abandoned the bottle; lovers disappointed in their hopes; flee to this powerful drug, either in its crude form, in the form of tincture, or some of its salts, to relieve their pain of body or mind, or to take the place of another repudiated stimulant. Such, too, is the morbid taste of these, that they think they require the soporific influence of opium to fill up the measure of their life enjoyment, just as the drunkard is wedded to his cups, or the tobacco-user to the weed.

The prevalence of this kind of indulgence is liable to increase in proportion as legal restrictions are placed upon the sale of alcoholic stimulants. By the so-called liquor laws, as enacted in some of the States, the responsibility of the sale of spirituous liquors is designed to be thrown into the hands of the druggist and apothecary; with him rests in great measure the necessary discrimination as to the sale of these powerful agents; he must endeavor to draw the line between the purchaser who seeks them for an undue indulgence in their intoxicating effects, and one who will apply them to legitimate uses in disease. That this is a difficult duty cannot be denied, and its observance implies the exercise of great care and tact as well as of moral courage.

Who would sell an ounce of laudanum to an applicant whose intention to commit suicide was apparent? And yet how often is it sold to individuals, who are only protracting their suicide by the demoralizing and dissipating habit of taking it in smaller and gradually increasing quantities?

The responsibility for many cases of habitual intoxication, both with alcohol and opium, rests with the physician. Almost every apothecary of large experience has met with instances in which the parties attribute their habit to the use of these agents, for the first time, under the advice of a physician, by whose direction it has been persisted in, in some chronic case, till it has become almost impossible to desist from the indulgence.

A habit among laudanum-takers, which evinces the care with which the practice is concealed from the apothecary, has fallen under my notice. A small well-washed vial is presented at the counter, and laudanum demanded; it is furnished, and labelled by the seller. The buyer consumes it all in a few hours, or days at most; he removes the label, cleanses the vial again, and presents it at another store, with the same request; and after it is used, he goes to a third, and so on perhaps to a dozen stores, till he comes to the first, again, in a few weeks after his original presentation; he may not be recognized at either place till months, or even years have rolled away, and his shrivelling skin, lemon-colored complexion, contracted pupil, and tremulous limbs mark him as a confirmed victim of this dangerous habit. The apothecary having found out his customer, remonstrates, but conscious of the fact that he will buy somewhere, and that acute pain and misery will be the consequence of abstinence, feels perhaps that it is justifiable, under the circumstances, to sell; and thus the days and weeks go on, till the habit and its victim alike disappear.

The quantity of laudanum that may be taken varies with different individuals. Those habituated to it consume from a few teaspoonfuls to an ounce or more per day. A medical friend informed me that a child less than two years old came under his observation, to whom was administered a dessertspoonful of laudanum per diem to keep it quiet, while the mother was engaged at her daily toil; this, of course, was the result of previous habit, originating in a small beginning.

Persons who have been addicted to the use of ardent spirits, are, perhaps, more apt to use laudanum in preference to the crude drug, or any of the salts of morphia. The cheapness of the tincture over the salts is a strong reason with others. We know of a lady whose bill for sulphate of morphia, during a single year, was ninety dollars, which, if we estimate it at the usual price, and take the daily average of the quantity consumed, would exhibit the enormous consumption of over 20 grains a day. And yet the victim of this slavery is able to attend, in some measure, to her daily pursuits, and has already attained middle age, without any evidence of organic disease.

Another lady, suffering from a uterine complaint, who had been for years in the habit of using opium, at first by the advice of a physician and subsequently from an impression of its value to her, continued it in gradually increasing doses, till the daily consumption of the gum and the tincture, taken alternately, amounted to many grains of the former, and half an ounce of the latter. In this case the patient was bedridden, and suffered a great deal of pain when the system was not directly influenced by the medicine.

A degree of restlessness and nervous irritability, amounting almost to spasm, when not under the effects of the drug, are characteristic in almost every aggravated case.

One colored woman, advanced in life, who had been advised, many years before, by her physician, to employ laudanum for the relief of the painful symptoms of a chronic disease, was known for several years to take invariably f℥iss of laudanum, which was purchased daily as required. A lady of my acquaintance, who I believe since recovered entirely from the habit, took for years a half grain powder of sulphate of morphia daily, sometimes perhaps twice a day. On one occasion, a man proposed to purchase at the counter a fluidounce vial of laudanum, and when the price of it was demanded, immediately swallowed the whole, as was supposed for the purpose of suicide. He was afterwards seen in the streets apparently in his usual health.

Dr. Garrod relates a case of a young man who took one drachm of Smyrna opium night and morning, and frequently from an ounce to an ounce and a half of laudanum in addition.

We are informed of an instance of a lady advanced to her threescore years and ten, who, from fear of the pains of death, from day to day kept herself under the influence of this narcotic. Such was the morbid mental influence which kept her unhappy in the anticipation of a result which has not yet occurred.

The moral responsibility connected with the question of prescribing and dispensing opium, may be greater than has been hitherto acknowledged; and the few remarks here presented are designed to awaken an interest among those who by position and pursuits are best qualified to exercise a wholesome influence upon its abuse.

CHAPTER IX.

THE GENERATION OF HEAT FOR PHARMACEUTICAL PURPOSES.

MANY of the processes directed in the *Pharmacopœia* may be conducted in an ordinary cannon stove—as making infusions and decoctions, syrups, some of the extracts, all of the ointments and cerates, and some of the plasters. The various kinds of cooking stoves are still better adapted to these purposes, each having its particular advantages, and nearly all offering facilities not only for performing the processes requiring the naked fire, but also being conveniently fitted with sand and water baths, and having ovens attached which answer the purposes of the drying chambers in regular pharmaceutical furnaces or stoves.

Permanent furnaces, fitted to the proper performance of every pharmaceutical process, are fully described in the work of Mohr, Redwood, and Procter, and in that of Prof. Morfit; a detailed account of these does not fall within the scope of the present work. A few notices of cheap and convenient forms of apparatus for generating heat, especially of a portable character, may be given.

The common clay furnace is much used in open chimney-places, or in the open air, charcoal being the fuel; a common bellows is employed when necessary to increase the intensity of the fire.

Similar furnaces are made of cast iron, but they possess no advantages for use with charcoal.

The small French hand furnace, Fig. 132, is light and portable, and preferable to the ordinary clay furnaces for table operations.

Many of the operations of the pharmaceutical laboratory are conveniently performed with lamps, alcohol being the fuel. A neat and elegant alcohol lamp is that shown in Fig. 130; it has a ground glass

Fig. 130.

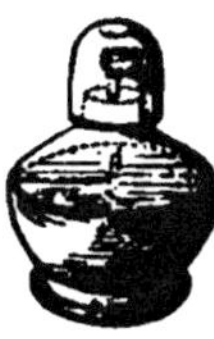

Glass spirit lamp.

Fig. 131.

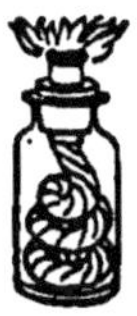

Extemporaneous glass lamp.

Fig. 132.

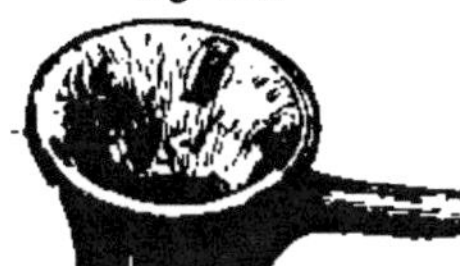

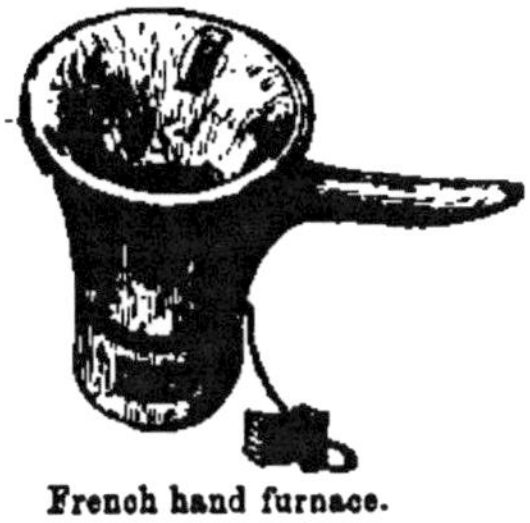

French hand furnace.

cap to prevent the waste of alcohol by evaporation. In the absence of such a lamp, a common glass bottle, with rather wide mouth, may be used; a perforated cork with a small glass tube about an inch long is inserted in the neck of the bottle, as shown in Fig. 131, and the wick is made to pass through this into the alcohol contained in the bottle.

A small tin alcohol lamp answers about as well as any for common purposes, with the exception of having no cap to prevent evaporation from the wick; such a one is here figured, Fig. 133 and 134, with a convenient stand in which to place it under a capsule or other vessel to be heated.

Fig. 133. Fig. 134. Fig. 135.

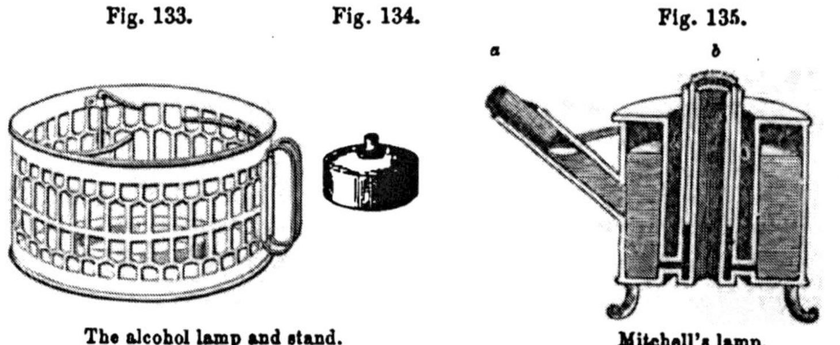

The alcohol lamp and stand. Mitchell's lamp.

Another kind of alcohol lamp, familiar to all chemical students, is Mitchell's argand lamp, shown in section in Fig. 135. In this, which is usually made of tin, an argand burner is placed in the centre of a cylindrical reservoir, *r*, with which it communicates at bottom by small lateral tubes; the reservoir is furnished with a tube near the top at *a*, for the introduction of the fluid; this is stopped with cork having a slight perforation, so as to admit the air as the alcohol is consumed. The cylindrical wick, *b*, which is inserted in the burner, is kept saturated with alcohol, owing to its communicating with the reservoir. When lighted at its upper edge, it burns freely, having a draft of air within as well as without the cylindrical column of flame, and generates a large amount of heat.

When no longer wanted for use, the lamp should be covered by a cap over the burner, or emptied of alcohol, otherwise waste will occur by continued evaporation from the wick.

Fig. 136 represents the argand burner on Mitchell's retort stand, in use; a great advantage is attained by the use of a chimney to surround and concentrate the flame; this may be set into the outer opening for draught between the reservoir *r* and the burner *b* (Fig. 135), so as to rest upon the little lateral tubes at the bottom; it should be long enough to project three inches above the top of the lamp.

Fig. 137 represents Berzelius's lamp; this is adapted to alcohol or oil; it is attached to a permanent stand, upon the upright rod of which it moves, being secured by a screw, which presses against the

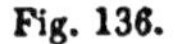

Fig. 136.

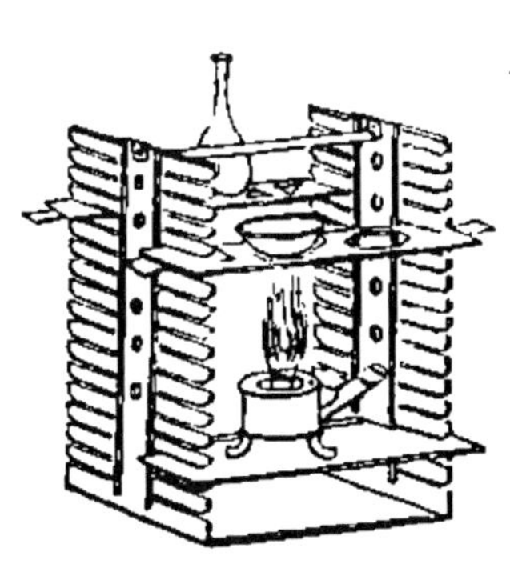

Mitchell's retort stand and lamp.

Fig. 137.

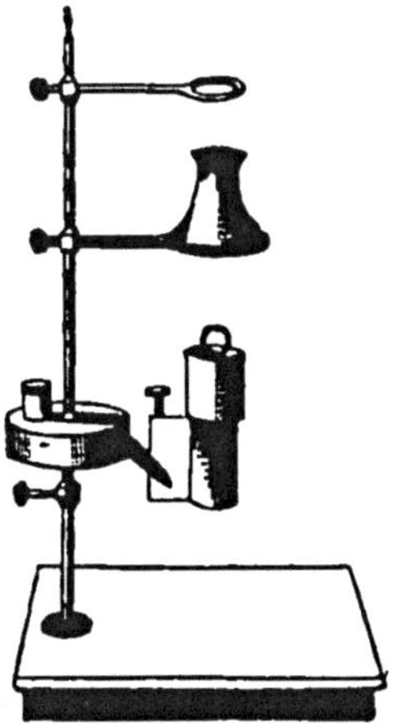

Berzelius's lamp.

rod; the reservoir is here separated from the burner, with which it communicates by a single tube. Another pattern has the burner in the middle of the reservoir, as in the case of Mitchell's lamp. A little screw is arranged alongside the burner to raise or depress the wick.

Fig. 138.

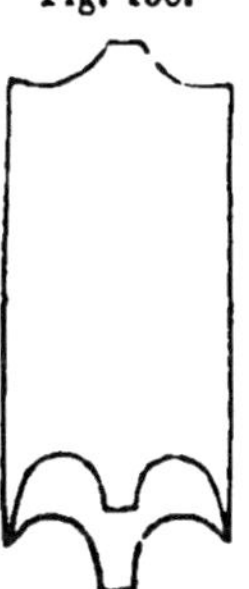

Lamp chimney.

Fig. 138 is a chimney, which is adapted to confine the flame within narrow limits, and to increase the draught, thus diminishing the tendency to smoke, and increasing the intensity of the heat. It may be applied either to Berzelius's or Mitchell's lamp.

One of the best contrivances for generating an intense heat for those few processes in pharmacy to which it is essential, and for fusing insoluble silicates in analytical processes, and for glass blowing and bending operations, and numerous other uses in chemical laboratories, is the lamp next figured, which is called the Russian lamp, or the alcohol blast lamp.

This is shown in Fig. 139. It consists of a double copper cylinder, *a*, inclosed at top and bottom, and surrounding an interior chamber, which extends somewhat below the bottom of the cylinder to a permanent copper bottom, as shown in the section. Near the top of the cylinder, an open tube of the same material is soldered on at *a*, for the purpose of filling it, and nearly opposite, on the other side, a tube *b*, also of copper, is inserted; this is bent, as seen in the drawing, and gradually tapering down to a small diameter, enters the internal chamber between the lower terminus of the cylinder and the bottom; it is now curved upward, and terminates with a small orifice at *c*; a movable top, *d*, is fitted with a handle, and so constructed as to fit tightly over the open top of the chamber. *E* represents a sheet iron stove or furnace in which the lamp may be placed when used, and which serves as a support for crucibles, dishes, &c. The mode of using this lamp is to fill the cylinder with alcohol by means of the tube *a* till it commences to run out of the jet *c*, then cork up the open

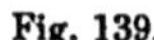
Fig. 139.

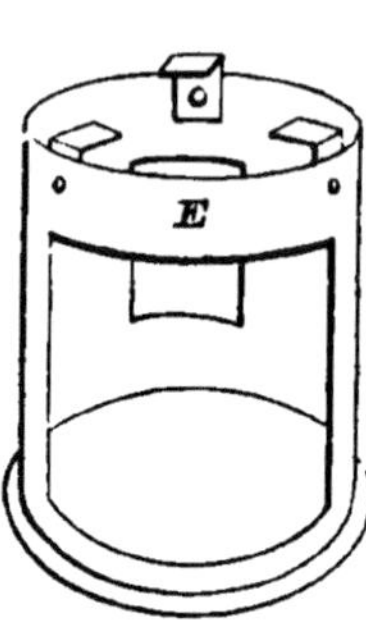

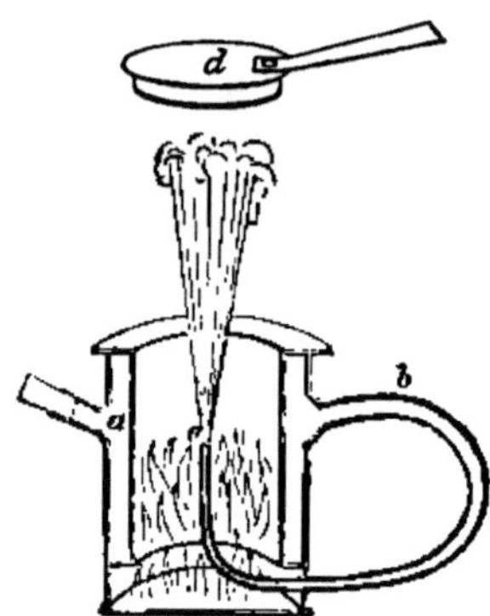

Russian or alcohol blast lamp and stove.

end of the tube *a*, observing not to secure the cork too tightly, for fear of explosions. About two fluidounces of alcohol are now poured into the central chamber, or sufficient to cover the bottom and rise to within an inch or two of the orifice at *c*. This spirit being now ignited by a match, quickly heats that contained in the surrounding cylinder, and, as this boils, the vapor formed is forced through the tube *b* in a powerful jet, which, as it escapes at *c*, is ignited by the flame playing upon the surface of that in the chamber, and thus forms a jet of flame possessing an intense heating power; should any obstruction occur in the tube *b*, or at the orifice *c*, the apparatus might explode, but that the cork at *a* would be likely to be thrown out. When it is desired to stop the flame, and whenever the apparatus is to be put out of use, the cover *d* is placed on the top.

For accomplishing fluxions with carbonated alkali, where a very intense heat is required, I have found this lamp an admirable arrangement, doing away with the necessity of a counter blowpipe. In order to apply this jet to the greatest advantage for the purpose named, a crucible jacket, *F* (Fig. 140), may be placed upon the projections on the top of the stove *E* (Fig. 139), immediately over the flame of the lamp. This is a sort of chimney made of sheet-iron, and serving the double purpose of keeping the crucible from all currents of air but those highly heated by the flame, and of returning the flame back, somewhat as in a reverberatory furnace.

Fig. 140.

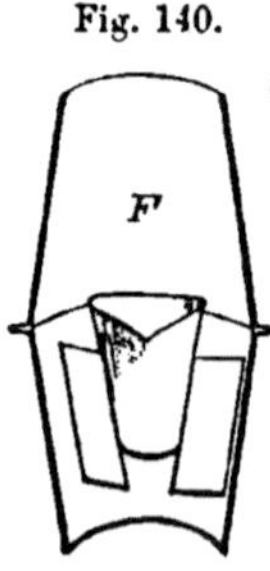

Crucible jacket.

The best fuel for pharmaceutical purposes is the coal gas now so freely and cheaply supplied in almost every considerable town.

The gas may be conducted by pipes into the

counter or table, and terminated at any convenient point just above its surface by a suitable burner; or, preferably, it may have soldered on to the iron pipe at its terminus a leaden one, which, being flexible, may be moved at pleasure to any desired part of the table. A very good portable apparatus, capable of being used in any part of the room, or in any room in the house, is shown in Fig. 141; it consists of a flexible tube of gum elastic material, which is terminated at one end by a cap to fit on to the burner of a common chandelier, pendant, or side light, such as

Fig. 141.

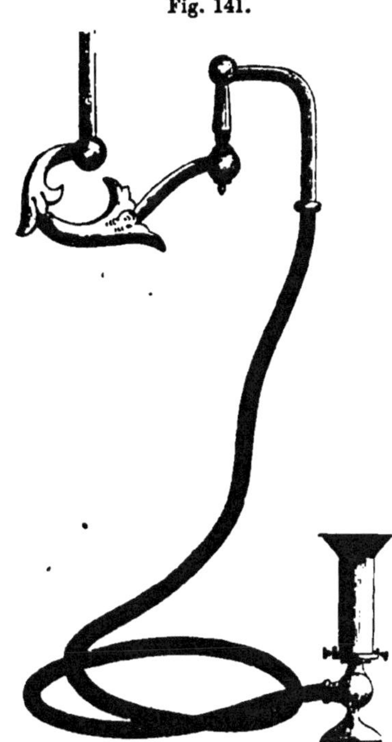

Fig. 142. Fig. 143.

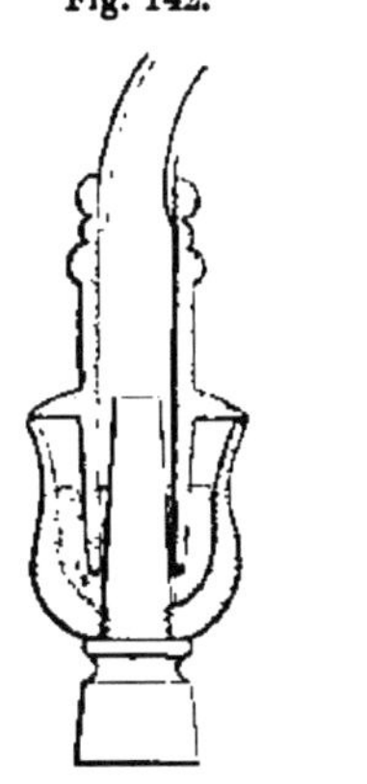

Gas burner with mercury cup and cap.

Ground gas burner and cap.

are suspended from the ceilings or walls of apartments for the purposes of illumination. To the other end of this tube is a little stand of metal surmounted by a burner to be adapted to some of the various kinds of gas furnaces to be described in the sequel.

Figs. 142 and 143 are sectional drawings to illustrate the different modes of connecting the flexible tube as above with the permanent pipe. Fig. 142 is the mercury cup arrangement; a small cup is screwed on to the burner at its base, into which is introduced a few ounces of mercury, and into this the cap of the conducting tube dips so as to form an air-tight joint, which is very readily shipped and unshipped; in this figure the cap is represented as having a flange covering the mercury cup, which, while it is in its place, protects the mercury from evaporation or from spilling out. When unshipped, however, the bath of mercury is unprotected, and becomes wasted, frequently requiring to be renewed, and leading to inconvenience. Fig. 143 is a ground burner and cap, such as is shown also in Fig. 141. The burner and cap are fitted and ground to each other, so as to make a direct air-tight connection when adjusted, and yet are removable at pleasure. The screws by which the burner is attached to the pipe, and the cap to the flexible tube above, and also the internal construction of the fish-tail burner, are shown in this section.

Fig. 144 represents the argand burner with rim; these were formerly much used with glass chimneys and shades, for illumination, but have been almost discarded on account of the great consumption of gas attendant on their use. The jet of gas is here through the small holes at the top of the hollow cylinder, the funnel-shaped appendage above being designed to spread the flame when used for illumination; the disk of brass screwed on below is used to support the chimney, and is perforated with holes so as to allow a draft of air around the flame, while the hollow cylindrical shape of the burner favors the draft through its centre. The argand burner is shown in Fig. 141, as covered by a gas furnace, to be described a few pages hence.

Fig. 145 is a kind of burner not much used in this country, but well adapted to applying a low gas flame to an extended surface, as in evaporation; *a*, is a cylinder of from 4 to 8 inches diameter, or more, with very fine orifices near each other, through which the gas

Fig. 144. Fig. 145.

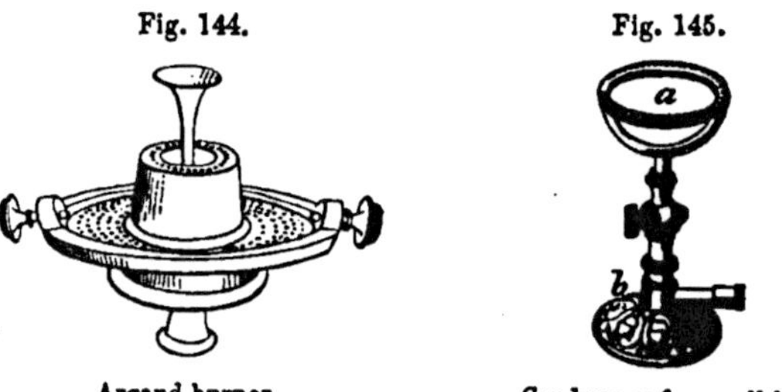

Argand burner. Gas burner for small jets.

is allowed to escape and inflame, the jet being controlled so as to avoid a deposit of soot, while a considerable amount of diffused heat is generated, owing to the extended surface inflamed. A cast-iron furnace containing a burner of this description, which I imported from England, has proved extremely useful in numerous processes requiring continued application of moderate heat.

Fig. 146 represents a cylindrical screen used to cover over either of the foregoing burners, the object being to confine the heat, to prevent the flame being affected by draughts, and to afford a support for the vessel being heated. The door is convenient, when the top is covered, to light the flame, and to see its elevation and depression during the process.

Fig. 147 represents a cylinder of sheet copper, iron, or tin (this may vary in length from 5 to 8 inches, and in diameter from 2¼ to 4 inches), with a ring of the same material about an inch wide, and just large enough to slide over the cylinder. A piece of copper or brass wire gauze, of about 50 apertures to the linear inch, and a little larger than the diameter of the cylinder, is stretched over the top, and secured by passing the ring over it, while the bottom is left open, and either supported on feet, or stood directly upon the table, the lower margin being, as in this case, scalloped, so as to allow the free passage of air into it. Prof. Boyé recommends iron wire gauze of 30 wires to the inch. The obstruction to the free passage of the mixed air and gas which fine gauze presents, he says, is the cause of the large amount of carbon in the flame of many of these furnaces. The gas accumulates in the top of the cylinder to the exclusion of the necessary proportion of atmospheric air. This gas stove, as thus constructed, is to be set immediately over a gas pipe, which may either be permanent or flexible, as in Fig. 141, or it may be open at the end, or terminated by an ordinary bat-wing, or fish-tail, or argand burner; preferably by the latter.

Fig. 146. Fig. 147. Fig. 148.

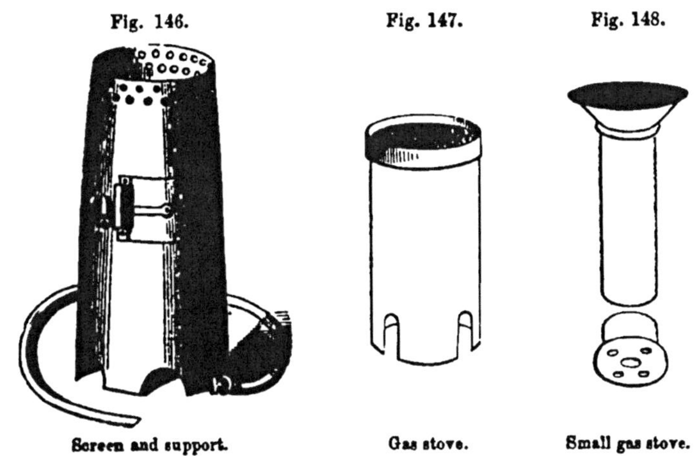

Screen and support. Gas stove. Small gas stove.

Fig. 148 is another form of gas furnace, of tin; the bottom being removed, it will fit the rim of the argand burner, and this is shown in Fig. 141, so arranged; the object of the little cap at bottom is to adapt it to an ordinary fish-tail or bat-wing burner. These are extensively introduced in Boston for family use; price 50 cents each. A great many restaurants, in the various cities, are also supplied with these, and their construction is often varied, so as to give support to the vessel to be heated. An iron tripod should accompany the gas furnace, when permanently fixed and used for a single object, but with a retort stand it may be adapted to a greater variety of operations when not in use.

The mode of using the stove is to place it over the burner, and to allow the gas to escape into it, and thus to become mixed with air, then to apply a light above the surface of the wire gauze. The gas which, under ordinary circumstances, burns with a bright yellow flame, indicating the presence of carbon in a state of incandescence, and depositing, in consequence, a large amount of soot upon any cold body brought in contact with it, may now be so completely diluted with air, by regulating the jet, as to burn with a light blue flame, containing no carbon. The combustion being much more complete, and spread over the whole surface of the gauze, gives an increased amount of heat, and so diffuses it over the bottom of the vessel as to diminish the liability to fracture. This kind of heating apparatus, when the fuel is accessible, is recommended by its cleanliness, as it is as free from any residue or sooty deposit as alcohol itself. Gas is far cheaper than alcohol, even in towns where the price reaches $4 00 per thousand feet. In Philadelphia it is but $2 25. It may be applied for an indefinite period without renewing, which in long evaporations is particularly desirable. It may, also, be regulated with perfect facility, and left burning during the absence of the operator, without the fear of a material increase or diminution of the flame, thus superseding, in many instances, the necessity for a sand and a water bath, to be described in a subsequent chapter.

In those instances where a gentle heat is required, and especially when the vessel to be heated is small, the stove may be dispensed with, and an argand burner being used, a small chimney of metal or glass is set on its rim, as shown in Fig. 149, and the jet of gas being small, and the object removed some distance above the flame, a steady and continuous heat is attained without a deposit of soot.

In some gas furnaces, the rim used to secure the wire gauze over the top is made to project for a half inch or more above the gauze, and the inclosure is filled with pieces of pumice-stone, or of brick, about the size of a chestnut; the advantages of this are, that the flame is not so liable to be blown out by a draught of air, the rim acting as a shield to it; the incombustible material becoming hot, radiates heat beside the direct heating effect of the flame. It also protects the wire gauze from corrosion by liquids accidentally spilled, and diminishes the liability to its becoming so perforated as that the flame may be communicated to the mixed gas in the interior of the stove, thus causing a slight explosion, similar to those which occur on a larger scale, on introducing a light into close apartments accidentally filled with a mixture, in large proportion, of gas and atmospheric air. If the cylinder rests on the table, and is short, so that the fire is brought near the top of the table, the heat will scorch, and may inflame it. To avoid this, elevate the top of the cylinder at least eight inches, or place it and the burner both on a plaster tile. The fashion of putting a wire gauze diaphragm between the gas burner and the top of the stove, with a view of mixing the gas and air more completely, though recommended in some of the books, is rarely followed.

Fig. 149.

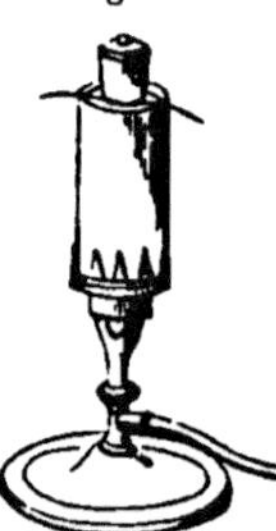

It is well to have two or three gas stoves of different sizes; the smaller will be useful in heating small capsules, and crucibles, in analysis, &c., while the larger will always be preferred for evaporating dishes, and other vessels of considerable diameter, used in manufacturing operations. Figs. 150 and 151 represent two of Shaw's patent aerified gas furnaces for laboratory use. Over the tube which contains a diaphragm of very coarse wire gauze, rises a finely perforated metallic chimney, which prevents the lateral escape of the products of the combustion of the gas, and determines an upward current in which

Fig. 150. Fig. 151.

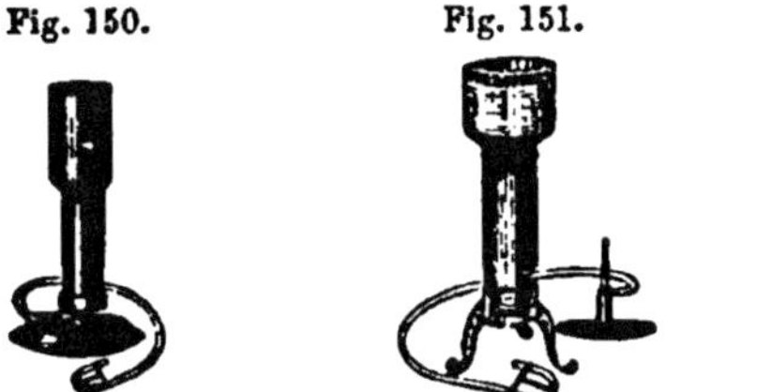

Shaw's patent gas furnaces.

Fig. 152.

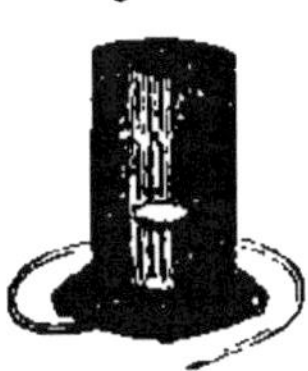

Shaw's gas stove.

the aldehyde and formic acid gas are completely consumed, adding to the heat of the flame, and obviating one of the chief objections to this mode of generating heat. Of all the forms of gas apparatus I have tried, these are the neatest and most perfect in their operation where a high heat is required. They reflect credit on the skill of the patentee, W. F. Shaw, of Boston, Mass., who has originated a variety of useful improvements in gas apparatus. Fig. 152 is a stove similar to that shown in Fig. 146; it contains a burner as above, and supersedes the necessity of a tripod or retort stand for holding the evaporating dish or kettle.

Fig. 153.

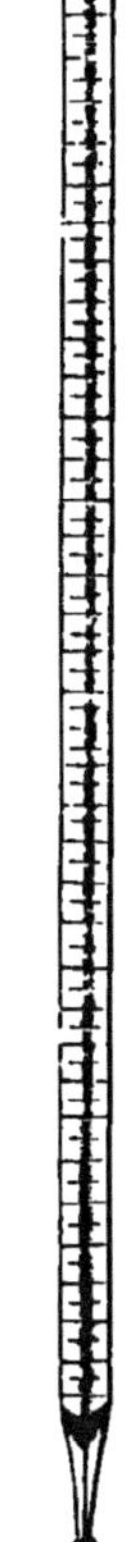

Thermometer.

The measurement of temperature, which is of practical importance in some heat operations, and in ascertaining the specific gravity of liquids, is effected by the use of a thermometer. These, as made for the measurement of ordinary changes in the temperature of the atmosphere, are of various cheap patterns, generally having a small range from a few degrees below zero of Fahrenheit, to about 120° above it. Fig. 153 represents a thermometer such as is convenient in a chemical or pharmaceutical laboratory. It is graduated from — 20° to + 640°.

In the United States and Great Britain, Fahrenheit's scale is universally used, but as the student is liable to see in works written in continental Europe, Centigrade and Reaumur's scales referred to, I append a description of these, with the mode of converting them into Fahrenheit's. The Centigrade scale is the best adapted to the wants of the scientific, by its decimal arrangement; in it the freezing point is zero, and the boiling point of water 100°, each degree being equal to 1.8 Fahrenheit's.

Reaumur's scale has the boiling point of water at 80° the zero being at freezing; it has been superseded, where it was formerly used, by Centigrade.

Fahrenheit's has the zero 32° below the freezing point, and 180° between freezing and boiling, so that the latter point makes 212°.

To reduce Centigrade to Fahrenheit's, multiply by 9, divide by 5, and add 32.

To reduce Reaumur's to Fahrenheit's, multiply by 9, divide by 4, and add 32.

The following diagram illustrates the relation of these three scales to each other:—

Fig. 154.

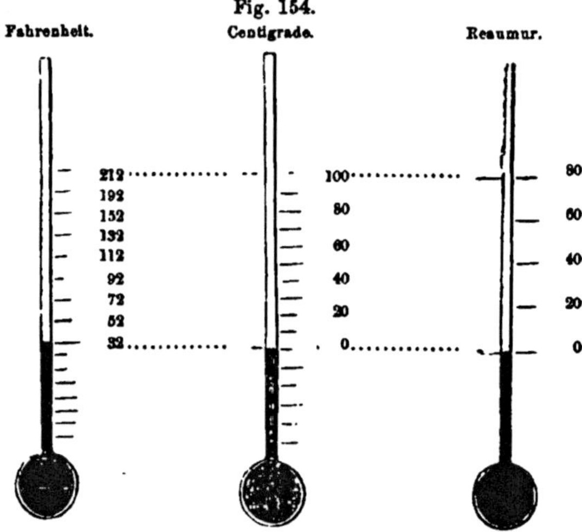

Diagram of different thermometers.

CHAPTER X.

ON THE MODES OF APPLYING HEAT FOR PHARMACEUTICAL PURPOSES, AND ON THE DECOCTIONS.

In most of the operations of the pharmaceutical shop and laboratory, the intervention of some conducting medium, between the fire and the vessel in which the operation is performed, is useful, either to prevent its too sudden elevation and depression of temperature, or to regulate the degree of heat applied. For these purposes sand, water, and steam baths are invented. As the scope of the present work is not such as to embrace a full description of these, as used in manufacturing establishments, the reader is referred to Prof. Procter's edition of *Mohr & Redwood's Pharmacy*, to *Morfit's Chemical and Pharmaceutical Manipulations*, and to the standard works on Technology, for full descriptions and illustrations of this kind of apparatus. My purpose is, merely to describe such simple means of regulating temperature as are compatible with the arrangements of a dispensing shop and country practitioner's office.

The Sand Bath.—This is used to prevent the sudden elevation and depression of temperature, and where arrangements for burning gas, such as are described in the last chapter, are at command, may be dispensed with in nearly all cases. A convenient sand bath, at all times ready during the winter season, is furnished by the top of an ordinary sheet-iron stove, such as is used with anthracite coal for warming apartments; a rim of sheet iron stretched around the top and projecting from three to four inches above it, makes a good receptacle for the sand, which becomes more or less heated according as the fire is increased or not, and may be used to digest infusions, to dry precipitates, and to evaporate any solutions, the vapors of which would not contaminate the atmosphere injuriously. For use with a common charcoal furnace, the best vessel to contain the sand is a shallow cast-iron pot, fitting, though not too closely, the top of the furnace; this is to be filled only so full of sand, as is necessary completely to cover the bottom of the vessel to be set in it; as a general rule, the greater the amount of sand, the greater will be the waste of heat. In introducing a vessel to be heated, it may be plunged into the sand, so as to cover the bottom and sides more or less, according to the degree of heat required; and when the diameter of the sand bath is greater than that of the fire below, there is a similar choice between placing it immediately over the source of heat, or in a less heated position near the edge of the bath.

The Water Bath.—A good extemporaneous water bath is prepared by procuring a rather shallow tin or copper cup, and an evaporating dish of just such size as will completely cover it, projecting slightly over its edge. Those glass evaporating dishes which have a projecting edge turned over and downwards, will fit more securely over the metallic vessel, without being pushed out of place by the force used in stirring. They are also convenient from not allowing the ready escape of steam round the edges: this being condensed, either passes back into the cup, or drops from the edge.

The outer vessel is to be nearly filled with water, and the substance to be heated placed in the evaporating dish, which being adjusted to its place, the whole is put over the fire, as shown in Fig. 155.

Now, the temperature of boiling water under ordinary circumstances of pressure being 212°, it is obvious that the contents of the evaporating dish cannot reach a higher point; it is found practically, that at least two or three degrees of heat are lost, in passing from the boiling water through the dish, so that when the water below is boiling, the temperature of the contents of the dish will not exceed 210°. Aqueous liquids will not boil in a water bath, but most of the solutions used for the preparation of extracts being alcoholic, undergo active ebullition at this temperature.

Fig. 155.

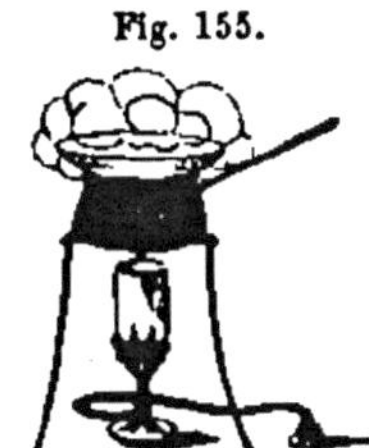

A disadvantage attending upon an extemporaneous arrangement, such as is shown above, arises from the rapid escape of steam from the lower vessel on all sides of the capsule: now the quantity of vapor which will be suspended in a given space in the atmosphere is constant at any given temperature, so that in proportion as such space is saturated with moisture, further evaporation becomes difficult.

A convenient water bath, less liable to the above objection, is here figured; it is constructed of tinned iron, or preferably of copper, and consists of an outer vessel or jacket soldered on to a shallow dish coated with tin, designed to contain the evaporating solution. The jacket is fed with water by the tube *a*, which may be fitted more or less tightly with a cork. It is tightly corked when the vessel is to be tilted in pouring off the contents of the upper part of the vessel, but loosely during the application of heat. In drying substances, and in all cases where it is desirable to prevent the escape of steam from the water in the jacket into the surrounding air, the cork may be perforated and fitted with a steam pipe of glass conducted into a vessel of cold water, *b*, into the flue of a chimney, or through a window. When put out of use, the water bath should be carefully dried by wiping out the upper or evaporating vessel, and placing it in such a position that the jacket will be completely drained of its moisture.

Fig. 156.

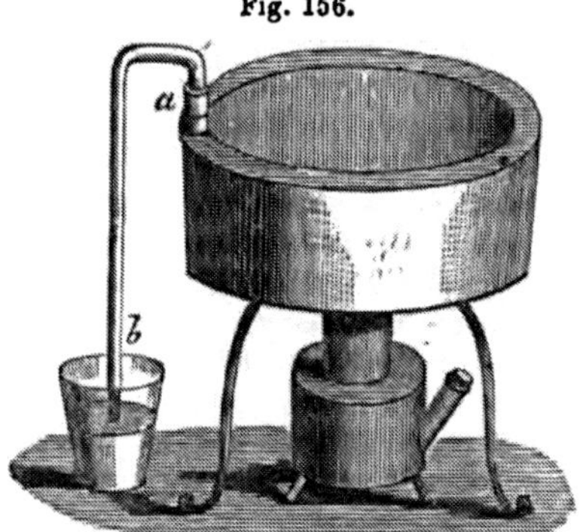

Fig. 157.

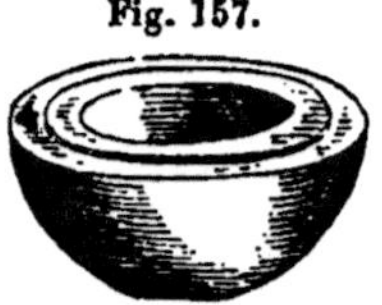

Porcelain water bath.

Fig. 158.

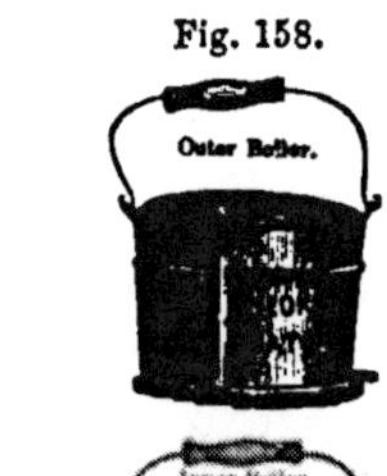

Fig. 159.

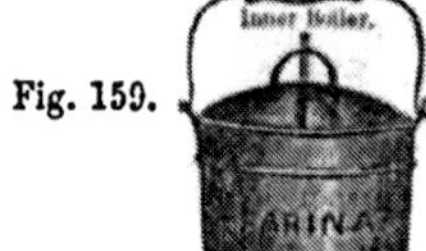

Fig. 160.

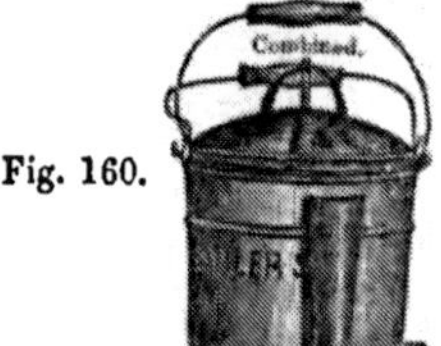

By adapting to the cork, as above, a tube of glass, and passing it into a vessel of mercury, steam may be obtained under pressure so as to raise the temperature of the bath somewhat above 212°, and this arrangement may be resorted to with advantage when a more rapid evaporation is desirable than that afforded by the ordinary water bath. Steam with regulated pressure is applied on a large scale in a variety of manufacturing processes. (See page 177.)

Fig. 157 shows a porcelain water bath sold

by the importers of Berlin ware, which is too small except for experimental purposes, or for the preparation of very small quantities of extracts or chemical products; it is, however, very convenient in these cases, and not liable to corrosion. Figs. 158, 159, and 160 represent the so-called Hecker's farina boiler, which is useful for the preparation of farinaceous articles of food, particularly where milk is employed; it obviates the danger of scorching, which is constantly experienced in heating milk over a naked fire. Fig. 158 is an outside tin vessel with a spout for the ready introduction of water. Fig. 159 is the inner vessel fitting into the above for containing the farinaceous substance, and Fig. 160 shows the two as fitted together.

Fig. 161 represents a little apparatus for applying the principle of the water bath to drying precipitates or filters; it consists of a kettle of water, surmounted by a steam jacket surrounding a funnel, which is closed at bottom, so that a substance laid into it is heated to about 212° when the water reaches the boiling point.

Fig. 162 illustrates the application of the water bath to filtering liquids while hot—Physick's jelly strainer, Fig. 92, operates on the same principle.

Fig. 161.

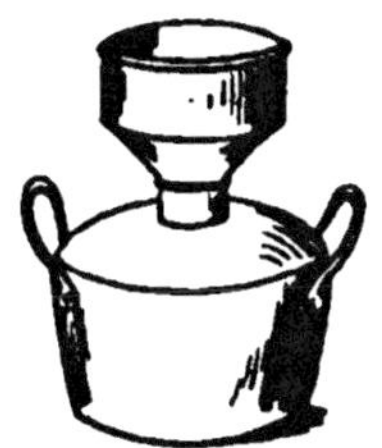

Water bath for drying filters.

Fig. 162.

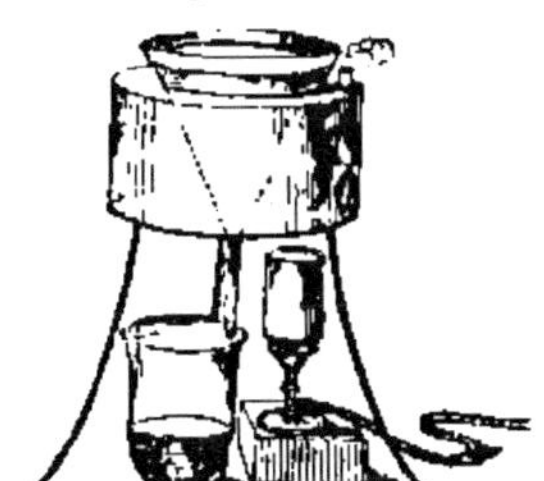

Apparatus for hot filtration.

PROCESSES REQUIRING HEAT.

Decoction.

In considering the processes of desiccation (Chap. I.), and of maceration and digestion (Chap. IV.), allusion has been made to the employment of artificial heat, and in the present and preceding chapters, the generation and application of heat in pharmacy have been specially treated of as far as deemed necessary to prepare the student for the consideration of the remaining processes of decoction, evaporation, distillation, &c., and of the Galenical preparations in preparing which they are necessary.

Decoction, or boiling, is a process to be applied with care to vegetable substances in contact with water; although boiling water, from its being permeated by steam, and from its being of less specific gravity, is more penetrating, and dissolves many principles which resist the action of water at a lower temperature. It is, nevertheless, liable to disadvantages as a menstruum for the preparation of Galenical solutions.

The boiling points of liquids, although constant under precisely the same circumstances, vary on account of increased or diminished atmospheric pressure, the greater or less depth of the liquid, and the nature of the containing vessel. Fluids boil at a lower temperature and more quietly in vessels with rough surfaces than in those which are polished; in glass vessels, especially, they display a tendency to irregularity of ebullition, and the boiling point of water, which, under ordinary circumstances, is at 212° F., rises sometimes as high as 221° in a vessel of pure and smooth glass.

The boiling points of infusions like those of saline solutions, rise in proportion to the amount of contained vegetable matter, and there appears to be a difference between the apparent temperature of a boiling solution, and the actual heating or scorching influence to which it is subjected by contact with the bottom and sides of the containing vessel. The steam generated at the point of contact being under heavy pressure in deep vessels, and temperature rising in proportion to pressure, it may be supposed at the moment of its formation to be much hotter than 212°, and if the portion of liquid immediately in contact with the heated vessel contains substances in solution liable to be burnt, it is reasonable to suppose that such a result may occur during the moment consumed in converting any portion into steam. In this way we may account for the well known injurious effect of boiling upon vegetable infusions.

Starch is a proximate principle, present in a large number of vegetables; being inert and soluble in water at a boiling temperature, it adds to the viscidity of decoctions, and renders them disagreeable to the patient, and yet it has generally no connection with their medicinal activity.

The extractive matter upon which depends the activity of some medicines, is more freely soluble in hot than in cold water, but the boiling temperature applied under ordinary circumstances produces the decomposition of this and other vegetable principles, or so modifies them as to impair their efficiency. The access of air seems to promote this result, and hence boiling in a covered vessel is preferable, except where the quantity of the solution is to be reduced by the process. In this case, by conducting the operation in a *still*, the surface of the liquid may be kept covered by the vapor, almost to the exclusion of the air.

A substance called *apotheme*, or by some *oxidized extractive*, is also apt to be deposited by vegetable solutions on long continued boiling with access of air; this may carry with it a portion of the active principles, and should not be rejected from the preparation.

If the plant under treatment contains a volatile oil which it is desirable to retain in the decoction, long boiling is inadmissible, especially in an open vessel.

Vegetable decoctions, if strained while hot, generally deposit a portion of insoluble matter on cooling, which may or may not contain active ingredients; but it is generally advisable to retain the precipitate and diffuse it through the liquid, stirring or shaking it up before taking each dose.

The proximate principle called vegetable albumen, which is soluble in cold water and alcohol, is coagulable at a boiling temperature, and hence is removed from decoctions on straining them.

The existence of starch and tannic acid together, in a vegetable substance, forbids the long-continued application of a boiling temperature, especially during exposure to the air, as a tannate of starch is formed which is insoluble, and probably nearly inert. The state of division of the drug is among the most important points to be observed in preparing decoctions; if too coarse, it is liable to be imperfectly extracted, while, by being too finely divided, it is rendered difficult to separate on the strainer. The use of the tobacco knife, Fig. 82, or of a pair of shears, furnishes a more uniform and convenient state of division than a mortar and pestle. In preparing decoctions of the vegetable astringents, the use of an iron or rusted tin vessel is to be avoided on account of the inky tannate of iron being formed.

The officinal directions for making decoctions vary according to the nature of the drug. They are all made by the direct application of heat, unless where a sand bath is more convenient, or where a steam apparatus is kept ready for use. Some are directed to be made by boiling the drug in the water for ten minutes, and straining the liquid. Others, by boiling from a pint and a half down to a pint; one, by boiling from twenty fluidounces down to a pint—directions which it is difficult to follow with any regard to accuracy, involving the necessity of a constant resort to the straining and measurement of the liquid till it reaches the required concentration, a care seldom observed in practice.

The ebullition should not be violent nor long continued, as simmering answers every purpose of more violent boiling. The vessel should be covered in all cases where the drug contains an essential oil or other volatile ingredient, but this is not compatible with the direction to boil down or concentrate from one measure to another. The importance of stirring the ingredient through the liquid from time to time during the process, should not be forgotten. The officinal direction in each case is given in the subjoined table, together with the proportions employed, and the medical properties of the drug. The usual dose of decoctions is the same as infusions, f℥ij, repeated several times a day. Some are given *ad libitum*.

Syllabus of Officinal Decoctions.

GROUP 1.—℥j to Oj.

Name.	Proportions.	Dose.	Med. Prop.
Decoctum chimaphilæ	℥j to Oiss; boil to Oj	Oj per diem	Alt. diaph.
" uvæ ursi	℥j to f℥xx do.	f℥ij repeated	Ast. diuretic.
" dulcamaræ	℥j to Oiss do.	"	Alt. sedative
" hæmatoxyli	℥j to Oij do.	"	Astringent.
" quercus alb.	℥j to Oiss do.	"	do.
" cinch. flav.	℥j to Oj, boil ten minutes	"	Tonic.
" " rub.	do. do.	"	do.
" cornus floridæ	do. do.	"	do.
" senegæ	℥j to Oiss, boil to Oj	"	Acrid expec't.
" hordei	℥ij to Oivss, boil to Oij	Ad libitum	Demulcent.

GROUP 2.—Exceptions to the usual proportions.

Name.	Proportions.	Dose.	Med. Prop.
Decoctum cetrariæ	℥ss to Oiss, boil to Oj	Oj per diem	Tonic demulc.
" taraxaci	℥ij to Oij do.	f℥ij repeated	Diuretic.
" sarsap. comp.	Sarsap. ℥vj, Sassafras, Guaiac, Liquorice, āā ℥j, Mezereon, ʒij } to Oiv, boil 15 min.	f℥iv	Alterative. Diaphoretic.

REMARKS ON THE ABOVE.

Care has been taken by the framers of the Pharmacopœia to select for this form of preparation those drugs least liable to deterioration by exposure to the influence of heat and the atmosphere. To this remark *the decoctions of cinchona* seem exceptions; these are even more objectionable than the corresponding infusions, letting fall a copious precipitate on cooling, which is apt to contain most of the alkaloids. They are improved by the addition of a little aromatic sulphuric acid, and should always be strained while hot, and shaken up when about to be administered.

Chimaphila and *uva ursi* are well adapted to this form of preparation, the coriaceous surface of the leaves resisting the action of water at a lower temperature. The *decoction of senega* is almost superseded by the syrup, which is a far more agreeable preparation, and is efficient in a much smaller dose. *Decoction of taraxacum* is eligible on account of the facility with which it may be prepared extemporaneously from the root, which may be gathered in abundance in almost every locality. The extract and fluid extract are most used for the cholagogue effect of the drug, while for its diuretic effect the decoction is preferable, owing to the amount of fluid contained in each dose.

Decoctum hordei, called barley-water, is peculiar in its mode of preparation, the directions requiring that the decorticated seeds, called pearl barley, should be washed with cold water to separate extraneous matters, then boiled for a short time in a small portion of water, which is to be thrown away: upon the seeds, which, by this process, are completely freed from any unpleasant taste, and are much swollen, the remainder of the water is poured boiling hot; it is now to be boiled down to two pints and strained. Various adjuvants are used to improve the taste of this, such as raisins, figs, liquorice root, &c., which are sometimes contra indicated. Its use is as a demulcent and nutritive drink in inflammatory and febrile diseases affecting the alimentary canal and the urinary organs.

Compound decoction of sarsaparilla, which is an imitation of the celebrated Lisbon diet drink, is also officinal in the British Pharmacopœias, and is much more extensively used in those countries than with us. It is often used along with or after a mercurial course. A modification of this used in Germany and occasionally prescribed with us, is as follows:—

Zittmann's Decoction (Stronger).

Sarsaparilla	12 oz.
Water	72 lbs. (5⅘ gals.)

Digest twenty-four hours, then add suspended in a bag—

White sugar,	
Alum, of each	6 drachms.
Calomel	4 drachms.
Cinnabar	1 drachm.

Boil down to 24 lbs., adding towards the end of the process—

Senna	3 oz.
Liquorice root	1½ oz.
Aniseed,	
Fennel seed, of each, ...	½ oz.

Finally, strain with pressure, and after some time decant the clear liquor. DOSE, a teacupful repeated.

The *weaker* decoction of Zittmann is made from the residue of the foregoing, with an additional portion of sarsaparilla and cinnamon, lemon peel, liquorice root, and cardamoms. It is not, I believe, prescribed in this country.

CHAPTER XI.

ON EVAPORATION AND THE EXTRACTS.

THIS process, which is employed in the preparation of most of the extracts, fluid extracts, and syrups, and in the concentration of solutions generally, differs from that of decoction in the degree of heat employed, and in the precautions necessary to success.

When the liquid under treatment is brought to a temperature above its boiling point, so that the formation of vapor is upon the inner surface of the containing vessel, and it escapes by its elasticity through the body of the liquid in the form of bubbles, the process is termed decoction; but when the liquid does not reach its boiling point, and the temperature and other circumstances are such that it is liberated without disturbance, in the form of vapor, directly from the surface exposed to the air, it is termed evaporation.

In decoction, the rapidity of the conversion of the liquid into vapor is in proportion to the extent of surface of the containing vessel exposed to the *fire*, while in evaporation it depends upon the extent of surface of the liquid exposed to the *air*. Viewed as processes for dissipating the volatile liquid ingredients from a solution, these differ chiefly in regard to the degree of heat employed, and the consequent rapidity with which the object is attained. For reasons hinted at in the last chapter, evaporation at a moderate temperature is generally preferred, and is indicated in the *Pharmacopœia*, for the preparation of most extracts. Many vegetable solutions, which would be greatly deteriorated by the long boiling necessary to reduce them to the condition of extracts, may be exposed to a temperature below their boiling point in a wide and shallow vessel until completely inspissated, with but little danger of losing their solubility, or their medicinal activity.

Extracts are, therefore, always evaporated in shallow vessels, which should be of porcelain, or well tinned iron or copper. Fig. 163 represents an evaporating dish of Berlin ware, which is the best material. The preparation of extracts is rendered tedious by the low temperature employed, the rapidity of evaporation being in proportion to the temperature, thus: at 180°, the rate of evaporation is only one-half what it is at 212°; and at 150°, it is only one-half what it is at 180°. The long exposure of a vegetable solution to a moderate heat, besides being so tedious, is liable to the objection of exposing the proximate constituents present for a long period to the oxidizing influence of the air, sometimes even allowing of the acetous fermentation.

Fig. 163.

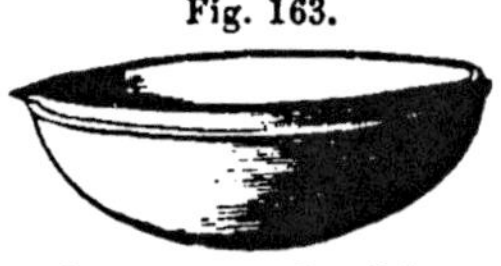

Large evaporating dish.

The liquid to be evaporated should be divided into comparatively small portions, and each reduced separately till it is highly concentrated: then the whole may be mixed. By this means, no one portion is kept a very long time under the unfavorable circumstances of an elevated temperature and exposure to the air.

A draught greatly facilitates evaporation by carrying off the air as fast as it becomes charged with moisture, and constantly furnishing a dry atmosphere to become saturated in turn with the escaping vapor. Constant stirring, by continually exposing a large surface of the heated liquid to the air, also increases the rapidity of evaporation.

The different modes of applying heat for the purposes of evaporation, are: 1st. Directly by exposing the containing vessel to the source of heat. 2d. By a sand bath. 3d. By a water bath. 4th. By a steam bath.

Fig. 164.

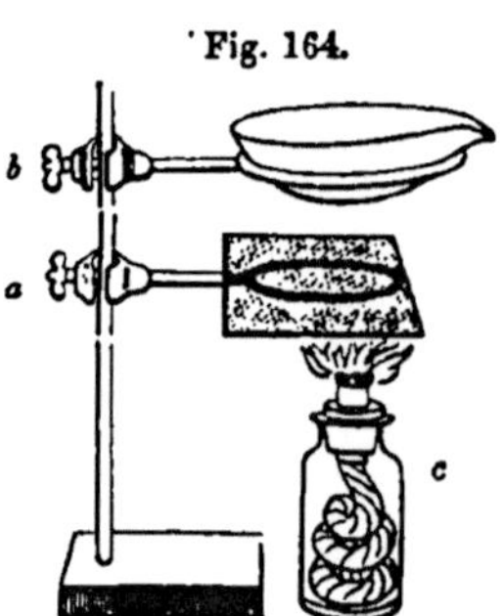

Application of radiated heat.

Whenever a vegetable solution is evaporated by a direct application of heat, it should be at such an elevation from the furnace or lamp, as not to be touched by the flame, so that the heat should be communicated by radiation. When the heat is under perfect control, as in a gas furnace, this plan is not objectionable, and may be substituted for the use of a water bath with the advantage of being raised to the boiling point, or depressed below it at pleasure.

Fig. 164 shows an arrangement for the direct application of radiated heat in evaporation; *a* is a diaphragm of wire gauze placed between the evaporating dish *b* and the source of heat *c*, which spreads the flame and prevents its contact with the dish, though brought closely together; the diaphragm *a* may be omitted in using a gas furnace, as the flame is then under control by regulating the jet.

As several retort stands have already been shown in the last chapter, and in that on displacement, and as the instrument as commonly constructed is sufficiently familiar, I shall here confine myself to describing an improvement in their construction which is worthy of notice. In the ordinary kind, it is necessary in adjusting apparatus, or when it is desirable to disconnect or alter the position of the rings for any purpose, to slide them up the whole length of the rod, and remove all above them, which is sometimes a very great inconvenience. In Wiegand's improvement, the casting that clasps the rod is open on one side to the diameter of the rod, so that by loosening the screw it may be slipped off laterally, and yet, when the screw is tightened so as to press firmly against the rod, it is sufficiently secure to bear any weight appropriate to such an apparatus. Fig. 165 gives a view of one of these separated from the rod, and in Fig. 164 the whole retort stand is shown in use, giving a front view of the improved clasp.

Fig. 165.

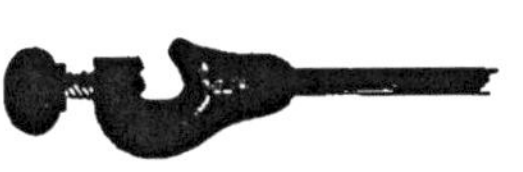

The sand bath is very little employed in the preparation of extracts, possessing no advantages over the carefully regulated direct application of radiated heat. The water bath is directed in all the officinal processes, for the preparation of extracts; its advantages are detailed on p. 169. Whatever means may be resorted to for effecting the concentration of vegetable solutions, with a view to the preparation of extracts, they should be finally evaporated to the proper consistence with great care, and a water bath furnishes a means of controlling the temperature, especially adapted to unskilful and inexperienced persons.

The steam bath is by far the most eligible means of applying heat for the purposes under discussion, although being out of the reach of a majority of pharmaceutists and medical practitioners, it is confined, for the most part, to the comparatively few who manufacture pharmaceutical preparations as a business. The difference between a steam bath and a water bath consists in the application of pressure to the steam boiler in the one case and not in the other. The temperature of steam bears a remarkable relation to the pressure under which it is maintained; steam under pressure of five pounds to the square inch is at a temperature of 226°, which is about as high as can be safely employed in making extracts; as the liquid will boil at this temperature, of course the evaporation is more rapid than ordinary surface evaporation, and yet the containing vessel is not so hot as to deteriorate the vegetable principles present.

By the regulation of the pressure, the temperature may be increased or diminished at pleasure, and its application may be suddenly stopped if required.

A steam boiler, by arranging pipes communicating with suitable forms of apparatus, and by adapting the fittings and safety-valve so as to regulate the pressure, may be made to supply the heat necessary for boiling, evaporating, digesting, distilling, drying, and even heating apartments.

In most public institutions recently erected, such as almshouses, prisons, insane asylums, and hospitals, arrangements are made for the introduction of steam pipes either directly into the apartments to be warmed, or preferably, into air chambers through which fresh air is made to pass by a system of ventilation into the several parts of the building. The boiler being located in a fire-proof basement, or at a suitable distance from the main building, the danger of conflagration is greatly lessened.

Since the introduction of steam apparatus into pharmaceutical laboratories, a great improvement has taken place in the pharmaceutical processes and products.

In the preparation of extracts by the use of these, the pressure is so regulated that, as the solution becomes inspissated, the degree of heat can be diminished. Near the conclusion of the process the extract is sometimes withdrawn, and poured in thin layers on plates of glass, which are placed in a drying room or closet till sufficiently hard.

The most perfect form of apparatus for the preparation of extracts, is a combination of the steam bath with a vacuum pan. A suitable air-tight boiler is connected with an air pump worked by machinery, which, by removing the pressure of the atmosphere from the liquid placed in it, lowers the boiling point, and greatly increases the rapidity of evaporation, even at a temperature much below 212°. The air being excluded, the principal objection to the long continued evaporation of vegetable solutions is also removed.

In all first-rate establishments for the manufacture of extracts, apparatus constructed upon this principle is employed, and the superiority of their products over those made by evaporation, under ordinary circumstances of pressure and exposure to the air, furnishes a clear proof of the advantage obtained by the steam and vacuum apparatus.

As the preparation of extracts is generally confined to those pharmaceutists who make it their chief business, a few words in relation to their physical characters, and the mode of distinguishing those of good quality, will be more useful to the student than a description of the processes and precautions to be observed in making them.

Extracts are classified in this work primarily, according to the menstruum employed in their preparation; and secondarily, according to their therapeutical properties, and both these ideas are kept in view in the syllabus presented below.

EXTRACTA, *U. S. P.*

CLASS I.

Narcotic Inspissated Juices, prepared by bruising or mashing the fresh plant into a pulp, and expressing the juice from this latter; then raising to the boiling point, to coagulate the vegetable albumen and green coloring matter, and separating these by straining; after which the clear liquid is evaporated to the proper consistence.

Officinal Name.	Med. Dose.	Remarks.
Extractum aconiti . . .	1 to 2 grs.	See Class I., Group 1, Tinctures, and Class II., Group 1, Extracts.
" belladonnæ . .	do.	
" stramonii foliorum	do.	See Class II., Ext. Stramonii seminis.
" conii	2 to 3 grs.	In practice, usually a smaller dose often repeated.
" hyoscyami . .	do.	Much used as a substitute for opium.

Good extracts of this class were formerly obtained almost exclusively from the English manufacturers, of which Squire, Allen, and Herring are the best known, although some nearly worthless were imported from Germany, and some produced by the Shakers. We now obtain some of them of fine quality from Tilden & Co., of New Lebanon, N. Y., to whose enterprise in this department of pharmacy a great improvement in the quality of medicinal extracts generally is due; they were the first manufacturers in this country who introduced the complete steam bath and vacuum pan in the evaporation of extracts, while, by the abundant cultivation of the herbs required, and the extensive arrangements of their factory, they are enabled to produce large quantities of these invaluable remedies at prices as low as the English can be imported. The enterprise of this firm has induced a spirited competition on the part of their old rivals, the United Brethren, or Shakers, who have improved the quality of their production within a few years.

The five extracts classed above form a remarkably natural group, therapeutically, pharmaceutically, and physically; as commonly prepared and imported, they have a more or less decidedly green color, and this feature was formerly regarded as a test of their having been prepared without scorching from the employment of too high heat; but inasmuch as the green coloring principle (chlorophylle) is associated with the inert and insoluble vegetable albumen, which the *Pharmacopœia* directs shall be first coagulated and separated, all strictly officinal extracts prepared by inspissating the juice of the green herbs are destitute of this, have a light brown color, and are soluble in water. Under the name of clarified extracts, Tildens offer an article answering this description.

The odor of extracts is one of the surest indications of the quality; it should, as nearly as possible, resemble that of the undried plant.

Extracts which are thus deprived of a portion of their inert constituents (clarified) are, of course, other things being equal, stronger than the kind formerly in use; and, hence, the doses stated in the books are generally rather above those usually prescribed. I have known of one instance of great inconvenience resulting from a physician ordering too large a dose of extract of belladonna, under a wrong impression as to the strength of the best commercial article. This impression was founded in part on his own experience with the inferior article which he had met with in country practice.

F. Mohr, starting from the fact that the activity of narcotic herbs belongs to principles which are soluble in both alcohol and water, a number of years ago proposed a method for preparing such extracts, the main features of which have been since adopted by the Prussian and other Pharmacopœias. It is the following: The fresh herb is expressed, mixed with about one-seventh of its weight of water, again expressed, the liquid raised to near the boiling point, and strained from the precipitated albumen, which has coagulated and thrown down the chlorophyll, it is then evaporated at from 120° to 130° F. to one-fourth the weight of the original material, mixed with an equal bulk of alcohol to separate gum and mucilage, strained, and with constant stirring evaporated to the proper consistence. This process furnishes very strong and reliable extracts; they are not so variable as those obtained by the inspissation of the juices, which vary much according to the locality and the season. The only principles here extracted are active, and the dose is correspondingly small. None of our manufacturers have as yet put this process in practice.

Extract of stramonium leaves is usually prepared from the whole herb, which yields about 18 per cent. of extract. (*Gray.*) It is the least employed of the group. Besides the uses to which the others are applied, this has been prescribed in spasmodic asthma. The ointment made from the extract is a popular remedy in piles.

Extract of henbane is the most extensively used internally of the series. The yield of the plant is about 5½ per cent. of extract. Its tendency to increase the secretions and to promote the action of the bowels renders it a particularly useful anodyne remedy.

Extract of belladonna is useful externally and internally as an anodyne in neuralgia, tic douloureux, &c., and as an antispasmodic in whooping-cough, and as a prophylactic in scarlet fever. It is much used in the treatment of diseases of the eye, and especially for the dilatation of the pupil before operation for cataract; for this purpose the extract is softened with water to the consistence of a thick liquid, and applied directly to the eyeball and painted on the upper and lower lids, a few hours before the operation. The fresh leaves yield about 5 per cent. of this extract.

Extract of conium, which is one of the most difficult of the extracts to prepare and preserve, is also one of the most useful. It is extensively employed in the treatment of glandular enlargement, scrofula, rheumatism, &c., as an alterative and anodyne, entering into the composition of numerous empirical preparations, and being very extensively prescribed in regular practice. The whole plant is usually employed in its preparations, though the Pharmacopœia directs the leaves only; the yield is about 3 to 5 per cent. Tilden's is generally reliable. It should have a strong and characteristic odor, and is readily tested by the following experiment: Take a small pellet of the extract, soften it into a thin paste with water, and add a drop of solution of potassa, or of carbonate of potassa; immediately a strong characteristic odor will be observed, resembling, when faint, the odor of mice. This is from the liberation in a gaseous form of *conia*, the active principle of the herb; and on holding near it a rod moistened with muriatic acid, a cloud of ammonia will be produced.

If the extract is very inferior, the experiment will not succeed, or will be only partially successful.

Extract of aconite is much employed in neuralgic affections both externally and internally. Its variable quality calls for care in its administration. The yield of the leaves is from 5 to 6 per cent. When of good quality, numbness and tingling result from its contact with the lips and tongue.

These extracts are to be ordered in prescription by the names given them above, and must be carefully distinguished from those to be now introduced.

CLASS II.

Hydro-Alcoholic and Alcoholic Extracts. By the preparation of tinctures with diluted alcohol, or with alcohol and water used separately, or alcohol alone, and subsequent evaporation to the proper consistence.

GROUP 1.—Narcotics, &c.

(Unofficinal in Italics.)

Name.	Dose.	Remarks.
Extractum aconiti alcoholicum	⅓ gr. to 1 gr.	Compare with class 1st of Extracts.
" belladonnæ "	do.	" " " Tinctures.
" stramonii seminis	do.	A reliable preparation.
" *digitalis alcoholicum*	¼ gr. to ⅓ gr.	To be used with great care.
" cannabis indicæ	⅓ gr. to 2 grs.	In the list of the *U. S. P.*
" conii alcoholicum	1 to 2 grs.	Alterative narcotic.
" hyoscyami "	do.	Laxative "
" nucis vomicæ	do.	Excito-motor.
" *ignatiæ amaræ*	½ gr. to 1 gr.	do.
" *lupulinæ*	3 to 6 grs.	Antiphrodisiac.
" *cimicifugæ*	do.	Sedative tonic.
" *valerianæ*	do.	Antispasmodic.

These correspond so nearly with the first class as to be conveniently studied in comparison with them. By the use of diluted alcohol with the dried leaves, a large amount of the extractive and albuminous matters are left behind, and, on evaporation, the active principles of the plant are obtained in a more concentrated form than when the thick expressed juice, containing also a portion of the cellular structure, is evaporated as in making the first class.

Recent investigations have strengthened the view that from the carefully dried plant an extract may be obtained, which, though less in quantity, is equally if not more active, than extracts prepared by the same process from an equivalent quantity of fresh herbs. Vielguth and Nentwich obtained from 10 pounds of fresh herb aconite, 4⅝ ounces of extract, containing 0.202 grammes, and from an equivalent quantity of dried herb 3¼ ounces, containing 0.322 grammes of nearly pure aconitine. Their process consisted in exhausting the plant with alcohol of .863 specific gravity, which leaves all deteriorating principles behind, and evaporating rapidly and with constant agitation at a temperature below 158° F.

These extracts have a brownish aspect; they should possess the odor of the plant, and be soluble in diluted alcohol.

As will be observed, their dose is about half that of the corresponding extracts of the first class.

They are seldom met with in commerce, but are designed to be prepared by the physician and apothecary, in the absence of reliable extracts of the first class. They may be obtained by the careful evaporation of the corresponding tinctures. They are seldom prepared, owing to the expense of obtaining the dried leaves in a state of perfect preservation, and the waste of alcohol. Extract of stramonium seed is an unexceptionable preparation, and might often be substituted for the extract of the herb with advantage.

Extractum Cannabis Indicæ.

Extract of Indian hemp, cannabis sativa, variety Indica, is imported in a crude state from the East Indies, and directed by the Dublin College to be purified by solution in alcohol, filtration and evaporation. The extract is also made extensively in England from the dried imported leaves, called in commerce gunjah, by steam displacement with alcohol, and evaporation. The dose of the extract under consideration varies very much with the quality, and ranges from a quarter of a grain to one or two grains; it is distinctly resinous and insoluble in water. Squire's is the best in the market. It is sometimes called *cannabine*, a name which might be advantageously applied to it to distinguish it from extract of apocynum cannabinum, also called Indian hemp, but a remedy of very different properties, and little used in regular practice.

Extract of nux vomica, though not properly a narcotic extract, is classed with the others for convenience; it may be prepared by the evaporation of the officinal tincture, and is an exceedingly powerful and efficient nervous stimulant much used in certain forms of dyspepsia connected with obstinate constipation.

Extractum Ignatiæ Amaræ Alcoholicum.

This preparation has been proposed as a "remedy" for dyspepsia, attended with nervous depression, and extensively advertised as such by a clergyman of Brooklyn, N. Y., who has been cured by it. The recipe, here given, is an improvement upon his, and is offered for the benefit of apothecaries who may be called upon to make it.

The beans of St. Ignatius, like nux vomica, have a very horny and
...rin and fixed oil), which renders it difficult

to powder them so as to extract their soluble matter. Professor Procter recommends the following process for their extraction. The beans are bruised in an iron or brass mortar, until reduced to small fragments or very coarse powder; they are then moistened with water in a covered vessel, and heated until the tissue of the pieces has become soft, and can be bruised into a pulpy mass. This is then mixed with twice its bulk of alcohol, sp. gr. .835, and allowed to macerate in a close vessel in a warm place for 24 hours, and then treated by displacement until 8 or 10 times the weight of the drug is obtained. The alcohol is then distilled off and the residue heated in a water bath until reduced to the consistence of a soft extract. By this process, about 10 per cent. of a brown colored, intensely bitter extract may be obtained. This extract is much stronger than extract of nux vomica, and is directed to be made into a mass with gum Arabic, in the proportion of 30 grains of the extract to 10 of gum, and divided into 40 pills (¾ grain in a pill), one of which is to be taken three times a day.

It is scarcely necessary to remark that the free use of a medicine of such power, containing one of the most poisonous of alkaloids, as a popular remedy, to be given without the advice and care of a physician, is most dangerous and unjustifiable.

Extract of Lupulin. W. W. D. LIVERMORE.

Take of Lupulin . . . . ℥iv.
" Alcohol . . . . f℥viij.

Mix in a percolator and allow it to stand an hour, then displace with

Alcohol . . . . q. s.

until two pints are obtained; pour this into a shallow dish and allow it to evaporate spontaneously. ℥j of lupulin yields about ℈ij of the extract, which is proposed as a substitute when prescribed in the pilular form. The dose being somewhat less than that of lupulin, is an advantage, besides its utility as a convenient and adhesive excipient with other substances.

Extractum Cimicifugæ.—This extract is made by evaporating separately a tincture prepared with 1 part of ether and 2 of alcohol, and one made with diluted alcohol, until they reach a syrupy consistence, then mixing these and finishing the evaporation over a water bath, with constant stirring. Eight grains of this represent ℨj of the root. —*Am. Journ. Pharm.*, vol. xxvi. p. 106.

Extractum Valerianæ.—Made as follows: Macerate the root in coarse powder, with twice its weight of strong alcohol, then displace with diluted alcohol, until exhausted. The first portion of the tincture is to be evaporated spontaneously, and reserved for addition to the extract formed by evaporating the diluted alcohol tincture. The addition of a portion of ether to the first portion of alcohol would facilitate the solution of the oil, and, also, the spontaneous evaporation of the menstruum.

GROUP 2.—Of the hydro-alcoholic extracts.

Officinal Name.	Dose.	Med. Prop.
Extractum hellebori	10 to 15 grs.	Cathartic.
" jalapæ	do.	do.
" rhei	do.	do.
" podophylli (May apple)	5 to 10 grs.	do.
" cinchonæ flav.	10 to 15 grs.	Tonic.
" " rub.	do.	do.
" sarsaparillæ	do.	Alterative.
" colocynthidis comp.	(Colocynth made into tincture and evaporated, aloes, scammony, soap, and cardamom added.)	Cathartic.

Of the above cathartics, each has its peculiar properties, adapting it to some peculiar use.

Extract of hellebore is used as an emmenagogue cathartic. In combination with aloes, myrrh, sulphate of iron, &c., it constitutes the celebrated Hooper's Female Pills.

Extract of jalap, and compound extract of colocynth, are combined with calomel and gamboge in the compound cathartic pill.

Extract of podophyllum is less used than it deserves, being equal to extract of jalap in its cathartic effect in half the dose.

Extract of rhubarb is rarely employed.

Extracts of cinchona and sarsaparilla are seldom used in practice in this country, although the latter is in good repute in England. These extracts of cinchona must not be confounded with the article called Wetherill's Extract, nor with extractum calisayicum, which are superior preparations.

Powdered Compound Extract of Colocynth.

The following formula has been suggested by Dr. E. R. Squibb, as a great improvement on that contained in the *Pharmacopœia* for the preparation of compound extract of colocynth. So inferior is the article, as found in commerce, that it becomes every pharmaceutist who values his reputation, and is really desirous to fill the responsible duties of his profession, to purchase it of Dr. Squibb, or some other reliable manufacturer who incorporates in it the full proportion of the active ingredients, or preferably to make it for himself.

Take of Colocynth . . A convenient quantity.
Alcohol . . Sufficient.

Form a tincture by maceration and expression, or preferably by displacement. Evaporate to dryness and powder, then

Take of Powdered Extract of colocynth as above	10½	drachms.
" Socotrine aloes . . .	34½	"
" Virgin scammony . . .	11½	"
" Cardamoms . . .	3	"
" Castile soap . . .	7½	"

The ingredients are to be thoroughly mixed in a mortar, passed through a fine sieve, and again well stirred together.—*Am. Journ. Pharm.*, vol. xxix. p. 97.

This furnishes the preparation in powder, which is its most convenient and uniform condition, and about 7 per cent. of water is sufficient to form it into pill mass.

Among the proposed changes in its composition, it is suggested to substitute resin of podophyllum (podophyllin) for the virgin scammony; it is cheaper and more accessible. This, however, might involve some changes in proportions used, and is not allowable until sanctioned in the *Pharmacopœia.*

CLASS III.

Extract made by Displacement with Cold Water and Evaporation.

(Unofficinal in Italics.)

Officinal Name.	Med. Dose.	Remarks.
Extractum gentianæ	10 to 20 grs.	Tonic.
" quassia	3 to 6 grs.	do.
" *chirettæ*	do.	do.
" dulcamaræ (bittersweet)	do.	Alterative narcotic.
" krameriæ (rhatany)	10 to 20 grs.	Astringent.
" juglandis (butternut)	do.	Carthartic.
" opii	1 grain.	Narcotic.

The great advantage of extracts of *quassia and chiretta* over extract of gentian in making pills, will be seen by comparing the dose. *Extract of rhatany* when well prepared, so as to be soluble in water, is a valuable substitute for kino and catechu, which it resembles in physical as well as medical properties. *Extract of opium* is added to eye-washes and astringent injections.

Syllabus of Extracts not belonging to either Class.

(Unofficinal in Italics.)

Name.	Dose.	Medical properties.
Extractum hæmatoxyli	10 to 20 grs.	Astringent.
" taraxaci	℈j to ʒj	Diuretic and cholagogue.
" colchici acet.	1 to 3 grs.	Diuretic and sedative.
" *lobeliæ* "	2 to 3 grs.	Sedative.
" *calisayicum*	2 to 3 grs.	Tonic.
" *pareiræ*	10 to 30 grs.	Tonic diuretic.
" *uvæ ursi*	do.	do.
" *ergotæ*	4 to 10 grs.	"Ergotine."

Extractum Hæmatoxyli (*logwood*) is made by decoction in water, straining and evaporating; it is highly esteemed as a very mild astringent, and is much used in the arts as a pigment.

Extractum Taraxaci (*dandelion*) is made by expressing the milky juice from the root and evaporating. No extract out of the narcotic series is so popular as this; it is much used in the treatment of liver complaint, habitual constipation, and as a diuretic in dropsy. Being soluble in water, it may be conveniently given in liquid form.

Extractum Colchici aceticum (*meadow saffron*) is made from vinegar saturated with colchicum, and evaporating. This most valuable preparation has been recently introduced; it is well adapted to combining with other ingredients in pilular form, and, with extract of digitalis, enters into the celebrated Lartique's Gout Pills. I usually obtain about 5 ounces of this extract from 10,000 grains of the root, near 25 per cent.

Extractum Lobeliæ Aceticum.—To prepare this, the powdered seed of lobelia are macerated, and then displaced with diluted alcohol, to the first portion of which has been added a small portion of acetic acid. This liquid is then to be evaporated to the consistence of an extract, which will be about one-eighth the quantity of the seed employed. (*Am. Journ. Pharm.*, vol. xiv. p. 108.) DOSE, from 2 to 3 grs. The object of the use of the acetic acid, is to form a soluble acetate of lobelina, less readily decomposable by heat than the native salt.

Calisaya Extract (Ellis).—Is made by boiling coarsely-powdered Calisaya bark in successive portions of water, acidulated with muriatic acid, precipitating the decoction with hydrate of lime, digesting the precipitate in hot alcohol till all taste is exhausted, and then evaporating the alcohol so as to leave an extract. The old-fashioned precipitated extract of bark was nearly identical with this, which is only objectionable on the score of expense.

It contains all the quinia and cinchonia contained in the bark, besides the amorphous quinia, or chinoidine, and is an admirable substitute for the celebrated Wetherill's extract, formerly much in vogue. Its dose is from 2 to 5 grs.—*Am. Journ. Pharm.*, vol. xx. p. 15.

Extractum Pareiræ is prepared from sliced pareira brava, by decoction with water, straining, and evaporating. A decoction is more frequently prescribed. DOSE, from 10 to 30 grs.

Extractum Uvæ Ursi.—The London College directs the preparation of this, also, by maceration and decoction with water. Its dose is the same as the foregoing, and they are both used as tonics and diuretics in chronic urinary disorders.

Ergotine.—Under this name an aqueous extract of ergot is sold in the shops, for which the following is the formula of M. Bonjean: Exhaust powdered ergot by displacement with cold water, heat the solution in a water bath and filter; evaporate to the consistence of syrup, and add rectified spirit to throw down the gummy matter; when settled, decant the clear liquid, and evaporate by water bath. One ounce of ergot yields about 70 grains. It is said to possess the hæmostatic without the toxic effects of ergot. DOSE, from 4 to 10 grs.

The *extracts of lettuce, poppyheads, and hops* are very weak narcotic extracts, occasionally prescribed, but less esteemed than lactucarium, opium, and lupuline, which are the more efficient products of their respective plants.

Chinoidine is the name given to an insoluble residuary extractive principle obtained in the manufacture of quinia, which will be adverted to under the head of alkaloids.

Extractum glycyrrhizæ is the name given in the list of the *Pharmacopœia*, to the common drug known as liquorice, imported from Italy and Spain. Until recently this was the only extract of liquorice used; our manufacturers now make a true and proper extract, which is made in either of two ways, as follows:—

1*st Process.*—Take of liquorice root, bruised, any convenient quantity, macerate in water, with the application of heat, until exhausted; strain, and evaporate to the consistence of an extract.

2*d Process.*—Take of liquorice (impure extract) any convenient quantity, lay the pieces of liquorice in a large displacer, or a barrel, in layers alternating with straw; macerate, and then percolate the mass with cold water, and evaporate the clear liquid that runs off. The pieces of liquorice will be found to have lost their saccharine extractive matter, although retaining their shape as before.

The extract has a yellow color, becoming brown by age, and, as made by the first process, has the taste of the root, and is deliquescent, so as to require to be kept in jars. One part of powdered liquorice root to sixteen of the extract will render it firm enough to keep in sticks. Tilden's extract of liquorice is made into sticks of a yellowish-brown color by admixture with gum Arabic; its taste resembles the root more decidedly than that of black liquorice.

The *physical properties of extracts* vary, according to their composition, age, and the circumstances in which they are kept.

The narcotic extracts of the first class, as vended by the manufacturers, are apt to be too soft for convenient use in the form of pills, and are disposed to deliquesce. This want of a firm consistence, which results from a disposition to preserve the more volatile ingredients from loss in the final concentration, causes no inconvenience when the extract is used with a considerable proportion of dry or hard ingredients. It may be obviated by combining with them powdered liquorice root, lycopodium, or tragacanth, when the additional bulk is no objection. The hydro-alcoholic extracts are seldom liable to this objection; they harden on exposure to the air, and when old are sometimes inconveniently dry.

The extracts of jalap and podophyllum are apt to become tough and unmanageable, so as to resist the action of the pestle either by trituration or contusion. Extract of jalap is ordered, in compound cathartic pills, in the form of powder, and this is in every respect its best form for use; it is conveniently kept in bottles, as other powders are, is readily weighed and incorporated with other substances, and becomes plastic by the addition of moisture. Few manufacturers push the evaporation so far as to produce the extract dry enough for powdering; but there is no difficulty in accomplishing it where steam is employed, and as a demand grows up for the article it will be more generally met with in the stores, although at a somewhat advanced price on the soft extract. Compound extract of colocynth is frequently brittle enough to powder, and is sometimes met with in this form. The addition of soap to its other ingredients prevents the liability to toughness, besides increasing its solubility.

Extract of rhatany is always pulverulent, and when properly made is nearly soluble in water.

The kind of jars usually employed for preserving extracts are here figured. Those with covers or tops are most eligible. In furnishing a shop where a good many are needed, it is well to reserve the canopy-top jars exclusively for ointments, the flat tops for extracts, for the sake of distinction. Extracts should never be put in gallipots or tie-overs, except for temporary purposes. Besides the cover, which fits loosely on the jars, there should be a piece of bladder, oiled paper, or preferably tinfoil, stretched over the open top before fitting on the lid.

Fig. 166.

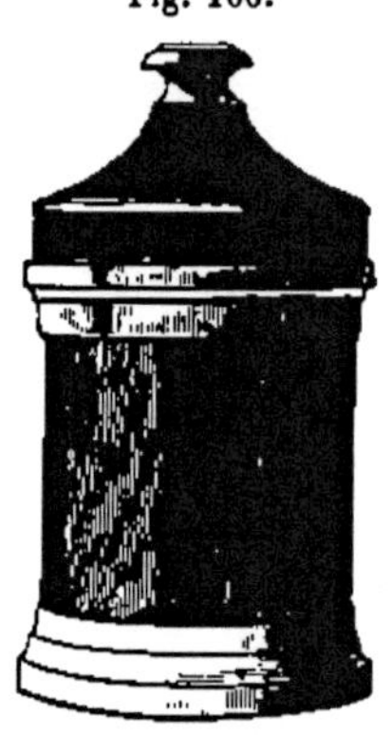

Canopy-top jar.

In the case of soft extracts, which have a tendency to mould, the occasional addition of a few drops of alcohol is found advantageous. Extracts put up in glass, wide mouth bottles, either with ground stoppers or corks, are preferable to jars in affording a more complete exclusion of the air, but the smaller sized bottles, having too narrow mouths to admit a spatula of ordinary width, are inconvenient.

Fig. 167. Fig. 168. Fig. 169.

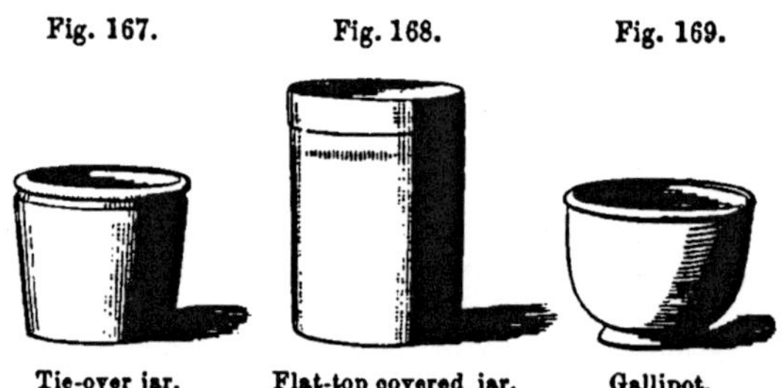

Tie-over jar. Flat-top covered jar. Gallipot.

The Uses of Extracts.—This class of preparations may be used either in the form of pills, solution, or mixture. They are chiefly prescribed in the pilular form, combined with other substances, and to this they are peculiarly adapted. One of the chief points in making pills is to increase or modify the effect in the highest degree, without a corresponding increase of bulk. Hence the utility of adding extracts to substances possessing no adhesiveness, choosing among them such as will most promote the therapeutic effect, while a plastic mass will be the result. Thus, in tonic pills, as of subcarbonate of iron or sulphate of quinia, extract of quassia, or of gentian would be preferable to an inert substance like conserve of rose or mucilage.

In dilute aqueous solutions, extracts are not generally preferable to the corresponding tinctures, but where the dose of the tincture would be large, the physician often avails himself of the extract in preference, as not containing alcoholic stimulus. Extracts are generally combined in *mixtures* containing sweet or viscid substances more than in *solutions* proper, although in cases where the quantity of the extract desired is large, and it is soluble in water, it may be employed to impart viscidity to a mixture, and to suspend insoluble substances without the necessity of using either gum or sugar.

In triturating an extract, particularly a hard one, with viscid liquids, as syrup or mucilage, or with lard in making ointments, considerable difficulty is experienced in dissolving or diffusing it equally throughout the mixture; to obviate this, it should be first softened with a few drops of water if aqueous, or alcohol if alcoholic, until it has about the consistence of thick honey or treacle, and then incorporated with the other ingredients. Frequently it will require a long and tedious trituration to accomplish the object thoroughly and effectually.

The aid of heat will greatly facilitate the softening of extracts, especially in making pill masses, which become dryer and more firm when rendered plastic by heat than when softened by a moist excipient.

CONCENTRATED EXTRACTS OR RESINOIDS.

The "concentrated remedies" of the so-called *eclectics* have within a few years obtained increased popularity, not only with practitioners of that school, but with physicians generally. Many of these, like resin of jalap and the new resin of scammony described below, belong to the class of resins proper, which are classified and described in their chemical and physical relations, under that head, in the third part of this work; others have no claim to a place among any class of proximate vegetable principles, and are to be regarded only as pharmaceutical preparations with more or less merit according as they are, or are not, prepared upon scientific principles.

I shall not attempt a full notice of all of these that have been proposed, but confine myself to such as are extensively known and esteemed.

Resin of Jalap. Jalapin of commerce.—This resin in its crude state is prepared, 1st, By digesting jalap root in boiling water for twenty-four hours, then slicing the root and further digesting with more water, which is afterwards boiled for ten minutes, stirring. The liquid is then expressed, and again boiled with fresh portions of water, and expressed two or three times. These decoctions, by evaporation, yield an *inferior* (aqueous) extract of jalap. The pressed root is now digested with successive portions of alcohol, the tinctures mixed, agitated with animal charcoal, filtered and evaporated, the alcohol being recovered. This product is a nearly colorless, friable resin, active as a cathartic in doses of from one to five grains.

The jalap resin of commerce is generally of a more or less dark color, having been prepared in copper or iron vessels, which discolor it. Frequently it is only a highly resinous extract of jalap, the dose of which would be from three to eight grains. The pure resin of jalap is insoluble in fixed oils and oil of turpentine, while common resins are soluble in those liquids. It is also insoluble in ether; powdered and thrown into cold water it does not dissolve, but forms a semi-fluid, transparent mass, as if it had been melted. Digested in a watch glass with a little sulphuric acid, a rich crimson colored solution is obtained, from which in a few hours a brown, viscid resin separates. About 13 per cent. of jalap resin consists of jalapic acid, which is the odorous principle of the root; it may be separated by adding an alcoholic solution of acetate of lead to a similar solution of the resin, throwing down the jalapate of lead. The lead may be then separated as sulphuret by a stream of sulphuretted hydrogen, and the acid collected by filtration and evaporation. It is a brownish, soft, greasy substance, soluble in alcohol and alkalies, and slightly so in ether. After the separation of jalapate of lead by this process, the pure resin remains in solution combined with acetic acid, traces of lead are to be separated by adding a few drops of sulphuric acid, and then the whole of the resin thrown down pure on the addition of five or six times its volume of water; this is dried by a current of warm air.

Jalap resin is an energetic cathartic in doses of from one to five grains, triturated with sugar or other diluents or correctives. (See Part III.)

Resin of scammony, prepared from the dried roots by the process of Dr. Williamson, of University College, London, is a similar preparation, and a great improvement on the common scammony of commerce. The roots are digested with water as in the above case, and with diluted acid, by which means they are deprived of all matter soluble in these menstrua, then with alcohol, which dissolves out the resin which is collected on the recovery of the alcohol by distillation. The roots are collected in Asia Minor, dried and shipped to London, where this improved scammony is now manufactured. The physical qualities of the scammony thus prepared differ considerably from that usually seen in commerce, and from virgin scammony, being non-porous, not producing a lather when rubbed with water, and, instead of possessing a musty or sour cheese-like odor, having an aromatic and fruity smell. In appearance, when in thin layers, it much resembles the scammony which is occasionally seen in the small shells (and regarded as the purest form of scammony), being transparent and of a yellow color. In composition it is almost entirely composed of a resin, which appears to bear the same relation to the root of convolvulus scammonia, as the foregoing does to jalap. Its dose is from four to twelve grains.

Resin of Podophyllum—Podophyllin.—This is the most popular and widely known of the whole class of "eclectic concentrated remedies." Of the several processes for its preparation which have appeared, the following, by F. D. Hill & Co., Cincinnati, is a modification of that of which I published the result in 1851, *American Journal of Pharmacy*, vol. xxiii. p. 329. It produces an article superior to that usually sold:—

"Exhaust coarsely-powdered mandrake root with alcohol by percolation. Place the saturated tincture in a still and distil off the alcohol; the residue will be a dark fluid of the consistence of molasses. Sometimes it is thicker; when this is the case add a small portion of it to water, and if it does not form a yellow-whitish precipitate, a small portion of alcohol must be added to it, enough to cause the light precipitate.

"Warm the thick residual liquid, and slowly pour it into three times its volume of cold water, which must be constantly agitated during the process. If poured in too fast, or without agitation, the fluid will fall to the bottom unchanged. Allow it to stand twenty-four hours, at which time nearly all the podophyllin will be precipitated. The addition of a sufficient quantity of muriatic acid will precipitate the remainder; the precipitated podophyllin of a whitish-yellow color, is now to be removed and placed on a linen filter, and washed several times with water. After this it is placed in thin layers on paper and dried in a room of a temperature between 65° and 90° F., or if in summer, at the natural atmospheric temperature. It becomes a shade or two darker by drying in this manner, but if artificial heat is employed to hasten the process, or a higher temperature, the resin becomes quite dark." According to my experiments, the root yields 3¾ per cent. of this substance. Another process for its preparation—the addition of a solution of alum to a concentrated tincture of the root—precipitates it of a greenish or olive tinge.

Podophyllin, as thus prepared, must not be confounded with the pure resinoid active principle of the drug, as first isolated by John R. Lewis, a graduate of the Philadelphia College of Pharmacy, and described in his inaugural thesis in 1847. The resin, as found in commerce, and prepared by the above process, has not, I believe, been analyzed; it probably contains a variety of principles, including both the resins, that soluble in alcohol and ether, and that insoluble in ether. It is insoluble in water and oil of turpentine, and only partially soluble in alcohol; it combines with alkali, forming a saponaceous compound.

Its medical properties are the subject of much comment in eclectic publications, and it is undoubtedly one of the most powerful remedies in use, acting, in doses of two to four grains, as a drastic cathartic, accompanied in its action with much nausea and griping. In smaller doses, ¼ grain to one grain, it operates as an alterative and cholagogue. It is claimed for this remedy that it is a regulator of almost all the secretions tending to restore them to normal activity, and that it completely substitutes mercury in all cases where it was formerly considered to be indicated, even to the extent, in some cases, of producing ptyalism. It is seldom or never employed alone, its effects being greatly increased, and its dose lessened, according to the testimony of practitioners accustomed to its use, by long trituration with four to ten times its weight of sugar or sugar of milk. Caulophyllin combined with it is said to materially lessen its painful and disagreeable effects. A compound of podophyllin, with ten parts of leptandrin and ten parts of sugar, is much esteemed as an alterative in dyspepsia, hepatitis, &c. (See *King's Eclectic Dispensatory*.)

Cimicifugin, or Macrotin, another eclectic resinoid, is prepared by forming a concentrated tincture of black snakeroot, diluting it with its bulk of water, and distilling off the alcohol. It is then collected from the bottom of this vessel and powdered. A modification of this process by Prof. E. S. Wayne, yields a more elegant and somewhat more active preparation. He directs that the strong tincture shall be allowed to evaporate spontaneously, until a solid mass is deposited, the remaining fluid is poured off and the mass dissolved in alcohol, slowly evaporated to the consistence of a fluid extract, and then placed in thin layers upon glass and allowed to dry.

As usually found in commerce, this is a dark-brown powder, of a faint odor, and a slightly bitter nauseous taste. It has not been analyzed, but appears to be an impure resin, which abounds in the root. I obtained $4\frac{3}{4}$ per cent. of it in my experiments. (See paper on Eclectic Pharmacy, *Am. Journ. Pharm.*, vol. xxiii. p. 329.) Its medical properties are described in Dr. King's *Dispensatory* as tonic, alterative, nervine, anti-periodic, with an especial affinity for the uterus. It does not, according to this authority, possess the narcotic properties of the root. Its applications in eclectic practice are very numerous; it is considerably used by practitioners generally, especially in the treatment of chorea. Of course, a great variety of combinations may be resorted to as occasion requires.

Leptandrin.—This is an impure resinoid, obtained from the root of *Leptandra Virginica*, or black root, an indigenous plant, formerly officinal in the *U. S. P.* It is prepared nearly like the foregoing, using high proof alcohol for the extraction of the root, as a small proportion of water present in the tincture prevents its successful precipitation. The character of the precipitate is also affected by the temperature, which should not exceed 180° F. Roots of the second year's growth are said to yield the most of this product.

Leptandrin, as thus prepared, is a jet black substance, resembling asphaltum, or sometimes has a gray or brown color, with a peculiar faint odor and taste. It is generally sold in powder. Though at first soluble in alcohol, it becomes less so by age; it dissolves in solution of ammonia and potassa, from which acids throw it down.

The remedy is highly valued by many practitioners as a cholagogue or stimulant to the hepatic secretion, without so decided a purgative action as usually pertains to that class of remedies. Like podophyllin, it is a leading article of production with several of the largest manufacturing pharmaceutists in the United States. The dose is two to four grains.

Hydrastin is the name applied in commerce to a concentrated remedy prepared from the root of *Hydrastis Canadensis*, golden seal, an interesting American plant of the family *Ranunculaceæ*. Prof. E. S. Wayne has given the following process for its preparation :—[1]

[1] See Hydrastia, Part III. of this work.

"Treat the powdered root of Hydrastis Canadensis by displacement with cold water, then acidulate the infusion with hydrochloric acid, which precipitates hydrastin and a gelatinous substance, collect the precipitate on a filter and wash with clean water; then dry it, dissolve the dried mass in alcohol, filter and set aside to crystallize."

Hydrastin, as thus prepared, is in yellow, translucent, acicular crystals, which are usually powdered before being sold. It is nearly insoluble in cold alcohol, ether, chloroform, oil of turpentine, and water, but is rendered more soluble in water by acetic acid, and in alcohol by ammonia and potassa. This is extensively used as a tonic remedy, especially adapted to treating dyspepsia and chronic inflammation of the stomach, and is said, combined with bitters, to have the effect of gradually removing the abnormal condition of the stomach in cases of intemperance, and in many instances of destroying the appetite for liquor. The dose for an adult is three to five grains, repeated three to six times a day. (See *Neutral Organic Principles*, Part III.)

Besides the above described preparation, there is another sold under the same name, which is said to be the *resinoid* principle, and possessed of similar though less active properties.

Sanguinarina and *sanguinarin* are two very different preparations from one of our most beautiful American plants, sanguinaria Canadensis or bloodroot, which belongs to the natural family papaveraciæ, the poppy tribe. Of the alkaloid *sanguinarina* mention is made in Part III. It is a powerful remedy, being used in doses of one-tenth to one-thirtieth of a grain, and should be carefully distinguished from the so-called "alka resinoid," which is chiefly used in the eclectic practice, and which contains an uncertain proportion of it.

Sanguinarin is thus prepared: Take of bloodroot, in coarse powder, a convenient quantity, and alcohol sufficient; make a saturated tincture, as in the case of the other resinoids; filter and add an equal quantity of water; distil off the alcohol and allow the residue to rest until precipitation ceases. Remove the supernatant liquid, wash the precipitate in water, dry it carefully by moderate heat, and pulverize it for use. As thus prepared, the powder is of a deep reddish-brown color, peculiar odor, and bitter, rather nauseous taste, followed by a persistent pungency in the fauces. It is insoluble in water, soluble in boiling alcohol, and partially soluble in alkaline solutions, acetic acid, and ether. This is given as a tonic in doses of from one-fourth to one grain, and as a hepatic and alterative from half a grain to two grains.

Caulophyllin.—This preparation, from the root of caulophyllum thalictroides, blue cohosh, is made by W. S. Merrill, of Cincinnati, by precipitation from the saturated tincture, similar to the preparation of podophyllin and cimicifugin, using, however, as small a quantity of water as possible to prevent waste, as the precipitate is soluble. Caulophyllin thus prepared is a neutral extractive or resinoid substance of a light brown color, with a peculiar, not unpleasant odor, and a slightly bitter taste, and some degree of pungency. It has not been analyzed. It is insoluble in ether, partially soluble in water, in alcohol more so;

the addition of solution of ammonia renders it completely soluble in either menstruum, and the solution becomes of a dark wine color. The following process for obtaining caulophyllin is by Dr. F. D..Hill of Cincinnati: Exhaust the root of caulophyllum with alcohol and obtain a thick fluid extract, add this to twice its volume of saturated aqueous solution of alum, and place it aside to rest for three or four days; then place it on a filter cloth, and allow the water to filter through; wash the product two or three times with fresh water, and let the residuum dry in the open air. When dry, it readily forms a powder of a light grayish color.

The ordinary dose of caulophyllin is from one fourth of a grain to one grain, three or four times a day; its therapeutic effect is exerted on the uterus, as a tonic and alterative. As a parturient it is given in doses of from two to four grains, at intervals of 15 to 30 minutes after actual labor has commenced.

Caulophyllin is prepared by some manufactures from an aqueous infusion of the root, decolorized by animal charcoal, and concentrated in vacuo, by adding infusion of galls, or 96 per cent. alcohol, collecting the precipitate, drying and powdering it. It is then sold as an *alkaloid*, although its properties are said not to vary much from those of the first, which is usually considered as a *resinoid.*

One of the evils growing out of this system of practice is the multiplication of these nondescript principles, which, while many of them may be valuable medicines, are prepared almost exclusively by a few manufacturers, each pursuing his own process, and liable to produce varying results; while under an imperfect system of nomenclature all are classed together.

They cannot with truth be called the active principles of the several plants from which derived, unless where these are purely resinoid, as in the case of podophyllum and jalap. In justice to the so-called eclectic practitioners, it must be admitted that they have been instrumental in introducing to notice some obscure medical plants which possess valuable properties; it is to be regretted that their disposition to run into pharmaceutical empiricism should have so long limited their usefulness and damaged their reputation.

CHAPTER XII.

FLUID EXTRACTS.

THE class *Extracta fluida* is found for the first time in the *Pharmacopœia* in the edition of 1850. Most of those at that time made officinal had been used and were esteemed standard remedies for several years previously, though two of them (the oleo resins) have not yet attained any great popularity. They are all made by displacement and evaporation.

Many of the large number of new remedies under this name are of very different characters, both as regards their strength, the menstrua employed in their preparation, and the antiseptic ingredient added for their preservation. It is scarcely practicable to reduce these to any regular system of classification; the object of the following tables and formulas is to render the subject as clear as it can well be made, and to furnish practical pharmaceutists facilities for producing these remedies for themselves.

The original idea of a fluid extract was to make it represent an equal portion of the drug, every ounce weight of the material from which prepared being converted into a fluidounce of the fluid extract. The result of this, if carried out, would have been to simplify the study of the doses of fluid extracts by stating the dose in each case to be the same as of the drug. This rule was early departed from, even in the *Pharmacopœia*, and the unofficinal formulæ published have in many instances been quite independent of any uniform rule of strength.

No effort will be made in the remarks which follow to include the fluid extracts issued by various manufacturers, according to their own arbitrary standards; these can only claim to be introduced into works on Pharmacy when their precise composition is made public.

Syllabus of Fluid Extracts.

Class I.—*Concentrated Syrups.*

Name.	Authority.	Proportions.	Adult Dose.	Adjuvants and Remarks.
Ext. sennæ fluid.	U. S. P.	f℥j—℥j leaves	f℥ss	Oil of fennel, added.
" rhei fluid.	"	f℥j—℥j root	fʒj	Oils and tinct. ginger.
" spigel. et sen. fluid.	"	{ f℥j—spigel. ʒiv senna ʒij	fʒj	Carb. potassa and oils.
" sarsaparillæ fluid.	"	f℥j—℥j comp.	fʒj	Sassafras, mezer., &c.
" *cinchonæ fluid.*	Jones	f℥j—℥ss bark	fʒj	Quinia as muriate.
" " "	Taylor	" "	fʒj	" as kinate, &c.
" *buchu fluid.*	Procter	f℥j—℥ss leaves	fʒj	See 2d class.
" " *comp.*	Parrish	" "	fʒj	Oil juniper, cubebs, &c.
" *hydrangeæ fluid.*	"	" root	℥ss	Butler's Oj—Hj.
" *rhei et sennæ fluid.*	Procter	{ f℥j—senna ʒvj rhubarb ʒij	℥ss	Bicarb. potassa, &c.
" *jalapæ fluid.*	"	f℥j—℥j root	♏xx	Carb. potassa and alc.
" *ergotæ fluid.*	Baker	f℥j—℥j rye	fʒj	Contains the F. oil.
" " "	Thayer	. . . .	fʒj	No ether used.
" *serpentariæ fluid.*	Savery	f℥j—℥ss root	fʒss	See 2d class.
" *anthemidis fluid.*	Procter	" flowers	fʒss	Anti-periodic, dos. fʒij.
" *cornus Floridæ fluid.*	Maisch	f℥j—℥j bark	fʒj	Subst. for cinchona.
" *scutellariæ lat. fluid.*	"	" herb	fʒj	Nervous sedative.
" *marrubii fluid.*	"	f℥j to ℥j "	fʒj	Tonic, adjuvant.
" *dulcamaræ fluid.*	"	f℥j to ℥j stalk	fʒj	Both sugar and alcohol.
" *uvæ ursi fluid.*	"	f℥j to ℥j leaves	fʒj	Tonic, diuretic.
" *sanguinariæ fluid.*	S. Campbell	℥j—℥ss root	♏x	Ext. by acetic acid.
" *pruni Virg. fluid.*	Procter	f℥j—℥ss bark	fʒj	HCy by emulsion of almonds.
" " *ferratum fluid.*	Warner	" "	fʒj	24 grs. cit. iron to f℥j.
" *hyoscyami fluid.*	C. Aug. Smith	" leaves	♏xx	℥ss ext. to f℥x aq.

Class II.—*Concentrated Tinctures.*

Name.	Authority.	Proportions.	Adult Dose	Adjuvants and Remarks.
Ext. valerianæ fluid.	U. S. P.	f℥j—℥ss root	fʒj	Oil ext. by ether.
" *buchu fluid.*	Procter	" leaves	"	See class 1st.
" " "	Weaver	" "	"	Oil ext. by ether.
Infus. cinchonæ spissat.	Ph. Lond.	. . . .	♏xx to f℥ss	Strained and evap.
Ext. serpentariæ fluid.	Taylor	f℥j—℥j root	♏xx	Strongest.
" *taraxaci fluid.* No. 1	Procter	f℥ss—℥j fresh	ʒj	Succus tarax. parat.
" " " No. 2	"	fʒvj—℥j "	"	From fresh root.
" " " No. 3	. . .	f℥j—℥j dried	"	" dried "
" " " No. 4	. . .	f℥j—℥ss ext.	"	Extemporaneous.
" *gentianæ fluid.*	Procter	f℥j—℥j root	"	Contains brandy.
" *gallæ fluid.*	Parrish	f℥j—℥ss galls	. . .	Use in dentistry.
" *lobeliæ fluid.*	Procter	" herb	♏v to xx	Acetic acid used.
" *cimicifugæ fluid.*	"	f℥j—℥j root	♏xxx	Ether and alc. used.
" *ergotæ fluid.*	"	f℥j—℥j rye	♏vx	Without the F. oil.
" " "	J. T. Watson	f℥iij—℥j "	fʒj	" " "
" *sumbul fluid.*	Procter	f℥j—℥ss root	♏x to ʒj	Substitute for musk.
" *lupulinæ fluid.*	"	f℥j—℥j leaf	♏v to xx	Nervous sedative.
" *ipecacuanhæ fluid.*	Stabler	f℥iij—℥j root	"	
" *calami fluid.*	Maisch	f℥iv—℥j "	. . .	Adjuvant.

Class III.—*Oleo-Resins*, made with Ether.

Name.	Authority.	Adjuvants and Remarks.	Dose in drops.
Ext. cubebæ fluidum	U. S. P.	Stim., diuretic.	5 to 30 drops.
" piperis "	"	Stim.	1 to 5 "
Piperoid of ginger		Carmin., in confectionery, &c.	" "
Oleo-resin capsicum		Too powerful for convenience.	?
Oil of male fern		Tapeworm.	20 to 40 "
" *of ergot*		In parturition.	" "
" *of Canada snakeroot*		Carminative.	?
" *of cardamom*		"	?
" *of parsley*		Diuretic.	3 or 4 "

General Remarks.

The preparation of what I have designated as the *first class* is accomplished as follows: A tincture is first prepared by displacement with a mixture of alcohol and water; after the strength is thoroughly extracted from the drug in this way, it is transferred to a capsule (preferably to a water bath), and evaporated to such a point as that, on the addition of sugar, it will make the quantity required. The proportion of sugar is made somewhat less than in the case of ordinary syrups, so as to prevent the preparation being too thick for convenience; and, to make up for this deficiency of sugar, alcohol, essential oils, or other antiseptics are added.

These preparations are generally the most eligible of their respective drugs. Their dose is comparatively small; they are mostly quite miscible with aqueous liquids. By dilution with simple syrup, the appropriate fluid extracts yield preparations nearly resembling the corresponding syrups, and, by dilution with water, the corresponding infusions. The proportions may be readily calculated by a comparison of the formulas.

The *second class* may be designated as those which contain alcohol as their chief or exclusive antiseptic ingredient. Some are scarcely different from strong tinctures, while others are made by first treating the powdered drug with a mixture of alcohol and ether by displacement, and allowing the ethereal tincture thus obtained to evaporate spontaneously, until the dissolved oleo-resin is left in solution in a small portion of the alcohol. While this evaporation is going on, the contents of the displacement tube are further treated with diluted alcohol, till a definite quantity of tincture has passed; to this the evaporated ethereal tincture first prepared is now added, and the mixture filtered. This process is best adapted to drugs containing volatile principles, and especially to stimulating substances, the action of which is aided by alcohol.

The *third class* or *oleo-resins* are not numerous, they do not seem to belong among the fluid extracts, though those in the *Pharmacopœia* are so classed.

These preparations are made by passing *ether* through the powdered drug in a covered displacement apparatus, and allowing this ethereal tincture to evaporate spontaneously. The resulting liquid is of a more or less oily consistence; usually of a dark color—brown, or with a tinge of green; extremely pungent, and reminding one of the drug. It consists of the essential oil holding in solution a portion of the waxy and resinoid principles associated with it in the drug. These are apt to be deposited in part, a circumstance which modifies somewhat the properties of different specimens of the same preparation. In the instance of fluid extract of pepper, the piperin is directed to be separated, and the oil of black pepper of commerce, which is similar to the fluid extract, is a residuary product of the manufacture of piperin. Cubebs yield from 12 to 28 per cent. of oleo-resin; black pepper about one-sixteenth of its weight; ginger from 6 to 9 per cent.

Owing to the solubility of fixed oils in ether, these, if present in the drug, are extracted, and are associated with the oleo-resinous preparations left after the evaporation. In the oleo-resins of cardamon and ergot the fixed oils are conspicuous though inert ingredients.

Some of the *formulas* which follow may appear conflicting, different writers having indicated different modes of treating the same drug, and directed different antiseptic ingredients to be associated with the active principles when extracted. I give all the recipes, because, in the present unsettled state of the subject, it would seem invidious to select those which appear best. In future revisions of the *Pharmacopœia*, there can be little doubt that authoritative directions will be given for the preparation of many medicines of this class, and those not made officinal will be more thoroughly tested by experience, and either come into general use or be forgotten and gradually omitted from our formularies. As has been before stated, they are all directed to be made by displacement and evaporation, but the latter process may be sometimes almost or entirely obviated by the skilful use of the former. When powders are sufficiently fine and uniform, and are treated by the process of Prof. I. J. Grahame, in a funnel, the resulting tinctures may frequently be obtained so strong as to require no concentration, except, perhaps, to adapt them to the further treatment by freeing them from alcohol, and in every preparation of the series, the chief aim of the pharmaceutist should be to manage the percolation so as to diminish the tedious and often injurious process of evaporation.

Laidley's Table showing the Proportion of each ingredient in the Officinal Fluid Extracts.

FLUID EXTRACT OF

f℥j of Fluid Extract represents of	Cubebs.	Black Pepper.	Rhubarb.				Senna.				Sarsaparilla.				Pink Root and Senna.					Valerian.
	Cubebs.	Black Pepper.	Rhubarb.	Tinct. Ginger.	Oil Aniseed	Oil Fennel.	Senna.	Oil of Fennel.	Hoffman's Anodyne.	(Sugar.)	Sarsaparilla.	Liquorice Root.	Sassafras.	Mezereon.	Pink Root.	Senna.	Carb. Potassa.	Oil Aniseed.	Oil Caraway.	Valerian.
♏ or grs.	480	960	60	4	1/16	1/16	60	⅜	¼		60	7½	7½	2¾	30	15	1⅛	⅛	⅛	30

Table showing the Officinal Fluid Extracts as compared with the other Preparations of the same Drugs.

f℥j Fluid Extract equal to	Cubebs.	Rhubarb.							Sarsaparilla.				Senna.			Valerian.		
	Tincture.	Infusion.	Syrup.	Aromat. Syrup.	Tincture.	Tinct. Rh. and Aloes.	Tinct. Rh. and Gentian.	Extract.	Infusion.	Comp. Syrup.	Comp. Decoction.	Extract.	Infusion.	Syrup.	Tinct. Sen. and Jalap.	Infusion.	Tincture.	Ammon. Tinct.
	f℥viij	Oss	℥iss	5½ oz.	1½ oz.	3 oz.	℥ij	ʒss	℥ij	¾ oz.	℥j	8 gr.	℥ij	℥j	℥ij	℥ij	℥ss	℥ss

FORMULAS FOR FLUID EXTRACTS.

Extractum Sennæ Fluidum, U. S. P. (*Fluid Extract of Senna.*)

Take Senna in coarse powder	. .	2½ pounds.
Sugar	. . . . .	20 ounces.
Oil of fennel	. . . .	1 fluidrachm.
Compound spirit of ether	.	2 fluidrachms.
Diluted alcohol	. . .	4 pints.

Mix the senna with the diluted alcohol, and, having allowed the mixture to stand for twenty-four hours, introduce it into a percolator, and gradually pour in water mixed with one-third of its bulk of alcohol, until a gallon and a half of liquid shall have passed. Evaporate the liquid, by means of a water bath, to twenty fluidounces, and filter; then add the sugar, and, when it is dissolved, the compound spirit of ether holding the oil of fennel in solution.

This preparation is greatly esteemed as an efficient cathartic, not disagreeable to children, to whom it is given in doses varying from a teaspoonful to a tablespoonful. It is apt to produce griping in its action, a symptom avoided, to a great extent, by the use of cold water alone, in the extraction of the senna, and evaporating in vacuo.

Extractum Rhei Fluidum, U. S. P. (*Fluid Extract of Rhubarb.*)

Take of Rhubarb in coarse powder	.	8 ounces.
Sugar	. . . . .	5 ounces.
Tincture of ginger	. . .	Half fluidounce.
Oil of fennel		
Oil of anise, each	. . .	4 minims.
Diluted alcohol	. . .	A sufficient quantity.

To the rhubarb, previously mixed with an equal bulk of coarse sand, add twelve fluidounces of diluted alcohol, until the liquor which passes has little of the odor or taste of the rhubarb. Evaporate the tincture thus obtained, by means of a water bath, to five fluidounces; then add the sugar, and, after it is dissolved, mix thoroughly with the resulting fluid extract, the tincture of ginger holding the oils in solution.

The dose of Fluid Extract of Rhubarb varies from half a teaspoonful to a dessertspoonful. It is too thick to pour with facility in cold weather, and is not an agreeable preparation. The formula would be improved by diminishing the proportion of rhubarb to one-half, and increasing the dose accordingly.

Extractum Spigeliæ et Sennæ Fluidum, U. S. P. (*Fluid Extract of Pink root and Senna.*)

Take of Pink root in coarse powder	.	1 pound.
Senna in coarse powder	. .	6 ounces.
Sugar	. . . . .	1½ pound.
Carbonate of potassa	. .	6 drachms.
Oil of caraway,		
Oil of anise, each	. . .	Half a fluidrachm.
Diluted alcohol	. . .	A sufficient quantity.

Mix the pink root and senna with two pints of diluted alcohol, and having allowed the mixture to stand for two days, transfer it to a percolator, and gradually pour upon it diluted alcohol until half a gallon of liquid has passed. Evaporate the liquid, by means of a water bath, to a pint; then add the carbonate of potassa, and, after the sediment has dissolved, the sugar, previously triturated with the oils. Lastly, dissolve the sugar with a gentle heat.

This is an admirable anthelmintic medicine, and is eminently worthy to replace the numerous nostrums so extensively sold as worm syrups. The dose is a teaspoonful, or somewhat less for young children; it requires no cathartic to be given after it.

Extractum Sarsaparillæ Fluidum, U. S. P. (*Fluid Extract of Sarsaparilla.*)

Take of	Sarsaparilla, sliced and bruised . .	16 ounces.
	Liquorice root, bruised	
	Bark of sassafras root, bruised, each .	2 ounces.
	Mezereon, sliced	6 drachms.
	Sugar	12 ounces.
	Diluted alcohol	8 pints.

Macerate all the ingredients together, except the sugar, for fourteen days; then express and filter. Evaporate the liquid, by means of a water bath, to twelve fluidounces; add the sugar to it while still hot, and remove from the bath as soon as the sugar is dissolved.

Sarsaparilla is so difficult to obtain in a proper condition for percolation, that maceration and expression are here wisely indicated. This is one of the best of the fluid extracts. DOSE, a teaspoonful.

Extractum Valerianæ Fluidum, U. S. P. (*Fluid Extract of Valerian.*)

Take of	Valerian in coarse powder .	8 ounces.
	Ether	4 fluidounces.
	Alcohol	12 fluidounces.
	Diluted alcohol	A sufficient quantity.

Mix the ether and alcohol, and, having incorporated the valerian with one half of the mixture, introduce the mass into a percolator, and gradually pour in the remainder; then add diluted alcohol until the whole liquid which has passed shall amount to a pint. Put the ethereal liquid thus obtained into a shallow vessel, and allow it to evaporate spontaneously until reduced to five fluidounces. Upon the mass in the percolator pour gradually diluted alcohol until ten fluidounces of tincture have passed. With this mix the five fluidounces left after the spontaneous evaporation, taking care to dissolve in a little alcohol any oleo-resinous matter which may have been deposited, and to add it to the rest. Allow the mixture to stand, with occasional agitation, for four hours, and then filter. The resulting fluid extract should measure a pint, and if it be less than that quantity, the deficiency should be supplied by the addition of alcohol.

This process of the *Pharmacopœia* has been found very satisfactory during a series of years. The addition of ether to the first liquid used in the percolation is designed to extract the essential oil and valerianic acid which are not dissipated during its spontaneous evaporation. DOSE, a teaspoonful.

Fluid Extracts of Cinchona.

Several formulas have been contrived for making fluid extracts of cinchona, the results of which vary in their physical and medical properties.

The first is that of M. Donovan, given in vol. xvii. p. 49, *Am. Journ. Pharm.*, and is chiefly objectionable as being complicated and difficult; besides, the liquid being made from the bark by repeated maceration in diluted alcohol, and by decoction with water, subsequently concentrated by evaporation, a rare salt, the dinoxalate of quinia, is added, in large proportion, to increase the strength of the preparation, and the whole is then formed into a very thick fluid extract, called, by Donovan, "Syrup of Bark."

As far as I am aware, this has not been prepared in this country; but the prevailing idea, that quinia and cinchona are not the only proximate principles of the cinchonia barks that give them their anti-periodic properties, and that the natural state of combination, in which the various principles exist, is to be preferred in certain cases, has led to several other formulas for fluid extracts of bark.

Infusum Cinchonæ Spissatum. (Ph. L.)

Take of Yellow bark, coarsely powdered	8 pounds.
Distilled water	6 pints (imperial measure).
Rectified spirit	A sufficient quantity.

Macerate the bark in four pints of the water for twenty-four hours and strain; then add the remainder of the water, macerate for twenty-four hours, and again strain; then mix the infusions. Evaporate by means of a water bath to one-fourth, and set apart that the dregs may subside. Pour off the clear liquor and filter the rest. Then mix, and again evaporate till the sp. gr. of the liquor becomes 1.200; into this when cold slowly drop the spirit, so that three fluidrachms may be added for every fluidounce. Lastly, set the liquor aside for twenty days, that it may become entirely clear. The dose of this is from twenty minims to half a fluidounce.

Isaac C. Jones, a graduate of the Philadelphia College of Pharmacy, in his inaugural thesis, proposed a fluid extract of cinchona to be made as follows:—

Take eight ounces of calisaya bark; exhaust it completely by displacement with water, acidulated with muriatic acid, in quantity not exceeding half a fluidounce. The infusion is now to be evaporated to nine fluidounces; and, while yet hot, fourteen ounces of sugar dissolved in it, which will bring it to measure a pint. Each fluidrachm of this fluid extract represents half a drachm of the bark, or about one grain of quinia. It becomes turbid on cooling, by the deposition of cinchonic red, which may be separated by straining or decanting it.

The preparation will then be clear; but it will be observed, it contains the quinia in the form of *muriate*, thus disturbing the natural state of combination existing in bark.

Some of our pharmaceutists prepare this, and furnish it when fluid extract of bark is prescribed.

Alfred B. Taylor has since communicated a formula, which was published in the *American Journal of Pharmacy*, vol. xxiii. p. 218, which presents the constituents of bark in an unaltered condition, although turbid, and less elegant in appearance than the foregoing. It is as follows:—

Take eight ounces (Troy) of calisaya bark, exhaust it completely by displacement with diluted alcohol; evaporate to nine fluidounces, then add fourteen ounces (Troy) of sugar; continue the heat until it is dissolved, and strain while hot, if necessary. This makes a pint, each fluidrachm of which represents half a drachm of bark, or one grain of quinia.

In the process of evaporating the tincture, as first prepared, in the last formula, a very copious precipitate, consisting of the cinchonotannates, and cinchonic red, is thrown down, coating the bottom and sides of the dish or water bath. It is designed to suspend this, by the aid of the sugar, subsequently added. I have found an advantage in varying the process, by pouring off the concentrated liquid into another vessel, and dissolving this precipitate in four fluidounces of alcohol. The sugar is now added, and becomes saturated with this alcoholic solution; the nine ounces of concentrated liquid, previously poured off, being now returned, and heat applied. The alcohol is nearly dissipated, while the sugar is dissolved. The result is a very complete suspension of the insoluble portion.

Fluid extract of cinchona is applicable to the cases in which the bark itself would be indicated; its dose, as a tonic, is usually about a fluidrachm. It is well adapted to admixture with other tonics, in the liquid form.

Fluid Extracts of Buchu.

Preparations of buchu have been used to some extent for many years. More than twenty years ago, Geo. W. Carpenter, of this city, advertised in his "Essays addressed to Physicians," a compound fluid extract of buchu, prepared by a secret formula, and recommended for diseases of the urinary organs, especially "gonorrhœa or clap, and gleets of long standing." Of latter time, since this valuable drug has come to be more generally known and appreciated, our *Pharmacopœia* has recognized an officinal infusion, and that of Dublin, a tincture. The fluid extract may be made so as to class it with the concentrated syrups; or may contain alcohol and thus be classed with concentrated tinctures. I shall proceed to give processes for both kinds, as also that for a compound fluid extract, which I have prepared for several years, and which has found favor with some. For the two next following recipes we are indebted to Prof. Procter.

The Syrupy Fluid Extract of Buchu.

Take of Buchu leaves	. . . .	8 ounces.
Alcohol	. . . . .	16 fluidounces.
Water	. . . . . .	A sufficient quantity.
Sugar	. . . . . .	8 ounces.

Reduce the leaves to coarse powder, moisten them in a covered vessel with twelve fluidounces of the alcohol, macerate for six hours and introduce the whole into a suitable displacer. When the clear liquid has ceased to drop, add the remaining alcohol mixed with four fluidounces of water, gradually, until the displaced alcoholic liquid amounts to twelve fluidounces, which is evaporated with moderate heat to four fluidounces. The residue in the displacer is then treated with a pint of cold water by maceration for twelve hours, and subjected to pressure, until a pint of aqueous liquid is obtained. (Displacement is ineligible, on account of the mucilaginous character of the marc.) This is evaporated to eight fluidounces and mixed with the four fluidounces of evaporated tincture previously obtained, and the sugar is dissolved in it by agitation. A pint of fluid extract is thus obtained from eight ounces of buchu, and a fluidrachm, the usual dose, represents half a drachm of the powdered leaves.

The Hydro-Alcoholic Fluid Extract of Buchu.

Take of Buchu leaves	. . . . .	8 ounces.
Alcohol	. . . . . .	16 fluidounces.
Water	. . . . . .	A sufficient quantity.

Reduce the leaves to coarse powder; moisten them with twelve fluidounces of the alcohol; macerate them for six hours, and introduce the whole into a suitable displacer; when the clear fluid has ceased to pass, add the remaining alcohol, mixed with four fluidounces of water, gradually, until the displaced alcoholic liquid amounts to twelve fluidounces, which is set aside until reduced to six fluidounces by spontaneous evaporation. The residue in the displacer is treated with water by maceration for twelve hours, and subjected to pressure until a pint of aqueous liquid is obtained. This is evaporated to ten fluidounces, mixed with the six fluidounces of evaporated tincture, and after occasional agitation for several days, may be filtered or strained, to remove the undissolved resinous and gummy matter. This is of the same strength as the preceding, and given in the same dose. It contains a little more alcohol, and no sugar.

The following recipe is an improvement on the foregoing, producing an elegant and very strong though less mucilaginous preparation.

Weaver's Fluid Extract Buchu.

Take of Buchu (finely powdered)	. .	8 ounces.
Ether	. . . . . .	4 fluidounces.
Alcohol	. . . . . .	12 fluidounces.
Diluted alcohol	. . . .	Sufficient.

Mix the ether and alcohol, and having packed the powdered buchu in a tall displacer, pass the mixture through it, then add sufficient diluted alcohol to obtain a pint of the tincture. Put the ethereal liquid, thus obtained, in a porcelain capsule, and allow it to evaporate to five fluidounces. Upon the mass in the percolator, pour, gradually, diluted alcohol until ten fluidounces of tincture have passed; mix this with the five fluidounces before obtained, and dissolve in a fluidounce of alcohol the oleo-resinous matter left in the dish and add it to the rest, after standing in a closed bottle for several hours, and occasionally shaking up: filter.

This is a dark-colored hydro-alcoholic liquid, with a tendency to the formation of globules of essential oil on the surface, and possessed in a very high degree of the characteristic odor and taste of the drug.

Parrish's Compound Fluid Extract of Buchu.

Take of Buchu in coarse powder . . 12 ounces.
Alcohol . . . . . 3 pints.
Water . . . . . 6 pints, or sufficient.

Treat the leaves by maceration and displacement, first with a portion of the alcohol, and then with the remaider mixed with the water; evaporate the resulting liquid by a gentle heat to 3 pints, and to this add

Sugar . . . . . . $2\frac{1}{2}$ pounds.

Continue the heat till it is dissolved, and, after removing from the fire, add—

Oil of cubebs,
Oil of juniper, of each . . One fluidrachm.
Spirit of nitric ether . . Twelve fluidounces.

Previously mixed; stir the whole together.

It will be perceived that this preparation, although it contains a portion of sugar sufficient to impart sweetness to the taste, does not owe its permanence to that ingredient. The oils of cubebs and juniper, and the spirit of nitric ether, are not only useful as therapeutic agents in the majority of cases in which cubebs would be used, but act as antiseptics, and would render the preparation permanent without the presence of alcohol or sugar.

It has been found a useful preparation, and is well adapted by its composition, to chronic maladies of the urino-genital organs, appearing to act topically in its passage through them.

Fluid Extract of Hydrangea.

The root of hydrangea arborescens, an indigenous plant found in many parts of the United States, was introduced to the notice of the medical profession by Dr. S. W. Butler, of Burlington, N. J., through the *New Jersey Medical Reporter*. Dr. Butler states that his father, who is connected with the mission to the Cherokees, learned of them the merits of this plant in the treatment of gravel and stone, and has himself, for many years, employed it in the course of an extensive practice among a people peculiarly subject to these complaints; he considers it as a most valuable medicine, and possessed, perhaps, of specific properties claiming for it a trial at the hands of practitioners. Dr. Butler's formula is as follows:—

Take of the Root of hydrangea	. . .	2 pounds.
Water	. . . . . .	12 pints.

Boil to four pints, strain, and add

Honey	. . . . . .	2 pints.

Boil further to two pints.

We have modified it thus:—

Take of Hydrangea	. . . .	16 ounces.
Water	. . . . . .	6 pints, or sufficient.

Boil the root in successive portions of water, mix them, and evaporate to half a pint; mix this with

Honey	. . . . . .	2 pints.

and evaporate to 2 pints. In the summer season push the evaporation somewhat farther, and add brandy, half a pint.

The dose is a teaspoonful twice or three times a day.

I have prepared fluid extract of hydrangea for several years, during which time I have dispensed it, under the direction of several practitioners, to numerous patients, and with general satisfactory results, in irritable conditions of the urethra, though its value as a specific remedy requires confirmation.

The plant is abundant in many localities; I have gathered it on the west banks of Schuylkill, about six to eight miles above Philadelphia.

Fluid Extract of Rhubarb and Senna.

The peculiar fitness of rhubarb and senna to be associated together in one cathartic preparation, so as to modify and assist each other, has led Prof. Procter to propose a fluid extract prepared as follows: (*Am. Journ. Pharm.*, vol. xxv. p. 23.)

Take of Senna, in coarse powder	.	Twelve ounces.
Rhubarb	. . . . .	Four ounces.
Bicarbonate of potassa	. .	Half ounce.
Sugar	. . . . .	Eight ounces.
Tincture of ginger	. . .	A fluidounce.
Oil of cloves	. . . .	Eight minims.
" aniseed	. . . .	Sixteen minims.
Water and alcohol, of each	.	A sufficient quantity.

Mix the senna and rhubarb (by grinding them together in a convenient way), pour upon them two pints of diluted alcohol, allow them to macerate 24 hours, and introduce the mixture into a percolator, furnished below with a stopcock or cork, to regulate the flow. A mixture of one part of alcohol and three of water, should now be poured on above, so as to keep a constant, but slow displacement of the absorbed menstruum, until one gallon of tincture has passed. Evaporate this in a water bath to eleven fluidounces; dissolve in it the sugar and bicarbonate of potassa, and after straining, add the tincture of ginger, holding the oils in solution, and mix; when done, the whole should measure a pint. The object in adding the alkaline carbonate in this fluid extract, is to prevent the griping which is apt to result from the use of the senna. The aromatics contribute to the same end. In making this and other fluid extracts, observe precautions under head of Evaporation.

Savery's Fluid Extract of Serpentaria.

The first published formula which appeared for a concentrated preparation of this valuable indigenous root was by John B. Savery, in his inaugural thesis in the *American Journal of Pharmacy*, vol. xxiii. p. 119. It is as follows:—

Take of Virginia snakeroot
Sugar, in powder, of each . Eight ounces.
Water
Alcohol, of each . . . A sufficient quantity.

The root is to be finely ground, and, after having macerated for a day or two in a pint of alcohol, is to be introduced into a displacer, and diluted alcohol poured on it until four pints shall have passed. The tincture thus obtained should be evaporated with a gentle heat and constant agitation, until it measures 12 fluidounces; the sugar is then to be dissolved, and the whole to be strained through flannel. This forms a clear, syrupy liquid (any resinous matter separated on mixing the more aqueous with the strong alcoholic tincture is dissolved on the addition of the sugar); it is free from the objection of containing an inconvenient quantity of alcohol, which pertains to the tincture, while the intense bitterness and powerful camphoraceous taste of the drug, are relieved by the presence of the sugar.

The dose is half a fluidrachm, representing 15 grains of the root.

Taylor's Fluid Extract of Serpentaria.

Alfred B. Taylor's process, vol. xx. p. 207, *Am. Journ. Pharmacy*, yields a preparation double the strength of the above, and belonging to the *second class* of fluid extracts. It is as follows:—

Take of Serpentaria, bruised . . Twelve ounces.
Alcohol
Water, of each . . A sufficient quantity.

Mix the serpentaria with 12 ounces of alcohol, and allow it to stand for twenty-four hours; then transfer it to a percolator, and pour alcohol gradually upon it, until a pint and a half of filtered liquor is obtained. Place this in an evaporating dish, and allow it to evaporate spontaneously, until reduced to six fluidounces. To the root, exhausted by alcohol, add water and displace till it is exhausted, or until about three pints have passed; evaporate this portion in a water bath to six fluidounces, mix the two parts together and filter. Each fluidounce of this represents one ounce of the root.

DOSE, from 15 to 45 drops.

Extractum Jalapæ Fluidum.—PROF. PROCTER.

In making a formula for this preparation it is necessary to use a menstruum that will dissolve the resin upon which its activity is to depend, and the liquid which is to remain in the preparation should possess the same solvent powers. Moreover, in reference to strength, it is best to take that of the fluid extract of rhubarb and of senna as the type—ounce to the fluidounce. Hence, it must be at least partially an alcoholic fluid extract, and not a saccharine one, as in the case of rhubarb. The following is the formula, from *Am. Journ. of Pharm.*, vol. xxix. page 108, viz:—

Take Jalap of good quality . .	Sixteen ounces (Troy).
Sugar	Eight ounces.
Carbonate of potassa . .	Half an ounce.
Alcohol	
Water, of each . . .	A sufficient quantity.

Reduce the jalap to coarse powder, pour on it one pint of a mixture of two parts alcohol and one water, and allow it to stand twenty-four hours. Then introduce it into a percolator, and pour ordinary diluted alcohol slowly on until half a gallon of liquid has passed. Evaporate this in a water bath, or still, till reduced to one half, then add the sugar and carbonate of potassa, and evaporate till reduced to twelve fluidounces. Put the liquid thus obtained, while yet warm, in a pint bottle, and add four fluidounces of alcohol, and mix by agitation.

The alkali forms a resinous soap with the jalap resin, greatly increasing its solubility in water, and at the same time renders the preparation less griping.

The object of the sugar is also to aid in the retention of the resinous matter in a fluid condition, as well as to mask the taste of the jalap. The dose will vary from fifteen minims to a fluidrachm according to the effect desired. By means of this preparation, the physician may prescribe jalap in mixtures with great facility, and avoid the large proportion of alcohol unavoidable when he resorts to the officinal tincture.

Fluid Extracts of Ergot.

This preparation was originally described by Jos. Laidley, of Richmond, Va., in a paper published in the *Stethoscope*, Jan. 1852, in which, however, the recipe for its preparation was not given in the usual way. Since that time, the following was published by T. Roberts Baker, of the same place. (See *Am. Journ. Pharm.*, vol. xxvii. p. 302.)

Take of Ergot, freshly powdered . .	2 lbs. com.
Ether	
Alcohol (80 per cent.)	
Water	
Simple syrup, of each . .	Sufficient.

1st. Displace the ergot with ether until it comes through nearly colorless, and evaporate spontaneously to procure the oil.

2d. Displace with alcohol to exhaustion, and evaporate by water bath (or regulated heat) to a thin syrupy consistence.

3d. Displace with water to exhaustion, and evaporate the resulting liquid as fast as obtained, to guard against chemical changes. Then strain to separate albumen, and mix the alcoholic extract, continuing the evaporation to a syrupy consistence. Incorporate the evaporated mixture first with the oil as obtained by the ether, and then with sufficient simple syrup to make up the measure of two pints. To each fluidrachm of this add one minim of oil of peppermint. The dose is f℥j, equal to ℈ij of the powder.

Prof. Procter's Fluid Extract of Ergot.

Take of Ergot, in powder, . . 8 ounces (Troy).
Ether,
Alcohol,
Water,
Diluted acetic acid, of each . A sufficient quantity.

Pack the ergot moderately in a suitable percolator, and pour on ether slowly, until a pint and a half of tincture has passed; and having spread the residue of the ergot on paper, suffer the adhering ether to pass off by evaporation. Meanwhile agitate well the ethereal tincture with two fluidounces of diluted acetic acid, and in a proper distillatory arrangement recover the ether by means of a water bath heat. Add two fluidounces of water to the oily residue, agitate, and, when subsided, decant the oil from the watery fluid, and set them separately aside.

Prepare a menstruum of two pints of water, half a pint of alcohol, and two fluidounces of diluted acetic acid, and having moistened the ergot residue with a pint of it, allow it to macerate two hours; introduce it into a percolator, and displace with the remainder of the menstruum, slowly, till exhausted. Mix this liquid with the acetic washings of the oil, and evaporate by means of a gentle heat (say 150° F.) till reduced to four fluidounces. To this when cold, add four fluidounces of alcohol, separate the gummy precipitate by filtering, and wash the filter with sufficient diluted alcohol to make the fluid extract of ergot measure eight fluidounces.

Fluid extract of ergot, thus prepared, is a laudanum colored fluid, thin consistence, a mild ergot odor and taste. A fluidrachm represents sixty grains of ergot, and the dose is from twenty minims to one-half of a teaspoonful, or by adding a teaspoonful to a tablespoonful of sweetened water, a teaspoonful of the mixture will equal ten or twelve grains of ergot.

The reason urged for complicating the process by the preliminary ethereal treatment is that ergot contains nearly, if not quite, a third of its weight in fixed oil, which shields the particles from the action of the watery menstruum, and obstructs its thorough action. If omitted, more care will be required in the exhaustion of the ergot with the menstruum directed. (*American Journal of Pharmacy*, vol. xxix. p. 543.)

Dr. Thayer has also published his process for fluid extract of ergot; he operates upon one hundred pounds of the coarsely powdered drug, preferring diluted alcohol as the menstruum, as a result of his experiments upon the residue left after its use, and after four or five days' maceration thoroughly extracts by displacement. The tincture being divided into different portions, the strongest is evaporated first, and afterwards the weaker portions of the displaced liquid, adding sugar to protect the extractive matter somewhat from the effects of heat, and to prevent its deposit on the bottom and sides of the pan. The temperature maintained in the vacuum pan during the evaporation ranges from 110° to 125°. At the close of the evaporation a portion of strong alcohol is added to the fluid extract, which dissolves the precipitates formed during its concentration.

Fluid Extract of Ergot. W. T. WATSON.

Take of Freshly powdered ergot . .	4 ounces (Troy).
Diluted alcohol (made by mixing one part of 95 per cent. alcohol with four parts of water) . .	1 pint.
Water	A sufficient quantity.
Alcohol	6 fluidounces.

Macerate the ergot in the diluted alcohol for four days, then transfer to a percolator, and when the liquid ceases to pass, pour on water until two pints have come through; by means of a water bath evaporate to six fluidounces, to this add the alcohol and mix; let it stand, with occasional agitation, for twelve hours, and filter. When finished, it is of a dark Madeira wine color, possessing a strong odor and taste of ergot. One fluidrachm or a teaspoonful of this extract represents twenty grains of ergot.—*Am. Journ. of Pharm.*, vol. xxviii. p. 519.

Fluid Extract of Taraxacum.

1st Process. By PROF. PROCTER, 1848.

Take of fresh dandelion root, collected in September or October, thirty-two ounces; slice it transversely, and reduce it to a pulp by bruising; mix this with one-sixth of its bulk of alcohol; macerate for twenty-four hours; then express strongly; add a pint of water containing a little alcohol, and again express; evaporate the liquid to twelve fluidounces; add four fluidounces of alcohol, and filter. A teaspoonful of this fluid extract represents half a drachm of extract of dandelion obtained from the fresh juice, which is several times the strength of that obtained by boiling the roots in water.

If alcohol should be objected to, eight ounces of sugar may replace it in the above, it being dissolved by agitation.

In this country, every one may obtain fresh roots of dandelion at the proper season, and may make the preparation but once a year; but where this is neglected, the carefully preserved dried root may be substituted, sixteen ounces being equal to thirty-two of the fresh. The dried root is to be powdered coarsely, and treated with alcohol and water by maceration, expressed, evaporated, and finished as directed.

2d Process. By PROF. PROCTER, 1853.

Take of Fresh dandelion root . . . 20 pounds (com.).
Alcohol (835°). . . . . 4 pints.

Slice the roots transversely, in short sections, and by means of a mill or mortar and pestle, reduce them to a pulpy mass; then add the alcohol, and mix them thoroughly. The mixture thus far prepared at the season when the root is proper for collection, may be set aside in suitable vessels (stoneware jars are appropriate), and extracted as the preparation is needed through the other seasons. After having stood a week, or until a convenient time, the pulpy mass is subjected to powerful pressure, until as much as possible of the fluid is removed. This is then filtered and bottled for use. It is necessary that sufficient time should elapse after the pulp is set aside for the alcohol to penetrate the fibrous particles and commingle with the natural juices, as well as for the woody structure of the root to lose its elasticity, that it may yield the juice more completely on pressure. When the pulp has stood six months in this, it yields the juice with great readiness, and is possessed of the sensible properties of the dandelion in a marked degree. When eight pounds, avoirdupois, of the root are thus treated, after standing several months, the practical result is about six pints of fluid with an ordinary screw press. This yield will vary in amount with the condition of the root when collected, and the length of time it is exposed afterwards, as well as the power of press used. Should the alcohol in this preparation be contraindicated, it might be partially removed by exposure in a water bath until the juice is reduced to five-sixths of its bulk; then for every pint of the residue, eight officinal ounces of sugar may be dissolved in it. The name *Succus Taraxaci Paratus* has been applied to this preparation, which resembles the English preserved juice.

3d Process.

Macerate four pounds of the recently dried root, in sufficient cold water, for twenty-four hours, expressing and evaporating to thirty-six fluidounces, to which liquid twelve fluidounces of alcohol is added; hence each fluidounce of the preparation represents an ounce of the *dried* root.

The evaporation of an aqueous solution of taraxacum is almost sure to have an unfavorable effect on its medical properties; it is well known that the solid extract, when prepared by the old process of decoction and evaporation in an exposed water bath, is greatly inferior to the best inspissated juice prepared in vacuo.

4th Process.

The only remaining process to be noticed is that for preparing the fluid from the solid extract, which is only employed where expedition is the desideratum. The following is the formula:—

Take of Extractum of dandelion, *U. S. P.* Four ounces.
Alcohol . . . . . . One fluidounce.
Water . . . . . . A sufficient quantity.

Triturate the extract with the water and the alcohol, and apply a gentle heat, till it is dissolved, taking care that the product measures just half a pint.

These processes yield a liquid which is substantially the same in physical and medical properties. The usual dose is a teaspoonful. It is a more convenient preparation for ordinary use than the solid extract, which is not well adapted to the pilular form, on account of the largeness of its dose.

Fluid Extract of Gentian. PROF. PROCTER.[1]

Take of Gentian, in coarse powder,	Sixteen ounces.
Water	A sufficient quantity.
French brandy . .	Six fluidounces.

Macerate the gentian in two and a half pints of water for twelve hours, and having introduced it into a suitable percolator, allow the infusion to pass slowly, adding water at intervals, until five pints of liquid have passed. Evaporate this to ten fluidounces by means of a water bath, add the brandy, and strain through cotton flannel; this fluid extract may be given in doses of half a teaspoonful to a teaspoonful, which represent half a drachm to a drachm of the root.

"When it is desirable to associate aromatics, they may be added in the form of tincture, in place of a part of the brandy, or the aromatics in substance may be extracted by the brandy, and the tincture thus formed added to the evaporated solution of gentian."—*Am. Journ. of Pharm.*, vol. xxvi.

Fluid Extract of Galls.

The following is for a preparation which has been occasionally used by dentists in Philadelphia; as it may be called for in the course of practice, it is introduced here:—

Take of Galls, in coarse powder .	℥viij.
Alcohol	Sufficient to make a pint.

Extract by displacement.

Used as a powerful astringent application.

Fluid Extract of Lobelia.

The chemical and pharmaceutical history of lobelia inflata, one of our most interesting and valuable indigenous plants, is connected with the labors of Wm. Procter, Jr., now professor of Pharmacy in the Philadelphia College of Pharmacy, and editor of the *American Journal of Pharmacy.* In 1837, he wrote his inaugural thesis for graduation in the institution with which he is now so honorably connected, on lobelia. In this paper, which was published in the *Journal* (vol. ix. p. 98), he gave a full chemical history of the plant, and proved the existence in it of a peculiar alkaline acrid principle, for which he proposed the name of *lobelina.*

Subsequently, in 1841, he called attention in a paper published in vol. xiii. p. 1, to lobelina and some other principles of the plant, and

[1] See also process of Thayer, *Peninsular and Independent*, Sept. 1858.

showed the advantage of fixing this alkaloid by the use of an acid, in making those preparations of lobelia requiring the application of heat.

In 1842, he again appears in the *Journal* in an article on some preparations of this drug, in which the principles already ascertained are applied in practice. The acetous extract, vinegar and syrup, there introduced, have not been made officinal, but the former is introduced under its appropriate heading in this work.

In 1852, the fluid extract of lobelia was proposed by Prof. Procter, and the following formula published in vol. xxiv. p. 207 of the *Journal*:—

Take of	Lobelia (the plant), finely bruised	Eight ounces.
	Acetic acid	One fluidounce.
	Diluted alcohol	Three pints.
	Alcohol	Six fluidounces.

Macerate the lobelia in a pint and a half of the diluted alcohol, previously mixed with the acetic acid, for twenty-four hours; introduce the mixture into an earthen displacer; pour on slowly the remainder of the diluted alcohol, and afterwards water, until three pints of tincture are obtained; evaporate this in a water bath to ten fluidounces; strain; add the alcohol, and, when mixed, filter through paper. Each teaspoonful of this preparation is equal to half a fluidounce of the tincture. The dose would vary from five drops, as a narcotic and expectorant, to twenty or thirty as an emetic.

Extractum Anthemidis Fluidum. PROF. PROCTER.

Take of	Chamomile flowers	Eight ounces (Troy).
	Sugar	Eight ounces.
	Alcohol,	
	Diluted alcohol, of each	A sufficient quantity.

Bruise the chamomile thoroughly, pour on it a pint of alcohol, and macerate for twenty-four hours, pack it moderately tight in a percolator, and pour on slowly diluted alcohol, until a pint of liquid has passed; then change the recipient, and continue the process until two pints more of tincture are obtained. Evaporate the first tincture by a gentle heat, or spontaneously, to six fluidounces, and the other in a water bath to four fluidounces, mix the liquids, add the sugar to them, dissolve by a gentle heat, and finally add alcohol until the whole measures a pint.

The dose of this preparation is from one to two teaspoonfuls as an anti-periodic, or half a teaspoonful as a tonic; a fluidrachm represents thirty grains of chamomile flowers.—*American Journal of Pharmacy*, vol. xxix. p. 111.

Fluid Extract Calamus.

A strong tincture of calamus was suggested by John M. Maisch, in his article on "The Use of our Indigenous Materia Medica," *Proceedings Amer. Pharm. Association*, 1857. To be made by treating four ounces of the root with a mixture of two parts of alcohol to one of water, so as to obtain a pint. This would be a convenient preparation, each fluidrachm representing fifteen grains of the root; it would scarcely come under the head of fluid extracts by any standard of strength as yet established for these preparations, and is introduced here as the only concentrated preparation of this root heretofore proposed.

Extractum Ipecacuanhæ Fluidum. Dr. R. H. STABLER.

Take of	Pulv. ipecac.	℥iiss.
	Alcoholis diluti	q. s.

Macerate the ipecacuanha in eight fluidounces of dilute alcohol for twelve hours, and displace with the same menstruum till exhausted, evaporate by a steam bath to seven and a half fluidounces; filter. Three minims are equal to one grain of ipecac.—*Proceedings Am. Pharm. Association*, 1857.

Fluid Extract of Sanguinaria. SAMUEL CAMPBELL.

Take of	Sanguinaria Canadensis	8 oz.
	Acetic acid, No. 8	2 oz.
	Water	10 oz.
	Sugar	8 oz.
	Diluted alcohol	q. s.

Reduce the root to a coarse powder, then incorporate it with the acetic acid, previously mixed with the water. After allowing it to macerate for forty-eight hours, transfer to a glass percolator, and exhaust by means of diluted alcohol. By means of a water bath evaporate the tincture to twelve fluidounces, then add the sugar, and, when dissolved, strain.

The preparation is of a deep red color, with an intensely acrid taste. Each fluidrachm represents thirty grains of the root.—*Amer. Journ. Pharm.*, vol. xxx. p. 221.

Fluid Extract of Wild Cherry Bark. PROF. PROCTER.

Take of	Wild cherry bark	24 oz. (Troy.)
	Sweet almonds	3 oz. "
	Pure granulated sugar	36 oz.[1] "
	Alcohol (88 per cent.),	
	Water, each	A sufficient quantity.

Macerate the powdered bark in two pints of alcohol for eight hours, introduce it into a percolator, and pour on it alcohol until five pints have passed, observing to regulate the passage of the liquid by a cork or stopcock. Introduce the tincture into a capsule, or distillatory apparatus, if the alcohol is to be regained, and evaporate it to a syrupy consistence; add half a pint of water, and again evaporate till the alcohol is entirely removed. Beat the almonds, without blanching, into a smooth paste with a little of the water, and then sufficient to make the emulsion measure a pint and a half, and pour it into a quart bottle previously containing the solution of the extract of bark, cork it securely and agitate occasionally for twenty-four hours, so as to give

[1] This may be substituted by sugar of milk, 8 ounces, and the preparation has then a less decidedly syrupy character.

time for the decomposition of the amygdaline. The mixture is then to be quickly expressed and filtered into a bottle containing the sugar, marked to hold three pints. Water should be added to the dregs and they again expressed till sufficient liquor is obtained to make the fluid extract measure three pints. The proportion of sugar, though less than that in syrup, is sufficient to preserve the preparation, aided by the preparation of the hydrocyanic acid.

The dose is a teaspoonful, which is equivalent to a wineglassful of the officinal infusion.—*Amer. Journ. Pharm.*, vol. xxviii. p. 108.

Ferrated Fluid Extract of Wild Cherry Bark. W. R. WARNER.

Take of Cortex pruni Virg. contus. . . . ℥xij.
Amygdalæ dulc. . . . . . ℥ij.
Ferri oxyd. hydrat. . . . . ℥ss.
Sacch. albi . . . . . . ℥xij.
Ferri citratis,
Alcoholis,
Aquæ font., āā . . . . . . q. s.

First exhaust the bark of its tonic principles with the alcoholic menstruum, and evaporate the resulting alcoholic tincture carefully to expel the alcohol, and then mix the residue with six ounces of water, and add the hydrated sesquioxide of iron; allow it to macerate for six hours, occasionally agitating, and filter into a bottle containing an emulsion of almonds (amygd. dulcis ℥ij., aqua pura ℥vj). When the reaction has ceased between the emulsin and the amygdalin, it is again filtered and the sugar added, and for every ounce thus to be prepared add 24 grs. of citrate of iron, previously dissolved in water sufficient to make the whole fluid extract measure twenty-four fluidounces. The addition of iron to the bitter principle and hydrocyanic acid of the simple extract of wild cherry, I think should render it much more efficient as a tonic, and greatly add to the value of the preparation.—*Am. Journ. Pharm.*, vol. xxx. p. 315.

Fluid Extract of Lupulin. PROF. PROCTER.

Take of Lupulin . . . Four ounces (Troy).
Alcohol,
Rectified ether, of each A sufficient quantity.

Put the lupulin in a glass displacer, pour upon it four fluidounces of ether, and then sufficient alcohol to gain six fluidounces by slow percolation, and set the liquid aside. Then continue the displacement with alcohol till ten fluidounces of liquid has passed. Evaporate this to two fluidounces and mix with it the ethereal tincture, and by means of a heat of 100° F., or spontaneously, let the ether evaporate, so that the resulting fluid extract shall measure four fluidounces. As a minim equals a grain of lupulin, the physician can easily regulate the dose.—*Am. Journ. Pharm.*, vol. xxix. p. 28.

Fluid Extract of Cimicifuga.

In an article on the pharmacy of cimicifuga, Prof. Procter proposes the following formula, which has been found very satisfactory both pharmaceutically and medically. (See *Am. Journ. of Pharm.*, vol. xxvi. p. 106.)

Take of		
	Black snakeroot (recently dried)	Sixteen ounces.
	Ether	Half a pint.
	Alcohol	One pint.
	Diluted alcohol	A sufficient quantity.

Powder the black snakeroot and introduce it into a displacer, suited to volatile liquids; pour upon it the ether mixed with the strong alcohol, closing the lower orifice, so that the liquid shall pass by drops. When the menstruum disappears above, immediately add diluted alcohol until the filtered tincture measures a pint and a half; set this aside in a capsule in a warm place until it is reduced to half a pint, and has lost its ethereal odor; meanwhile continue the percolation with diluted alcohol until two pints more tincture are obtained. Evaporate this in a water bath to eight fluidounces, and mix it gradually with the first product, so as to avoid as much as possible the precipitation of the resin from the latter. After standing a few hours, the fluid extract should be filtered, and, if it does not measure a pint, add sufficient alcohol to make that measure. If the amount of resin precipitated is considerable, it may be separated by a cloth strainer, re-dissolved in a little alcohol, and added to the solution, which should then be filtered.

As thus prepared, the fluid extract has a dark, reddish-brown color, like laudanum; is transparent, and possesses the bitter disagreeable taste of the root, in a marked degree. A fluidrachm represents about a drachm of the root. The dose usually given is from thirty to sixty drops.

Fluid Extract of Uva Ursi. By J. M. MAISCH.

Take of		
	Leaves of uva ursi	℥xvj.
	Alcohol and water, each	A sufficient quantity.
	Sugar	℥xij.

Reduce the leaves to a moderately fine powder, pour upon them ten ounces each of alcohol previously mixed, and after macerating for 24 hours, displace slowly with a mixture of three parts water to one of alcohol, until the powder is exhausted. Then evaporate to one pint and strain.

Fluid Extract of Hyoscyamus. C. AUG. SMITH.

Take of		
	Hyoscyamus leaves (garbled)	Eight ounces (Troy).
	Diluted alcohol	A sufficient quantity.
	Sugar	Eight ounces (Troy).

Reduce the hyoscyamus to a coarse powder; pour over it a pint of diluted alcohol; allow it to macerate twenty-four hours; put it into a suitable percolator, and, when carefully packed, pour gradually upon it diluted alcohol, until three pints of tincture has passed. The flow should be very slow, so that thorough exhaustion of the leaves shall take place. The tincture is then evaporated to ten fluidounces—the sugar dissolved in it while hot, and when cold, two fluidounces of alcohol (.835 sp. gr., or as much as is sufficient to make the whole measure a pint) is added, and the fluid extract passed through a fine muslin strainer.

This preparation affords an admirable means of prescribing henbane in fluid preparations. The alcohol of the tincture is avoided, and the trouble of incorporating the solid extract superseded. It is of the same proportional strength as the fluid extract of valerian, and the dose varies from fifteen drops to half a teaspoonful, the latter dose being equivalent to two or three grains of extract.

When the apothecary has in possession solid extract of hyoscyamus of ascertained good quality, a fluid extract of similar strength may be obtained by triturating half an ounce of the extract with ten fluidounces of water, till dissolved; eight ounces of sugar dissolved in it, and, finally, sufficient alcohol in it to make it measure a pint, and strain. Practically, henbane yields but 5 per cent. of extract; the above recipe assumes it to be 6¼ per cent., a difference altogether proper in view of the possible injury to the juices in preparing the extract originally.

Fluid Extract of Cornus Florida.

Notwithstanding the almost universal assent of the medical profession to the value of this tonic, its general employment as a domestic remedy, and the belief of many that in its effects it is nearly allied to cinchona bark, there has not yet been generally introduced a single liquid preparation except the officinal decoction, the employment of which is avoided, as it should be. Maisch has prepared a fluid extract by exhausting sixteen ounces of the powdered bark with diluted alcohol, evaporating to about a pint, dissolving twelve ounces (officinal) of sugar, and completing the process by evaporating to sixteen fluidounces. A teaspoonful of this represents a drachm of the bark. A small proportion of the exterior skin of the fresh orange-peel may be added to advantage.

Fluid Extract of Scutellaria Laterifolia.

Skullcap, though not much prescribed by regular physicians, is greatly esteemed by the eclectic practitioners, who employ it in several different preparations in the treatment of nervous irritation. The mode of preparation indicated by Maisch is to exhaust sixteen ounces of the powdered herb by the use successively of diluted alcohol, and a mixture of four parts of water and one of alcohol, then to evaporate the mixed liquids to about a pint, add one pound (officinal) of sugar, and further evaporate to one pint.

Fluid Extract of Marrubium Vulgare.

Horehound ranks as a tonic, and is much used in the form of syrup, candy, and hot infusion as a domestic remedy for *colds*, incident to our changeable climate.

The fluid extract may be made exactly as the foregoing, substituting horehound for the skullcap.—*Proceedings Am. Pharm. Assoc.*, 1857.

Fluid Extract of Dulcamara.

Among the contributions of J. M. Maisch to this branch of Pharmacy, is the excellent formula which follows for one of our most valuable though neglected alterative narcotics.

Macerate sixteen ounces of bittersweet stalks with a mixture of two parts of alcohol and one of water, then exhaust it thoroughly by percolation. Evaporate the resulting tincture on a water bath to about one-half, then mix with two drachms of acetic acid, and continue the evaporation till all the alcohol is driven off, adding eight ounces of sugar, and discontinuing the evaporation when the liquid measures twelve fluidounces, strain it through close flannel, to separate a little chlorophyl and resin, and while still warm, add four fluidounces of alcohol, to make it measure one pint. Each fluidrachm of this represents a drachm of dulcamara, a full dose. The acetic acid is used to render the *solanine* soluble in the aqueous menstruum, which predominates as the alcohol is dissipated.

Fluid Extract of Sumbul. PROF. PROCTER.

Take of	Musk-root	Four ounces.
	Ether	Four fluidounces.
	Alcohol and water, of each . . .	Sufficient.

Bruise the root, moistened with a little alcohol, until reduced to a coarse powder. Mix the ether with twice its volume of alcohol, pour it on the musk-root, macerate in a covered vessel for 24 hours, and introduce into a suitable percolator. The absorbed tincture, which has a light-brown color, is displaced slowly by alcohol (sp. gr. .835), until twelve fluidounces are obtained, when the process is continued with a mixture of equal parts of alcohol and water, until a pint has passed. Water is then poured on the residue until a pint of liquid has filtered. The ethereo-alcoholic tincture is suffered to evaporate in a warm place until reduced to two fluidounces; the hydro-alcoholic tincture is concentrated on a water bath to the same bulk; and the watery infusion evaporated to one fluidounce. The two last liquids are now mixed, three fluidounces of alcohol added to the first (ethereal) liquid, to dissolve the oleo-resin, and the other mixture added gradually with agitation, so that the whole will measure eight fluidounces, the mixture afterwards shaken occasionally for 24 hours. A portion of oleo-resin, and some gummy extractive remain undissolved, and must either be removed by filtration or left as a sediment.

When the ethereo-alcoholic tincture is evaporated to one-sixth, nearly all the oleo-resin separates, and hence the necessity of redissolving this by alcohol before adding the other liquids.

The dose of this is fifteen minims to f℥j. It has the odor of musk and the antispasmodic effects of valerian. The root is used in Russia in delirium tremens, and has been somewhat prescribed in Philadelphia and elsewhere in a variety of nervous affections.—*Am. Journ. Pharm.*, vol. xxvi. p. 233.

Fluid Extracts of the Third Class. Oleo-Resins.

See Syllabus, page 196.

Cubebs, pepper, ginger, capsicum, filix mas, asarum Canadense, cardamom, parsley, ergot, and mustard yield more or less fluid, oily extracts, on the spontaneous evaporation of their ethereal tinctures. These have been but little introduced as yet, and there has been very little written about them.

Extractum Cubebæ Fluidum, U. S. P. (*Fluid Extract of Cubebs.*)

Take of Cubebs, in powder . . . . . A pound.
Ether . . . . A sufficient quantity.

Put the cubebs into a percolator, and, having packed it carefully, pour ether gradually upon it until two pints of filtered liquor are obtained; then distil off, by means of a water bath, at a gentle heat, a pint and a half of the ether. Expose the residue in a shallow vessel, until the whole of the ether has evaporated.

This preparation varies with the quality of the cubebs employed, being more or less pungent and fluid, according to the amount of essential oil it contains. Cubebs yield about one-sixth its weight of the oleo-resin. Dose, five to thirty drops, on sugar, or in the form of mixture or pill.

Extractum Piperis Fluidum, U. S. P. (*Fluid Extract of Pepper.*)

Made as the foregoing.

It deposits piperin in crystals as the ether evaporates, and the officinal directions require this ingredient to be removed by expression through a cloth. Black pepper yields a little over 6 per cent. of the oleo-resin. The oil of black pepper of commerce, which is a residuary product of the manufacture of piperin, is chiefly substituted for this, with which it is nearly identical. The dose is one or two drops. Its chief use is as an adjuvant to pill masses.

Oleo-Resin, or Piperoid of Ginger.

Treat powdered ginger by displacement, with a mixture of one part of alcohol and four of ether, until nearly exhausted of its taste and odor; expose this ethereal tincture to spontaneous evaporation, until deprived of the odor of ether. The resulting oleo-resin is a dark-brown, transparent, oily liquid, extremely pungent, insoluble in water, but soluble in ether and strong alcohol. Ginger is said to contain about 1½ per cent. vol. oil, and $3\frac{8}{10}$ per cent. soft resin. The proportion yielded by the root, treated as above, varies with the commercial variety of ginger. A commercial pound of African ginger yielded, by this process, one and a half ounces, or 9.3 per cent., while the same quantity of the Jamaica variety yielded only one ounce—6.2 per cent. That from the African was darker in color, thicker, and somewhat less pleasant than the other. One ounce of the piperoid added to twenty pounds of melted sugar, make "ginger drops" of about the usual pungency.

Oleo-Resin of Capsicum.—Capsicum owes its intense fiery taste, and its powerful stimulating properties to a peculiar principle soluble in ether, about four per cent. of which is said to exist in the fruit deprived of seeds. The preparation named above is an impure form of this. It is too powerful for convenient use.

Oil of Male Fern.—Oil of filix mas, usually extracted from the powdered rhizome, is used as a remedy for tapeworm. It is extracted by ether, which is afterwards allowed to evaporate spontaneously, and leaves a dark-green colored oily liquid, having the odor of the plant. The dose directed to expel *tænia* is eighteen grains, or from ten to twenty-five drops at night, and repeated in the morning. It should be made into an emulsion.

Oil of Asarum Canadense.—Canada snakeroot or wild ginger is prepared in the same way; it is used chiefly as a perfume; it is also gratefully stimulant in small doses, being not unlike ginger in its properties.

Oil of cardamom, prepared in the same way with ether, is an impure oily fluid, containing both the fixed and volatile oil of the seeds, and esteemed a powerful carminative stimulant; it is little known to practitioners.

Oil of parsley is a diuretic remedy, sometimes called *apiol.* It is prepared by treating parsley seeds with strong alcohol, and subsequently with ether or chloroform; these menstrua are then distilled off, and the oil may be further purified if desired. It is also prepared by the spontaneous evaporation of an ethereal tincture, as in the other cases. It is highly charged with the odor of the plant, of which it is probably the chief active constituent. DOSE, 3 or 4 drops in a day.

Oil of Ergot.—Under this name a brown colored, acrid, oily liquid is sold in the shops, which is obtained by treating powdered ergot with ether, or a mixture of ether and alcohol, and evaporating off the menstruum. Its most bulky ingredient is the peculiar bland fixed oil, which, according to the experiments of T. Roberts Baker, is nearly isomeric with castor oil. My friend, Ambrose Smith, informs me that he has found oil of ergot, when made with pure ether, to become inconveniently thick—almost solid; which difficulty is obviated by adding a portion of alcohol to the ether employed. Although the pure fixed oil is destitute of any of the effects of ergot, this preparation, owing to its other ingredients, is more or less active. Its dose, in cases of labor, to promote uterine contractions, is from 20 to 50 drops.

CHAPTER XIII.

OF SYRUPS.

THE term syrup is applied to any saturated or nearly saturated solution of sugar in water, and there are numerous simple, medicated, and flavored syrups used in medicine and pharmacy, both officinal and unofficinal. The kind of sugar used in the officinal preparations is that named on the list of the *Pharmacopœia*, saccharum, and called commonly white, sometimes loaf sugar, or, as more commonly met with now, broken down or crushed sugar. This, as supplied to our markets by the refineries, is nearly chemically pure cane sugar, and requires no further preparation for pharmaceutical use. It is soluble in less than half its weight of water; to a less extent in alcohol, and insoluble in ether. It crystallizes from its solution in the form of oblique rhombic crystals, containing water, and called, as found in the shops, rock candy. (*See* PART III.)

The advantages of the use of sugar in pharmaceutical preparations are, 1st. Its agreeable taste. 2d. The viscidity and blandness of its solution. 3d. Its conservative properties, when in sufficient proportion. It is chiefly objectionable in cases where, from want of tone in the digestive organs, it is liable to produce acidity of stomach, with its attendant symptoms.

Syrups are most used as expectorants, and in the treatment of the diseases of children, with whom a sweet taste goes far to reconcile otherwise disagreeable properties of a medicine. They are, also, much used with other and more active medicines, as adjuvants and vehicles. The first of this class to be noticed, is

Syrupus, U. S. P. (*Simple Syrup.*)

Take of Sugar . . Two pounds and a half (officinal.)
Water . . One pint.

Dissolve the sugar in the water by the aid of heat.

Syrup is a viscid liquid, constituted of two-thirds sugar and one-third water, and having a specific gravity, when boiling hot, of 1.261 (30° Baumé); or when cold, 1.319 (35° Baumé). Syrups prepared from the juices of fruits, or others which contain much extractive matter, mark about 2° or 3° higher on Baumé's scale. It is of a pure sweet taste, without odor, when freshly prepared. The boiling point is 221° F.

The proportion of sugar in syrup is a matter of primary importance, as, owing to the presence of minute quantities of nitrogenized principles, which are apt to be accidentally present, even in simple syrup, fermentation will be set up, unless the syrup has very nearly the full officinal proportion, which is about two parts, by weight, of sugar, to one of water (14,400 to 7,290 grs.).

My experience coincides with that of some others in preferring to make syrups with a very slight excess of water, and I prefer the following formula not only on account of the very great advantage gained in weighing large quantities by the substitution of the common commercial weights for the officinal, but also because it gives, on the whole, more satisfactory results. There is always some waste of the fluid by evaporation where heat is applied, and when the full officinal proportion is used (2½ lbs. officinal equal 14,400 grs.), a portion of sugar is liable to crystallize out on standing, and thus by abstracting sugar weakens the remainder.

Recipe for Simple Syrup.

	To make 2 pints.	To make 10 gallons.
Take of Sugar . .	2 lbs.	80 lbs. (commercial).
Water . .	1 pint	5 gallons.

Dissolve by the aid of a gentle heat.

The two pounds of sugar, when dissolved, are about equivalent to one pint of the liquid, by measure, so that the syrup resulting from these quantities would just about measure as above. It is, then, important to bear in mind the rule, which may be thus abbreviated: *Two parts of sugar are required by one part of water, and make two parts of syrup.*

The following curious rule is given by Dr. Ure for ascertaining the quantity of sugar in syrup: "The decimal part of the number denoting the sp. gr. of a syrup multiplied by 26, gives the number of pounds of sugar it contains per gallon very nearly." This appears to refer to the commercial and not the officinal weight.

In the absence of extraneous, and particularly of nitrogenized principles, a syrup will keep well enough in cold weather, without reference to its proportions; but in a majority of instances of medicated syrups, it is absolutely necessary to observe the above well-established rule, which insures a nearly saturated saccharine solution.

If impure or brown sugar is employed, it is necessary to boil the syrup until the proper specific gravity is attained; skimming or straining off the scum which contains the impurities; but when the sugar is pure, this is unnecessary.

If impurities are diffused in the liquid, which will not readily rise as scum, it is well to add, before applying heat, a little white of egg, previously beaten up with water, which, by its coagulating at the boiling temperature, forms a clot, inclosing the impurities, and facilitating their removal. A richer and more elegant syrup is produced by the use of Havana sugar, clarified in this way, than from the best refined sugar, and some of our most careful pharmaceutists use this process for their mineral water syrups, on account of its superior product, though so much more troublesome.

In some of the medicated syrups, a boiling temperature is directed, in order that the vegetable albumen contained in the medicinal ingredient may be coagulated, and thus separated. This should be done before adding the sugar, and the liquid should then be filtered so that a perfectly clear syrup may be obtained from the first. Syrups may be discolored by filtration through animal charcoal, and to obtain perfect transparency should be strained slowly, after they are partially cooled, through two or three thicknesses of flannel. In many instances, the presence in the drug, or in the menstruum employed, of antiseptic properties, insures the permanence of the preparation. Syrup of squill is an instance, in which, owing to the presence of the antiseptic element, acetic acid, in the menstruum, we are enabled to reduce the proportion of sugar somewhat below that necessary in other instances. Among the articles added to syrups, to prevent fermentation, the following may be mentioned:—

Essential oils, which, of course, greatly modify the taste and other properties of the preparation, as in compound syrup of sarsaparilla. *Brandy*, which is much used with aromatics; or, preferably to this, a small proportion of pure alcohol, which is directed by the London Pharmacopœia. *Glycerin*, which does not alter the taste or other properties of the preparation, but has not been sufficiently tried to speak with confidence of its eligibility. About 4 per cent. of *sugar of milk*. *Sulphite of lime*, a small proportion of which will effectually prevent or arrest fermentation, though it is liable to impart an odor unless afterwards subjected to heat. *Hoffmann's anodyne*, which is one of the very best antiseptics, though liable to the objection of imparting an ethereal odor and taste. It should, however, be added in small quantity only; one part, by measure, to seventy-five of syrup, which is stated to be proper, seems to me unnecessarily large. One fluidrachm to a pint has generally answered the purpose.

It must not be forgotten, in attempting to restore syrups that have fermented, that they have lost sugar in proportion to the amount of acetic acid produced, and this must be restored when they are heated, besides the addition of the antiseptic. Syrups should be kept in a cool, though not in a cold, place; those most liable to ferment, in small and well stopped bottles.

After these preliminary observations, the medicated syrups, classified with reference to their mode of preparation, may be introduced; those in the *Pharmacopœia* do not require the publication of the formulas, and are therefore separated in the syllabi.

SYRUPI, *U. S. P.*

1ST CLASS.—*Infusions or Decoctions rendered permanent by Sugar.*

Officinal Name.	Preparation.	Use.	Dose.
Syrupus aurantii corticis	By maceration with b. water	As an adjuvant	
" sennæ (with fennel)	By digestion with hot water	Laxative	f℥j to f℥ij.
" krameriæ	By displacement with cold water	Astringent	f℥ss.
" pruni Virginianæ		Sedative and tonic expectorant	"
" senegæ	By decoction	Stim. expectorant	fʒj to ʒij.
" scillæ comp.	"	"	♏ 20 to fʒj.

We have, in the above class, instances of three processes. In the treatment of orange-peel and senna, heat is applied below the boiling point, so as to form hot infusions. In the case of rhatany and wild cherry, cold infusions, by displacement, are directed, while seneka, and the mixed seneka and squill, are to be boiled in water, and the decoctions, after being strained and evaporated, are, like the others, made into syrup by the requisite addition of sugar.

In *syrup of orange-peel*, the fresh rind of the sweet, or Havana orange, is preferred to the bitter orange-peel prescribed in the various tonic preparations, this syrup being used for its flavor rather than for any medicinal effect. (See *Orange Syrup*.)

Syrup of senna is generally superseded by fluid extract of senna, which is preferred, owing to the comparative smallness of its dose.

Syrup of rhatany leaves nothing to be desired for its particular use; it is readily prepared, and is an elegant and efficient preparation.

Syrup of wild cherry is one of the most popular and really valuable of remedies, being much used in pulmonary affections, connected with an atonic condition of the systen. The preparation of this syrup requires the precaution of subjecting the powder to the action of water previous to displacement, as directed in the *Pharmacopœia*. I have also observed that the infusion acquires richness of flavor and color by standing until a precipitate begins to form in it, before adding the sugar. In this instance, less than the full proportion of sugar directed for syrups, generally, is sufficient to preserve it, owing to the production of hydrocyanic acid by the reaction of its proximate principle, this being an excellent antiseptic.

F. A. Figueroa has suggested the addition of glycerin to the water used in this preparation. He is thus able to diminish the quantity of sugar without endangering its permanency. He adds two fluidounces of glycerin to the pint, and then dissolves in the infusion only six ounces of sugar.

Syrup of seneka, and compound syrup of squill, are made either by the process of decoction, as above, when haste is an object, or otherwise, by the use of alcohol, as in the 2d Class, now to be introduced.

CLASS II.—*Extracted with Alcohol and Water, by displacement, concentrated by evaporation, and completed by the addition of Sugar.*

Officinal Name.	Proportion.	Use	Dose.
Syrupus ipecacuanhæ	℥ss in Oj of the syrup	Expectorant	fʒj to f℥ss.
" senegæ (2d process)		"	fʒj to fʒij.
" scillæ comp.	Squill and seneka, + tart. emetic, gr. j to f℥j		gtt. xx to fʒj.
" rhei	℥j in Oj of the syrup	Laxative	f℥ss to f℥iv.
" sarsaparillæ comp.	Sarsaparilla, guaiacum, roses, senna, liquorice root, and oils of sassafras, anise, and partridge berry	Alterative	f℥ss

The simplest statement of this process for making syrups, is the following: Of the drug, properly powdered, make a tincture by displacement; evaporate this in a capsule, to the point named in the *Pharmacopœia*, thus getting rid of the alcohol contained in it. Now add sugar, in the proportion of two parts to one of the liquid, and dissolve it dy the aid of heat.

Of this important class each individual should be carefully studied; the *Pharmacopœia* should always be in hand in preparing these and other officinal preparations, and, in making them, the officinal directions must be accurately observed. The importance of the use of officinal weights, or their equivalents in the commercial weights, need hardly be insisted upon. (*See* Chapter on Weights and Measures.)

Syrup of ipecac, as it is now generally called, although not a strong preparation, is one of the most useful expectorants we have, and in domestic practice is perhaps the most popular in Philadelphia. It is particularly adapted to the treatment of the catarrhs of children. The dose may be so regulated as to produce a gentle relaxing, or, in the case of children, a powerful emetic effect, with the advantage of causing neither stimulating nor depressing after-effects.[1]

Syrup of seneka is the most acrid of its class; its use is indicated in chronic catarrh not accompanied by inflammatory action; it is seldom urged so as to produce its emetic effect, except in combination with other remedies.

Coxe's hive syrup (syrupus scillæ compositus) has been for many years a very common remedy in croup. As originally prepared, it contained honey, which, being by many objected to from its alleged liability to ferment, was changed in the *Pharmacopœia* of 1840 to sugar, and the preparation was thus removed from mellita to syrupi. As now prepared, it is not popular either among physicians or pharmaceutists, the former regarding it as therapeutically, and the latter as pharmaceutically, objectionable. The officinal process for preparing it would be improved by the substitution of diluted alcohol for the weak alcoholic menstruum directed in preparing the tincture in the first part of the process. The precaution should not be neglected in this instance, as also in syrup of senega, of boiling this diluted alcoholic preparation during the evaporation, and filtering, before adding the sugar. A copious coagulation of the vegetable albumen takes place at the boiling temperature, the removal of which on the filter obviates, to some extent, the tendency to fermentation in the resulting syrup. The solution of the tartar emetic in the syrup should

[1] The process for making it may be varied, according to the suggestion of Joseph Laidley, of Richmond, Va., as follows: Make a concentrated tincture of ipecacuanha with strong alcohol, and evaporate it so that two fluidounces shall represent an ounce of the root; add a fluidounce of this to half a pint of simple syrup; evaporate to six fluidounces, and add eight fluidounces of syrup and two of water, which, when mixed, will constitute one pint of syrup of ipecac of the officinal strength. I do not recollect to have met with any difficulty in keeping this syrup in midsummer, when prepared strictly by the officinal formula.

be accomplished while it is hot, by trituration in a mortar, as prescribed under the head of Solution.

The liability of this preparation to ferment renders it one of the most troublesome of the syrups to the pharmaceutist. Of the numerous suggestions for its improvement, that of Wm. Hodgson, jr., to add fʒj of acetic acid to each, if inserted in the *Pharmacopœia* would perhaps be the most satisfactory. The addition of a few drachms of glycerin to each pint of the liquid employed, before adding the sugar, has a tendency to prevent fermentation.

In cases of croup, it is customary to increase the dose of hive syrup very much above that mentioned in the books, or to repeat it every fifteen or twenty minutes till the patient vomits. The dose for a child one year old may be ten drops, for one of two years fifteen, of three years twenty-five drops, and so on, repeated as above.

Simple syrup of rhubarb is very extensively used as a mild cathartic for children. Its mode of preparation is precisely that indicated for the class; its dose is from fʒj to f℥ss for children; that given in the Syllabus is adapted to adults.

Compound syrup of sarsaparilla is manufactured in very large quantities by regular pharmaceutists, and, after many fluctuations, has an extended reputation among practitioners of medicine, as well as the public at large. Its chief use is in skin diseases, and in syphilitic and scrofulous cases, in which it is used both alone and combined with mercurials, iodides, &c. Its composition is similar, though not identical, with the fluid extract; it contains, besides the soluble principles of sarsaparilla, those of guaiacum-wood, red roses, senna, and liquorice-root, extracted by diluted alcohol, evaporated, and made into a syrup, as before indicated for the syrups of this class. For the improvement of its flavor, and as antiseptics, the oils of anise, sassafras, and partridge-berry are directed to be added. The extensive range of diseases to which sarsaparilla is applicable, and the harmless character of the remedy, have made it a great favorite with empirics, so that there are an immense number of quack medicines sailing under its name, and not a few called alteratives and panaceas, which contain it as one of their ingredients. So numerous and so generally popular were these several years ago, that the period of their greatest popularity, from 1845 to 1850, has been called among druggists the "sarsaparilla era." Many of these, as the notorious Townsend's, the chief merit of which was its great dilution and the large size of the bottles in which it was put up, have gone into disuse, while a few are yet in demand.

It is greatly to be regretted that educated physicians should so frequently lend their influence to the empiric by countenancing, and even recommending, these medicines, some of which may no doubt be found useful in their hands, but, besides the disadvantage of our being ignorant of their composition, they are generally inferior to the officinal and other published preparations, in medicinal virtues.

CLASS III.—*Syrups containing Acetic Acid.*

Syrupus Allii. By maceration of garlic in dil. acet. acid, sugar being afterwards added. Antispasmodic. Dose, f℥j.
" Scillæ. Vinegar of squill Oj + sugar ℔ij. Expectorant. Dose, f℥j.

Of these, the first is but rarely used; but the second is an extremely common expectorant, used both by itself and in combination with camphorated tincture of opium, tincture of digitalis, syrup of ipecac, and with other medicines. The presence of the acetic element takes from this preparation the cloying character which belongs to the syrups generally.

CLASS IV.—*Having Simple Syrup as a base.*

Officinal Name.	Preparation.	Use.	Dose.
Syrupus acidi citrici	ℨj to Oj + oil of lemon ♏ij	Adjuvant & vehicle	
" krameriæ	(Second process) ext. ℥j to Oj	Astringent	f℥ss.
" tolutanus	(*U. S. P.* 1840) tinct. f℥vj to Oj	Adjuvant	
" zingiberis	(*U. S. P.* 1840) " f℥ss to Oj	"	
" rhei aromaticus	(See page 227).	Carminative & laxative	fℨij to f℥j.

Citric acid syrup is used as a substitute for lemon syrup, and, when the ingredients are of good quality and well prepared, is a far pleasanter article; it is much used largely diluted with water, in which form it is called lemonade. It is also well adapted to use as an excipient in extemporaneous prescription.[1]

Syrup of rhatany, which has been introduced among the first class, may also be made extemporaneously, as above, from the officinal extract, by dissolving it in syrup by the aid of heat.

Ginger and Tolu syrups are made, according to the last edition of the *Pharmacopœia*, by impregnating sugar with the proper proportion of the tincture, stated in the syllabus, and driving off the alcohol by heat, after which the sugar is dissolved in the requisite quantity of water. This process is troublesome, and its only advantage is that the syrup thus prepared is somewhat clearer than that by the old process of adding the tincture directly to hot simple syrup, which plan is satisfactory for common purposes.

These two syrups have been made the subject of comment by several pharmaceutists: first, by the late John D. Finley, in an inaugural thesis; afterwards by Joseph Laidley; and more recently by Professor Procter. They agree in preferring the trituration of a concentrated tincture with carbonate of magnesia and a small portion of sugar, thus making an aromatized water, which is rendered clear by filtration and converted into a syrup by the addition of sugar in the usual

[1] See Mineral Water Syrups.

way. The same plan is recommended for making syrup of orange-peel.

Spiced syrup of rhubarb (syr. rhei aromat.) is the most familiar remedy for the so-called summer complaint of children, the form of diarrhœa, usually connected with teething, so extremely prevalent and fatal in our large cities during the intense heat of summer. It has the advantage of being a warming tonic or stomachic, as well as a very mild laxative, and is given in doses from a teaspoonful for an infant of a year old to a tablespoonful or more for older children and adults. The formula for its preparation, reduced so as to make one and a half pints of the syrup, and somewhat modified in phraseology, is as follows:—

Take of	Rhubarb	Five drachms.
	Cloves and cinnamon, each .	One drachm.
	Nutmeg	Half a drachm.

Reduce to a uniform coarse powder, pack them into a small percolator, and pour upon them gradually diluted alcohol, frequently repassing the first portion until half a pint of clear tincture is obtained; then evaporate to four fluidounces, and add syrup (while hot) one and a half pints.

An old recipe for this preparation, credited to the late Dr. James, and preferred in practice by my father, the late Dr. Joseph Parrish, and some contemporaneous practitioners, prescribes a considerable portion of French brandy, not to be evaporated, but retained in the syrup when finished. To meet this preference, the rhubarb and aromatics may be displaced with brandy, which may be mixed with a somewhat smaller proportion of syrup, the evaporation being dispensed with altogether.[1]

UNCLASSIFIED SYRUPS.[2]

Syrupus Amygdalis	1 p. bitter almonds, 3 p. sweet almonds	Demulcent.
" Limonis	Lemon-juice Oj, sugar ℔ij	Adjuvant and vehicle.
" Acaciæ	Gum ℥j, sugar ℥vij, water f℥iv	Excipient for pills.

Almond or orgeat syrup is a most delightful preparation for use as a drink with water, or with carbonic acid water; it is frequently modified by the addition of orange-flower water, vanilla, or other flavoring materials, which, however, do not improve it. It is occasionally prescribed in large doses frequently repeated, in gonorrhœa. Its process involves, 1st, the blanching of almonds (depriving them of their skins by maceration in warm water, and then pressing out the kernel from the skin between the fingers); 2d, the beating of these into a paste with a portion of sugar; 3d, the formation of a milky mixture or emulsion by trituration with successive portions of water; and 4th, the solution in this of the required quantity of sugar, which should be done without the aid of heat.

[1] See Syrup of Blackberry Root.

[2] See Fruit Syrups.

Lemon syrup is more acid than syrup of citric acid; its quality is mainly dependent on the freshness of the lemon-juice.

Syrup of gum Arabic, of the *Pharmacopœia*, must be distinguished from the French *Sirop de Gomme*, which, diluted with water, is a favorite demulcent drink. Our syrup is a saturated solution of gum and sugar designed to be permanent; it is very viscid, so much so as to be only fitted for suspending insoluble substances, and for combining unadhesive materials in pill. The use of well-selected gum Arabic not powdered, insures a clearer and more elegant syrup than can be made from the ordinary powdered gum.

Unofficinal Syrups.

In this division, I shall include an account of the following syrups, grouped according to their resemblance to the foregoing classes:—

Class I.—Syrups of Chamomile, Pipsissewa, Uva Ursi, Sweet Gum Bark, the Compound Syrups of Blackberry Root and of Carrageen.

Class II.—Syrups of Poppies, Frostwort, Bittersweet, and Gillenia.

Class IV.—Syrup of Sulphate of Morphia.

Unclassified.—Jackson's Pectoral Syrup, Syrups of Manna, Galls, Assafœtida, Lactucarium, Williams's Sarsaparilla Syrup, and the Mineral Water and Fruit Syrups.

Syrup of Chamomile. (*Syrupus Anthemidis.*)

The following formula by the author was published in the *American Journal of Pharmacy*, vol. xvi. p. 18, and although not an active medicinal agent, has been acceptable to some of the many admirers of chamomile.

Take of Chamomile flowers, in coarse powder One ounce.
Cold water . . . . Twelve fluidounces.
Refined sugar, in coarse powder . Twenty ounces.

Make an infusion by displacement of the chamomile flowers and water, remove the residue from the apparatus, and place the coarsely powdered sugar in its stead; on this, pour the infusion until it is entirely dissolved.

The dose might be stated at a tablespoonful.

Syrup of Pipsissewa. (*Syrupus Chimaphilæ.*)

Formula by Prof. Procter, published in *Am. Journ. Pharm.*, vol. xv. p. 70.

Take of Pipsissewa, (Chimaphila, *U. S.*) . Four ounces.
Sugar . . . . . . Twelve ounces.
Water . . . . . . A sufficient quantity.

Macerate the pipsissewa, finely bruised, in eight fluidounces of water for thirty-six hours, and then subject it to displacement, until one pint of fluid is obtained; reduce this by evaporation to eight fluidounces, add the sugar, and form a syrup in the usual manner.

The long preliminary maceration is rendered necessary by the coriaceous character of the leaves, which impedes their easy saturation by the menstruum.

On account of this property, some have preferred boiling them in successive portions of water, mixing the decoctions, evaporating, and, after the sugar has been dissolved, adding a small portion of alcohol to obviate the proneness to decomposition, common to most syrups made in this way.

One fluidounce of this syrup represents two drachms of the leaves. Syrup of pipsissewa is an elegant preparation of one of our most valuable and abundant indigenous tonic and alterative medicines. DOSE, a tablespoonful.

Pipsissewa is also much used in combination with sarsaparilla and other alteratives, and enters into numerous private recipes of that description.

Syrup of Uva Ursi. (*Syrupus Uvæ Ursi.*)

Formula by Duhamel and Procter, published in *American Journal of Pharmacy*, vol. xi. p. 196.

Take of Bearberry leaves (Uva Ursi, *U. S.*) Four ounces.
Water . . . . . . A sufficient quantity.
Sugar . . . . . . One pound.

To the finely bruised uva ursi, add water till it is thoroughly moistened, then place it in a displacement apparatus, and operate by percolation till it is exhausted of all its soluble active principles; then evaporate to ten fluidounces; add the sugar, and form a syrup, marking 31° Baumé.

The dose of this might be stated at a tablespoonful. Like the foregoing, this syrup is a good preparation of a valuable medicine, and one much in vogue. The two may often be advantageously associated in diseases of the urinary organs.

Compound Syrup of Carrageen.

The following recipe has been in use for some 15 years in our establishment, and the syrup has been pretty extensively used as a popular cough medicine. It does not keep well in summer, unless in a cool place.

Take of Horehound (Marrubium, *U. S.*) . . 1 ounce.
Liverwort (Hepatica, *U. S.*) . . 6 drachms.
Water . . . . 4 pints.

Boil for 15 minutes, express, and strain, then add

Carrageen (Chondrus, *U. S.*) . . . 6 drachms.

Previously well washed with cold water. Boil again for 15 or 20 minutes, strain through flannel, and add

Sugar, 1 lb. (commercial) to each pint by measure.

The dose of this agreeable medicine is a tablespoonful occasionally; it is a good demulcent, without sedative effects.

Compound Syrup of Blackberry Root. (*Syrupus Rubi Villosi Comp.*)

This is another hitherto unpublished formula. Its object is to furnish a substitute for the spiced syrup of rhubarb, where that remedy is deficient in astringency. It has been used chiefly as a popular medicine in domestic practice. The astringent virtues of blackberry root are almost universally known, and it is much used in the form of decoction and syrup throughout the country, both as a domestic remedy and in regular medical practice. The experience of some ten years past has proved the eligibility of this old-fashioned formula.

Take of Blackberry root, well bruised[1] . . 8 ounces.
Cinnamon,
Cloves, and
Nutmegs, of each . . . . . 3 drachms.
Sugar . . . . 4 pounds.
Water . . . . 4 pints.

Boil the root and the aromatics in the water for one hour; express and strain; then add the sugar, form a syrup, and again strain; then add

French brandy . . . . . . 6 fluidounces.
Oil of cloves, and
Oil of cinnamon, of each . . 4 drops.

Dose, from a teaspoonful for a child of two years old, to a tablespoonful for an adult, repeated till the symptoms abate.

Syrup of Sweet Gum Bark.

Dr. Charles W. Wright, Professor of Chemistry in the Kentucky School of Medicine, recommends a syrup made from the bark of *liquidambar styraciflua*, or sweet gum tree of our forests, as a remedy in the diarrhœa so prevalent among children in our large cities in hot weather, and which frequently terminates in cholera infantum. His formula is that of the officinal syrup of wild cherry, merely substituting one bark for the other. The advantage claimed for it is that of being retained by an irritable stomach when almost every other form of astringent medicine is rejected; the taste is very agreeable. The dose for an adult is a fluidounce after each operation of the bowels; children may take from a fluidrachm to half a fluidounce.

Syrup of Frostwort.

Rock rose, frostwort, and frost weed, are common synonyms of the herb which is officinal in the secondary list of the *Pharmacopœia* as helianthemum, the herb of helianthemum Canadense; but more familiarly known as cistus Canadensis, the name given to it by some botanists.

[1] Dewberry root (rubus trivialis) will answer equally well.

Having for some years prepared a syrup of this plant, which was used with much success by my brother, the late Dr. Isaac Parrish, in scrofulous affections of the eyes, and also by several other practitioners in diseases of the scrofulous type, I insert the formula for the information of such as are disposed to make a trial of this valuable indigenous alterative:—

Take of Frostwort (the herb)	4 ounces.
Water, and	
Alcohol, of each	A sufficient quantity.
Sugar	16 ounces.

Macerate the bruised herb in eight fluidounces of diluted alcohol, for twenty-four hours; displace with a mixture of one part of alcohol to three of water, till the liquid comes over nearly free from the taste and color of the plant; then evaporate to one pint, add the sugar, boil for a minute or two, and strain.

The dose of this syrup is a fluidrachm three times a day.

Syrup of Poppies (*Syrupus Papaver*).

This syrup, which, as usually prepared, is extremely liable to ferment, and on that account is a very troublesome preparation to apothecaries who have occasional calls for it, may be conveniently made by the following process of Professor Procter, so as to be permanent:—

Take of Poppy-heads	16 ounces.
Diluted alcohol	4 pints.
Sugar	30 ounces.

Deprive the poppy-heads of their seeds; bruise them thoroughly, macerate them in twice their weight of diluted alcohol for two days, express powerfully, add the remainder of the diluted alcohol, and after twenty-four hours again express; evaporate the liquid to one pint, strain, and add the sugar, and dissolve by the aid of a gentle heat.

The proportion of the capsules, though somewhat smaller in this than in the formula of the London *Pharmacopœia*, is larger than those of most of the continental authorities; the dose may be stated to be from a fluidrachm to a half fluidounce. There is considerable difference in the strength of this syrup, if the weight of the capsules is taken before the removal of the seeds, as implied in this recipe, instead of afterwards, as implied in the recipe of the London College. The London College directs its preparation with boiling water, and the subsequent addition of alcohol to prevent fermentation, a very inferior process to that recommended above.

Syrup of Bittersweet. (*Syrupus Dulcamaræ.*)

The following recipe, from the same source as the foregoing, furnishes a syrup which is adapted to use by itself, or in combination with those of sarsaparilla and other alteratives in cutaneous and rheumatic diseases:—

Take of Bittersweet, coarsely powdered	.	4 ounces.
Water	. . . . . .	12 ounces.
Alcohol	. . . . . .	4 fluidounces.

Mix the liquids, pour on the powder in a displacer until one pint of tincture is obtained, adding water to displace the mixed alcohol and water; evaporate to half a pint, add fifteen ounces of sugar, and make a syrup. Dose, a tablespoonful.

Syrup of Gillenia.

The high price which ipecacuanha has so long sustained, has led to inquiries for a good substitute growing on our own soil, and always attainable. "Gillenia trifoliata," Indian physic, is a common indigenous herb, the root of which has long been known to possess very decided nauseant and emetic properties. It cannot be claimed for it that it very closely resembles ipecacuanha in therapeutical action, although sufficiently allied to it to be used in many cases, particularly of catarrhal affections, as a substitute. The following syrup I have contrived with a view to remove one of the chief objections on the part of the physician to the trial of indigenous drugs, namely, the absence of suitable preparations. As far as it has yet been used, it gives promise of answering a good purpose:—

Syrup of Gillenia.

Take of Gillenia	. . .	℥ij.
Diluted alcohol	. .	Oj.
Sugar	. . .	℔iiss.
Water	. . .	Sufficient.

Reduce the gillenia to coarse powder, treat it by displacement with diluted alcohol till Oj is obtained. Evaporate to f℥vj, filter, and add sufficient water to make the liquid measure Oj, then add the sugar and dissolve by the aid of heat.

This syrup has twice the proportion of the medicinal ingredients contained in syrup of ipecacuanha; it is less agreeable to the taste. The dose is fℨj.

Syrup of Sulphate of Morphia.

I believe there is no published recipe for this except one that is given in Griffith's *Formulary*, credited to Cadet, which prescribes one grain of the salt to four fluidounces of syrup. Under the head of Syrup of Poppies, in the *U. S. Dispensatory*, Dr. Wood suggests the use of a syrup made by dissolving four grains of the sulphate of morphia in a pint of syrup (a quarter of a grain to the ounce, the same as Cadet's) as a substitute for the syrup of poppies, which, made by the old recipe, is so prone to ferment.

Notwithstanding that we have no officinal or other recognized recipe (that of Cadet being almost unknown in this country), physicians frequently prescribe syrupus morphiæ sulphatis, and generally, as far as I have inquired, under the impression that there is a syrup corresponding in strength with the officinal liquor morphiæ sulphatis, one grain to the ounce, and hence the habit has grown up with apothecaries of making this preparation extemporaneously of that strength. This is more remarkable, from the fact that the syrups of acetate and muriate of morphia of the *Dublin Pharmacopœia* are in the proportion of one grain to four fluidounces.

This discrepancy in practice cannot, I think, be remedied by the further publication of unauthorized recipes, and physicians should not fail to indicate the proportions designed in prescribing the salt in solution in syrup. Should there not be an officinal preparation with such a distinctive name and authorized proportions as would remedy so serious a departure from uniformity?

Jackson's Pectoral Syrup.

Alfred B. Taylor, in the *American Journal of Pharmacy*, vol. xxiv. p. 34, holds the following language:—

"A prescription of Prof. Samuel Jackson, of Philadelphia, familiarly known as his 'pectoral syrup,' has obtained considerable reputation from its beneficial action in cases of coughs, colds, &c. We believe the prescription was originally given to Mr. E. Durand, but as the syrup has for some time been a standing preparation with many of our druggists, we have thought that a published formula would be acceptable both for the purpose of giving its benefit to those who may not be familiar with its composition, and of promoting uniformity among those who may already be accustomed to prepare it. Dr. Jackson has furnished us with the following recipe:—

℞.—Sassaf. medullæ	ʒj.
Acaciæ	℥j.
Sacchari	℔j½.
Morphiæ muriat.	gr. viij.
Aquæ	Oj, or q. s.

"The sassafras pith and gum Arabic are to be put into the water and allowed to stand ten or twelve hours with occasional stirring. The sugar is to be dissolved, cold, in the mucilage, which, after being strained, should be made to measure two pints by the addition of water; lastly, the muriate of morphia is to be dissolved in the syrup."

In the recipe which I have used for a number of years, half a grain of sulphate of morphia is prescribed in place of a quarter of a grain to the ounce as in the above, and to this is added about half a drachm of Hoffmann's anodyne, and a drop of oil of sassafras to each pint.

A recipe used by some pharmaceutists is as follows:—

Take of Syrup of gum Arabic . . .	One pint.
Muriate of morphia . . .	Four grains.
Oil of sassafras	Four drops.

Mix.

The adult dose of this syrup is a teaspoonful.

Syrup of Manna. (*Syrupus Mannæ.*)

This is often directed by practitioners, without a very clear idea of what they are prescribing, since neither of the British pharmacopœias, nor our own, contain any mention of it. The following recipe, taken from the *Pharmacopie Universelle*, I have used with satisfactory results:—

Take of Flake manna . . . Ten ounces.
Water . . . . . Twelve ounces.
Make a solution, strain, and add
Sugar . . . . . One pound.
Which dissolve by the aid of heat.

This is an elegant laxative, where not contraindicated by debility of the digestive organs, and is chiefly prescribed for children and pregnant women.

When extemporaneously prepared, there seems no necessity of adding the sugar at all, as a simple solution of manna in water is sufficiently agreeable, besides being stronger than the above. The peculiar sugar of manna is not fermentable.

Syrup of Galls. (*Syrupus Gallæ.*)

This old and esteemed recipe is attributed to several eminent physicians of the last generation. It is used in chronic diarrhœa, and obstinate cases of dysentery.

Take of Bruised galls . . . . . ℥ss.
Brandy . . . . . . f℥viij.

Introduce into an f℥viij vial, digest in hot water for half an hour, and filter; then pour it into a saucer, and inflame the spirit with a lighted taper; add sugar ℥ij, by melting it in the flame on a fine wire support, and allowing it to drop into the brandy, which must be stirred till it ceases to burn, and a syrup is formed. Then introduce it again into the f℥viij vial, and fill it up with water.

Dose, a teaspoonful to a tablespoonful; for infants from 10 to 20 drops. Some recipes direct that cinnamon and nutmeg, of each ʒij, shall be digested in the brandy, which is an improvement on the foregoing.

Williams's Sarsaparilla Syrup.

This preparation was much prescribed by the late Dr. J. K. Mitchell, who furnished the following formula:—

Take of Compound syrup of sarsaparilla . Oj.
Corrosive chloride of mercury . gr. ij.
Extract of conium . . . ʒj.

Triturate the corrosive chloride with a little alcohol and water till dissolved, then incorporate it and the extract of conium with the syrup. DOSE, a tablespoonful.

Syrup of Assafœtida.

Richard Peltz, while a student of the Philadelphia College of Pharmacy, proposed the following formula, which, with specimens of the syrup prepared by it, were presented to the college, at a pharmaceutical meeting, in the spring of 1852. The object is to furnish a preparation of assafœtida, free from alcoholic stimulus, and yet tolerably permanent. Although an old specimen of this syrup has a more fetid odor than a recent one, yet the change takes place much less rapidly, and to a less extent, than in the case of the milk or mixture of assafœtida, for which it may be substituted by the physician when it is not convenient to prepare the former:—

Take of	Assafœtida	One ounce.
	Boiling water	One pint.
	Sugar	Two pounds.

Rub the assafœtida with part of the boiling water, till a uniform paste is made; then gradually add the rest of the water, strain, and add the sugar, applying a gentle heat to dissolve it. DOSE, a tablespoonful, containing seven grains and a half (15 grains to the ounce) of assafœtida.

By adding one part of tincture of assafœtida to four parts of syrup, and evaporating off the alcohol, a good substitute for the foregoing may be prepared.

Syrup of Lactucarium.

This elegant sedative remedy I have found very satisfactory when made according to the following formula of T. S. Weigand:—

℞.—Lactucarium in coarse powder	grs. 64.
Carbonate of potassa	grs. xxxii.
Distilled water	Sufficient.
Sugar	4 oz.

Grind the lactucarium with carbonate of potassa, and continue the trituration till the two are thoroughly mixed; add sufficient water to moisten it completely, allow it to stand for twelve hours, and displace slowly till two fluidounces are obtained; then add the sugar: dissolve with a gentle heat. Each fluidrachm of this syrup contains two grains of lactucarium.—*Am. Journ. Pharm.*, vol. xxv.

GLYCEROLES.

Glyceroles are preparations in which glycerin is used to substitute sugar wholly or chiefly, in the preparation of remedies for internal use. Glyceroles used externally are called "Plasma," Liniments, Lotions, &c., and several of these are mentioned among the topical remedies. Of those used internally one or two will be found among the chemical remedies. The special uses of glycerin in Pharmacy are, *first*, as a solvent, in which capacity it has very numerous applications. *Second*, as an antiseptic, for which it is well adapted. *Third*, as an emollient in irritable and inflammatory conditions of the mucous surfaces and in skin diseases; and *fourth*, as a bland nutritive material to substitute oils and fats. The chief objections to its use are founded on its high price, and the fact that the glyceroles are not usually as agreeable in taste as corresponding syrups.

The solvent power of glycerin is, in general, between that of water and alcohol, and generally substances may be said to be more soluble in glycerin, the more they are so in alcohol. A high temperature greatly increases its solvent power. The following statement shows some of the more important chemical substances freely soluble in glycerin: Iodine, iodides of potassium, iron and sulphur, sulphurets of potassium and calcium, biniodide of mercury, corrosive sublimate, sulphate of quinine, tannin, salts of morphia, veratria, brucia, atropia, tartar emetic.

Glycerole of Lactucarium. (*F. Stearns.*)

Take of	Lactucarium . . .	One ounce.
	Diluted alcohol,	
	Boiling water, of each	Sufficient.
	Glycerin . . .	Twelve fluidounces.
	Citric acid . . .	Fifteen grains.
	Orange-flower water .	Two fluidounces.

Reduce the lactucarium to a moderately fine powder; moisten with one fluidounce of diluted alcohol and pack into a small displacer. After macerating twelve hours, pour upon it gradually diluted alcohol until the filtrate measures sixteen fluidounces, or until it passes without taste. Evaporate this on a water bath nearly to dryness, then boil this residue with six fluidounces of water; pour this off from the undissolved residue into a filter placed over a bottle containing the glycerin; add four fluidounces of water to the undissolved residue, boil, and filter into the first portion. Then evaporate the whole on a water bath to fourteen fluidounces, and when cool, add the orange-flower water in which the citric acid has been previously dissolved. Each fluidounce represents a half drachm of lactucarium. Dose, one to three teaspoonfuls.

Mineral-Water Syrups.

These are used for flavoring mineral water, and in the manufacture of pleasant refrigerant drinks. Some of the remarks which follow are compiled from an article by Ambrose Smith, in the *American Journal of Pharmacy*, vol. xxii. p. 212, and are, in part, the result of my own experience in regard to their preparation and uses.

As some of the subjects have already been introduced among the officinal syrups, the remarks which follow may be considered as supplementary, and are somewhat more in detail.

Lemon Syrup.

This is now almost universally made from citric or tartaric acid, oil of lemon, instead of lemon juice. Some of the confectioners, when they are overstocked with lemons, make them into syrup, but from the use of fruit that has partially spoiled, and from the syrup being made in such large quantities at once as to become more or less altered by keeping, before it is consumed, the article thus made is inferior to that made from acid and oil of lemon. A very fine flavoring syrup may, however, be made by using fresh lemons and making the syrup in small quantities, with the proper precaution spoken of under the general head of Syrups.

Citric acid is preferable to tartaric for preparing a syrup. When made with the former acid it has a more agreeable flavor, which it retains longer unimpaired. The syrup made with either acid, when long kept, is liable to throw down a white granular deposit of grape sugar. Its flavor changes gradually on keeping long, even when made with citric acid. This is probably due to a change in the oil of lemon, by which the syrup acquires a terebinthinate flavor. This turpentine taste is very common in the lemon syrup which is manufactured and sold wholesale, and may frequently be due to the employment of old or impure oil of lemon. A common adulteration of this oil is the admixture of recently distilled oil of turpentine or camphene, and the adulterated oil may contain a considerable portion of it without its being perceptible by taste or odor while new, but as the camphene becomes resinous, the turpentine flavor is developed. But even pure oil of lemon degenerates in flavor and odor, when long kept; therefore, it is better to prepare the syrup in small quantities, so that it will be consumed before there is any change in its quality. The following formula furnishes a pleasant mineral-water syrup, which can be made in a few minutes:—

Take of Oil of lemon . . . . . ♏xv.
Citric acid . . . . . ʒx.
Simple syrup . . . . . Cong. j.

Rub the oil of lemon first with a little powdered sugar, and afterwards with a portion of syrup, dissolve the citric acid in an ounce or two of water, and mix the whole.

A more delicate flavor of the lemon may be obtained by macerating the outer portion of lemon-peel in deodorized alcohol, allowing this to evaporate spontaneously, and, when it is nearly all dissipated, adding it to sugar to be incorporated with the syrup, or triturating with magnesia, adding water, filtering, and making a syrup; not forgetting to add the requisite proportion of citric acid.

The simple syrup may be made in the proportion of six commercial pounds of sugar to half a gallon of water. This recipe directs rather more acid than the officinal *syrupus acidi citrici.* Some prefer the use of a little tartaric acid; citric acid ℥j, and tartaric acid ʒij, is a good proportion to the gallon. A few fresh lemon-peels thrown into the hot syrup is a good substitute for the oil of lemon, though giving it a slight bitter taste.

Lemonade.

Mix Lemon syrup	. . .	Oj.
Water (iced)	. . .	Cong. ij, or q. s.

Stir them well together.

Orange Syrup.

Take of oranges, the fresh fruit, a convenient number, grate off the yellow outside peel, cut the oranges and express the juice, to each quart of which add

Water	. . . .	1 pint.
Sugar	. . . .	6 lbs. com.

Mix the sugar with the grated peel, add the mixed water and juice, and apply a gentle heat till it is dissolved, then strain.

One dozen oranges will make one and a half to two gallons of syrup.

The flavor is more delicate, and free from a certain "musty" taste that the juice is apt to acquire if the acid taste is supplied by the addition of a small portion of citric acid, say forty-five grains to each pint, and the syrup of the outer rind as above.

The following elegant process for syrup of orange-peel is extracted from the *Am. Journ. Pharm.*, vol. xxvi. p. 298.

Take of Peel of sweet oranges, recently dried	.	2 ounces.
Carbonate of magnesia	. . . .	½ ounce.
Sugar, in powder	. . . . .	2½ pounds.
Deodorized alcohol,		
Water, of each	. . . . .	Sufficient.

Reduce the orange-peel to coarse powder, put it in a small glass percolator, and pour deodorized (Atwood's) alcohol slowly on it till six fluidounces of tincture have passed; evaporate this spontaneously to two fluidounces; triturate this with the carbonate of magnesia; an ounce of sugar and half a pint of water gradually added; pour this on a filter, and when it ceases to pass, add water till a pint of filtrate is obtained; to this add the sugar, dissolve with a gentle heat, and strain if necessary.

If a pure and fresh article of oil of orange can be obtained, the syrup may be made by the following formula:—

Take of Syrup	. . . .	Oij.
Oil of orange	. . . .	♏v.
Tartaric acid	. . . .	ʒj. Mix.

Ginger Syrup.

The formula of the *Pharmacopœia* makes a syrup of about the proper strength for use with mineral water. It is usually made in considerable quantities, and it will be found most convenient to prepare the simple syrup somewhat more dilute than the officinal, and, while it is hot, to pour on the surface the tincture of ginger, allowing the alcohol to evaporate before mixing with the syrup. If the tincture is mixed directly, the syrup will be cloudy. On the other hand, if it is allowed to remain too long on the surface of the hot syrup before mixing, the resin separates in globules, which cannot afterwards be thoroughly diffused through the syrup. The tincture should be allowed to evaporate from the surface of the syrup until the vapor ceases to ignite on the approach of flame, then mixed immediately. The method of making ginger syrup, prescribed in the *Pharmacopœia*, is to pour the tincture on to the sugar, which is to be exposed to the air until the spirit has evaporated, and then made into syrup. This plan is more operose, however, and does not answer better than the one indicated above. The introduction of the whites of two or three eggs, before boiling and straining, makes the syrup much clearer. Some druggists prefer to boil ginger in water, which extracts a large amount of starchy matter, and makes a richer and more frothy mineral-water syrup. The following is the recipe:—

Take of Ginger, bruised . . . . 3 ounces.
Water . . . . 2 pints.
Boil for half an hour in a covered vessel, strain, and add
Sugar . . . . 4 lbs. com.
Continue the heat until it is dissolved.

Capsicum Syrup.

Take of Simple syrup . . . . . . Oij.
Tincture of capsicum . . . . . f℥j.
Proceed as for ginger syrup.

This is a fine stimulant, which is used to advantage in mineral water, in intensely hot and debilitating weather, when the relaxed condition of the digestive organs seems to contraindicate the use of cold drinks.

Sarsaparilla Syrup for Mineral Water.

As this syrup is intended for making a pleasant beverage, it is made much weaker of sarsaparilla than the compound syrup of the *Pharmacopœia*, and the senna, guaiac, &c., which enter into the composition of the latter, are very properly omitted.

The following is the formula of Ambrose Smith:—

Take of Sarsaparilla, finely bruised,
Liquorice root do. each . . 2 lbs. (com.)
Sugar . . . . 30 lbs. (com.)
Oil of anise, wintergreen, and sassafras,
of each . . . . 40 drops.
Oil of cinnamon . . . . . . 5 drops.
Water . . . . q. s.

Digest the roots 12 hours, with 2 gallons of warm water, then put into a displacer and displace, adding sufficient water until 2 gallons of infusion are obtained. In this dissolve the sugar with the aid of heat, and to the syrup when cooled add the oils, previously rubbed up with a little sugar.

The following formula is employed by some of the druggists of this city:—

Take of Sarsaparilla, liquorice root, each . . . 1 lb.
Cinnamon, sassafras, each, ... 6 oz.
Cloves, anise, coriander, each . . . . 2 oz.
Red saunders, cochineal, each . . . . 1½ oz.
Alcohol . . . . 2 pints.
Water . . . . 2 gallons.

Digest the above for 4 days, strain, and make a syrup with 27 lbs. (com.) sugar. It is also frequently made by diluting the compound syrup with twice its measure of simple syrup, and adding the essential oils. The fluid extract of sarsaparilla, if mezereon enters into its composition, does not answer, as the persistent acrimony of this bark is so perceptible even in the diluted syrup as to make it unpalatable.

The following is our own formula:—

Take of Simple syrup . . . . Oij.
Comp. syrup of sarsap. . . . . . f℥ij.
Caramel . . . . fʒvj.
Oil of gaultheria, and
Oil of sassafras, of each . . . . . 3 drops.

Mix by shaking up in a bottle.

Orgeat Syrup.

This corresponds with the officinal syrupus amygdalæ (see p. 227), with the addition of some more decided flavoring substance, as orange-flower water, bitter almond oil, or vanilla.

The following formula is sometimes prepared, as requiring less time and trouble in its preparation:—

Take of Cream syrup,
Vanilla syrup, each . . . . . . 1 pint.
Oil of bitter almonds . . . . . . gtt. iv.

Mix well together, observing not to make more than sufficient for one day's sales.

Fruit Syrups.

To make one gallon of strawberry, raspberry, or blackberry syrup:—

Take of the fresh fruit	. . . . . .	4 quarts.
Water	. . . .	Sufficient.
Sugar (refined)	. . . . . .	8 lbs. com.

Express the juice and strain, then add water, till it measures four pints, dissolve the sugar in this by the aid of heat, raise it to the boiling point, and strain. If it is to be kept till the following season, it should be poured while hot into dry bottles, filled to the neck, and securely corked.

Fig. 170 represents the straining bag; and Figs. 171 and 172 the

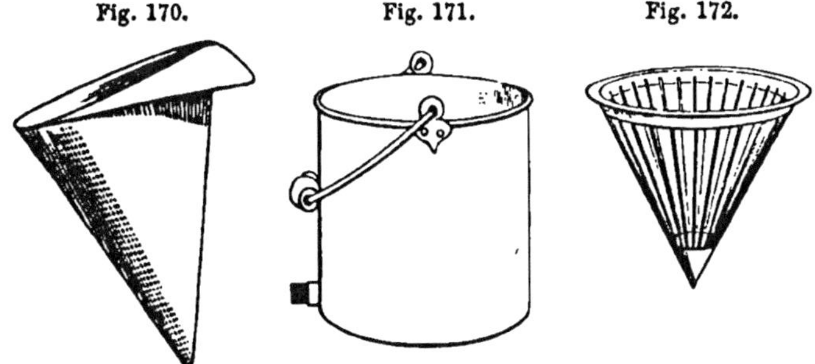

Fig. 170. Fig. 171. Fig. 172.

apparatus for straining and expressing, by means of a square piece of flannel or muslin.

Strawberry syrup is made by first inclosing the ripe fruit in a strong bag—coarse linen is well adapted to the purpose—then apply a gradual pressure by means of a screw or lever press, if the quantity operated upon is large; for small quantities it may be pressed sufficiently by hand. The juice is now diluted, if necessary, mixed with sugar, and transferred to a kettle, in which it is heated to the boiling point, and then strained while hot.

Another way to prepare this syrup, where a fine and very delicate flavor is desired, is to macerate the ripe berries in layers interspersed with powdered sugar, one and three-quarter pounds of sugar to a pound of the picked berries for twenty-four hours, in a cellar, and then throw them on a sieve or perforated capsule for the syrup to drain off. This juice is to be put into a bottle, loosely corked, set into a vessel of water, and heated to the boiling point; after which it is to be tightly sealed and laid away in a cool place.

Raspberry Syrup is made by the same process; the juice is richer in pectin and more liable to glutinize than the foregoing, so that it bears a larger dilution; it improves the flavor of this syrup to use a small proportion of pie-cherries, or currants—say a pound to four quarts of the raspberries.

16

With the object of removing pectin from the juice of raspberries and other fruits, the *Prussian Pharmacopœia* directs the production of incipient fermentation. The following is the recipe for *cherry syrup*, which is the type of the class:—

Take of fresh sour cherries a convenient quantity, bruise them with the stones and let them stand for 3 days, then express the juice and set aside until, after fermentation, it has become clear. To 20 ounces (weight) of this filtered juice add of sugar 36 ounces, and make into a syrup by raising to the boiling point.

The raspberry (and other fruit) juice, as it is frequently imported into this country from France and Germany, is, or ought to be, the juice prepared in the above way; it is devoid of the mucilaginous principles (pectin, &c.), contains a small quantity of alcohol, and keeps well in sealed bottles; exposed to the air, of course it undergoes acetous fermentation.

Blackberry syrup does not differ from the other fruit syrups in its mode of preparation, except in the usual addition of a small proportion of French brandy, say f℥j to Oj of syrup. The proportions for these three syrups are the same, and, as they yield variable quantities of juice, the degree of dilution may be so regulated as that every quart of the fruit will yield a quart of syrup.

Blackberry brandy contains a much larger proportion of brandy and less sugar, with some infusion of aromatics, as cinnamon and cloves.

The following recipe was furnished me by Dr. P. B. Goddard:—

Aromatic Blackberry Syrup.

Take of Blackberry juice	Oij.
Sugar	℔j.
Nutmegs, grated	No. vj.
Cinnamon, bruised	℥ss.
Cloves	ʒij.
Allspice	ʒij.
Brandy	Oj.

Mix and make into a syrup.

The astringent properties of blackberry juice adapt it particularly, in combination with carminatives, to the treatment of bowel complaints.

Raspberry Vinegar.

Take of Raspberry syrup	Oij.
Acetic acid	f℥ss.

Mix them.

Added to iced water according to taste, this is one of the most delightful of refrigerant drinks.

The following formula, though not recommended as a substitute for the true fruit syrup, will be found a tolerable approximation to it:—

Artificial Syrup of Raspberry.

Take of		
Take of	Orris root (selected)	1 oz.
	Cochineal	2 dr.
	Tartaric acid	2 dr.
	Water	1 quart.

Powder the orris root coarsely together with the cochineal, infuse in the water with the acid for twenty-four hours; strain, and add four pounds of sugar; raise to the boiling point and again strain.

Pineapple Syrup.

Take of the fruit a convenient number, pare them and mash them, without slicing, in a marble or porcelain mortar, express the juice, and take for each quart—

Water	1 pint.
Sugar	6 lbs. com.

The water and sugar may be placed on the fire and heated to near the boiling point before adding the juice, after which, continue the heat till the syrup boils, then remove from the fire, skim, and strain. Preserve this as the foregoing.

Vanilla Syrup.

Take of	Vanilla	6 drachms.
	Boiling water	4½ pints.
	Sugar	8 lbs. com.

Reduce the vanilla to fine powder by trituration with a portion of sugar, boil this with water two hours in a covered vessel; then strain.

Coffee Syrup.

Take of	Roasted coffee	4 oz.
	Boiling water	2 pints.
	Sugar	4 lbs. com.

Digest the coffee in coarse powder in the boiling water, in a covered vessel, filter, or clarify with white of egg, strain, and add the sugar.

Wild Cherry Syrup is a popular and wholesome flavor for mineral water; the officinal article can hardly be improved upon.

Cream Syrups.

These are mixtures of highly flavored syrups with fresh cream. They must be made fresh every few days, and may contain equal parts of their ingredients, or, preferably, two parts of the flavored syrup to one of cream.

Some pharmaceutists prefer to make syrup of cream, and to flavor this by the addition of strong fruit and other syrups in the glass on drawing the mineral water.

Simple Syrup of Cream.

Take of	Fresh cream	1 pint.
	Powdered sugar	1 lb. com.

Mix and shake well together. To be kept in bottles not exceeding a pint. The formula of A. B. Taylor directs equal parts of cream and milk with the same proportion of sugar. That of O. S. Hubbell directs fourteen pounds of sugar to each gallon of cream.

Nectar Cream is variously made from cream syrup and flavored syrups. The following is a good mixture:—

Take of	Simple syrup of cream	1 part.
	Vanilla syrup	3 parts.
	Pineapple syrup	1 part.
	Lemon syrup	1 part.

Mix.

Hubbell's formula directs the addition of sherry wine, against which objections might be urged as tending to promote a taste for alcoholic stimulants. A great variety of fancy names are given to these combinations of cream syrup with alcoholic and other flavoring ingredients.

Factitious Cream Syrup.

Take	Ol. Amygd. Dulcis (recent)	f℥iij.
	Pulv. Acaciæ	℥ij.
	Aqua	℥ix.
M. ft.		
	Emulsio et adde,	
	Sacchari albi	℔j.
	Albumen Ovi	No. ij.

Dissolve the sugar by a gentle heat, and strain; fill small bottles and keep in cool places, well corked. This preparation will keep for a long time. For use, mix one part with eight of any of the ordinary syrups, or add about a drachm to every glass. It forms an imitation of *orgeat* by mixing two drachms or more with two ounces of simple syrup, and flavoring with bitter almond and orange-flower water.

CHAPTER XIV.

OF PULPS, CONSERVES, CONFECTIONS, ELECTUARIES, PASTES, LOZENGES, AND CANDIES.

PREPARATIONS having pectin, the sugar of fruits, as their basis, or containing medicinal substances suspended in a semi-solid form by the aid of honey and syrup, are variously termed as above. The first class to be taken up, as named in the *Pharmacopœia*, is the following:—

PULPÆ, *U. S. P.*

Pruni pulpa . . . . 10 parts = 12 of the fruit; softened by steam and pressed through a sieve.
Tamarindi pulpa . . . 7 parts = 12 of the fruit; digested with water, strained, and evaporated.
Cassiæ fistulæ pulpa . . 5 parts = 12 of the fruit; digested with water, strained, and evaporated.

In straining these, the chief object is to remove the seeds, skin, and stringy portions, and, in the case of cassia fistula, the fragments of pods, and to obtain a smooth, soft mass, which, in small quantities, is agreeable, and, in the case of tamarind pulp, is pleasantly acid. These are rarely prepared, except by the manufacturers of confection of senna, some of whom use them in the fabrication of that article.

CONFECTIONES, *U. S. P.*

This class naturally subdivides into two, which are nearly alike in their properties, but quite unlike in their mode of preparation.

1ST CLASS.—*Conserves.*

Confectio Rosæ (by an unofficinal process), 1 part to 3 sugar.
" Aurantii corticis, *U. S.*, 1 part (grated) to 3 sugar.
" Amygdalæ (*Lond. Ph.*), sweet almonds, gum, and sugar.

By beating with powdered sugar a fresh, moist substance, as undried rose petals, or the rind of a fresh orange, or a fruit rich in oil, and naturally moist, like the almond (which should be previously blanched), we obtain a true conserve. The trituration should be continued till a smooth and uniform firm paste is produced, which will generally be permanent if kept in a well-covered vessel, except in the instance of the almond, which will generally be rendered unfit for use by long keeping, and hence the confection has been omitted in the recent edition of the *U. S. Pharmacopœia.*

Confection of rose is more frequently made, according to my observation, by the above process, with the common hundred-leaved and damask rose petals, than by that of the *Pharmacopœia*, in which the powdered red-rose petals are directed to be made into an electuary; so that Confectio Rosæ, as usually met with, is not decidedly astringent.

Confection of orange-peel is made chiefly from the rind of the common sweet orange, so abundant in our market, and not from bitter orange-peel, as sometimes supposed by physicians.

Confection of almonds is made from the blanched almonds, triturated through a fine sieve, and thoroughly incorporated with the gum and sugar, thus forming the whole into a mass. It furnishes a ready mode of forming almond mixtures.

2D CLASS.—*Electuaries.*

Confectio Rosæ, *U. S. P.* Powd. rose 2 p., sugar 15 p., honey 3 p., rose water 4 p.
Confectio Aromatica. Arom. powd. 5½, saffron ½, syr. orange-peel 6, honey 2.

Confectio Opii (1 gr. in 36). Opium powd. 4½, aromat. powd. 48, honey 112.
Confectio Sennæ. P. senna and coriander, added to a syrup of liquorice-root and figs, to be triturated with equal parts of pulps of prunes, tamarinds, and purging cassia.

All of this division of confections are made from dried and powdered materials, incorporated mechanically with a saccharine solution into mass.

Confection of rose is used as a vehicle in the preparation of pills, which is almost its only use.

Aromatic confection and *confection of opium* are somewhat used as vehicles; the latter is prescribed in old recipes, and sometimes in prescriptions, as *Theriaca Andronica.* It enters into the composition of a celebrated fever and ague mixture introduced among extemporaneous preparations.

Confection of senna is a fine laxative, and, when properly prepared, is one of the most agreeable remedies of its class. If given in large enough quantities to purge actively, it is liable to disagree with the stomach when there is a want of tone in that organ, and to become distasteful to the patient. It constitutes the basis of the next preparation to be noticed.

Hæmorrhoid Electuary.

The following recipe has been in use for many years as a remedy for piles, and, from the numerous cases in which it has afforded relief, is believed worthy a place among our unofficinal formulæ:—

Take of Supertartrate of potassa,
Powdered jalap,
Powdered nitrate of potassa, of each half an ounce.
Confection of senna . . . . an ounce.

Make an electuary with syrup of ginger.
Dose, a piece the size of a marble three times a day.

Confection of Black Pepper (*Confectio Piperis, Ph. L.*).—*Ward's Paste.*

The following is the recipe from the *London Pharmacopœia* for this celebrated preparation, which is not unfrequently prescribed for piles; it is said to require to be used continuously for some months to realize good results:—

Take of		Reduced.
Black pepper,		
Elecampane, each	1 pound	℥j.
Fennel (seeds)	3 pounds	℥iij.
Honey,		
Sugar, each	2 pounds	℥ij.

Rub the dry ingredients together into a very fine powder, and keep them in a covered vessel; but, whenever the confection is to be used, add the powder gradually to the honey, and beat them until thoroughly incorporated. Dose, ʒj to ʒij, three times a day.

PASTES.

Medicines having sugar and gum for their basis, of a firm yet flexible consistence, intermediate between confections and lozenges, are called *Pastes*. These are usually sold in sheets, or in small squares, each of which is of suitable size to be taken at one time into the mouth, and covered with powdered sugar, or, in the case of jujube paste, with oil, to prevent their adhering together.

The object proposed in their preparation is the production of an agreeable demulcent and expectorant form of medicine; as their pleasant qualities are to a great extent lost by age, they should be freshly prepared.

The transparent kinds are allowed to cool and harden spontaneously, while the opaque varieties are stirred and beaten as they cool. A few recipes for pastes are appended:—

Jujube Paste. (Transparent Gum Paste.)

Take of Gum Arabic . . . . 6 ounces.
Water . . . . 8 fluidounces.

Bruise the gum, and make it into a clear mucilage, which may be conveniently done by inclosing it in a bag of coarse gauze suspended near the top of a vessel of cold water; introduce the mucilage into an evaporating dish, and add—

Syrup . . . . 7 ounces (by weight).

Evaporate to a very thick consistence, adding, towards the last—

Orange-flower water . . . 2 fluidrachms.

Let it cool, remove the crust which will have formed on the surface, and run the paste into shallow tin pans, which lay away in a warm place to dry. In order to turn out the paste, some are in the habit of slightly greasing the cans; but, this oil sometimes becoming rancid and giving unpleasant properties to the paste, it is suggested by Dorvault to make use of tin pans prepared by spreading with a rag a globule of mercury over the whole inside surface, and then wiping it well. The moulds need to be gone over with the mercury only once in eight or ten times. The French Codex directs the addition of a decoction of jujube; but this, which was the original practice, and gave name to the preparation, is now generally abandoned. The use of orange-flower water is generally substituted in this country by oil of lemon or rose, and, where the latter is used, a red color is imparted to the paste for the sake of distinction. Other flavors may be used.

Marshmallow Paste. Opaque Gum Paste. Pate de Guimauve.

Take of Gum Arabic (white),
Sugar, of each . . . . ℔j.
Water . . . . Sufficient.
Orange-flower water . . . . . f℥iij.
White of eggs . . . . . . No. x.

Bruise the gum, dissolve it in the water, and strain; put the gummy solution upon the fire in a deep, wide pan, add the sugar, stirring continually until it has the consistence of thick honey, carefully regulating the temperature. Then beat the eggs to a froth, add them and the orange-flower water gradually to the paste, which must be constantly stirred; continue to beat the paste until, in applying it with the spatula upon the back of the hand, it does not adhere to it, then run it out upon a slab, or into pans covered with starch.

Formerly this contained marshmallow; now it is, properly speaking, only an opaque paste of gum.

The *Iceland moss paste*, so extensively advertised of latter years, may be closely imitated by this process, slightly varying the flavor. The asserted presence of *Iceland moss* in it improves it only in name.

Carrageen Paste. (*Mouchon.*)

Take of Carrageen	℥j.
Water	Ovj.

Boil the carrageen (previously soaked) first in four pints, and then in the remainder of the water, and mix the liquids; to this add—

Pure gum Arabic,	
Sugar, of each	8 ounces.

Strain, evaporate to a very thick consistence, cool it, and separate any crust, and run it out into pans or on a slab.

Iceland Moss Paste. (*French Codex.*)

Take of Iceland moss	℥ij.
Gum Arabic	℥x.
Sugar	℥viij.
Water	Sufficient.

Wash the Iceland moss in boiling water, and, having rejected this water, boil it in an additional portion of water during an hour. Express and strain, add the gum and sugar, and evaporate till a drop does not adhere to the back of the hand; then cool it on a marble slab.

Trochisci.—Lozenges.

The manufacture of lozenges, as of confections, and of some syrups, pertains to the confectioner, in common with the pharmaceutist, and is principally confined to the former; yet the obvious eligibility of this form of preparation, for certain expectorant and other medicines, particularly for children, makes a knowledge of them desirable both to the physician and pharmaceutist.

The process for preparing them is quite simple, and so well adapted to all insoluble, tasteless, and agreeable medicines, that we may with propriety resort to it for ordinary purposes in prescribing.

The author has repeatedly made up medicines in this form extemporaneously by physician's prescription, and with considerable advantage, as compared with the usual pharmaceutical forms.

The lozenges to be described are of two classes:—

First Class.—Those which consist of white sugar combined with a medicinal substance, and made up by the addition of mucilage. The dry ingredients are first to be thoroughly reduced to powder and mixed together; then beaten in a suitable mortar, with sufficient mucilage of tragacanth or gum Arabic to form a tenacious and tolerably firm mass; this mass, being dusted with a little powdered sugar (not starch, which is sometimes used), is to be rolled out upon a suitable board, or marble slab, to the required thickness, previously ascertained; and then, with a small punch, either round, oval, stellate, or cordate to suit the taste of the maker, cut out singly, and laid away to dry on a suitable tray or sieve

Fig. 173 represents a simple apparatus used for rolling and cutting this description of lozenges; the rolling-board is adjusted as follows: Having a punch of a certain diameter, a small portion of the mass is rolled and cut out, and its weight ascertained; if it be too heavy, the cake is rolled thinner, and so on until adjusted to the required weight; a strip is now tacked on to each side of the board, within the range of the roller, and corresponding in thickness with the cake, so that the roller, when passed over, will reduce the medicated mass to the right point. A board arranged in this way should be kept for each kind of lozenges, as the weight of different materials varies, and, in adjusting it, a small allowance must be made for the moisture present in the soft mass, which increases its bulk. In dividing a mass extemporaneously, it is convenient to roll the whole out into a square or oblong cake of suitable size, and then, with a spatula, divide it equally into a definite number of square masses.

Fig. 173.

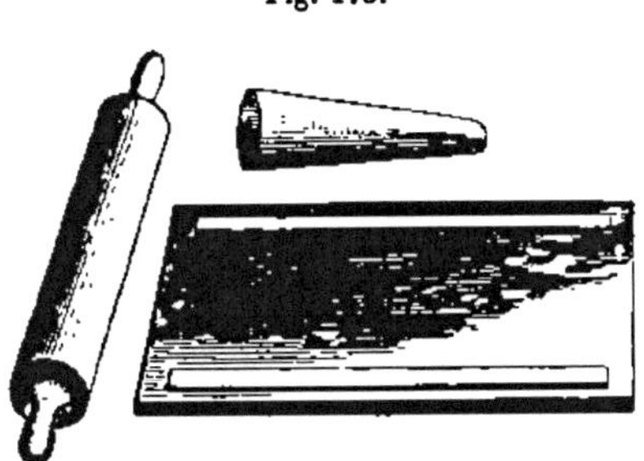

Board, roller, and punch, for making lozenges.

Some manufacturers have, independently of their cutting punches, a stamp bearing the name of the base of the lozenge, or the card of the manufacturer, which they impress upon each lozenge; for white lozenges, the punch is sometimes dipped in an infusion of cochineal. The cutting punches are sometimes so made as to combine cutting and marking in one operation.

In order to have lozenges nicely cut, it is important to clean the cutting punch frequently by steeping it for a moment in water, then wiping it dry.

In lozenges made of vegetable powders, as, for instance, those of ipecacuanha, the use of thick mucilage is advised to prevent the extractive matter from coloring the product.

The mucilage used is nearly always made of gum tragacanth, but some pharmaceutists prefer that of gum Arabic, as giving them a more translucent appearance; white of egg is recommended for the same purpose.

The quantity of mucilage necessary to thicken substances varies somewhat; it is greater for lozenges which contain dry powders than for those made of extractive substances. It may be remarked that lozenges containing a large proportion of mucilage become very hard by time.

Mucilages are sometimes made with simple water, and sometimes with aromatic waters, or the latter are replaced by essential oils added directly to the mass, or to the dry powders.

M. Garot mentions a German method which confectioners sometimes make use of to aromatize lozenges extemporaneously after their desiccation. It consists in dissolving a volatile oil in ether, and pouring this solution upon the lozenges contained in a bottle with a large mouth, shaking them well, then pouring the lozenges upon a sieve, and instantly placing them in a stove to dispel the ether. This method is very convenient, as it permits the preparation of a large quantity of inodorous lozenges, which may be flavored as they are needed.

Second Class.—This embraces those which consist of adhesive, saccharine, and mucilaginous materials, softened by water and beaten into a mass with flavoring and medicinal ingredients, and then rolled into lozenges, generally of a different shape from the others.

Although there are an immense number of lozenges in use, the following syllabus embraces all those recognized in the *Pharmacopœia*:—

TROCHISCI, *U. S. P.*

CLASS I.—*Each lozenge weighing* 10 *grains.*

Officinal Name.	Proportion.	Adjuvants.	Med. Prop.
Trochisci cretæ . .	3½ grs. in each	Powdered nutmeg	Antacid, astringent.
" magnesiæ .	2½ "	"	Antacid and laxative.
" sodæ bi-carb.	" "		Antacid.
" ipecac. .	¼ gr. "	Arrowroot	Expectorant.
" menthæ pip.	$\frac{1}{10}$ ♏ "		Carminative.

CLASS II.—*Each lozenge weighing* 6 *grains.*

Trochisci glycyrrhizæ et opii	Opium, 1 gr. in 10 lozenges Sugar, liquorice, gum Arabic, and oil of anise	Sedative. Expectorant.

Before describing the preparation of the only officinal lozenge of the second class, it will be proper to introduce to view the following unofficinal lozenges of my own invention:—

Iron Lozenges. (*Trochisci Ferri Carbonatis.*)

I have prepared these for several years, and, without the stimulus of newspaper puffing, or the employment of any unprofessional means, they have grown into general favor and enjoy a wide-spread reputation both in and out of the profession, furnishing an answer to those who assert the necessity of illegitimate aids to the successful introduction of a popular remedy. The following is the formula:—

Take of		
	Subcarbonate of iron	5 ounces.
	Vanilla	1 drachm.
	Sugar	15 ounces.
	Mucilage of tragacanth	q. s.

Triturate the vanilla with a portion of the sugar into a uniform powder; mix this with the remainder of the sugar, in powder, and the carbonate of iron, then beat the whole into a mass with the mucilage, and divide into round lozenges, each weighing twenty grains.

Each lozenge contains five grains of subcarbonate of iron, the usual dose for a child; an adult might take two or three for a dose three times a day. They have been used with success in the early stages of chorea, in anæmia, and in cases, generally, in which this well-known and popular chalybeate salt would be indicated.

The use of carbonate of iron as an anthelmintic is worthy a more general trial. From experience with these lozenges, I believe they are better adapted to meet the popular demand for worm medicines than any of the numerous pink-root preparations sold in such vast quantities.

Phosphatic Lozenges.

Take of		
	Phosphate of lime	10 ounces.
	Phosphate of iron	2 ounces.
	Phosphate of soda	6 drachms.
	Phosphate of potassa	2 drachms.
	Sugar, in powder	17 ounces.
	Piperoid of ginger, or	
	Powdered ginger,	
	Syrup of phosphoric acid, of each sufficient.	

Mix the phosphates of lime and iron, with the sugar and ginger, by passing through a fine sieve; then, by the aid of heat, dissolve the phosphates of soda and potassa in the syrup of phosphoric acid, and make into a mass with the mixed powders. Roll this into a cake of the proper thickness, dusting it with a sifted mixture of one part of phosphate of iron and eight parts of sugar, and cut out the lozenges, each weighing fifteen grains.

The syrup of phosphoric acid is made by dissolving one drachm of the glacial acid in eight fluidounces of syrup. Each lozenge contains five grains of phosphate of lime, one grain of phosphate of iron, and half a grain of the mixed phosphates of soda and potassa. It is necessary that the phosphates of potassa and soda should be used only in small proportion, to avoid imparting a decidedly saline taste to the lozenges.

The use of the phosphates, particularly phosphate of lime, has recently been highly recommended abroad, and adopted, to some extent, in this country, as supplying elements to the system which are exceedingly apt to be deficient, particularly among children, in large cities. It is asserted that this salt not only aids in the building up of the bony structure, when it is deficient, but assists in maintaining the irritability, without which assimilation and nutrition are always lacking. My friend, Dr. W. E. Brickell, now of Vicksburg, Miss., used these lozenges, with great success, in an asylum for friendless children, in this city, in treating the glandular swellings, sore heads, and other forms of scrofulous disease prevailing among that class. He also reports a case of secondary syphilis, and another of sciatica benefited by their use.

Lozenges of the Hypophosphites.

The complete solubility and disagreeable taste of the salts usually entering into the compounds of the hypophosphites, renders these unfit for use in the form of lozenges, except diluted largely with sugar and flavoring ingredients. In the following recipe I have contrived to cover up the taste very satisfactorily:—

Take of Hypophosphite of Lime . .	25 grains.
" Potassa . .	19 grains.
" Soda . .	19 grains.
" Iron . .	10 grains.
Sugar	20 ounces.
Powdered red rose leaves . .	1 ounce.

Make lozenges of each fifteen grains, containing one grain of the mixed hypophosphites; 2 to 3 is a dose for a child, three times a day.

Catechu Lozenges.

These are particularly adapted to cases of relaxation of the uvula, irritation of the larynx, and to diarrhœa.

Take of Catechu	2 ounces.
Tragacanth	½ ounce.
White sugar	12 ounces.
Rose-water	Sufficient.

Make into ten grain lozenges; to be used *ad libitum.*

Wild Cherry Tablets.

Under this name, several manufacturers vend compounds of sulphuret of antimony, morphia, &c., flavored with oil of bitter almonds. Wm. R. Warner first suggested a really scientific lozenge of wild cherry, formed by mixing an alcoholic extract of the bark with powdered sweet almonds, and incorporating with sugar and gum. His recipe, as published in the *American Journal of Pharmacy*, vol. xxxi., page 22, was defective from omitting sugar, the chief ingredient. The following I have found to produce a fine preparation, retaining the sedative virtues of the drug as concentrated as is safe, in this form of preparation:—

Take of Wild cherry bark (powdered) .	℔j. (officinal.)
Alcohol	q. s.

Make a tincture by displacement, evaporate to dryness, and powder the extract—to this add

Powder of blanched almonds . .	℥iij.
Gum	℥iv.
Sugar	℔iij–℥iv.

Make a mass, and divide into oval lozenges, of each ten grains. The uses of these will be obvious. They develop hydrocyanic acid when introduced into the mouth, and should be used with care.

Wistar's Cough Lozenges.

In the second class of the foregoing syllabus, but one officinal preparation is placed, which is that commonly known as Wistar's cough lozenges. These are known and esteemed throughout the United States, and are almost as familiar to the public at large as to the physician and pharmaceutist. The recipe, which originated with the late Professor Wistar, of the University of Pennsylvania, has been considerably modified by most manufacturers, although retained nearly in its original form in the *Pharmacopœia*. In giving that employed in our own establishment, I may preface it by the remark that most pharmaceutists and physicians prefer buying them to attempting their preparation. The formation of a mass possessing the requisite softness and pliability, and yet firm enough to retain the shape given to it, is a matter of considerable difficulty, even with those who are somewhat accustomed to it, while those who are not often waste their material, as well as their time, in the manipulation. This remark, however, lessens in force when the quantity manipulated with is small.

Take of Powdered liquorice,	
" gum Arabic,	
" sugar, of each . .	5 ounces.
Oil of aniseed	30 drops.
Sulphate of morphia . . .	12 grains.
Water, and	
Tincture of Tolu, of each . .	A sufficient quantity.

Dissolve the sulphate of morphia in one fluidounce of water, and add the oil of aniseed, with sufficient powdered gum Arabic to incorporate it thoroughly. To this add one fluidounce of water, or a sufficient quantity; add this, now, to the powder, and beat thoroughly into a mass of the proper consistence. This is to be divided into lozenges, each weighing six grains, and these, after they are dry, are to be varnished with tincture of Tolu.

The mode of rolling and dividing these, and, consequently, their shape, is different from that indicated for the previous lozenges. After beating the ingredient into a mass, portions of 168 grains each are weighed out, and each of these being rolled between two smooth pieces of board, into a cylindrical stick, 28 inches in length, is laid away upon a smooth drying board, until nearly dry and brittle, and then cut with a sharp knife or scissors into 24 equal lozenges, each about $1\frac{1}{8}$ inch in length, and weighing 6 to 7 grains.

The dose is one, taken occasionally. About twelve lozenges contain an ordinary adult dose of sulphate of morphia. Made by this recipe, they are less liable to constipate the bowels, and are less bitter to the taste than the officinal.

Spitta's (Coryza) Lozenges.

These are unofficinal but popular lozenges, for cold in the head, particularly for the painful sense of tightness and obstruction in the nasal fossæ. They will frequently cure sore-throat and hoarseness, the cubebs they contain adapting them to these complaints by its local stimulant effect. They are generally made into the same shape as Wistar's, and in very much the same way, but they are larger, each lozenge containing 10 grains, and not so palatable.

Take of Powdered cubebs	4 ounces.
" extract of liquorice	16 ounces.
" gum Arabic	8 ounces.
Oil of sassafras	40 drops.
Syrup of Tolu	sufficient.

Beat the ingredients together into a uniform mass, and divide into lozenges of 10 grains each.

These may be taken almost *ad libitum*, the lozenge being allowed to dissolve gradually in the mouth.

Dr. Jackson's Pectoral Lozenges.

This formula was first published by A. B. Taylor, who obtained it directly from its distinguished author. It is anglicized as follows:—

Take of Powdered ipecacuanha	10 grains.
Precip. sulphuret of antimony	5 grains.
Muriate of morphia	6 grains.
Powdered gum Arabic	of each 11 drachms.
" sugar	
" ext. of liquorice	
Tincture of Tolu	4 drachms.
Oil of sassafras	4 drops.

To be made into a stiff mass, with simple syrup, and divided into 200 lozenges, or into lozenges of 10 grains each. Each lozenge contains $\frac{1}{20}$ grain of ipecac, $\frac{1}{40}$ grain of the antimonial, $\frac{1}{33}$ grain of morphia. They are usually rolled into flat cakes, and cut out with a round punch, as described under the head of the officinal lozenges.

Dr. Jackson's Ammonia Lozenges.

Take of Muriate of ammonia	1½ drachms.
" morphia	3 grains.
Powdered elm bark	6 drachms.
" gum Arabic	of each 7 drachms.
" sugar	
" ext. of liquorice	
Tincture of Tolu	3 drachms.
Oil of partridgeberry	4 drops.

To be made with syrup into 180 lozenges, or into lozenges of 10 grains each, containing $\frac{1}{2}$ grain muriate of ammonia, and $\frac{1}{80}$ of a grain of the morphia salt.

These are used for somewhat similar affections with the foregoing, and are made into the same shape.

Parrish's Cough Lozenges.

We have been in the habit, for the last seven or eight years, of preparing a pectoral lozenge not unlike that of Dr. Jackson. The recipe, which is as follows, was contrived with the aid of a medical friend, and has proved a useful one, producing a comparatively active preparation:—

Take of Powdered ipecacuanha	50 grains.
Kermes mineral	100 grains.
Sulphate of morphia	16 grains.
Pow'd sugar	of each 3 ounces.
" gum Arabic	
" extract of liquorice	
Oil of anise	40 drops.
Syrup of Tolu	Sufficient.

To be made into a mass and divided into 320 lozenges, each containing about $\frac{1}{6}$ grain of ipecacuanha, $\frac{1}{3}$ grain of Kermes, $\frac{1}{20}$ grain of morphia salt.

The dose of these is one three times a day.

Candy and Drops.

Various kinds of candy are used in medicine for the well-known expectorant or demulcent properties of the sugar alone, or for the effects of such medicines as may be conveniently combined with it. The manufacture of these pertain almost exclusively to the confectioner, who prepares a thick semifluid mass by using with the sugar a small portion of water, and boiling till it is brought to such condition as that a small portion removed from the fire upon a glass rod will solidify into a transparent candy on cooling; it is then poured out upon a marble slab. If the coloring or flavoring ingredient is in powder, as, for instance, tartaric acid used in making lemon drops, it is worked in with the melted candy on the slab; otherwise it must be added before testing its hardness and removing from the fire. The sheet of melted candy being smoothed upon the surface, if designed for secrets, a very common form, is partially cut through into squares, and then, when brittle, broken off; if designed for drops, the candy requires to be run into moulds upon a machine constructed for the purpose; if for sticks, it is rolled and drawn out to the required thickness.

By kneading and working this material while soft, its whiteness is increased. The principal art in making candies is in removing them from the fire at just the right moment before *caramel* begins to be formed, and not until the whole of the uncombined water is driven off; besides the proximate mode, with a glass rod, given above, the elevation of the boiling point to exactly a certain point is an indication that the candy is finished.

The fruit essences, so called, prepared by artificial processes from *fusel oil*, have been much used of late to flavor drops. Lemon and ginger drops are also much in vogue; the latter are best prepared from the piperoid, or oleo-resin of ginger (see p. 218).

The following recipes are appended, as of utility to the pharmaceutist, who may procure the admixture of the medicinal ingredients, with candy at the confectioner's for a few cents per pound advance on the cost of the sugar.

Ginger Drops.

To ten pounds of the melted candy add one ounce of piperoid of ginger, and, by means of an appropriate apparatus, run it into drops the size of cherry-stones.

Medicated Secrets, or Cough Candy.

To ten pounds of melted candy add the following mixture, and divide into secrets:—

Take of Tincture of squill	. . . . . .	f℥iv.
Camphorated tincture of opium / Tincture of Tolu	of each	f℥ss.
Wine of ipecacuanha	. . . . .	f℥j.
Oil of gaultheria	. . . . . .	♏viij.
" sassafras	. . . . . .	♏vj.
" aniseed	. . . . . .	♏iij.

Used *ad libitum* in ordinary coughs.

CHAPTER XV.

ON DISTILLATION AND SPIRITS.

This process, the reverse of evaporation in its applications, is, like it, designed to separate the volatile from the fixed ingredients in a solution. While in evaporation the object is to dissipate and reject what is volatile, preserving and retaining what is comparatively fixed, in distillation the volatile ingredient is to be secured. To distil a solution, it is first converted into vapor by the application of heat, and the vapor is then condensed in a separate part of the apparatus.

In a work of the design and scope of the present, any elaborate description of the apparatus used in distillation, and the mode of conducting the process on a large scale, would be quite out of place. The uses of the still in the manufacture of spirituous liquors and the spirit of turpentine of commerce, and in the rectification of these into alcohol and camphene, and in various other branches of manufacture, are among the most important subjects connected with chemical technology, and occupy a prominent place in works on that subject. In the present chapter, I shall have reference chiefly to the use of distillation in Galenical pharmacy, referring to another part of the work an account of its application to some of the small chemical processes falling within the range of the pharmaceutist and country practitioner. The dry distillation of solid substances, which are unaltered by the heat employed, is called *sublimation*. In Galenical pharmacy, this is applied to the separation of benzoic acid; in chemistry, to the manufacture of calomel, corrosive sublimate, &c. When this is accomplished in close vessels by a degree of heat which decomposes the substances acted on, it is called *destructive distillation*, as in the manufacture of acetic acid.

Apparatus for Distillation.

Fig. 174 exhibits a copper still and block-tin condensing worm, such as may be conveniently used for the distillation of liquids which are not liable to corrode metallic vessels. Such an apparatus is particularly adapted to distilling water for pharmaceutical use, also rose-water and the alcoholic solution of essential oils, called spirits. The physician or pharmaceutist is, however, more frequently supplied with retorts, which are usually made of glass; they are adapted to make distillations sometimes without, and sometimes with, condensing arrangements attached. The plain retort is almost superseded by the tubulated, which is represented in the accompanying figure, Fig. 175. Formerly, the retort was nearly always connected with a *receiver*, which is a glass globe with a wide mouth and neck, into which the beak of the retort is inserted, either loosely or by the aid of a cork, or as in Fig. 176, with the use of an *adapter*. The retort here represented is of the kind called plain; the receiver *b* is tubulated; *a* is the adapter. The use of a vial of appropriate size and shape, with the bottom and rim, or lip of the neck, cracked off, furnishes a tolerable substitute for the adapter.

Fig. 174.

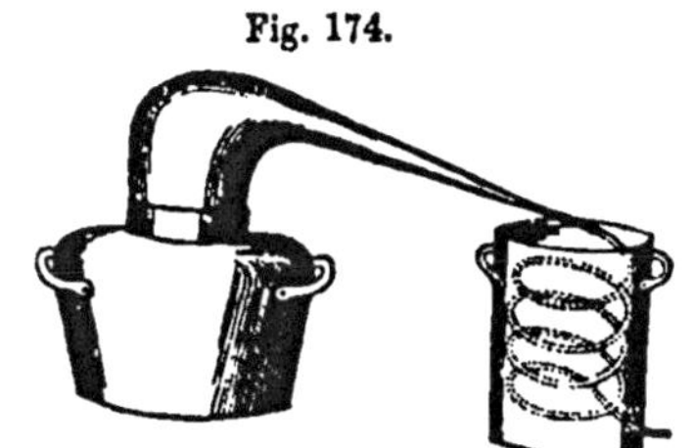

Fig. 175.

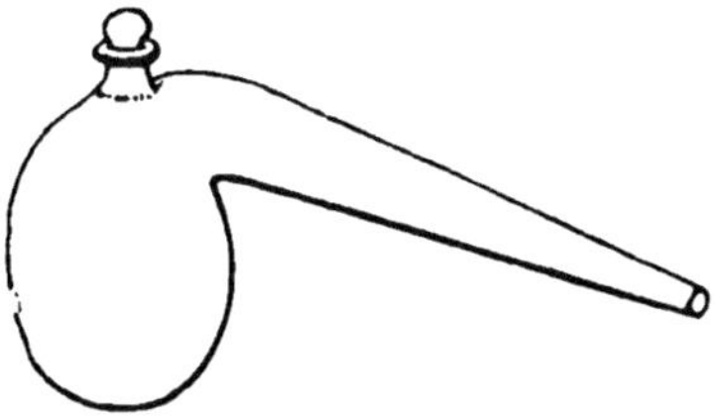

Tubulated retort.

17

Fig. 176.

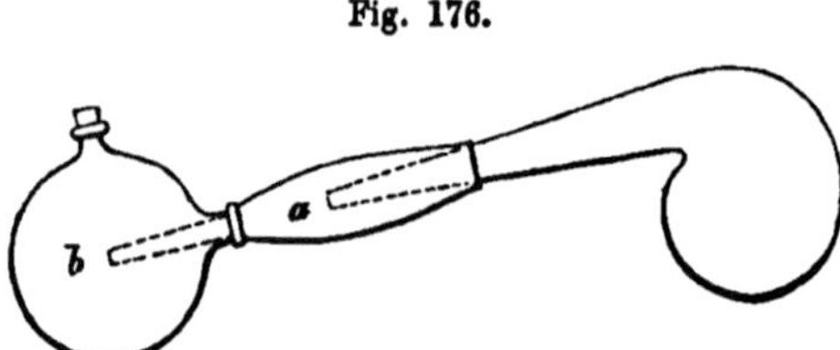

Plain retort, tubulated receiver, and adapter.

The substance to be distilled being introduced into the retort and heat applied, the vapor given off passes at once into its beak or neck, and, if this is not refrigerated, into the receiver. In some cases, particularly in treating very volatile liquids, it is found more convenient to apply cold directly to the beak, as in Fig. 177, in which pieces of linen or cotton cloth, folded several thicknesses and laid lengthwise on the beak, are kept constantly wet by the dropping of water from a filter suspended above it. At the point *a*, below the lower edge of the wet cotton, a piece of lamp-wick, or other suitable string, is tied tightly round the beak, to conduct off the descending warmed water. The receiver here shown, though not tubulated as in the other plate, is quilled or drawn out into a fine tube, which enters the receiving vessel below; this being fully refrigerated, insures the complete condensation of the liquid.

Fig. 177.

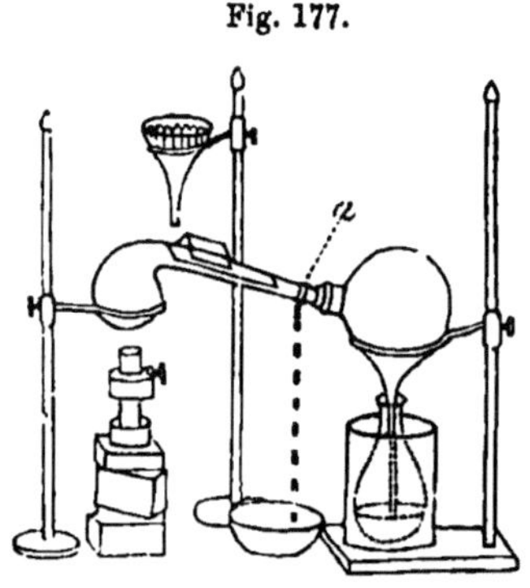

Retort with quilled receiver.

When the liquid to be distilled is condensed at a moderate elevation of temperature, the mode of refrigeration last mentioned is conducted without the use of a receiver, the distillate being collected directly from the beak of the retort, from which it drops as fast as it accumulates. Sometimes the receiver is refrigerated, and not the beak of the retort, and this is perhaps the most common arrangement for retort distillation. It is rather roughly shown in Fig. 178, which represents a plain retort, a plain receiver, and a funnel from which the cold water is supplied. Where this arrangement is adopted, care should be taken not to secure the beak of the retort tightly into the neck of the receiver, in which case the expansion of the

Fig. 178.

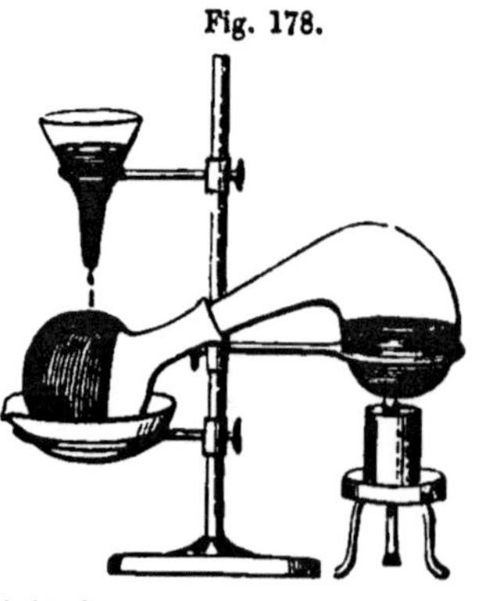

Distillation with plain retort and receiver.

heated air and vapors, on commencing the operation, would lead to a rupture of some part of the apparatus.

Fig. 179 represents a vessel of tinned iron, which I have contrived as a convenient substitute for a glass retort in all operations in which no corrosive or acid substance enters into the liquid to be distilled. Near the top of a deep tin vessel is soldered on a small gutter, so arranged on

Fig. 179.

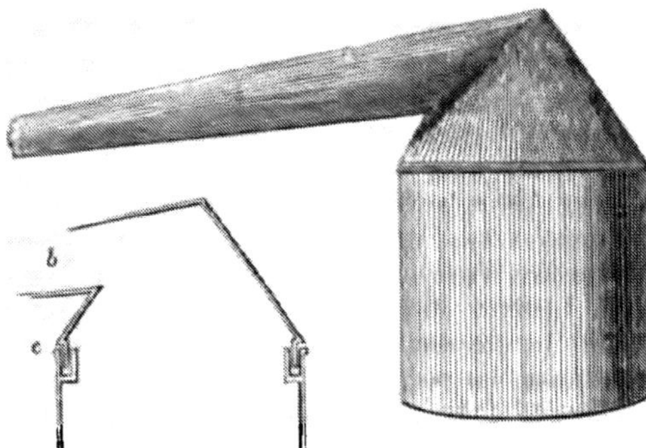

Tin retort with water joint.

its inside as not to reach quite up to the level of the sides of the vessel. The top, *b*, has a rim projecting downwards, which sets into this gutter, as shown in the section. When about to use this, after charging it with the substance to be distilled, the little gutter is filled with water and the top fitted on. The water joint thus formed prevents the escape of any portion of the vapor, while it is prevented from becoming empty by the moisture condensed on the inside of the conical top dropping into it as it descends.

Fig. 180 represents a well-known form of condensing apparatus

Fig. 180.

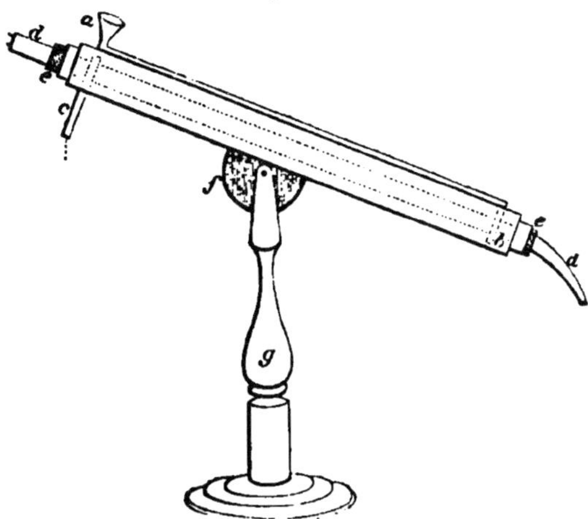

Liebig's condenser.

which has almost superseded the arrangements before figured. This is constructed on a variety of patterns, and of different materials. That represented, Fig. 180, is one I have had in use for several years, and prefer on several accounts to the more expensive and complicated kinds. It consists of a tin tube 18 inches long and 2½ inches in diameter, and having the ends reduced to 1¼ inch to suit the largest size of good corks that are readily attainable. The funnel *a*, is the upper termination of a very small tin tube, which, passing down the whole length of the apparatus, enters it near the lower extremity, where it is extended by a bent leaden tube, as shown by the dotted lines, to the very bottom, at *b*. A short piece of thin lead pipe, *c*, leads from near the apex of the condenser, and, passing out through a perforation into which it is soldered, terminates about two inches below. *d d* is a glass tube 1 inch in diameter, drawn out and bent at its lower end, which passes through the whole length of the apparatus, being secured by the perforated corks *e e*, at either end. These corks must be perfect, and as soft as can be obtained. A smooth and even perforation may be made by a brass cork borer, Fig. 181, or rat-tail file, Fig. 182, or both, so as to constitute a water-tight joint. *f* is a stout piece of sheet copper soldered on to the main tube, and made to work by a screw upon the wooden upright *g*.

Fig. 181.

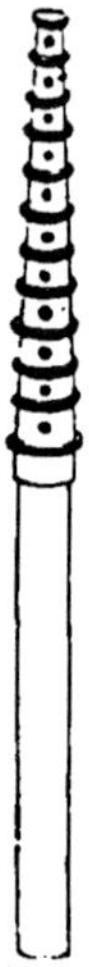

Cork borer.

Fig. 182.

The use of cement or luting to surround the corks is necessary if they are not very perfect and very completely fitted, and as no alcoholic liquids will come in contact with them, dissolved sealing-wax is found to answer an excellent purpose. With one or more retorts, and an apparatus of this kind, most of the processes requiring distillation can be satisfactorily accomplished. The expense of a condenser, such as here described, is from $3 50 to $5. The bottom of the wooden stand should be grooved on the under side and filled in with melted lead, to prevent the ill effects of warping, and to give solidity to the whole.

Fig. 183 represents a condenser supported on a retort stand, having freedom of motion in every direction; *x* is a cast-iron foot, in which is fixed a solid rod of iron *z*. The condenser, as here represented, is designed to be made of brass, with a glass tube fitted into it with corks, as in the other case; the comparative size of the outer tube, as here shown, is much smaller, which requires a much more rapid passage of the cold water through it, especially in distilling very volatile liquids. The Gay Lussac holder *a*, and the rings, are usually made of brass in this arrangement.

Fig. 184 represents a Liebig's condenser and flask attachment made entirely of glass, and such a one as a pharmaceutical student might readily fit up for himself; the tube for the ingress of cold water and the egress of the warm, here enters through the same corks as are perforated for the tube containing the condensing vapor; this tube is

Fig. 183.

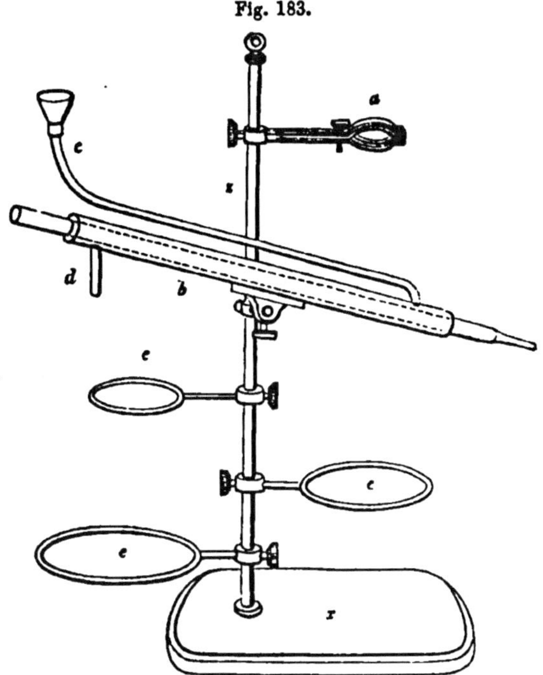

Brass Liebig's condenser in retort stand.

continuous from the neck of the flask to the other end of the apparatus. In the absence of a large glass tube suitable for this apparatus, which is not always to be had, a tin tube, as, for instance, an adhesive plaster can, with the ends taken off, may be substituted.

Fig. 184.

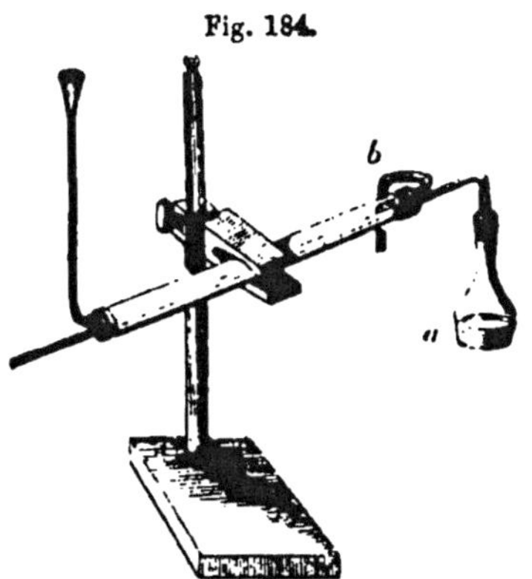

Small glass condenser and flask.

A mechanical support for the retort and for the refrigerating apparatus, is, of course, absolutely necessary in the arrangement of a distillatory apparatus; at least *one retort stand* is quite necessary, even in connection with the Liebig's condenser, Fig. 183; in which case one of the rings might have a sufficiently long handle, connecting it with the screw that clasps the upright rod, to hold a retort or a flask at a sufficient distance from the condenser, to be adjusted to it for use; but this is not the case with any that I have seen, and would render the whole apparatus unsteady when loaded with the liquid.

Fig. 185 will give an idea of the arrangement of the retort and vessel for supplying the condenser with water, and that for catching

Fig. 185.

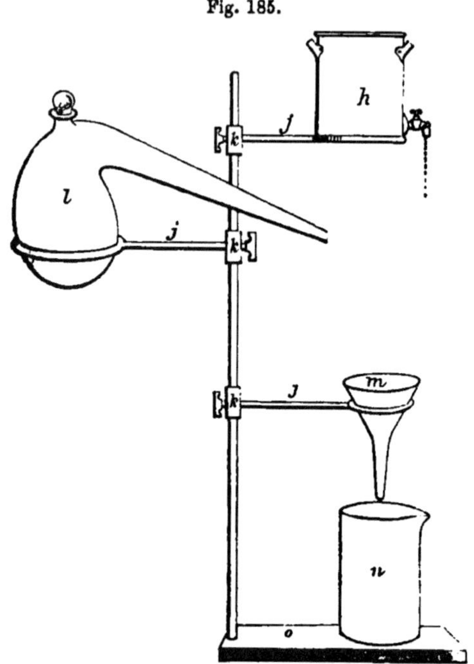

Retort stand for use in distillation.

the waste water upon one retort stand, which, however, must be in due proportion to the size of the condenser.

In Fig. 177, it will be seen that as many as three retort stands are used in a small operation.

When put together, the apparatus for distillation will be complete as arranged in Fig. 186. The tin bucket *h* has a small brass cock, which is so regulated in using the apparatus as to drop the water either slowly or rapidly as the warming of the water in the condenser may require.

The only use of the funnel *m*, is to prevent the splashing of the water as it falls from the condenser. By placing the heavy *receiving* vessel *n* on the wooden base of the retort stand, it is rendered solid, and the weight of the retort *l* is counterbalanced.

A flask with perforated cork and glass tube, as shown in Fig. 187, may be substituted for the retorts before described, an arrangement well adapted to distilling very volatile liquids, and those which boil with great violence. This figure also shows a tube for introducing fresh portions of the liquid without removing the cork; the tube,

Fig. 186.

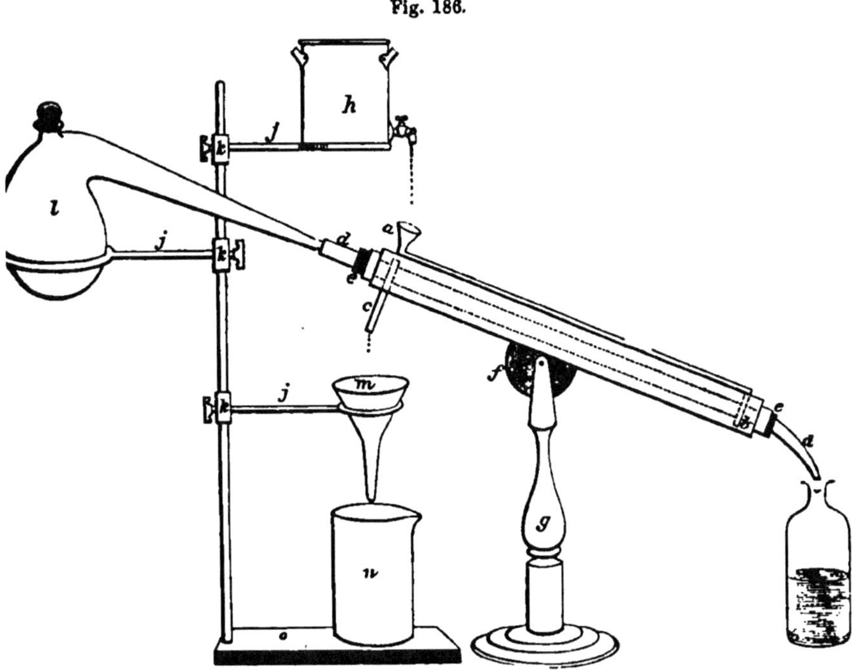

Complete apparatus for distillation.

being bent, retains a portion of liquid in the bulb and adjacent curve, which prevents the escape of vapor from the interior. It is designed to extend only a little below the cork. In case of any stoppage in the apparatus by which an accumulation of vapor might take place in the flask or retort, these tubes would serve as a safety valve, and the liquid being forced out would allow of the escape of the accumulated steam.

Fig. 187.

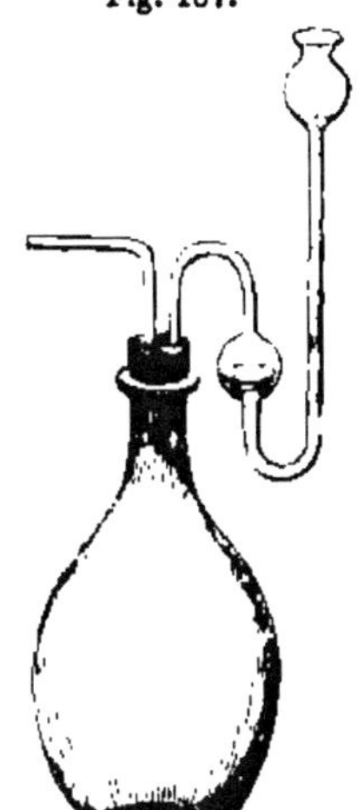

Flask and safety tube.

The pharmaceutical still is the name given to an old-fashioned and cheap form of apparatus, in which the condenser is immediately over the heated liquid, and the distillate is collected by means of a ledge or gutter on its lower surface.

Fig. 188 represents a section of this still, which may be made of tinned iron, and of any required size. *A* is a deep tin boiler, with a rim soldered round its top at *a a*, forming a gutter for the water joint, by which it is connected with the dome or head *B*. This is the refrigerator, on the inner sur-

Fig. 188.

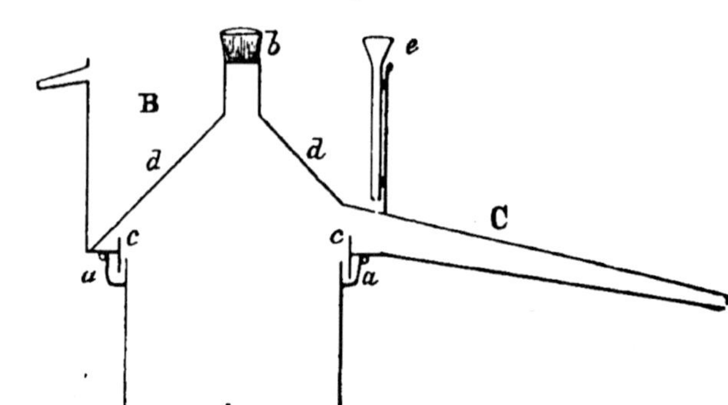

Section of pharmaceutical still.

face of which the condensation occurs; *C* is the neck or tube for carrying off the distillate; *c c* is a circular rim soldered on to the base of the head *B* in such a position as that the upper projection forms a gutter for conducting the condensed fluid as it runs down on the under surface of the cone *d d* into the neck *C*, while the lower part projects downward into the gutter *a a* to form the water joint.

The course of the circular rim *c c* is of necessity inclined downwards toward the under edge of the neck *C*, as indistinctly shown in the section, in order to determine its liquid contents in that direction.

b is an opening in the top of the condenser, stopped by a cork, for inspecting the progress of the distillation, and adding to the contents of the boiler; *e* is a funnel tube into which a current of cold water is directed during distillation, while as it becomes warm it ascends and escapes by the tube on the other side. The water joint is to be nearly filled at the commencement of the operation, and effectually prevents the escape of the vapor.

The Process of Distillation.

From the description and illustration of apparatus now given, the reader will have a pretty good idea of the process as conducted on a small scale. A volatile liquid or mixture containing a volatile ingredient being introduced into a retort or flask connected as before described, and heat applied, the volatile ingredient will rise in vapor, and, being cooled by contact with the neck of the retort, the receiver, or the glass tube of the Leibig's condenser, will be condensed, and may be collected in a liquid and generally a pure condition.

One of the chief practical difficulties in distilling arises from the irregularity of the boiling of liquids in glass vessels, occasioning violent bumping, and sometimes the fracture of the vessel. In treating resinous substances in this way, and in numerous chemical processes, especially as in the preparation of hydrocyanic acid, where a large amount of heavy precipitate is present in the liquid, this renders the operation one of great difficulty and annoyance. The best remedy for this is found in the diffusion of the heat over the sides of the retort, and indeed over the whole surface in contact with the liquid, and in the interposition of small angular fragments of insoluble material, such as rock crystals, flint, or broken glass, among the particles of the liquid, and it is entirely prevented by a glass rod or a metallic wire reaching from the bottom to the surface of the liquid, which serves to diffuse and equalize the heat, and thus to remove the cause of these concussions. Advantage is also gained by covering the bottom of the glass vessel with wire gauze, which diffuses the heat of the flame, or preferably by coating the retort with metallic silver on its inner surface, which may be done by reducing a solution of ammonio-nitrate of silver, by boiling it in the vessel to be plated with oils of cinnamon and cloves, in solution in alcohol. Silver forms the most eligible metallic coating, next to platinum. Flasks may be coated on the outside with metallic copper so as to answer an excellent purpose. This is done by the aid of a battery. (*See* Mohr, Redwood, and Procter, p. 457.)

The application of heat must of course be regulated by the volatility and inflammability of the liquid treated. Strong alcoholic or ethereal liquids, being volatilized at low temperatures, may be heated by a water bath or a sand bath, not too hot, which, besides preventing the excessive boiling of the liquid, will diminish the danger from a fracture of the glass vessel used.

In distilling from flowers or herbs for obtaining essential oils or medicated waters, there is great liability to scorching, from the contact of masses of the solid material with the heated surface of the still, thus producing empyreumatic principles which quite destroy the agreeable fragrance of the product. A false bottom or perforated diaphragm, a few inches above the point of contact with the flame, is a preventive of this, adopted in large operations. In some cases even this is not sufficient, and, as in preparing oil of bitter almonds, it will be found necessary to introduce the pulpy mass upon a layer of straw over the bottom or upon the diaphragm; by this means the contact of the material with the spot where the heat is applied is effectually prevented. The application of carefully regulated steam heat is, of course, in this as in most other heat operations on a large scale, a great improvement.

The pharmaceutical still, Fig. 188, is well adapted to recovering the alcohol from tinctures to be made into syrups, fluid extracts, or extracts; the alcohol obtained, even though impure and below standard strength, is suited to preparing the same tincture again; and the saving of alcohol by this means, in a large establishment, will be very considerable. The long-continued application of a pretty high heat, which is necessary in this case, involves an expense which, if gas, or even charcoal fuel is employed, may approach the value of the alcohol recovered, so that in the winter time it is well to avail ourselves of the stove used for heating the apartment by fitting the still to it, and distilling slowly at the moderate heat thus obtained. The advantage gained by the exclusion of the atmosphere in distillation is not to be overlooked when vegetable preparations are being concentrated. The head of the still becoming full of steam excludes the air, for the most part, and the condensation of the steam brings about a partial vacuum which favors evaporation at low temperatures.

The proper refrigeration of the condensing surface, whether of the retort beak, receiver, Leibig's condenser, or pharmaceutical still, requires pretty free use of cold water; and the application of this has direct relation to the degree of heat required to vaporize the liquid being distilled. An indication by which the operator may always judge when the refrigeration is insufficient, is the escape of uncondensed vapor. When this is observed, he should diminish the heat applied, and increase the application of cold to the condensing surface; this precaution is very important when the vapor is inflammable. The methods indicated in the drawings for the continuous application of cold water by a funnel, and by a small cock, near the bottom of a tin bucket, are well adapted to the several kinds of apparatus figured.

The processes in Galenical pharmacy requiring the use of the still, are chiefly limited to those articles prepared on a large scale, and the apparatus is not commonly in use in retail pharmaceutical establishments, or in those of country practitioners; yet, I have fitted a number from time to time for medical students leaving the school of practical pharmacy, who have found in using them, both for experiment and manufacture, an agreeable and profitable employment during the tedious process of "getting into practice."

Officinal Preparations made by Distillation.

Aqua Destillata, *U. S.* (*Distilled Water.*)

This is directed to be used in a great many preparations in the *Pharmacopœia.* In some, its employment seems called for, while in others the river or spring water, so freely supplied in nearly all towns and cities, answers every purpose.

The inorganic impurities imparted to spring waters by the rocks through which they permeate, are in the highest degree important in connection with solutions of delicate chemical substances, and the same may be said of the organic substances which contaminate some of the natural sources of water, and form precipitates with nitrate of silver, tartrate of antimony and potassa, and a few other very delicate chemical agents. It is, however, generally sufficient, that water should be pure enough for safe and wholesome drinking, to be fit for use in preparing the Galenical and even many of the chemical preparations.

One of the most important uses to the apothecary and physician, of the apparatus for distillation figured and described on the foregoing pages, is to enable him to prepare and keep at hand for special occasions, *aqua destillata.*

OLEA DESTILLATA, *U. S.*

The distilled oils are prepared by mixing the bruised herb or other part containing the oil with a small portion of water in a still, when, after macerating for a suitable length of time, and adjusting the apparatus, heat is applied. The oil, though its boiling point is always much above that of water, is readily diffused in the steam; and when this is condensed in the refrigerated part of the apparatus, the oil, if in excess, separates, and if specifically lighter, collects on the surface of the distilled water; or, if heavier, it settles to the bottom, and may be separated; the mode of preparing the officinal *aqua rosæ*, and other common distilled waters, corresponds with this, the proportion of water being so adjusted as that no excess of the oil beyond what is soluble in the water shall be present.[1]

SPIRITUS, *U. S.*

Alcoholic solutions of essential oils are usually called spirits or essences; they are sometimes prepared by distilling alcohol from the fresh herb, which thus gives up its essential oil, and on its condensation retains it in solution; they are also prepared by dissolving the oil directly in alcohol, as in the tinctura olei menthæ piperitæ, tinctura olei menthæ viridis, called essences of peppermint and spearmint, and tinctura camphoræ, called spirits of camphor. For the preparation of all spirits by solution, fresh volatile oils ought to be selected, to impart the flavor in its purity; old resinified oils should be rejected for this purpose, or if used, a subsequent distillation, with the previous addition of a little water, is advisable; thus the oils will be purified, empyreuma of the resin prevented, and the flavor of the spirits be considerably improved; to this circumstance is due the superiority of *distilled* spirits. The officinal class *spiritus* consists of some which are made by distillation, and some which are simple solutions or mixtures of essential oils and alcohol.

Syllabus of Spiritus.

The following syllabus represents the composition and mode of preparation of each of the officinal class:—

GROUP 1.—Made with diluted alcohol.

Spiritus myristicæ	Nutmeg ℥ij to diluted alcohol 1 gallon	By distillation.
" juniperi comp.	Oils of juniper ʒiss, caraway ♏x, and fennel ♏x	By solution.
" pimentæ	Oil of pimenta fʒij, in diluted alcohol 1 gallon	do.

GROUP 2.—Made with strong alcohol.

Spiritus rosmarini	Oil fʒiv to 1 gallon of alcohol		Solution.
" lavandulæ	Flowers ℔ij to " "		Distillation.
" " comp. (lavender compound)	Cinnamon ℥j Cloves ʒij Nutmeg ℥ss Saunders ʒiij	to spt. Lavender Oiij and spt. Rosemary Oj	Maceration or displacement.

[1] See Part III., Chapter on Essential Oils, Camphors, and Resins.

The simple spirit of lavender prepared by distillation is one of the pleasantest of perfumes. That made by solution from the recipe given on page 272 is dependent on the freshness and fine quality of the oil for its value as a perfume. The cultivated or garden lavender yields a much better oil than the common wild plant; the finest quality oil of garden lavender comes from England, and commands a comparatively high price.

The only preparation of this series which is much prescribed, is the last named. This is very often directed by practitioners as a flavoring and coloring ingredient in prescription. The choice of saunders as the coloring agent is, however, unfortunate from the resinous deposit which is apt to separate by dilution with water and on long standing. Cochineal is a much brighter and handsomer coloring ingredient, and the compound tincture of cardamom is, on that account, to be preferred to the lavender compound as a coloring ingredient in solutions.

The following recipe of George Coggeshall is preferred by many practitioners for *Compound Spirit of Lavender.*

Take of Lavender flowers	. . .	12 ounces.
Rosemary leaves, / Cinnamon (bruised)	. each	4½ ounces.
Nutmeg (bruised) / Cloves (bruised)	. . each	6 drachms.
Coriander (bruised) / Red saunders (rasped)	each	3 ounces.
Powdered turmeric	. . .	1 drachm.
Alcohol	. . . . . .	6 pints.
Water	. . . . . .	5¼ pints.

Mix and digest for fourteen days, and filter.

Essences for Perfumery.

Besides the use of fragrant essences for the mere gratification of the sense of smell, they serve a good purpose in headache, and as grateful refrigerant applications in dry and hot conditions of the skin. I append a few recipes for agreeable and ready spirituous perfumes. The art of perfumery has attained a perfection in France towards which most of our manufacturers make but a faint approximation. The French recipes call for so many ingredients not readily obtained in this country, and altogether derived from their own gardens and manufactories, that they require considerable modification to make them practicable to us. I shall, therefore, confine myself to inserting a few good recipes which constitute a pretty good assortment of essences.

Cologne Water.

Eau de Cologne, as imported from Cologne, and from Paris, is a highly rectified spirituous perfume obtained by distillation from a variety of fragrant plants. Of the numerous Farina colognes imported, all are highly rectified and apparently distilled from the plants, while, as prepared in this country, Cologne water is almost always made from essential oils dissolved in alcohol. This may be very good, if the oils are fresh and combined with reference to their relative strength and accord.

Best Cologne Water. (*No.* 1.)

Take of Oil of bergamot	. . .	f℥ij.
" neroli	. . .	fʒij.
" jessamine	. . .	f℥ss.
" garden lavender	.	fʒij.
" cinnamon	. . .	♏j.
Benzoated tincture	. .	f℥iij.
Tincture of musk	. .	fʒss.
Deodorized alcohol	. .	Cong. j.
Rose-water	. . .	Oij.

Mix, and allow the preparation to stand a long time before filtering for use.

Common Cologne Water. (*No.* 2.)

Take of Oil of lavender	. . .	℥iss.
" rosemary	. .	℥ss.
" lemon	. . .	℥j.
" cinnamon	. .	gtt. xx.
Alcohol	. . . .	Cong. j. Mix.

Much cheaper than the foregoing.

Benzoated Tincture for Colognes, &c.

Take of Tonqua beans	. . .	℥j.
Vanilla	. . . .	ʒij.
Nutmegs, grated	. . .	No. j.
Mace	. . . . .	ʒij.
Benzoic acid	. . .	gr. x.
Alcohol	. . . .	Oj.

Macerate the solid ingredients, in coarse powder, in the alcohol *ad libitum*, and filter.

TOILET WATERS.—(*Substitutes for Eau de Cologne.*)

Rose Geranium.

Take of Essential oil of citronella (India)	. .	f℥ij.
" " lemon grass "	. .	f℥ss.
" " bergamot	. . . . .	f℥ss.
" " lavender (French)	. .	fʒij.
Extract of jessamine (from pomade)	.	f℥j.
Benzoated tincture	. . . . .	f℥ij.
Alcohol (95 per cent. deodorized)	. .	Cong. j.

Mix and reduce with water which has previously been saturated with oil of citronella by trituration, after the manner of the officinal medicated waters, as long as it can be done without precipitating too much of the essential oils; let it stand for a few days and filter.

Orange Blossom.

Take of Essential oil of neroli (petal bigarade No. 1) . f℥j.
" " orange peel (bigarade No. 1) . gtt. xl.
" " rosemary (from flowers only) . f℥ss.
" " bergamot . . . . f℥j.
Extract of orange flowers (from pomade),
" jessamine (from pomade), of each . f℥ij.
Alcohol (95 per cent. deodorized) . . . Oiv.
Distilled orange-flower water . . . . . Oj or q. s.

Mix, and proceed as before.

Putcha Pat. (*Patchouly.*)

Take of Essential oil of Patchouly . . . . . f℥ij.
" " copaiva . . . . . f℥ss.
" " orange peel (bigarade) . . ♏v.
" " valerian . . . . . ♏ij.
" " rosemary (from flowers only) ♏xv.
Tincture of ginger . . . . . . ℥iss.
Benzoated tincture . . . . . . f℥ss.
Alcohol (95 per cent. deodorized) . . . Cong. j.
Patchouly water (made with oil of patchouly, after the method of medicated waters, as in rose geranium) . . . . . . Oj. or q. s.

Rose.

Take of Balsam Peru . . . . ♏xxv.
Essential oil of bergamot . . . . . f℥iij.
" " santal . . . . . . ♏xl.
" " neroli (bigarade petal No. 1.) . ♏xx.
" " rosemary (aux fleurs) . . f℥iss.
" " rose (kisamlic) . . . f℥ij.
" " citronella (India) . . . f℥iss.
Extract of rose (from pomade) . . . . f℥ij.
Alcohol (95 per cent. deodorized) . . . Ovj.
Rose-water, distilled . . . . Oj.

Add the last, after the mixed oils and alcohol have stood two or three days, and filter the whole.

Lavender.

Take of Essential oil of lavender (aux fleurs) . f℥iss.
" " lemon . . . . fʒiij.
" " lemon thyme . . . f℥j.
" " orange peel, *sweet* . . fʒj.
" " nutmeg . . . . fʒj.
" " sage . . . . fʒss.
Tincture of musk . . . . . . fʒvj.
" benzoin (Piesse) . . . f℥j.
Sweet spirit of nitre . . . . . f℥ij.
Alcohol (95 per cent. deodorized) . . Cong. ss.
Lavender water (made from the oil and water)Oj.

Millefleur.

Take of Balsam Peru . . . . fʒiij.
Oil of bergamot . . . . . . fʒvj.
" cloves . . . . fʒiij.
" neroli (*pet. gr.*) . . . . . fʒvj.
Extract of musk . . . . . . f℥iij.
Orange-flower water . . . . . Oiss. or q. s.
Alcohol (deodorized) . . . . . Ovj.
Mix.

Frangipanni.

Take of Essential oil of rose . . . . . . ♏xx.
" " neroli (bigarade) . . . . ♏x.
" " melisse . . . . . ♏v.
" " bergamot . . . . . f℥j.
" " santal wood . . . . f℥ij.
Extract of vanilla (Piesse) . . . . . f℥ss.
" magnolia (from pomade) . . . f℥j.
Tincture of santal wood saturated,
Alcohol, āā . . . . Cong. ss.
Sandal water from oil . . . . . q. s to dilute.
Mix.

Essence of Patchouly.

Take of Oil of copaiva . . . . . . gtt. xx.
" orange . . . . gtt. iij.
" valerian . . . . . . gtt. j.
" rosemary . . . . . . gtt. j.
Tincture of Tolu . . . . . . gtt. xx.
Alcohol, ginger, āā . . . . . . q. s.
Mix.

Verbena Water.

Take of Oil of balm melisse . . . . . f℥iij.
Deodorized alcohol . . . . . Oij.
Water. . . . . Sufficient.
Make a clear solution.

This may be made somewhat stronger, though of a less pure verbena favor, by the addition of a little oil of lemon. Oil of balm melisse is imported, though its smell seems identical with our garden lemon trifolia.

Lavender Water. (*Simple Spirit of Lavender.*)

Take of English oil of garden lavender . f℥ij.
Deodorized alcohol . . . . Oj.

Make a solution.

A little fresh calamus root macerated in the above improves it.

Aromatic Vinegar.

A pungent and reviving perfume, formerly esteemed a preventive of contagion.

Take of Acetic acid, very strong,
Camphor, in powder,
Oil of cloves, of each a sufficient quantity.

Mix them, and secure in a strong and well stoppered bottle.

Tincture of Musk.

Take of Musk . . . . ʒij.
Water . . . . Oss.
Macerate twenty-four hours and add—
Solution of potassa, *U. S.* . . . . f℥ij.
Macerate twenty-four hours and add—
Alcohol . . . . Oss.

Let it stand at summer temperature for one month and decant.

Perfume for adding to Mouth Washes.

Take of Asarum Canadense . . . . . ℥ss.
Orris root . . . . . . ℥ss.
Strong alcohol (Atwood's) . . f℥viij.
Make a tincture and add—
Tincture of musk . . . . f℥j.
Essence of millefleurs . . . f℥ss.
" patchouly . . . gtt. xx.

Superior Mouth Wash.

Take of Old white Castile soap . . . . ʒij.
Alcohol . . . . f℥iij.
Honey . . . . ℥j.
Perfume, as above . . . . f℥iv.

Dissolve the soap in the alcohol, and add the honey and perfume.

PART III.

ON PHARMACY IN ITS RELATIONS TO ORGANIC CHEMISTRY.

CHAPTER I.

LIGNIN AND ITS DERIVATIVES.

THIS work is designed mainly for a class little versed in the intricacy of organic chemistry, and whose object is to acquaint themselves with the practical parts of pharmacy rather than with its theory. Some may study it in connection with a course of experimental manipulations, while others, perhaps, will use it as a guide in the daily routine of a dispensing office or shop. To such it is adapted by an arrangement, which, without any claim to a scientific basis, is recommended by simplicity, and a gradual advancement from the easy to the more difficult manipulations.

Abandoning for the present this arrangement of subjects, it is designed, in Part III., to present to view some matters which could not be conveniently introduced in the previous portions of the work, and yet are important in a scientific point of view, and appropriately considered before approaching the succeeding Chapters on Extemporaneous Pharmacy.

Although a more scientific classification of subjects than that heretofore observed is called for in this connection, and some chemical knowledge on the part of the reader is presupposed, the effort will be made, by simplicity of language, to adapt it as far as possible to the class for which it was designed.

The pharmaceutical classification of materia medica is primarily into organic and inorganic medicines. Of these, the organic will be brought into view in Part III.

The study of these in their chemical relations has, of latter years, become an object of great interest, and has developed the germs of a system of classification of plants founded on their chemical composition.

All plants are composed of a collection of organic proximate principles, which, when further resolved, are found to consist of carbon, oxygen, and hydrogen—the two latter elements frequently combined in the proportion in which they exist in water; some of these princi-

article on the same subject, by John P. Maynard, of Dedham, Mass., in which he claims to have been the first to use the preparation as an adhesive plaster, and proceeds to detail its advantages, as proved by a number of experiments made by himself, and by numerous physicians and surgeons in Boston. In the same number of the *Journal* appears an editorial notice, which recommends the collodion, as it is there named, in terms of approval, and in relation to its adhesiveness, says: "Nothing known to us will compare with it in this respect." Of its mode of preparation, both these writers left us in the dark, although Dr. Maynard's formula for preparing it was placed in the hands of Maynard & Noyes, druggists, Boston, who commenced the manufacture of it, and measures were taken to introduce it throughout the United States.

On the first introduction of Maynard & Noyes' article in Philadelphia, my lamented friend, W. W. D. Livermore, then an assistant in my store, and myself, jointly pursued a series of experiments in its preparation, the result of which we announced in a paper published in the *American Journal of Pharmacy*, vol. xx. p. 181, stating the best formula that we had tried for the preparation of this solution. It prescribed the mixing of equal portions of nitric and sulphuric acids, and the maceration in it of clean bleached cotton for twelve hours. The proper strength of the nitric acid was then known to be a matter of importance, the acid of 1.5 sp. gr. furnishing the most satisfactory results.

This cotton, after washing and thorough drying, was to be dissolved in a certain proportion of ether, free, or nearly free, from water.

The recipe was accompanied by such practical suggestions as our experiments led to, and although some of the views advanced in that paper were afterwards abandoned, the recipe, with slight modifications, has continued to give us satisfaction to this time, and is that now most generally used.

In the following year an article appeared in the same journal, extracted from the *London Medical Gazette*, in which a formula of M. Mialhe was offered as more uniformly satisfactory.

He directed of finely powdered nitrate of potash, 40; sulphuric acid, 60; carded cotton, 2 parts, to be treated as follows: Mix the nitre with the sulphuric acid, in a porcelain vessel, then add the cotton and agitate the mass for three minutes, by the aid of two glass rods; wash the cotton, without first pressing it, in a large quantity of water, and, when all the acidity is removed (indicated by litmus-paper), press it firmly in a cloth; pull it out into a loose mass, and dry it in a stove at a moderate heat.

The proportions of ether and prepared cotton directed for the preparation of collodion in this recipe are omitted, as they were, I think, inadvertently wrong.

Much discussion occurred in the journals about this time in regard to this new and attractive preparation; some chemists preferring the process by mixed acids, and others getting better results by M. Mialhe's.

In the fourth number of the *Am. Journ. of Pharm.*, 1849, I published the result of further experiments upon the new adhesive solution, giving a modified formula, which was strongly recommended, as allowing the preparation of a much larger quantity at one time, and with far less trouble; as avoiding the exposure of the operator to corrosive acid fumes, while stirring the cotton with the semi-fluid mass, which, in the other case, makes it necessary to work either in a well-ventilated apartment, or in the open air; and as facilitating the washing of the product, which comes out from the mixed acids with no solid crystalline ingredient contaminating it, and may be purified with the utmost facility.

This, as slightly modified, is here given.

Parrish's Formula.

Take of Fuming nitric acid,	
Sulphuric acid, of each . . .	Four fluidounces.
Clean carded cotton[1]	Half an ounce.
Ether	Three pints.
Alcohol	Sufficient.

Thoroughly saturate the cotton with the acids, previously mixed, and allowed to become cool; macerate for twelve hours; wash the nitrated cotton in a large quantity of water; free it from water by successive washings in alcohol, and dissolve it in the ether.

The present officinal process, which is a modification of that of Mialhe, is here introduced—

The U. S. P. Formula, 1850.

Take of Cotton, freed from impurities,	
and finely carded . . .	Half an ounce.
Nitrate of potassa, in powder,	Ten ounces.
Sulphuric acid	Eight fluidounces and a half.
Ether	Two pints and a half.
Alcohol	A fluidounce.

Add the sulphuric acid to the nitrate of potassa in a wedgewood mortar, and triturate them until uniformly mixed; then add the cotton, and by means of the pestle and glass rod, imbue it thoroughly with the mixture for four minutes; transfer the cotton to a vessel containing water, and wash it in successive portions by agitation and pressure until the washings cease to have an acid taste, or to be precipitated on the addition of chloride of barium. Having separated the fibres by picking, dry the cotton with a gentle heat, dissolve it by agitation in the ether previously mixed with the alcohol, and strain.

The recent essays on this subject, which have appeared in the journals, have not materially altered its aspect. C. Caspari, in the *Trans. Md. Col. Ph.*, June, 1858, direct that where the mixed acids are used,

[1] There is an asserted advantage in macerating the cotton in solution of nitrate of potassa and drying it previous to treating it with the acids. Paper is said to produce a better collodion for photographic purposes.

they should be allowed to cool to 110° F. before introducing the cotton. He also recommends the use of hot water in washing the cotton as prepared by the officinal process, so as to remove more thoroughly all traces of sulphate of potassa. In the use of the mixed acid process he has macerated as much as nine days, so as to produce a pefectly soluble product. He says, that the use of Nordhausen acid, with nitric acid or nitrate of potassa, produces an excellent gun-cotton, (Pyroxylin); but it is too insoluble for use in collodion.

A. P. Sharp, in the same journal, Sept., 1858, adverting to the deficiency of the commercial acids in strength, gives a formula which is a combination of Mialhe's and my own, and obviates the noxious fumes liberated in the first, and the asserted liability to failure from deficiency in material in the second. He takes of commercial nitric acid, sp. gr. 1.40, eight fluidounces; sulphuric acid sixteen fluidounces; nitrate of potassa four ounces, and fine cotton one ounce; dissolves the nitrate of potassa in the nitric acid, and then adds the sulphuric acid; mixes well together, and while warm immerses the cotton for three minutes, transferring to a basin, washing well with water, drying, and dissolving.

Oliver G. Sherman, in his inaugural thesis, submitted to the Philadelphia College of Pharmacy in the spring of 1848, and published in the Journal the same year, details some experiments to show the different solubilities of prepared cotton made from the mixed acids of different strengths, and immersed at different temperatures.

From the strong acids in equal parts he obtained a large increase in the weight of the cotton—56⅔ per cent. It was soluble, though not completely and rapidly, in ether and a mixture of five parts of ether to three of alcohol. The addition of a small portion of water to the acids before mixing produced the effect of partially dissolving the cotton and furnishing a very soluble inexplosive product. Immersion of cotton in five parts of sulphuric to three of nitric, produced a still greater increase of weight, nearly 70 per cent.; the product being nearly insoluble, and highly explosive.

The importance of temperature in this preparation was tested by immersing the cotton in a mixture of the refrigerated acids which only reached 112° F. after being mixed; the product was found to have increased 40 per cent. in weight, but was comparatively insoluble. In another case, the cotton was immersed after the cooling of the mixed acids, as directed in the foregoing recipe; the product gained 50 per cent., was slightly explosive, and partially soluble. In no case was long maceration resorted to, and the trials were hardly so numerous as to justify the conclusions stated in the paper, that the acids, before mixing, should have the temperature of 65° F., to which they should be brought, artificially, in the winter, and that at the time of immersing the cotton the thermometer should indicate about 130° F. I have seen a large quantity of cotton completely consumed under nearly these circumstances, with the liberation of immense volumes of nitrous fumes.

Prof. Procter published, in 1857, *Am. Journ. Pharm.*, vol. xxix. p. 105, an essay calling attention to the advantage of long maceration in making collodion, and directing that the cotton should be exposed four days to the mixed acids. He gives preference at the same time to the process with the mixed acids over that of the Pharmacopœia, which, taken in connection with the evidence of its superiority, so abundantly furnished from all sources, leaves no room to doubt the superior claims of this, the original process.

Washing and Drying.—It now remains to notice, in connection with the process of preparing soluble gun-cotton, the best mode of washing and drying it. The cotton should be removed, when the reaction is complete, into a funnel or other suitable support, and the stream from a hydrant turned upon it; or, if this is not convenient, let it be thrown into a vessel of water, and teased out with two sticks or glass rods, so as to be thoroughly permeated by the water, then collected into a compact form, and the acidulated water decanted, to be renewed once or twice, or as often as necessary to purify the prepared cotton. This is now found to be white, tasteless, inodorous, and, if dried, harsh and almost crystalline in its texture. The object of drying is to free it from the water absorbed by it in washing; and here I would notice the elegant expedient directed in the formula; it was suggested to me by the late W. W. D. Livermore: to drain off the water by pressure, and then to macerate the cotton a few minutes in alcohol, which, by its affinity for the water, rapidly extracts it, and then may be sufficiently separated by expression, as it is not incompatible with the ethereal solution, which, in fact, it improves. Rehn's patent for this process of washing prepared cotton for collodion dates long since this suggestion, and even since its public announcement by me in the Philadelphia College of Pharmacy.

Straining and expressing collodion are often necessary when it contains a large amount of undissolved fibre, as the last portions in a bottle from which the clear liquid has been from time to time decanted; a slight precaution may save the operator a great deal of trouble and mortification from his hands becoming coated with it beyond remedy. When about to squeeze the strainer, or to thrust the hands into the liquid for any purpose, be careful to have a towel at hand, and instantly, on removing them, wipe them thoroughly dry before time is allowed for evaporation and the consequent deposit of the pellicle. This plan will be found effectual.

The contraction of the collodion pellicle in drying is a decided objection to its use in some cases. C. S. Rand proposes Venice turpentine as the best addition to obviate this effect.

Rand's Modified Collodion.

Take of Prepared cotton . . . . . . ʒij.
Venice turpentine . . . . . . ʒij.
Sulphuric ether . . . . . . ℥v.

Dissolve, first, the cotton in the ether; add the turpentine, and, by slight agitation, complete the solution.

The resulting collodion, when applied to the skin, forms a transparent pellicle, more difficult to remove than that of ordinary collodion. Being more pliable, it yields to the motion of the skin, and will not crack even after several days' application. It might be supposed that the turpentine would render it more irritating, but this does not seem to be the case, owing to the absence of that mechanical stimulus so powerfully displayed in ordinary collodion. The addition of two drachms of mastic to the above may be at times advisable, if the pellicle be required of great toughness and strength; but it dries more slowly, and remains opalescent longer than that containing Venice turpentine alone. This preparation is more suitable for the purpose of a varnish than as an application to the skin, and is especially adapted to coating labels on vials, which it renders impervious to cold and hot water and alcohol. *Castor oil* has also been found to be an excellent addition to collodion for the prevention of this contraction.

Properties.—Collodion is a clear, colorless liquid, of a syrupy consistence, becoming thinner by age, with a strong odor of ether; when applied to a dry surface, it evaporates spontaneously, yielding a transparent pellicle without whiteness, possessed of remarkable adhesiveness and contractility, and quite impervious to moisture or to the action of any ordinary solvents, ether excepted.

"A piece of linen or cotton cloth covered with it, and made to adhere by evaporation, to the palms of the hand, will support, after a few minutes, without giving way, a weight of from 20 to 30 lbs. Its adhesive power is so great that the cloth will sometimes be torn before it gives way. Collodion is frequently not a perfect solution of cotton; but contains, suspended and floating in it, a quantity of vegetable fibre which has escaped the solvent action of the ether. The liquid portion may be separated from these fibres by decantation or straining, but it is doubtful whether this is an advantage for surgical use. In the evaporation of the liquid, these undissolved fibres, by felting with each other, appear to give a greater degree of tenacity and resistance to the dried mass, without destroying its transparency.

Mode of Preservation—Collodion is one of those liquids which, owing to extreme volatility, it is objectionable to use from a large bottle, not only from the waste by evaporation every time the stopper is drawn, and the consequent inspissation of the liquid; but, also, from the explosive nature of the vapor of ether when it comes in contact with flame; it should, therefore, be put up in small vials, from which it may be used with economy and safety.

Formerly the manufacturers usually put it in ground stoppered vials, of one or two ounce capacity; but an improvement has been made in the substitution for these of common cork stoppered, one ounce vials.

Cork, by its elasticity, can be made to fit the neck of a vial more tightly than the best glass stopper, and is, therefore, less liable to be thrown out on an elevation of temperature of the contained volatile liquid.

Collodion is generally applied by the aid of a camel's-hair brush, but if one of these is allowed to dry, after being immersed in the liquid, it is apt to be too stiff to use again. To obviate this disadvantage, a contrivance, such as is shown in the accompanying figure, is resorted to; it consists of a long f℥j vial, with a cork stopper, which is perforated with the smallest cylinder of the cork borer, or with the rat-tail file (see Figs. 181 and 182, p. 260), and into this perforation a thin piece of wood with a turned cap about the diameter of the cork is tightly inserted; this plug of wood has the diameter of the quill of a camel's-hair brush of medium size, and it is long enough to project below the cork so that the quill will fit on to it and be secure. The bottle being now nearly filled and the cork inserted, the brush will dip into the collodion, and, by constant immersion, will keep moist and always ready for use. For further particulars in regard to the application of this principle to the administration of medicines, the reader is referred to the chapter on Dispensing.

Fig. 189.

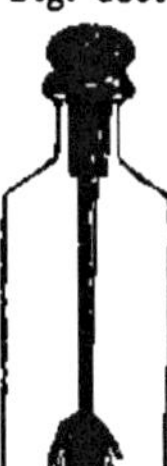

Collodion vial.

I have observed that where, from exposure, a part of the ether has evaporated, the addition of more ether will serve to redissolve the gelatinous residue, unless it has dried beyond a certain point, at which it becomes quite insoluble.

Uses of Collodion.—The chief use of this interesting liquid is in photography, which has already extended so as to become one of the most important of the modern arts. In medical practice its principal application is to ordinary superficial sores, as cuts and abrasions of the skin, and also to some skin diseases, where the indication is to protect the part from external irritating influences, and where violent itching is one of the most troublesome symptoms. Prof. Simpson, of Edinburgh, recommends it for sore nipples, which it completely protects without interfering with the sucking of the infant; for this purpose, it would seem that Rand's preparation would be best suited. It was first principally recommended for the application of bandages, and is used in France as a substitute for dextrin in permanent splints, which, by its use, may be applied over a less extended surface without diminishing the strength and permanence of the dressing.

In cases of burns, where the cuticle has been removed and the symptoms of acute pain allayed by suitable applications, collodion is capable of one of its most useful applications, though for this purpose its contractility should be obviated by adding Venice turpentine or castor oil, as before indicated.

By combining collodion with the ethereal tincture of chloride of iron, a compound is produced which is said to furnish a much more resisting and pliable, though thinner pellicle, and one adapted to the treatment of erysipelas.

The following combinations have been proposed by James T. Shinn, of Philadelphia, for adapting collodion to useful therapeutic applications.

Iodinal Collodion.

Take of	Iodine	Half an ounce.
	Canada balsam	Half an ounce.
	Collodion	A pint.

Dissolve the iodine and balsam in the collodion.
Used as a substitute for iodine ointment.

Belladonnal Collodion.

Take of	Select belladonna leaves, powdered	Eight ounces.
	Ether	Twelve fluidounces.
	Alcohol (95 per cent.)	Sufficient.
	Canada balsam	Half an ounce.
	Collodion wool (prepared cotton) .	A drachm.

Macerate the leaves in the ether with four fluidounces of alcohol, for six hours, pack in a percolator, and pour on alcohol till a pint of tincture is obtained; in this dissolve the cotton and balsam. This is a desirable substitute for belladonna plaster. It may be made free from color by dissolving atropia in collodion.

Aconital Collodion may be made from aconite root by a similar formula. (See *Blistering Collodion.*)

The composition of collodion has excited much discussion, and some ingenious hypotheses. The discovery by Prof. Leidy, of this city, of a beautiful crystalline deposit in inspissated collodion, and a similar and independent observation in London, are among the most remarkable facts bearing upon the composition and chemical relations of the group of principles to which lignin belongs.

The action of nitric acid on cotton appears to result in the substitution of nitric acid for hydrogen, or nitric acid for water, in the formula of cotton. According to Porret & Teschemacher, the formula for true pyroxylin (gun-cotton) is $C_{12}H_8O_8+4N,O_5$, or $C_{12}H_8O_{12}+4NO_4$. According to this formula 2 equivalents of water in the cotton are replaced by 2 of nitric acid, and this compound is combined with 2 equivalents of nitric acid. *Gladston, Pharm. Journal*, xi. 481, gives the composition of the soluble prepared cotton thus, $C_{24}H_{17}O_{17}3NO_4$. If this is correct, the inference is warranted that 3 equivalents of nitric acid enter into this compound, and it seems probable that there is a relation not yet fully established between the explosiveness of the product and the amount of nitric or nitrous acid entering into its composition. That there is also a relation between explosiveness and solubility is established by the experience of practical men; the real pyroxylin is insoluble in ether, xyloidin is freely soluble, and from one extreme to the other there seems every grade of solubility. A careful study of the increase of weight in the preparation of specimens of different degrees of solubility, might lead to clearer ideas upon the composition of this as yet uncertain preparation.

M. Reschamp, Professor in the School of Pharmacy at Strasburg, has succeeded in reproducing cotton from pyroxylin, by heating it at the temperature of 212° with a concentrated solution of proto-chloride of iron. The chloride deepens in color, and very soon there is a disengagement of pure nitric oxide. When this has ceased, and the cotton has been washed with hydrochloric acid, to remove the peroxide of iron impregnating it, the cotton is found to have lost the properties of pyroxylin. In the same way, amidon has been produced from xyloidin.

PRODUCTS OF THE DISTILLATION OF WOOD.

By the distillation of the purer kinds of wood in close vessels, a variety of interesting compounds are produced, which are useful in the arts and in medicine. Of these, charcoal (carbo ligni, *U. S.*), acetic acid (acidum aceticum, *U. S.*), and pyroacetic and pyroxylic spirit, and creasote (creasotum, *U. S.*), may be mentioned as of special interest to the physician, and a short notice of each is appended.

Carbo Ligni and Carbo Animalis, U. S.

The former of these two kinds of charcoal is used in medicine, while the latter is most employed in chemical processes as a decolorizing agent.

Willow charcoal, the variety most used in medicine, is chiefly obtained from the manufacturers of gunpowder, who devote much attention to the production of a pure and fine powdered article.

Charcoal is wholly insoluble, tasteless, and inodorous; it absorbs moisture and gases from the air, and contains a small portion of the incombustible saline materials of the wood, from which it may be freed by digestion in diluted muriatic acid, although this precaution is not necessary as a preparation for medicinal use.

The dose of powdered charcoal as an absorbent disinfectant, is about a teaspoonful or less; as an aperient, a tablespoonful, or somewhat less, mixed with magnesia.

Animal charcoal, or *bone-black*, is made from bones by calcination, and, besides carbon, contains phosphate and carbonate of lime in abundance; these important constituents have much to do with the peculiar porosity which gives to this substance the power of absorbing coloring matter and gases, and adapts it for the various uses in the arts and in pharmaceutical chemistry to which it is applied. It is not very convenient to use in fine powder, and is hence generally prepared in a granular condition.

Carbo animalis purificatus, *U. S.*, is among the preparations designed to be made by the apothecary. It is prepared by digesting a pound of animal charcoal with twelve fluidounces each of muriatic acid and water, for two days, at a moderate heat, pouring off the liquid and washing the charcoal thoroughly with water.

This is adapted to many uses to which the unpurified powder would be unsuited, owing to its saline ingredients.

In the preparation of the alkaloids, gallic acid, and numerous other chemical substances, animal charcoal is used to absorb the associated coloring matters; but it should not be forgotten that the same property which adapts it to take up the coloring matter also occasions, to some extent, the absorption of the alkaloid or other principle, so that the loss by the decolorizing process is considerable, unless means are resorted to for the subsequent extraction of the absorbed portions.

To its absorbent property animal charcoal owes its utility as a disinfectant and antidote to the powerful vegetable poisons, which, as proved by Dr. B. H. Rand, may be rendered innoxious in their effects by a large admixture of this inert but porous powder.

Charcoal Dentifrice.

Take of Recently-burnt charcoal, in fine powder . 6 parts.
Powdered myrrh,
Powdered cinchona bark (pale), of each . 1 part.
Mix thoroughly.

Charcoal Tooth-paste.

Take of Chlorate of potassa . . . . . A half drachm.
Mint water . . . . . . 1 fluidounce.
Triturate to form a solution, then incorporte with—
Powdered charcoal . . . . . 2 ounces.
Honey . . . . 1 ounce.

A charcoal prepared from areca nuts is much esteemed as a dentifrice in England.

ACIDUM ACETICUM, *U. S.*

The acid liquid distilled over when charcoal is prepared from wood, in close cylinders without access of air, contains this valuable acid in a very impure state. By subjecting this to further distillation, the liquid is collected which is known as wood vinegar, or pyroligneous acid. By saturating this acid with lime, acetate of lime is produced, which, by decomposition with sulphate of soda, furnishes sulphate of lime and acetate of soda; the latter salt being crystallized in a state of purity, yields, by distillation with sulphuric acid, pure hydrated acetic acid in solution in water.

The officinal acetic acid is directed in the *Pharmacopœia* to have a specific gravity of 1.041, which, however, is a less satisfactory assurance of its strength than its saturating power, which, as before stated under *Aceta*, is such that 100 grains saturate 60 of crystallized bicarbonate of potassa, and contain 36 grains of monohydrated acid.

Acetic acid is now so cheaply and abundantly produced for use in the arts, that it is placed in the *Pharmacopœia* among the articles of materia medica; the process above given is selected from a variety in common use. Acetate of lead is one of its sources of production.

Under the name of *glacial acetic acid*, the Dublin Pharmacopœia directs a concentrated acid, which, at the temperature of 40° F., deposits crystals. It may be prepared by exposing finely powdered acetate of lead (previously dried at a temperature of about 300° F., until it ceases to lose weight) to an atmosphere of dry hydrochloric acid in a flask or retort, until nearly the whole of it exhibits a damped appearance, then connecting it with a Leibig's condenser and applying heat by means of a choride of zinc bath, until the whole of the acid shall have distilled over. The specific gravity of this acid is 1.065; it contains about 98 per cent. of hydrated acetic acid, is volatile, colorless, inflammable, and dissolves camphor, resins, volatile oils, &c. Its chief use is in perfumery for forming a very pungent perfume for smelling-bottles.

Acetic acid is also produced by the oxidation of alcoholic liquids, especially cider and wine, and in this impure and diluted form is called vinegar; in chemical works it is generally classed among the derivatives of alcohol.

Much of the vinegar of commerce is largely adulterated or sophisticated, although, according to the experiments of W. W. D. Livermore, the use of sulphuric acid is less common than has been supposed. Of sixteen specimens of commercial vinegar obtained from different sources, none were adulterated with sulphuric acid. Tested for malic acid, gum, and extractive matter, believed to be always present in cider vinegar, all but two gave evidence of containing one or more of these products by throwing down a precipitate with subacetate of lead, soluble in nitric acid.

The strength of the different specimens was ascertained by him as follows. The numbers represent the number of grains of bicarbonate of potassa saturating 100 grains of vinegar:—

No.	Grains	No.	Grains
No. 1	9 grains.	No. 10	4 grains.
" 2	4 "	" 11	$5\frac{6}{10}$ "
" 3	8 "	" 12	8 "
" 4	$4\frac{4}{10}$ "	" 13	$8\frac{4}{10}$ "
" 5	6 "	" 14	$5\frac{6}{10}$ "
" 7	8 "	" 15	$8\frac{3}{10}$ "
" 8	$8\frac{7}{10}$ "	" 16	$7\frac{8}{10}$ "
" 9	6 "		

The normal saturating power is about $7\frac{1}{2}$ grains of the bicarbonate to 100 grains of vinegar.

Camphorated Acetic Acid.

Take of Camphor	. .	Half ounce.
Acetic acid	. .	$6\frac{1}{2}$ fluidounces.

Pulverize the camphor by means of a few drops of spirits of wine, and dissolve it in the acetic acid. Used as a fumigative in fevers, an embrocation in rheumatism, and a refreshing and pungent perfume.

Acetone, or Pyroacetic Spirit, C_3H_3O, and Pyroxylic Spirit, or Wood Naphtha, $C_2H_4O_2$.

These are products of the distillation of wood, which are separated from the acid liquors, after they are saturated with lime, by simple distillation and rectification.

They are both colorless, or slightly yellow, inflammable, volatile, pungent liquids, closely resembling each other in sensible and medical properties, nearly always impure, and generally confounded with each other, in commerce; they may be known apart by their reactions with chloride of calcium.

While pyroacetic spirit does not dissolve or mix with a saturated solution of the chloride, pyroxylic spirit instantly mixes when dropped into it.

The normal specific gravity of each is about the same, .792 to .798; but, as found in commerce, they oftener reach .820 to .846.

Under the name of methylic spirit, hydrated oxide of methyl ($C_2H_3O + HO$), pyroxylic spirit is extensively used in England as a cheap substitute for alcohol, and is sometimes substituted for it in the preparation of chloroform. Dr. Hastings, of London, introduced it several years ago as a remedy for consumption, and both this and pyroacetic spirit are sometimes prescribed, though not so much as formerly, in connection with cough medicines. DOSE, about 10 to 40 drops.

CREASOTUM, *U. S.*

This is a secondary empyreumatic product of destructive distillation which the *Pharmacopœia* describes as being obtained from tar. As found in commerce, it is an oily liquid obtained indiscriminately from various kinds of tar, especially that from bituminous coal, and varies in composition.

Pure creasote is colorless and transparent, having a high refractive power and oleaginous consistence. Its ordor, when diffused, is peculiarly smoky, its taste burning and caustic; its specific gravity is about 1.057. It is freely soluble in alcohol, ether, acetic acid, caustic potash, and in water to the extent of six or ten drops to the ounce.

The article now generally sold as creasote, is quite different from what was formerly met with under that name. It is now imported from Germany, and is much cheaper than the kind which formerly came from England, and was obtained from wood tar. The present article, which is remarkable for readily assuming a brown color on exposure to the light and air, is prepared from coal tar. It has a specific gravity of 1.062, and boils at 386°. A slip of pine wood dipped first into this, and then into hydrochloric acid, becomes blue, which is not the case with the true wood-tar creasote. In an article on this subject, in the *New York Journal of Pharmacy*, Oct., 1853, Professor Edward N. Kent has given a method of manufacture and purification which has proved successful in his hands, and expresses the opinion that carbolic acid, as he considers it, is creasote in a purer form than that obtained from wood tar. It is certainly less disagreeable for use.—(See *Phenylic Acid.*)

The most important property of creasote is that of coagulating albumen, which renders it powerfully antiseptic and caustic. Placed in contact with a suppurating surface, it whitens the cuticle and destroys it, like nitrate of silver.

Its principal use internally is in the form of creasote water, to check nausea. For this purpose, about two drops may be dissolved in an ounce of water, and a little gum and sugar added. DOSE, a tablespoonful (equal to one drop), frequently repeated.

Dropped upon a fragment of cotton, after dilution with alcohol, ether, or chloroform, and inserted into the cavity of a tooth, it relieves toothache when the pain is occasioned by the exposure of the nerve, and is popularly regarded as the most certain remedy.

From very frequent experiment and practice, I believe that any of the highly pungent essential oils, as of cloves and cinnamon, are equally efficient, while tannic acid and chloroform, which are much less offensive, are nearly always successful. Very painful and distressing accidents are liable to occur from attempting to drop any of these liquids into the cavity of a tooth from a vial.

As an external caustic, creasote may be applied, undiluted, with a camel's-hair pencil; but for other purposes it is usually prepared in the form of ointment (unguentum creasoti, *U. S.*), or in solution in water. In hemorrhages, it acts as a most efficient styptic, and is successfully applied in solution, in the proportion of about six drops to the ounce of water.

Creasote is one of the remedies which the apothecary is most frequently called upon to prescribe and apply. Large quantities are also consumed by dentists.

CHAPTER II.

ON FARINACEOUS, MUCILAGINOUS, AND SACCHARINE PRINCIPLES.

STARCH, $C_{24}H_{20}O_{20}$, having the same composition as lignin, differs from it widely in physical properties; it exists in various parts of plants, especially in seeds, tubers, and bulbous roots, in minute cells, which may be distinguished by a microscope of moderate power. The size and shape of these have been made special subjects of investigation by pharmacologists, and their study has been found to aid in the recognition of the different varieties of fecula, and in detecting adulterations. The envelop of these starch granules is insoluble in cold water, but is ruptured by the application of heat, so that the contents are exposed and become dissolved. Hence, starch is said to be insoluble in *cold*, but soluble in *hot* water. By the action of heat, and a very small proportion of strong infusion of malt, starch is converted into *dextrin*, a soluble form having the same composition, and so named from its power of causing the plane of polarization to deviate to the right. This object is also attained, as in the case of lignin, by the action of dilute acids, which also ultimately convert it into *grape sugar*. One of the most striking characteristics of starch is its reaction in cold solution with iodine, with which it

Fig. 190.

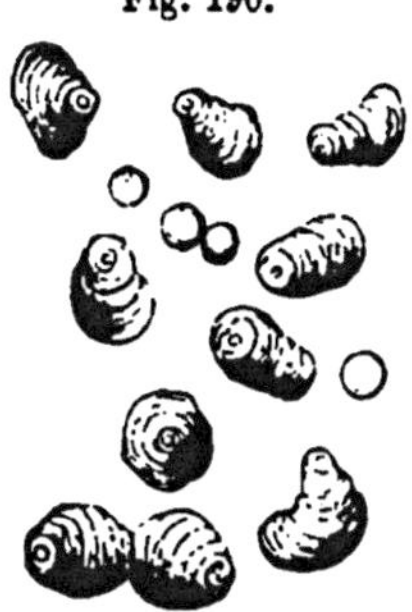

Starch granules as seen under a microscope.

forms a rich blue colored iodide, which loses its color by heat. These two substances thus become tests for each other. With bromine it produces an orange-colored precipitate, which cannot be dried without decomposition.

Lichenin from cetraria, *carrageenin* from chondrus, *inulin* from inula helena, and other sources, are closely allied to starch, but are distinguished from it and from each other by physical peculiarities, and by the fact that while lichenin turns blue with iodine, inulin becomes yellow or brownish with that test, and carrageenin is not affected by it, though differing from gum in solubility and in certain chemical relations.

GUMS differ from starch chiefly in the absence of the granular condition, and their partial or complete solubility in cold water. They are obtained from certain plants in amorphous masses, mostly exuding spontaneously or upon a puncture of the bark. A solution of gum is not affected by iodine, but the most common varieties are precipitated in a very insoluble form by subacetate of lead, $2PbO,\overline{A}c$. A solution of gum is also precipitated by alcohol.

The different varieties of gum are as follows:—

Arabin is derived largely from the acacias; it is extremely soluble in water, forming a clear and colorless though viscid solution, almost free from taste. It may be considered the type of the class, and exists nearly free from impurities in the finer qualities of gum Arabic.

Bassorin is an insoluble variety, swelling with water and dissolving in alkalies. This predominates in gum tragacanth, and, according to some, in salep.

Pectin and Pectic Acids.—Many plants contain, in different organs, especially in succulent roots and acidulous fruits, a body called pectose, which, through the influence of a peculiar ferment called pectase, the organic acids and light and heat, undergoes a change into other bodies of the same relative combinations.

Pectin, parapectin, and metapectin	$C_{64}H_{40}O_{56}+8HO$.
Pectosic acid	$C_{32}H_{20}O_{28}+3HO$.
Pectic acid	$C_{32}H_{20}O_{28}+2HO$.
Parapectic acid	$C_{24}H_{15}O_{21}+2HO$.
Metapectic acid	$C_{8}H_{5}O_{7}+2HO$.

The unripe fruits contain only pectose; while ripening, pectin and parapectin, and subsequently metapectic acid are formed, so that the change of the consistence of the fruits is less dependent on a change of the cellulose, than owing to this transformation. Green fruits exhale oxygen in daylight; with the alteration of pectose, the formation of sugar sets in, carbonic acid is exhaled, the green color disappears, and the free acids (citric, malic, tartaric, &c.) become neutralized by potassa, lime, &c., or their taste is masked by the increase in the quantity of sugar.

Pectin is the cause of the gelatinizing of the juices of currants, raspberries, &c., and of gentian, dandelion, rhubarb, and other roots. The salts of the above acids are uncrystallizable; those with the metallic oxides are mostly gelatinous precipitates, while those with alkalies are soluble in water, but gelatinize on cooling.

Cerasin is the name given to the insoluble ingredient in cherry-tree gum; it much resembles Bassorin, but requires investigation.

Mucilage, which exists in the mallows, in flaxseed, and in salep, is soluble, but forms a less clear solution than Arabin; it is distinguished chemically by being precipitated by neutral acetate of lead, PbO,Ac.

Mezquite is a name proposed for a gum, to which attention has been called by Dr. Geo. Shumard, produced abundantly in Texas and New Mexico—parts of our own country as yet but little explored; it is extremely soluble, and differs from Arabin principally in not being precipitated by subacetate of lead, 2PbO,Ac.

SUGARS.

Sugars are of several kinds, which are closely allied to each other and to the foregoing ternary principles in composition. They are distinguished by a sweet taste, and a more or less distinctly crystalline form. They are mostly soluble in water and somewhat soluble in alcohol.

The following table exhibits the composition, sources, and chemical properties of the different varieties:—

(1.) *Carbohydrates. Sugars of the Composition* $C_{12}H_xO_x$.

a. Directly fermentable.		
Grape sugar, Glucose $C_{12}H_{12}O_{12}+2HO$	In grapes, the fruit of rosaceæ, &c., in diabetic urine, from starch by the action of sulphuric acid.	Deviates polarized light to right;[1] soluble in 1½ parts cold water, insoluble in alcohol; with NO_5, yields oxalic acid.
Fruit sugar, uncrystallized sugar s. Chulariose $C_{12}H_{12}O_{12}$	In fruits, honey, &c.	Rotating left; easily soluble in water and diluted alcohol.
b. Fermentable by being converted first into fruit sugar by yeast.		
Cane sugar $O_{12}H_{10}O_{10}+HO$	In sugar-cane, Chinese sugar-cane, corn-stalks, beets, sugar maple, several palms, &c.	Rotating right; easily soluble in water, little in alcohol; yields oxalic acid with NO_5.
Melitose $C_{12}H_{12}O_{12}+2HO$	In Australian manna from eucalyptus mannifera.	Rotating right; crystallizes in needles; reactions similar to cane sugar.

[1] Polarization of light, which is stated as characteristic in the case of the several sugars, consists of a change produced upon light by the action of certain media and surfaces by which it ceases to present the ordinary phenomena of reflection and transmission. Instruments employed to exhibit this change are called *polariscopes*. By the use of these, differences may be readily detected between substances which are nearly identical in chemical properties.

c. Not fermentable by yeast.		
Melezitose $C_{12}H_{11}O_{11}$	In the exudation of the larch, larix communis (Fr. *mélèze*)	Rotating power right; sweet like glucose; very soluble in water, almost insoluble in alcohol; ferments easily after treatment with diluted SO_3.
Mycose $C_{12}H_{11}O_{11}+2HO$	In ergot.	Rotating power right; easily soluble in water, almost insoluble in alcohol.
Eucalyne $C_{12}H_{12}O_{12}$	In Australian manna, accompanying melitose.	Uncrystallizable; even after treatment with SO_3, not susceptible of fermentation.
Inosite (Phaseomannite) $C_{12}H_{12}O_{12}+4HO$	In muscular flesh, and in the unripe kidney bean. Phaseolus vulgaris.	Efflorescing; soluble in water, little soluble in alcohol; not altered by diluted acids; otherwise similar in behavior to grape sugar; with NO_5, nitro-inosite.
Sorbin $C_{12}H_{12}O_{12}$	In the berries of Sorbus aucuparia.	Rotating power left; soluble in ½ water, little in boiling alcohol; hard crystals, not altered by diluted SO_3; yields oxalic acid with NO_5; reduces oxide of copper.
Lactin, sugar of milk $C_{12}H_{10}O_{10}+2HO$	In milk.	Rotating power right; very hard prisms; soluble in 6 parts cold water, insoluble in ether, slightly soluble in alcohol; by dilute acids, converted into lactose, and then fermentable; yields mucic acid with NO_5.

(2.) *Sugars of the Composition* $C_{12}H_xO_{x-2}$.

Not fermenting.		
Mannite $C_{12}H_{14}O_{12}$	In manna, mushrooms, &c.	No rotating power; soluble in 5 parts cold water, scarcely in cold alcohol, with NO_5, saccharic and oxalic acids.
Dulcose, Dulcin $C_{12}H_{14}O_{12}$, or $C_{14}H_{14}O_{12}+2HO$	From an unknown plant in Madagascar.	No rotating power; easily soluble in water, with difficulty in alcohol; yields mucic acid with NO_5.
Quercite $C_{12}H_{12}O_{10}$	In acorns.	Sublimes in needles; with nitric acid, yields oxalic acid.
Pinite $C_{12}H_{12}O_{10}$	In pinus Lambertiana.	Rotating power right; very sweet; readily soluble in water; nearly insoluble in boiling alcohol.
Melampyrite $C_{12}H_{15}O_{13}$	In melampyrum nemorosum.	No rotating power; soluble in 25 parts water, 1362 parts alcohol; not altered by diluted SO_3, with NO_5, mucic and oxalic acids.

(3.) *Sugars of other Composition.*

Not fermenting.		
Glycerin $C_6H_7O_5+HO$	The basic principle of fats.	Oily liquid; miscible with water and alcohol; insoluble in ether; with NO_5, yields glonoin.
Erythromannite $C_{12}H_{15}O_{12}$, or $C_{11}H_{14}O_{11}$	Product of decomposition of erythrin.	Supposed to be identical with phycite.
Phycite $C_{12}H_{15}O_{12}$	In protococcus vulgaris *Algæ*.	No rotating power; easily soluble in water, with difficulty in alcohol; with NO_5 oxalic acid.
Glycyrrhizin $C_{36}H_{24}O_{14}$	In glycyrrhiza glabra, and echinata.	Uncrystallizable and yellowish; scarcely soluble in cold water, soluble in cold alcohol.

Remarks on the Sugars.

Cane sugar is one of the sweetest of the sugars; when pure it is white or crystallized in translucent double oblique prisms, soluble in alcohol but not in ether. It is soluble in ⅓ its weight of water; its solution heated in contact with salts of copper, mercury, gold and silver, decomposes them. Its watery solution with yeast undergoes the vinous fermentation; sugar forms both a soluble and insoluble compound with oxide of lead; lump sugar is permanent in the air, and phosphorescent in the dark when struck or rubbed. Its tendency to crystallize or form a translucent candy is prevented by the addition of cream of tartar. By the application of heat it melts and cools to a glassy amorphous mass (barley sugar); long boiling diminishes its tendency to crystallize and increases its color.

Preparation.—The juice of the cane is extracted by pressure between iron rollers, after which it is collected and boiled with quicklime, strained, and reduced by evaporation to a thick syrup, when the whole is cooled and granulated in shallow vessels; it is now raw sugar of commerce. By purification or refining, which is accomplished by the aid of animal charcoal, it is obtained as loaf, or more commonly as broken-down or crushed sugar—the condition in which it is mostly preferred for use in pharmacy.

In the granulation of raw sugar, the uncrystallizable portion which remains is drawn off and constitutes molasses of commerce. Molasses, by careful manipulation, is made to yield a further portion of sugar, and thus constitutes sugar-house molasses, or, as it is called abroad, treacle.

Rock candy is a very pure and pleasant form of cane sugar, prepared by crystallizing it slowly upon a string from a strong solution; it is preferred for coughs from the slowness with which it dissolves in the mouth, and is very generally used to sweeten mucilaginous and acid drinks used in catarrhs.

The peculiar brown coloring matter called *caramel*, which is identical in composition with cane sugar in combination, is produced by heating that substance to a temperature at which it loses four equivalents of the elements of water, and becomes quite altered in its properties; it is freely soluble in water, and has a bitter and not disagreeable empyreumatic taste. It is much used to color liquors, as in the fabrication of brandy, and is a useful addition to soups; as this substance is not without practical importance, and is little known to pharmaceutists, I append a formula which I have found to answer very well for its preparation:—

Take of Sugar	1 pound.
Tartaric acid	1 drachm.

Mix them in a porcelain capsule, and apply a gradually increasing heat, not over 430° F., till the sugar melts and burns a little, and the whole assumes a dark brown color, then add water.

Mannite.—This interesting variety of sugar is much called for of latter years as a vehicle for other medicinal substances, as well as for its own valuable properties; its intense and agreeable sweetness is one of its most important characteristics, fitting it to disguise the taste of nauseous medicines.

It may be prepared from manna by several processes: *First.* By digesting manna in boiling alcohol, and filtering while hot. As the liquid cools it precipitates the mannite in tufts of slender colorless needles; these may be purified if necessary by re-solution and crystallization.

Second. By mixing manna with cold water in which the white of an egg has been beaten, boiling for a few minutes, and straining the syrup through linen while hot, the strained liquid forms a semi-crystalline mass on cooling; this is to be pressed strongly in a cloth, then mixed with its own weight of cold water and again pressed, then mixed with a little animal charcoal and dissolved in boiling water, and filtered while hot into a porcelain dish over the fire; the solution is now to be evaporated till a pellicle forms, and set aside to crystallize in large transparent quadrangular prisms.

Third. By dissolving manna in water, precipitating gummy and coloring matters with subacetate of lead, removing lead from the filtrate by carefully dropping into it sufficient sulphuric acid, though not in great excess, evaporating and crystallizing.

Mannite fuses between 320 and 330° F., and crystallizes again at about 284.° In sealed tubes mannite may be heated to 482° without altering, except that a small portion turns into mannitan $= C_{12}H_{12}O_{10}$ (anhydrous mannite), which may be obtained by many processes calculated to abstract the water of crystallization: it is a neutral syrupy sweetish substance, scarcely liquid, insoluble in ether, slowly soluble in anhydrous alcohol, freely soluble in water; in contact with air it absorbs water, liquefies and crystallizes to ordinary mannite.

Though mannite is not fermentable under ordinary circumstances, it may be converted into fermentable sugar, by leaving it in contact under peculiar circumstances with animal tissues. (See *Am. Journ. of Pharm.*, vol. xxix. p. 450.)

Mannite is generally believed to be destitute of purgative properties, but this is incorrect; it is now known to have the cathartic properties of manna without its disagreeable taste. It is even used with success in obstinate constipation, and is especially esteemed in Italy, where it is largely manufactured for exportation. The dose for children varies from one to four drachms; for adults an ounce may be given. (See *Extemporaneous Pharmacy.*)

Sugar of milk is not manufactured in this country, but is said to be chiefly imported from Switzerland, where it is made on a large scale from whey; it is crystallized upon sticks or strings in masses not unlike stalactites in appearance. The greatest consumption of this is by the homœopathists, who use it as a vehicle for almost all their medicines in the form of powders and pillets. It is said by them to have the least action upon the system of any substance they have experimented with; and hence its employment as a diluent for the infinitesimal doses, which, according to their theory, are increasingly powerful in proportion to their dilution. Its physical condition of hardness or resistance to mechanical action adapts it to develop the latent efficiency of those medicines which they assert are only rendered active by long attrition. Recently, powdered sugar of milk has come into use in regular practice, as a food for infants in teething, less apt to produce acidity than cane sugar.

As already stated, by the action of diluted acids upon lignin and starch, they are converted into a soluble form called dextrin, and ultimately pass into grape sugar; this change may be produced by long boiling alone; it is also produced in starch by nitrogenized ferments, especially by that peculiar substance known as diastase. By the same means, cane sugar is spontaneously converted into fruit sugar, and this into alcohol, and ultimately into acetic acid; and, in fact, the alcoholic and acetic liquors of commerce are produced in this way from the various starchy and saccharine vegetable products used in their manufacture.

Glucose or grape sugar is a variety produced in grapes and in different fruits; it is readily obtainable from old and inferior raisins, on which it is deposited as a white powder. It is also deposited by honey, from which it may be obtained in considerable quantities by straining off the uncrystallizable sugar. It abounds in apples, pears, currants, gooseberries, &c. It constitutes also the *sugar of diabetes.* The most economical method of obtaining it is by acting on starch or lignin with sulphuric acid.

Testing for Grape Sugar, or Diabetic Sugar, in Urine.

Under this head the several processes for testing the presence of grape sugar are introduced; they are particularly applicable to the examination of urine. When urine has a high specific gravity, and other symptoms of diabetes appear, the physician finds it of the utmost importance to make a chemical examination. The pharmaceutist is very liable to be called on for this, and will find it an advantage to be supplied with a reliable urinometer (see page 69), a test rack and tubes, and the necessary chemical reageuts.

Horsley's.—Five or six drops of diabetic urine produce a deep sap-green coloration in a boiling solution of chromate of potassa containing free alkali.

Maumene's.—Chlorine at a temperature at and above boiling water causes a brown color, deepening to black on drying. Organic substances of a similar composition with sugar, such as lignin, hemp, linen, cotton, starch, &c., suffer a similar decomposition. A strip of white woollen, merino (which is not altered), is saturated with a solution of perchloride of tin and dried; a single drop of a saccharine or similar solution put on the strip, and heated over a lamp to a little above the boiling point of water, instantly effects a black stain. Even ten drops of diabetic urine in ten cubic centimetres of water produces a brownish-black color.

Boettger's Test for Diabetic Urine.—A tablespoonful of urine and of soda solution, containing one part of crystallized carbonate of soda to three parts of water, are boiled with as much officinal nitrate of bismuth as will cover the point of a knife; glucose imparts a grayish or black color to the nitrate. Albumen is to be previously separated by coagulation, cane sugar and all organic substances usually present in urine are without action.

Mulder's.—Indigo is dissolved in strong sulphuric (better Nordhausen) acid, the liquid over-saturated with carbonate of potassa, to render it alkaline. This, when used, is sufficiently diluted to be of a light blue color and boiled; if now a trace of grape, or fruit sugar be added, the blue color is changed to green and purple; from a larger proportion of sugar, the color passes through red into yellow. If afterwards the liquid is shaken, the purple passes through green into blue, but the yellow through the above shades into green or greenish-blue.

Heller's Test.—The urine is mixed with solution of caustic potassa, the mixture divided in two test-tubes of equal width, one of which is heated to boiling. The presence of sugar is indicated by a darker color, which is ascertained by comparison with the unheated liquid.

Trommer's test is based on the reduction by grape sugar of oxide of copper to suboxide, for which purpose a solution of sulphate of copper in caustic potassa is employed. The way to apply it is to mix the urine or other saccharine liquid with some caustic potassa in a test-tube, and then add a diluted solution of sulphate of copper, drop by drop, and constant agitation, until the occasioned precipitate just commences to remain undissolved; the mixture is then raised to the boiling point, and if it contains grape sugar deposits the orange-red hydrated suboxide of copper, which, while the solution gradually loses its blue color, settles in considerable quantity in the tube.

Fehling's Quantitative Test for Grape Sugar.—The test liquid is prepared by dissolving 40 grammes of crystallized sulphate of copper in 160 grammes of distilled water, and mixing this solution with 160 grammes of neutral tartrate of potassa dissolved in a little water; from 600 to 700 grammes of solution of caustic soda, specific gravity 1.12, are then added, and sufficient water to make the whole measure at 60° F. (15° C.) 1154.4 cubic centimetres. As 1 equivalent of glucose ($C_{12}H_{12}O_{12}$) reduces 10 equivalents of oxide of copper to suboxide, 1 litre of the above solution requires 5 grammes, and 10 cubic centimetres .05 grammes of grape sugar.

A saccharine solution for the quantitative determination of sugar is diluted until it contains not over 1 per cent. of grape sugar. 10 cubic centimetres of the test are diluted with 4 cubic centimetres of water, heated to boiling, and the saccharine liquid gradually added until it ceases to produce a red precipitate of suboxide of copper; the quantity of the liquid used contained .05 gramme of sugar. The quantity of sugar may likewise be calculated from the amount of suboxide of copper obtained, which is separated by filtration, well washed and dried. 10 equivalents of protoxide (CuO) yield 5 equivalents of suboxide (Cu_2O); the weight of equivalent of the latter being 71.2, 5 equivalents weigh 71.2×5=356; the equivalent of grape sugar ($C_{12}H_{12}O_{12}$) weighs 180, and if we express the ascertained weight of suboxide of copper by *s*, the weight of grape sugar=*x* is calculated by the following proportion—356: 180=*s*: *x* or by adding one-half and $\frac{1}{18}$ part of the weight of the suboxide.

Fehling's test is not affected by pectin, tannin, or mucilage, but when several weeks old it is acted on by acetic, tartaric, oxalic and the aromatic acids. In small, well-corked vials, if protected from contact with the air, it keeps well for some time, but it is always safest to prepare it when wanted for use; the copper solution may be kept ready for mixing with a freshly prepared solution of the tartrate, and with the caustic soda, preserved in well-stoppered vials. Free uric acid reduces the test liquid, which fact must not be lost sight of in analysis of urine, which ought to be used quite fresh.

Cane sugar and starch cause no reaction with the test, but when they have been previously converted into grape or fruit sugar by a continued boiling with diluted sulphuric acid, the oxide of copper will be reduced, and from the ascertained quantity of grape sugar 95 per cent. indicates the weight of cane sugar ($C_{12}H_{11}O_{11}$), and 90 per cent. that of starch ($C_{12}H_{10}O_{10}$).

The test is likewise applicable to milk sugar, which reduces for each equivalent 7 equivalents of oxide of copper, so that 1 litre of the test liquid requires 7.143 grammes of sugar of milk for its reduction.

It has been ascertained by Professor Brücke, that grape sugar is a normal ingredient of urine, and it is, therefore, necessary to determine its quantity in disease; for this purpose Fehling's test is applicable, the inaccuracy of which arising from the presence of uric acid may be removed by precipitating the urine with oxalic acid or with $\frac{1}{25}$ of its measure of muriatic acid of 1.10 specific gravity, setting it aside for twenty-four hours in a cool place, after which time it contains but traces (.0001 p.) of uric acid.

Owing to the ammonia contained or readily formed in urine, which keeps some suboxide of copper in solution, Trommer's test does not show the small proportion of sugar in healthy urine, but it generally reacts with the urine of pregnant or nursing women. Minute quantities of sugar are not indicated by Boettger's test, if the black color of bismuth should be owing to the formation of sulphuret; a black coloration will also be obtained by digesting the urine with levigated litharge. Heller's test is the most reliable for detecting very small proportions of sugar, but in a deeply colored urine, the change produced by boiling may not be visible, and another experiment with Boettger's test be advisable.

Remarks upon the Principal Farinaceous, Mucilaginous, and Saccharine Medicines.

The starch group contains, besides the starches, all the cereal grains, which owe their immense utility as articles of food to the presence of starch mingled with a due proportion of a nitrogenized principle, gluten. In many drugs, starch exists to an extent which interferes with their convenient preparation for use in medicine, while it is an important element in certain demulcent and nutritious articles used in medicine, as food for infants, &c.

Arrowroot, maranta of the Pharmacopœia, derived from maranta arundinacea of the West Indies, is considered the best form of pure starch for infants.

The commercial varieties of this fecula used in this country, are Bermuda, which commands the highest price, Jamaica, Liberia, Florida, and Georgia arrowroot; these all appear to possess the same wholesome and nutritive properties, provided they are well prepared and well preserved. There are few articles more liable to deteriorate by improper modes of preservation than this; a musty taste is imparted to it by exposure to moisture, and it readily acquires the odor of drugs with which it is placed in contact. It should be kept in glass bottles, tin cans or wooden boxes, such as are made for the purpose. See an able article on the culture and preparation of arrowroot in the United States, by Dr. Robert Battey, in the *Proceedings of the American Pharmaceutical Association*, for 1858, p. 332.

Arrowroot is an important diet for young children. When fresh and pure, it forms one of the most wholesome and nutritious articles of food in the dietetic category. Great care is necessary in its preparation, and the reader is referred for instructions upon the subject to the article on diet for the sick in the appendix.

Corn fecula has lately been introduced, and largely manufactured in this country. It is made from maize, and is an admirable substitute for arrowroot for table use, being much cheaper, and equally free from unpleasant odor and taste. It is much sold in England under the name of Oswego prepared corn.

Amylum is the officinal name given to wheat starch; this is a very useful article in domestic economy and in the arts, but is not adapted to use in medicine or for food.

Canna, or tous les mois arrowroot, is derived from the tubers of canna edulis, a plant of the natural order *marantaceæ*. It is prepared in the island of St. Kitts, but very little of it seems to reach our markets of latter years. The jelly yielded by this species is said to be more tenacious, but less clear and translucent than that of other arrowroots. Owing to the large size of the starch granules, they exhibit a glistening and satiny appearance, which is quite characteristic.

Curcuma arrowroot is an East India variety which, however, does not reach this country: in England it is said to be used for the purpose of adulteration.

Potato starch, called in England British arrowroot, is also used for the purpose of adulteration, and a test is given by Hassell, by which to distinguish it from *maranta:* it is as follows—mixed with twice its weight of concentrated muriatic acid, maranta yields an opaque paste, while potato starch yields a transparent jelly. There are several other starches used to adulterate arrowroot, but the only reliable mode of distinguishing them is by the microscope, which exhibits characteristic differences in the size and other appearances of the granules.

Sago and *tapioca*, owing to their mode of preparation, are partly soluble, the least soluble parts having properties somewhat resembling those of tragacanth. Their physical condition seems to diminish the tendency to become musty, which is so common a difficulty with arrowroot, while their preparations are better adapted to the taste of adults generally, than the more fluid arrowroot pap.

Of the materials used as food, which owe their utility to containing starch, I need only refer to such as are commonly prescribed in the sick-room.

Reference has been made elsewhere to *pearled barley*, and the mode of using it as directed in the *Pharmacopœia*, is mentioned under the class Decocta. *Barley flour* is a fine preparation of this.

Rice is a very bland and nutritious farinaceous seed, which, like barley, comes into commerce decorticated, ready to be prepared by boiling. Several of its preparations are mentioned with the recipes inserted under the head of diet for the sick; these are nutritive, demulcent, and somewhat astringent in their effect upon the bowels. Rice, by long boiling in water, becomes nearly dissolved, forming a jelly, which is one of its most useful forms of administration in disease.

Oatmeal is distinguished from either of the above in powder by containing the husk ground with the seed. Unlike the foregoing, it is adapted to relieve constipation. It is easily digested, and exceedingly nutritive. Oatmeal may be given to infants when there is no tendency to diarrhœa, and very generally to females after parturition.

Orrisroot, which consists chiefly of starch, is much used as an infant and toilet powder, for which it is adapted by its whiteness and delicate though persistent odor. Its use in dentifrice powders is well known.

Mucilaginous or Gummy Group.—Gum is associated in some plants with resin; and gum resins, a remarkably natural class of drugs, will be hereafter referred to in treating of resins.

Variously associated with other proximate principles, gum is present in a great variety of vegetables, and like starch, it plays an important part in the physiology of the plant; it enters as an element into a great number of articles, both of food and medicine. In its important relations to the art of prescribing and compounding medicines, we shall have occasion to refer to it frequently throughout the subsequent parts of the work, and now introduce it only for the purpose of calling attention to a few medicines, into which it enters in some of its modified forms.

Salep and *tragacanth* are modified gums which seem adapted to nutritious combinations, and enter into Castillon's powders, introduced among articles of diet. Tragacanth is much used for making paste for common adhesive purposes.

The chief use of *carrageen* in medicine has been adverted to under the head of compound syrup of carrageen, but it remains to refer to it as furnishing a most agreeable article of diet, known as *blanc mange*, for which a recipe is given under the appropriate head. The only difficulty in making agreeable preparations of carrageen arises from its salt-water taste, which may be removed by long soaking in water previous to subjecting it to preparation.

Iceland moss contains a bitter principle, adapting it to use as a tonic demulcent.

Elecampane, *burdock*, and *comfrey*, and the root and flowers of *marsh-mallow*, enter into a variety of domestic expectorant remedies.

Flaxseed contains, with its mucilaginous ingredient, a large amount of fixed oil; under the head of Infusions, the well-known demulcent drink called flaxseed tea is introduced. Infusion of *sassafras pith* is mentioned in the same syllabus; its chief use is as a bland application to inflamed eyes. Coarsely powdered *elm bark* and flaxseed are much used as poultices or cataplasms. *Poppyheads*, beaten into a mass, are adapted to the same uses.

The well-known fact that flaxseed meal, particularly that abounding in oil, becomes very acid by age, is well accounted for by M. Pelouze, who finds that whenever a seed containing an oil is crushed so as to break up the cells, and to bring the oil in contact with the associated ferments, acidification almost immediately commences, and goes on till frequently the whole of the oil is decomposed with the liberation of its appropriate oil acid.

The kind of powder called cake meal, which is made from the flaxseed cake after the expression of the oil, and so much used for feeding cattle, is preferred to ordinary flaxseed meal for making poultices in the Pennsylvania Hospital, where great quantities are consumed for that purpose. The cake meal forms a firmer poultice, and one less liable to adhere to the skin than the more oily material which is usually sold in the shops and preferred by many practitioners as more emollient. Dr. R. P. Thomas informs me that he finds the use of one-third bran with the latter kind an improvement. The most approved powder in the Paris hospitals is a mixture of flaxseed meal with cake-meal.

In *buchu* and *carrot*, mucilage is associated with an essential oil which adapts these drugs to use as diuretics.

Quince seeds are much used for making bandoline for the hair, a preparation which is sold extensively by the perfumers. The consistence of its mucilage, and its property of continuing moist for a long time, adapt it to this use.

The *sesamum*, or *benne plant*, grows readily in gardens in our climate, and might be generally introduced with advantage. The seed yields a bland fixed oil.

Benne leaves have been quite popular for several years as an excellent demulcent and nutritive article for infants, prostrated by the so-called summer complaint, which is so fatal to this class in our large cities; the mucilaginous principle they contain is readily dissolved out by macerating a leaf in a glass of water for a few minutes. The dried leaf furnishes a much less agreeable mucilage than the fresh.

Honey is a mixture of uncrystallizable and grape sugar; by long standing, the latter constituent is apt to be deposited in a granular form; it also generally contains a volatile odorous principle and wax. Honey is a favorite remedy in sore throat, which it will often cure when used singly; it is very commonly associated with astringents in gargles. Many persons find honey to produce flatulence and diarrhœa to an extent that forbids its use as an article of diet, while others thrive upon it. As a domestic remedy, it is used for irritable conditions of the mucous surfaces. It may not be generally known that the honey so extensively sold in the cities in tin cans holding a quart or more, and in bottles of somewhat less capacity, by the druggists and grocers, is a factitious article made on a large scale from Havana sugar; this fact, which has only recently come to light, will surprise many who have been favorably impressed with the article as remarkably pure and agreeable honey.

Genuine honey is quite apt to be very impure, and to require clarifying. This is accomplished by heating it in a suitable vessel to a very moderate degree, and maintaining the temperature till it ceases to separate a scum, which is to be skimmed off as it rises to the surface.

Liquorice root, and the extract prepared from it, and known in commerce as liquorice ball, or Spanish juice, are drugs used exclusively for their saccharine principles; the latter is so impure as to be well substituted by an extract for which two formulas are given under the head of Extracts.

Raisins are used almost exclusively for their sugar, while *prunes* and *figs*, although the former contains a vegetable acid, and both, perhaps, purgative principles, seem well associated with the saccharine group.

Syllabus of Starchy, Mucilaginous, and Saccharine Medicines.

Acacia, *U. S.*, gum Arabic. Concrete juice of A. vera, and other species.
Althææ radix, *U. S.*, marshmallow root. Contains starch, mucilage, asparagin.
" **flores**, *U. S.*, " flowers. " " " "
Amylum, *U. S.* The fecula of the seeds of triticum vulgare.
Avenæ farina, *U. S.*, oatmeal. Meal of avena sativa. Contains the hulls.
Buchu, *U. S.*, leaves of barosma crenata, &c. Contains mucilage and ess. oil.
Carota, *U. S.* The fruit is officinal, but it is the root that contains pectin.
Cetraria, *U. S.*, Iceland moss. Contains lichenin and a bitter principle.
Chondrus, *U. S.*, carrageen, chondrus crispus. Contains carrageenin, pectin.
Cydonium, *U. S.*, quince seeds. Seeds of cydonia vulgaris; mucilaginous.
Ficus, *U. S.*, the fig. Dried fruit of ficus carica. Sugar; laxative.
Glycyrrhiza, *U S.*, root of glycyrrhiza glabra. Peculiar sugar, glycyrrhizin.
Hordeum, *U. S.*, barley. Decorticated seeds of H. distichon; farinaceous.
Inula, *U. S.*, elecampane. Root of inula helena; inulin.
Iris florentina, *U. S.*, orrisroot. Starchy rhizome.
Lappa, *U. S.*, burdock. Root of lappa minor. Contains inulin.
Linum, *U. S.*, flaxseed. Seeds of linum usitatissimum; mucilage, with fixed oil.
Manna, *U. S.* The concrete juice of cornus Europæa.
Maranta, *U. S.* The fecula of the rhizoma of M. arundinacea.
Mel, *U. S.*, honey. A liquid prepared by apis mellifica.
Oryza sativa, rice. The seed deprived of hulls; farinaceous.
Papaver, *U. S.*, poppyheads. Ripe capsules of papaver somniferum; mucilaginous.
Prunum, *U. S.*, prunes. Dried fruit of prunus domestica; laxative principle.
Sago, *U. S.* The prepared fecula of the pith of sagus rumphii.
Sassafras medulla, *U. S.* Pith of sassafras officinale; rich in mucilage.
Sesami folia, *U. S.*, benne. Leaves of sesamum indicum and orientale; mucilaginous. Seeds rich in fixed oil.
Symphytum officinale, comfrey. Root rich in mucilage.
Tapioca, *U. S.* The fecula of the root of janipha manihot.
Ulmus, *U. S.*, elm bark. The interior bark of ulmus fulva; highly mucilaginous.
Uva passa, *U. S.*, raisins. Dried fruit of vitis vinifera; contain grape sugar.

CHAPTER III.

ON ALBUMINOUS AND SIMILAR PRINCIPLES, AND CERTAIN ANIMAL PRODUCTS.

Albumen, *fibrin*, and *legumin*, or *casein*, are, like the fixed oils and fats, common to vegetable and animal bodies. They contain nitrogen, and, according to some, consist of a hypothetical radical, protein,[1] $C_{40}H_{31}N_5O_{12}$, with varying proportions of sulphur and phosphorus. Whether this view, which has been disputed, be true or not, it affords a convenient grouping under which to arrange them, and the present chapter will be devoted to presenting these, with *gelatin*, which is naturally associated with them, in some of their medical and pharmaceutical relations.

These compounds are of great interest in a physiological point of view, as existing, according to some, in all really nutritious food, whether animal or vegetable; as they are found much more largely in animal than in vegetable organisms, they are most conveniently considered in their practical relations in connection with some of the more familiar articles of animal food.

Albumen, in its natural condition, is soluble in cold water, but coagulable at a temperature of about 169° F.; it is abundant in many vegetable juices, as those of the fleshy narcotic plants, and in a solid form in nuts, almonds, mustard seed, &c. It is seen separating as a flocculent precipitate from the cold infusions or tinctures of senega, ipecac, and other medical roots, on submitting them to the action of heat. In the animal organism, it is a large constituent; like the other quaternary organic substances, it is prone to putrefy and to produce fermentation in starchy and saccharine preparations, and, on that account, its removal is provided for in a number of the formulas for permanent preparations given throughout this work. There seems a close connection between the green coloring matter of plants, chlorophylle, and this coagulable principle, so that the green color is readily separated from many vegetable juices by heating and straining them.

[1] *Protein* has recently been prescribed by physicians as a nutritive tonic causing an increased appetite and improved health generally. In the treatment of eczema and impetigo capitis it has been used with asserted advantage, the disease disappearing without untoward symptoms supervening. Dose for young children 3 to 5 grains three times daily. A process is appended by which it may be prepared. As the existence of such a principle is disputed by many chemists, it would, perhaps, be better to follow Gregory and others, and call it *pure insoluble albumen*. The process is as follows: Mix white of egg with its own bulk of water, filter and evaporate at 104° F., to the original bulk; then add a concentrated solution of caustic potash; the whole soon forms a translucid, yellowish, elastic mass, this is to be broken up, exhausted by cold water, avoiding exposure to the air, then dissolve it in boiling water or boiling alcohol, and precipitate the solution by acetic or phosphoric acid.

Albumen is coagulated by corrosive sublimate, ferrocyanide of potassium, creasote, alcohol, infusion of galls and most acids. Analogous to albumen, are the principles named emulsin and myrosyn, existing respectively in bitter almonds and in black mustard-seed, and which, by their reaction with amygdalin, a neutral crystallizable principle in almonds, and a peculiar sulphuretted principle in black mustard, form important and interesting essential oils.

The physician has frequent occasion in the examination of urine to search for albumen and mucus (which is modified albumen), among the abnormal constituents of that secretion.

To test urine for albumen, it should be heated in a test-tube to boiling. Unless the urine is very alkaline it will coagulate and separate in flakes. The precipitate may consist of phosphates, which will readily dissolve in a little nitric acid, though if the acid is added in excess, it will, after dissolving the phosphates throw down albumen if present. If a precipitate is produced by nitric acid and none by boiling, an excess of uric acid is probably present. If the urine was alkaline this precipitate may be albumen, as an excess of alkali prevents its precipitation by heat.

Fibrin exists in vegetable juices, and is apt to separate spontaneously as a slight coagulum. It exists in nearly all seeds, and is a large constituent of gluten, the nutritious principle associated with starch in wheat flour. It is insoluble in water, and is the chief constituent of lean meat. By the action of neutral salts aided by a little alkali, fibrin is dissolved and then has the properties of albumen.

Casein, or legumin, is found most abundantly in peas, beans, &c. It is not coagulable by heat, which, however, causes a scum on the surface of solutions containing it. It is coagulable by acids, even very dilute. Casein exists largely in milk, and separates as a curd on the formation of lactic acid by the fermentation of its associated saccharine principles.

Ovum, U.S. *The Egg of Phasianus Gallus, or Common Dunghill Fowl.*

Eggs are well known to consist of three parts: ovi albumen, the white; ovi vitellus, the yolk or yelk; and ovi testa, the shell.

The *white of egg* consists of nearly pure albumen and water; it comprises about 60 per cent. of the whole. It is very coagulable, forming a firm, rather tough mass upon long boiling. The completely coagulated albumen of eggs is considered rather indigestible. Three minutes immersion of the egg in boiling water is sufficient to bring it to a proper condition intermediate between its natural glairy consistence and a tough coagulum.

The *yelk* contains a yellow oil suspended in water by the aid of albumen; it is inclosed in a sac, and comprises about 29 per cent. of the whole egg. By heat, it is coagulated and dried into a granular solid, from which the fixed oil may be obtained by expression.

Oil of Eggs.—Under this name a preparation is prescribed in some-parts of England, and on the continent of Europe, as an emollient for sore nipples, and excoriations, and it is sometimes called for in this country. It may be prepared by gently heating yelks of eggs until they coagulate and the moisture evaporates; then breaking into fragments, digesting in boiling alcohol, which is filtered while hot and evaporated. The Paris Codex directs the yolks to be exhausted with ether. A dozen eggs yield about an ounce. This oil contains sulphur and was formerly used to "cut" mercury.

The *shell*, or *testa*, consists of carbonate of lime so intimately mingled with animal matter that the inorganic particles are thoroughly isolated. Powdered and levigated, they are more acceptable to delicate stomachs than other forms of the carbonate.

Eggs, owing to their universal diffusion as common articles of food, are available for emergencies in which albumen is needed in medicine, or especially as an antidote for poisons. The white of egg is the antidote usually prescribed for corrosive sublimate and sulphate of copper, with which it combines, and it is useful in all cases of poisoning by corrosive or acrid poisons. The yelk is adapted to a similar use by its demulcent and sheathing properties. In suspending oily matters, both parts are used, the yelk being perhaps the best, although the white is recommended, by absence of color; for most purposes, there is no objection to mixing them. The use of white of eggs to clarify syrups has been already spoken of. For clarifying, the white of egg, separated from the yelk, is to be beaten up with a small portion of water and well mixed, cold, after which the liquid being raised to the boiling point, the albumen is coagulated and collects as a scum, suspending the impurities; it may then be separated by skimming or straining. (See *Articles of Diet*, Appendix.)

Eggs are often desired by the sick and convalescent, and are sometimes allowable. There are one or two forms of acute disease in which they may sometimes be used with advantage. In cholera infantum, the stomach being irritable and the digestive process exceedingly imperfect, the yelk of an egg that has been boiled till it is dry (say fifteen minutes or more), and reduced to a fine powder, may be readily appropriated by the infant without aggravating the intestinal irritation, care being taken to administer it in divided portions. In those cases of dysentery of a low type, which frequently occur in malarial districts, where the patient is visited with fearful prostration, and the demand for support is imperative, and the stomach rejects the ordinary nutriment, the cessation of vomiting and nausea may be brought about by the administration of the yelk of an uncooked egg, taken in an unbroken state from the shell and dipped in a wineglass containing a little iced water or brandy and water.

No article of the Materia Medica could be classed as *fibrinous*. Fibrin is, however, especially interesting to the physician from its existence in a liquid form in the blood, while it forms also a solid element of muscular fibre. By long-continued boiling, fibrin becomes partly dissolved, and is hence present in most soups. As a constituent of the various cereal grains and of animal flesh, it enters largely into the food of the human race. Farinaceous materials containing gluten serve a good purpose as antidotes to acrid poisons.

Lac. Lac Vaccinum. (*Cow's Milk.*)

This contains casein, in common language known as curd; an oily ingredient in semi-opaque globules, which imparts to milk its opacity and color, and which, when separated, constitutes butter; lactin, or sugar of milk, which, in solution in water, is the chief ingredient in the serum of milk; and alkaline and earthy salts.

The relative proportions of these ingredients vary according to the age of the cow, the time after calving, food, weather, and time of milking, but they are approximately shown in the following table:—

MM. O'Henrie and Chevalier.		Prof. Poggiale.	
Casein	4.48	Casein	38.0
Butter	3.13	Butter	43.8
Lactin	4.77	Lactin	52.7
Salts	0.60	Salts	2.7
Water	87.02	Water	862.8
	100.00		1000.0

By examination under the microscope, the oily ingredient, in exceedingly minute globules, is seen floating in the serous-looking white fluid; being lighter than the liquor in which they are suspended, a portion of these rise to the surface by standing, carrying with them some casein and whey, and forming *cream.*

The quantity of cream varies from 5 to 22 per cent. by measure; the milk from which cream is separated is called *skim-milk.*

Buttermilk approaches skim-milk in composition, but contains even less of the fatty globules. Dr. Gloninger, of Philadelphia, informs me that he has found it a valuable corrective of nausea, as in the case of drunkards; its use was first suggested to him by Dr. Wm. Ashmead, who also uses it in the treatment of dysentery. Its use as an application to "sunburn," is well known to country people.

Curds and whey are made up of all the elements of milk, but the form in which they exist is changed by the addition of the rennet; the curd contains most of the fatty globules, while the whey consists of the sugar of milk and salts in solution.

Cream cheese consists of the moist curd which has been deprived of the greater portion of the whey by pressure.

Ordinary cheese, which contains little or much of the oily ingredient of milk, according as it is made from skim or from whole milk, is made by precipitating the curd, and subjecting it to great pressure.

The *lactometer* is an apparatus for telling the specific gravity of milk, which, although it varies from 1.008 to 1.031, should reach nearly 1.030. Skim-milk is, however, a little heavier, so that it will bear dilution with a little water to bring it to the normal specific gravity. The absence of the cream is, however, so easily detected by the blue tinge of color, and want of the characteristic rich taste, that this variation in the instrument is of little account. The specific gravity is not usually given on the instrument, but the degree of dilution, which, of course, is only approximative. The microscope forms the best test for the purity and richness of milk, showing the proportion of the oil-globules.

Full directions for its quantitative analysis, and tables of its relative richness as modified by circumstances, will be found in Dr. Hassell's work on Adulterations in Food and Medicine.

Solidified milk having been extensively introduced to public notice, the following account of its mode of preparation and uses is extracted from the *American Medical Monthly*, by whose editor it was written, after a visit to the extensive manufactory and pasture lands in the State of New York, where it is made:—

"To 112 lbs. of milk, 28 lbs. of Stuart's white sugar were added, and a trivial proportion of bicarbonate of soda, a teaspoonful, merely enough to insure the neutralizing of any acidity, which in the summer season is exhibited even a few minutes after milking, although inappreciable to the organs of taste. The sweet milk was poured into evaporating pans of enamelled iron, imbedded in warm water heated by steam. A thermometer was immersed in each of these water baths that, by frequent inspection, the temperature might not rise above the point which years of experience have shown advisable.

"To facilitate the evaporation, by means of blowers and other ingenious apparatus, a current of air is established between the covers of the pans and the solidifying milk. Connected with the steam engine is an arrangement of stirrers, for agitating the milk slightly whilst evaporating, and so gently as not to *churn* it. In about three hours the milk and sugar assumed a pasty consistency, and delighted the palates of all present; by constant manipulation and warming, it was reduced to a rich, creamy-looking powder, then exposed to the air to cool, weighed into parcels of a pound each, and by a press, with the force of a ton or two, made to assume the compact form of a tablet (the size of a small brick), in which shape, covered with tinfoil, it is presented to the public."

Solidified milk is extensively introduced into commerce by the American Solidified Milk Establishment. It was formerly met with in tablets, as above described, but is now sold put up in tin boxes, in a granular condition, and dissolves with facility in warm water. The milk produced from it is quite superior to much that is met with on shipboard and elsewhere, and is found to be an exceedingly useful article, especially for infants disordered by ordinary milk, or, from other causes, requiring to be weaned.

One pound will make three quarts of rich pure milk. For tea, coffee, or chocolate, it can be put upon the table and used as sugar, but should be allowed to dissolve in the cup a moment before being stirred, as the cream-globules will then remain unbroken. For young children, a tablespoonful dissolved in a teacupful of water is sufficient.

The *uses of milk* are so numerous and well known as to require no detail in this place. The bread and milk poultice is one of the most familiar of domestic remedies. Various applications of milk to the preparation of diet for the sick, and for infants, will be found in the Appendix.

Butyrum, butter.—Many druggists have private recipes for the preparation of compound ointments of red oxide of mercury, sold under various names, such as fresh butter ointment, tetter ointment, &c.; these preparations generally keep much better than the red precipitate ointment made with lard or simple ointment. Recently, butter has been proposed as an excipient for this officinal ointment, which is said to keep well when prepared with it. Butter likewise makes a beautiful citrine ointment of a proper consistence and permanent color. Though prepared in this manner by some pharmaceutists for several years, it was not until the year 1858, that J. R. Mercien, of Jersey City, first drew public attention to it. (See *Amer. Journ. of Pharm.*, vol. xxx. p. 103.)

Oil of butter is the name given to a good emollient, perhaps slightly astringent preparation, well adapted to treating the summer complaint of children. It furnishes a suitable vehicle for the small doses of calomel, or mercury with chalk, and opium, so much prescribed in that complaint.

It is made by warming butter floating on water, and when it is fluid skimming it off for use.

As an antidote, *milk* has the same applications as the albumen of eggs, and the gluten of flour. As a demulcent, it is a valuable substance in irritation of the pulmonary and digestive organs. It is also used on account of its demulcent properties in the preparation of the bread and milk poultice.

Wine whey (serum lactis vinosum) is described elsewhere; when taken warm and combined with sudorific regimen, it acts powerfully on the skin, and is valuable in febrile disorders. Cold, it is used as a gentle stimulant and nutritive diet.

Bile (*Fel*).—This is a yellow-greenish, viscid, oily liquid, with a bitter taste, followed by a sweetish after-taste, which is separated from the blood of animals by the liver, and collected in the gall-bladder. It is entirely miscible with water, and its solution froths like one of soap. Its composition varies with different animals, but it consists mainly of two salts of soda in which that base is combined with two remarkable nitrogenized substances, choleic and cholic acids: another constituent is a peculiar crystallizable fatty substance, called cholesterin.

Inspissated ox-gall (*Fel bovinum*) is occasionally prescribed in dyspeptic affections connected with habitual costiveness. It is prepared for use by being heated and strained, and then evaporated in a water bath, or by well-managed radiated heat, to a pilular consistence. The dose, when thus inspissated, is from five to ten grains.

Ox-gall is also much used as a detergent, and in a refined or clarified condition is adapted to the use of landscape painters as a delicate green pigment.

Pepsine is the name given to a neutral principle obtained from the gastric juice of animals, and which, associated with lactic and muriatic acids, has the property of digesting certain kinds of food. As it would be impossible to collect the gastric juice from living animals for the purpose of extracting the pepsine for use in medicine, recourse is had to the little tubes upon the inner surface of the stomach, in which it is secreted. The process of Boudault applies to the rennet-bags of sheep, that of Vogel to the porous parts of the stomach of the hog. As they nearly resemble each other, the latter only need be given; it is as follows:—

Preparation of Pepsine.—The porous parts of the stomach of the hog, freed from the glandulous membrane, are cut, and repeatedly macerated with water for twenty-four hours; the filtered liquors are precipitated by sugar of lead, the precipitate washed with water, decomposed by sulphuretted hydrogen, filtered, evaporated by a very gentle heat, to syrupy consistence, and mixed with alcohol; pepsine is slowly precipitated as a white voluminous mass, which is washed with alcohol and dried. As thus prepared, it is a yellowish tough mass with a peculiar animal odor, disagreeable taste; it is not altered by influence of air, has a slight acid reaction on account of a little acetic acid.

M. Boudault, who has prepared this largely as a remedy for indigestion, after evaporation to a syrupy consistence, a little lactic acid being added, stirs in such a quantity of dry starch as that 15 grains will digest a drachm of dry fibrin at the temperature of the body. Boudault's pepsine, as thus produced, is a fawn-colored powder, with a peculiar odor and taste, yielding to water, the pepsine and lactic acid producing a solution with the color, odor and taste of gastric juice. As thus prepared, pepsine is precipitated by salts of mercury and lead, and these, when decomposed by sulphuretted hydrogen, yield it again with its physiological properties. Tannin and strong alcohol destroy its activity, and at a temperature of 120° F., its digestive power is entirely destroyed.

The dose of Boudault's pepsine is 15 grains taken at meal times, between thin slices of bread or in tepid soup.

GELATINE is obtained from bones, animal membranes, &c.; although it has no existence in the vegetable kingdom, it is conveniently considered in its practical bearings in connection with the foregoing; its distinguishing character is that of dissolving in hot water and forming a jelly on cooling, in its impure form, as prepared from hoofs and hides, it is called *glue;* its purest natural form is *isinglass*, which is found in commerce, prepared from the swimming bladder of the sturgeon and other fish. Gelatine is the basis of a variety of artificial preparations used as food; it is precipitated in an insoluble form by tannic acid, for which it is a test. Osseine is the name given to this principle by chemists, the term gelatine being applied to the product of boiling it with water.

Ichthyocolla. (*Isinglass.*)—A variety of articles are met with in our markets under this name. One of the cheapest is that called *fish glue*, used almost exclusively for clearing coffee, as a substitute for white of egg; this, I believe, is identical with the New England isinglass described as being prepared from the air-bladder of the common hake (gadus merluccius), which being macerated in water a little while, is then taken out and passed between rollers, by which it is pressed into thin ribbons of several feet long, from an inch and a half to three inches in width. It is an inferior variety, unfit for internal use. (See Report by C. T. Carney, *Proceedings Am. Pharm. Assoc.*, 1857.)

Russian isinglass is met with principally in the form of sheets, or folded into compact and twisted forms, called staples. Sometimes it is in fine shreds. In sheets and shreds it is esteemed the best, but is very expensive, and on that account mostly superseded by the articles next to be described.

Gelatine exists largely in bones and in the skins of animals, from which it is prepared for use in making the various popular forms of jelly. In this country, the principal kinds of common gelatine are: "Cooper's refined American isinglass," the transparent French gelatine, and Coxe's gelatine. The former comes in sheets 9 inches long, and 3½ wide, and about ⅛ inch thick, in a very light opaque form, nearly white color, and marked with the nets on which they have been dried; sometimes these are cut up into small pieces.

The *French* is in cakes which are rather smaller, very thin, and quite transparent, similarly marked by the drying nets; sometimes it is imported in shreds, put up in boxes with directions for use. My experience is in favor of the French, over Cooper's. It is more readily clarified, and makes an equally good jelly. Sometimes the French is colored red. Coxe's sparkling gelatine is a superior article, put up in packages, and extensively introduced throughout the United States.

The principal cause of failure in the preparation of jellies from these is using a deficient quantity, which fault is due to the indefinite character of the printed circulars accompanying the commercial articles, also to a deficient soaking of the gelatine previous to making the jelly; this is made necessary by the slight taste it acquires at the surface or point of contact with the air and moisture. It should be soaked at least an hour in cold water, which should then be thrown away, and the gelatine, after draining a little, is fit for use.

Calves' feet are still in request by many who believe gelatine, as manufactured from ordinary animal tissues, to be altogether inferior. The *extract of calves' feet*, prepared by John Mackay, of Edinburgh, though not at first furnishing so clear a jelly as some others, is, when clarified by white of egg, exceedingly brilliant, and possesses a peculiar softness and richness upon the palate, which connoisseurs recognize as that of the true calves' foot jelly.

Isinglass plaster is now made by several manufacturers in this country. The mode of preparing it is generally kept a secret. From some experiments with the article now in the market, I am convinced it is made by coating sheets of silk with a solution of common New England isinglass, or fish glue. It is a very popular and good article, despite the tendency to decompose which has been charged against it; when this takes place, which is perhaps seldom, it produces inflammation of the exposed surface to which it is applied. *Court-plaster* is made by a similar process; the old recipes direct calves' feet for its preparation; but on a large scale, it is probable some other form of gelatine is applied. The chief difference between it and the isinglass plaster, which is sold in sheets seven inches wide, rolled and inclosed in boxes, is in the shape in which it is put up for sale.

The original Liston's isinglass plaster, or gum-cloth, was made by spreading several coats of strong solution of isinglass in very diluted alcohol over the surface of animal membrane, previously prepared for the purpose from the peritoneal membrane of the cæcum of the ox.

To make Court-Plaster or Isinglass Plaster.

Take of Isinglass	℥j.
Water	f℥viij.
Dissolve with heat—	
Benzoin	ʒij.
Alcohol	f℥ij.

Dissolve, strain, and mix the two solutions together, and, with a brush, apply several coats of this mixture, while it is kept fluid by a gentle heat to silk stretched on a frame; each successive coat being allowed to dry before applying the next. Then paint a layer of the following solution on the other side of the silk:—

Venice turpentine	℥j.
Tincture of benzoin	f℥ij.
Mix.	

Black and flesh-colored silk are both used for court-plaster.

Os, U. S. (*Bone.*)—Bones are officinal for their uses in the preparation of bone phosphate of lime, and the phosphates of soda and ammonia; they are also used in preparing animal charcoal. Bones consist of gelatinous tissue, into which earthy and saline matters have been deposited until they have acquired solidity and firmness. By soaking in muriatic acid, the phosphates and carbonates are dissolved, and the gelatine is left as a tough, flexible, nearly transparent mass, having nearly the same form as the bone.

CHAPTER IV.

FERMENTATION, ALCOHOL, AND THE ETHERS.

Fermentation is the process, whether spontaneous or artificially induced, by which the ternary compounds considered in Chapter II. are decomposed, and resolved into more stable and unorganized forms. It has been stated, in describing these, that under the influence of diastase, a peculiar principle found in germinating seeds and buds, the insoluble principle, starch, becomes converted into the more soluble dextrin and grape sugar; also that, under the influence of chemical agents, a similar change may be made to take place in lignin.

Cane sugar, under the influence of any causes predisposing to fermentation, undergoes a change into the same proximate principle, which, in its relations to fermentation, is the most interesting and important of its class.

Associated with these ternary principles, we find constantly in plants, nitrogenized or quarternary principles treated of in the last chapter, which, by inducing these changes, are continually tending to the production of grape sugar and to its further metamorphose into alcohol and carbonic acid.

The circumstances necessary to produce fermentation, are, a solution containing starch or sugar, at a moderate elevation of temperature, say from 70° to 90° F., which, however, rises as the process proceeds; and a ferment, or nitrogenized principle itself in a state of decomposition or growth. The juice of the apple furnishes one of the most familiar illustrations of the presence of these conditions. We have in that liquid the ternary compounds associated with vegetable albumen, a nitrogenized material capable of playing the part of a ferment, and at the season of the year when the juice is extracted, the requisite elevation of temperature. As a consequence, fermentation takes place. The vegetable albumen absorbs oxygen from the air, runs into decomposition, sets the whole of the starchy and saccharine constituents of the juice to fermenting, and they are converted first into grape sugar, and then into alcohol, which is present in the resulting cider, and carbonic acid which is given off, producing the well-known frothing of the liquid.

In the production of wine, we have another instance of spontaneous fermentation—the expressed juice of the grape set aside in large casks, undergoes spontaneously the necessary change; if the sugar is in excess, and the azotized matter deficient, a sweet wine is produced; if these proportions are reversed, and the whole of the sugar is changed into alcohol, a dry wine results. If the wine is bottled before the alcohol has been produced in sufficient proportion to coagulate the albumen, the process goes on after it has been corked up, the carbonic acid is confined, and a sparkling wine results.

The composition of alcohol is expressed by the formula $C_4H_6O_2$, and its production by the decomposition of grape sugar is thus explained; one equivalent of grape sugar $= C_{24}H_{28}O_{28}$, is broken up in 4 of alcohol, $C_4H_6O_2 + 8$ of carbonic acid, $CO_2 + 4$ of water, HO, thus—

$$\begin{array}{lcl} 4C_4H_6O_2 & = & C_{16}H_{24}O_8 \\ 8CO_2 & = & C_8\quad\;\; O_{16} \\ 4HO & = & \quad\;\; H_4O_4 \\ \hline & & 24\;\; 28\;\; 28 \end{array}$$

Or, adopting the view of Mitscherlich and Soubeiran, that fermentable sugar has the composition when perfectly dried, represented by $C_{12}H_{12}O_{12}$, it may break up into $2C_4H_6O_2$ and $4CO_2$, without the production of water.

In this reaction, the ferment appears to communicate the molecular change taking place among its particles to the starch and sugar in solution, which are here seen to suffer no increase nor diminution of the number of atoms they contain by the contact or its results.

The *acetic* fermentation consists in the oxidation of alcohol by long exposure to the air in a very divided condition, or in contact with ferments, as when cider is allowed to remain in open casks until it passes into vinegar. Under the head of *aceta*, the preparation of vinegar for use as a menstruum in pharmacy is spoken of, as also its substitution by diluted acetic acid.

The *lactic* and *butyric* fermentations are produced in milk by the action of the nitrogenized principle, casein, upon sugar present in the whey. (See, also, *Malic Acid.*)

The *viscous* fermentation takes place in certain complex saccharine and mucilaginous mixtures by the action of ferments; its results are carbonic acid, hydrogen, alcohol, lactic acid, and mannite.

Fermentation is artificially produced in the process of manufacturing most of the spirituous liquors and beer; the insoluble yellowish viscid matter deposited from the infusion of malt in the process of making beer, called yeast, *fermentum cerevisiæ*, is the best substance for producing the "catalytic" effect in starchy and saccharine solutions. Added to an infusion of rye and Indian corn, it produces, by fermentation, rye whiskey; to potatoes ground to pulp and mixed with hot water, potato spirits; to molasses, rum, &c. In each case a portion of malt is used to facilitate the process by furnishing diastase.

Malt is barley which has been steeped in water till much swollen and softened, and then piled in heaps, to undergo a species of fermentation, or rather germination, during which a portion of its starch has passed into sugar and become soluble, and the peculiar ferment before mentioned as diastase is produced; the seed is then kiln-dried, to destroy its vitality.

The so called neutral sweet spirits, or neutral spirits, is whiskey, which, without being redistilled, has been rectified by passing through charcoal; it ranges from first to fourth proof in strength.

Holland gin is manufactured from malted barley, rye meal, and hops, and distilled from juniper berries, to which it owes its flavor. The Schiedam Schnapps, now so extensively advertised, is understood to be Holland gin, of good quality, though an inferior counterfeit article is also sold under that name. Common gin is rectified from turpentine. Arrack is the spirit from the fermentation of rice; it is not met with in our commerce.

The origin of alcohol and other spirituous liquors which have apparently no foreign odor, can be found out by agitation of about two fluidounces of the liquor with five grains of caustic potassa dissolved in a little water, and subsequently evaporating until about 1½ to 2 fluidrachms remain, which residue is to be mixed with about seventy minims of dilute sulphuric acid, when the characteristic odor will be immediately diffused; the spirit obtained from grain is thus unmistakably discovered.

Malt liquors are obtained by subjecting malt to infusion with water, mixing this with a due proportion of hops, which give the taste and tonic properties, and subjecting to the requisite fermentation. Under the head of *Medicated Wines*, a recipe was given for wine of tar, or Jew's beer, a medicated, fermented liquor.

The following recipe furnishes a very good and wholesome summer beverage, which, without intoxicating, furnishes an agreeable stimulus in the debilitating summer weather of our climate.

Ginger Beer.

Take of Race ginger (bruised) . . . Four ounces.
Bitartrate of potassa . . . Three "

Mix them.

Directions.—Add to these ingredients five pounds of loaf sugar, two lemons (sliced), and five gallons of boiling water. Let it stand twelve hours; then add a teacupful of yeast to the mixture, and bottle immediately and securely. In a day or two it will be ready for use.

Pipsissewa Beer.

The virtues of this excellent alterative diuretic are obtained in an agreeable form, by the following process:—

Take of Pipsissewa (chimaphila, *U. S.*) . Six ounces.
Water . . . . . . One gallon.

Boil, strain, and add—
Brown sugar . . . . . One pound.
Powdered ginger . . . . One-half ounce.
Yeast . . . . . . A sufficient quantity.

Set it aside till fermentation has commenced; then bottle it for use. DOSE, a small tumblerful three or four times a day.

In the same way, sarsaparilla, sassafras, uva ursi, and other medicinal substances, may be made ito *Cerevisiæ*, or beers.

Table of the Proportion, by measure, of Alcohol, sp. gr. .825, *contained in* 100 *Parts of the Liquids named.*

WINES.		WINES.	
Port (strongest)	25.83	Cincinnati	9.00
" (weakest)	19.00	Currant wine	20.55(?)
Madeira (strongest)	24.42	Gooseberry "	11.84
" (weakest)	19.24	Orange "	11.26
Sherry (strongest)	19.81	Elder "	8.79
" (weakest)	18.00	Cider (strong)	9.88
Teneriffe	19.79	" (weak)	5.21
Lisbon	18.94	Burton ale	8.88
Malaga	17.26	Edinburgh ale	6.20
Claret (strongest)	17.11	Brown stout	6.80
" (weakest)	12.91	London porter	4.20
Malmsey	16.40	Small beer	1.28
Sauterne	14.22	Brandy	55.39
Burgundy	14.57	Whiskey (Irish)	52.20
Hock	12.08	Rum	53.68
Champagne	12.61	Gin	51.78

These figures, which are compiled from the tables of Brande and others, are of course only approximative. They are believed, by pretty good authority, to be generally too high.

Alcohol.

This is obtained from spirituous liquors by distillation, which process has for its object the separation of the alcohol from the less volatile impurities associated with it in these liquids. These are chiefly coloring matters, water, and, in the case of whiskey, fusel oil. The rectification of alcohol has of latter years become a very extensive branch of business, and has undergone great improvements; so that the product is both cheap and good as compared with the foreign article. Whiskey, as procured from the farmers, is generally the product of the distillation of fermented infusion of Indian corn, mixed with rye; the smallest proportion of the latter ingredient that answers well is one part to two of the corn. A few distillers of alcohol make their own whiskey, but those in the large cities usually buy it. I am told that, in the western States, much of the whiskey is produced by the fermentation and distillation of the refuse from flour or grist-mills. The whiskey is inspected by an officer appointed by the State government, whose business it is to fix the value of every lot by ascertaining the proportion of alcohol it contains; all below 50 per cent. of absolute alcohol being below proof.

The terms first, second, third and fourth proof spirits, apply to the relative strength of specimens, according to arbitrary standards fixed by law, but varying in the several States. The standard of the U. S. custom houses is fixed by the tables of Prof. R. S. McCulloh, published by order of Congress, entitled, "Report of the Computation of the Manual of Tables to be used with the Hydrometer," and "the Manual for Inspectors of Spirits."

The standard of *proof* is fifty per cent. by volume or measure of absolute alcohol, and fifty per cent. of water, sp. gr. .936. This is 15 per cent. weaker than London proof spirits. *Second proof* has 52½ per cent. alcohol, sp. gr. .931. *Third proof* is 55½ per cent. alcohol, sp. gr. .925. *Fourth proof*, 58 per cent. alcohol, sp. gr. .920, this is London proof.

The instrument used for testing the sp. gr. of spirits, sometimes called an alcoholmeter, is a modification of the ordinary hydrometer, made by Luhme & Co., and Greiner, of Berlin, and sold by importers of chemical apparatus. These have thermometers in the bulb to indicate the changes of temperature, and consequent variations in specific gravity.

Considerable uncertainty exists in stating the proportion of alcohol in spirits, owing to some tables being founded on the percentage by weight, and others the percentage by volume; the alcoholmeters above referred to have two scales indicating both.

The rectification of alcohol is accomplished in appropriate apparatus, consisting chiefly of large *stills*, some capable of taking a charge of 60 gallons. These are chiefly made of copper, and consist of the body and head, which are connected with a furnace, and the worm, which is inclosed in an appropriate refrigerating tub. The whiskey being turned into the body, and the apparatus closed, heat is applied, the vapor formed passing into the cooler, is condensed and runs out at the lower end. The first and last portions that come over are collected separately from the rest as of inferior quality, and the main body of the distillate is transferred to barrels which have been charred on the inside, and constitutes commercial alcohol.

This, the most common variety in this country, is called *druggists' alcohol.* It varies with the care used in its preparation, and especially with the heat employed. Sometimes, by urging the process too rapidly with a hot fire, the alcohol has too strong an odor of fusel oil, and is too weak; the former may be detected by its odor, which reminds of whiskey, and the latter, by its sp. gr., which exceeds the standard, .835. Sometimes it is discolored from deficient charring of the cask.

Besides this quality, the common or old sort of *deodorized alcohol* is made. For preparing this, the whiskey is submitted to extensive filtration through long tubes containing charcoal, and is then distilled from a fresh portion of charcoal, which is placed with it into the body of the still; the charcoal is suited by its property, noticed in a previous chapter, of absorbing odor and coloring matters, for abstracting the fusel oil, and hence rendering the whiskey free from that impurity, while, by careful distillation, it is highly rectified and adapted to the purposes of the perfumer. Another quality is the so-called *absolute alcohol.* This term properly applies to the anhydrous article, but is used commercially to designate the strongest kind sent out by the manufacturers. The peculiarity in the preparation of this is the moderate heat employed, and the consequent very slow distillation. It usually has from 90 to 95 per cent. of alcohol, and is very useful as a solvent of some articles which resist the ordinary commercial article. Castor oil is one of these; when the alcohol is in small proportion, a perfect solution will not result, unless the so-called absolute alcohol is used.

Atwood's patent, which is now used by several manufacturers, is a fine improvement in the preparation of alcohol. It requires the rectification of druggists' alcohol, by distilling it from manganate of potassa, which effectually purifies it, decomposes the fusel oil and renders it unexceptionable.

The chemical tests for fusel oil commonly prescribed are: 1st. A weak solution of nitrate of silver (1 part in 40 parts of water) is added to the alcohol, in the proportion of 25 minims to 4 fluidounces, and the liquid exposed to a bright light for twenty-four hours. If any fusel oil is present a black precipitate will separate. This being separated in a filter, which has been previously washed with diluted nitric acid, and again exposed, if the alcohol is reasonably pure will form no precipitate, though if in excess, a further separation of the black oxide will be produced. 2d. To a test-tube half filled with alcohol, slowly add an equal bulk of sulphuric acid; if the spirit be pure it will remain colorless, otherwise the amount of impurity will be shown by the depth of the tint produced.

In the *American Journal of Pharmacy,* vol. xxx. p. 1, Dr. E. R. Squibb published an elaborate article on the purification of alcohol and other liquids in the state of vapor, and figures an apparatus used by him in the Louisville Chemical Works, in which this principle is very successfully carried out.

For some of the pharmaceutical facts in regard to alcohol, the reader is referred to the chapter on *Tinctures*, page 130.

ÆTHEREA, *U. S.* ETHERS.

This class of organic derivatives is produced by the action of various chemical agencies on alcohol. Ethers are usually considered as exclusively artificial products, but numerous analogies lead to the idea that similar influences at work in the organic world, especially in the ripening of fruit, give birth to some of the delightful flavors so familiar in the vegetable kingdom. There is a familiar instance of the spontaneous production of a peculiar ether in the ripening of wines, under the influence of the slow and gradual fermentation which takes place, especially after the production of a considerable proportion of alcohol in the fermenting juice; in this case, the presence of an excess of tartaric acid may be concerned. The peculiar ether here formed, called œnanthic ether, or bouquet of wine ($C_{18}H_{18}O_3$), has been isolated and examined by Liebig and Pelouze.

The artificial essences of banana, jargonelle pear, pineapple, &c., are instances of the attempted imitation of natural volatile principles by artificially prepared ethers.

The type of the class of ethers was called in our *Pharmacopœia* of 1840, *æther sulphuricus*, but is now, for the sake of brevity and simplicity, named as follows:—

Æther, U.S. (*Sulphuric Ether.*)

This is directed to be prepared by mixing alcohol and sulphuric acid in a glass retort or flask adapted to a suitable condenser, and applying a gentle heat; the very volatile ether, contaminated with a little alcohol, is driven over at a low temperature, and collected in the receiver. This is the case as long as the requisite proportions are maintained; but when the acid is largely in excess, which soon comes to be the case unless a continuous supply of alcohol is kept up, the boiling point rises, and other products are produced, among which is ethereal oil, to be referred to again as one of the constituents of Hoffmann's anodyne.

The highly volatile and inflammable nature of ether makes its preparation dangerous, except in establishments where every convenience and safeguard is provided. The direct application of flame to the retort or flask is attended with great danger, and in the event of a fracture or leakage occurring either in the retort or receiver, the proximity of fire might entail the most disastrous consequences. The ether of commerce is made exclusively by manufacturing chemists, who produce it on a large scale. It is generally pure enough for most of the uses to which it is applied, though not for inhalation. Where alcohol is an impurity, it may be readily separated by shaking up the ether with water, which unites with the water, allowing the mixed water and alcohol to subside, and pouring off the ether, it will now be what is called in commerce *washed ether*, or hydrated ether. This contains a small percentage of water, and is the kind adapted for making tannic acid from galls. It is also pure enough for inhalation, as the presence in its vapor of the small proportion of vapor of water is no disadvantage to it. Hydrated ether is, however, not suited to dissolving gun-cotton, nor to most of the uses of ether, as a solvent.

To separate the water from it requires its redistillation from a solution of lime or potassa, which is also adapted to neutralizing any free acid which may have come over with it, or may have formed in it by the oxidizing action of the air.

The sensible properties of ether are familiar to most; it is colorless, very volatile, limpid, with a high refracting power, pungent taste, and a peculiar rather fragrant odor. Its proper specific gravity, when of standard purity, is .750; it may be reduced as low as .713. It is remarkable for the comparatively great specific gravity of its vapor, which is 2.586.

It causes intense cold by its evaporation; the greatest reduction of temperature yet produced is from its admixture with solid carbonic acid. When ignited with air or oxygen, it explodes violently. Pure ether, when evaporated on the hand, should have no odor. The great volatility of ether, the highly inflammable nature and high specific gravity of its vapor, combine to make it a most dangerous substance to handle, or even to decant, in the vicinity of flame. It should be kept in bottles of not exceeding a pound capacity, in cold situations, as cellars where fire is never kindled, and should always be decanted by daylight. Many disastrous accidents have happened from neglecting this precaution.

Besides its property of dissolving a small proportion of water, it is dissolved by water to the extent of ten per cent., and the *Pharmacopœia* test directs that, when shaken with an equal bulk of water, it shall lose about $\frac{1}{10}$th its volume.

Ether dissolves most of the volatile oils and resins, and the fixed oils and fats, also, iodine, bromine, phosphorus, corrosive sublimate, sesquichloride of iron, and some of the alkaloids, which it separates from their aqueous solutions; it dissolves also caoutchouc to a limited extent, and xyloidin and etheroxylin to an indefinite extent.

The empirical constitution of ether is C_4H_5O. Much uncertainty has rested upon the manner in which these elements are grouped. This seems settled by the discovery, by Dr. Frankland, of a compound radical ethyle, which has the composition C_4H_5, of which ether is undoubtedly the oxide, while alcohol is the hydrated oxide. The result of the action of sulphuric acid upon alcohol is then the separation, from each equivalent of alcohol, of one equivalent of the elements of water.

$$\begin{aligned} \text{Alcohol} &= C_4\,H_5\,O,\ HO, \\ \text{Ether} &= C_4\,H_5\,O, \\ \text{Ethyl} &= C_4\,H_5. \end{aligned}$$

The complex reactions which take place during the passage of alcohol into ether under the influence of sulphuric acid, will be found fully described in chemical works; they do not fall within the scope of this.

Oleum Æthereum, U. S. (*Heavy Oil of Wine.*)

This officinal product of the decomposition of alcohol is rarely met with in commerce. It is a volatile liquid, neutral to test paper, resembling an essential oil in consistence, having a yellow tint, a penetrating aromatic odor, bitter taste, sp. gr. 1.096. It is insoluble in water, but dissolves readily in alcohol and ether. It has anodyne effects similar or superior to those of ether, and is officinal in the *Pharmacopœia* only with reference to the preparation of Hoffmann's anodyne. Some specimens I have met with were evident sophistications.

Dr. Squibb has experimented and written upon ethereal oil and Hoffmann's anodyne, and to his thorough investigation of the officinal process and its resulting preparation, we owe much of our knowledge of them. The reader is referred to his article, *American Journal of Pharmacy*, vol. xxix. p. 197. Dr. Squibb has also recently introduced this article into commerce, of standard purity.

Spiritus Ætheris Compositus, U. S. (*Hoffmann's Anodyne.*)

Take of		
	Ether	Half a pint.
	Alcohol	One pint.
	Ethereal oil . . .	Three fluidrachms.

Mix them.

Hoffmann's anodyne is rarely made by this formula. This important preparation is made by a process which, in its very nature, is certain to give varying results. In the distillation of ether, as already stated, the resulting liquor is liable to vary according to the proportions of the ingredients in the retort. If the alcohol be in due proportion, and the boiling point consequently low, a tolerably pure ether will pass over; but when the acid ingredient comes to be in large excess, sulphurous acid, water, and ethereal oil will come over. Now it is usual with the manufacturers to push the process as far as possible in the first instance, getting a product which contains ether, alcohol, and water, contaminated with a very small portion of ethereal oil. This is rectified by a second distillation, the first portion (as long as it comes over at or below 54° Baumé), being reserved as rectified ether. The less volatile products are now driven over, and are found to consist of ether, alcohol, and water, impregnated with ethereal oil. This is now made into Hoffmann's anodyne by mixing it with ether, alcohol, or water, as may be required to give it nearly the sensible properties of a standard specimen kept on hand. These properties, however, furnish a very poor criterion of quality to the manufacturer or to the consumer; the milkiness occasioned by dilution with water is varied by the relative proportions of alcohol and ether. If too much alcohol is present, this milkiness is deficient. If too much ether, the opalescence is not diffused, the oil-globules having a tendency to run together, and thus varying the appearance. Professor Procter analyzed five specimens of Hoffmann's anodyne, four from leading chemical manufacturers, and one made by the officinal recipe. These

be found to differ in sensible properties, in specific gravity, and in composition.

While the *U. S. P.* specimen marked .8151, one of the others had a sp. gr. .8925, the others being intermediate; one of the manufactured specimens contained very little ether, being chiefly alcohol and water; another contained less alcohol, but more ether; a third had less water than the others, but more alcohol than one, and more ether than the other; while the fourth approached nearer the officinal proportions, though neither of them contained the full proportion of ether. The proportion of heavy oil of wine was not ascertained, as there is no known practicable method of estimating this. It was proved, however, that all the specimens but that by the officinal recipe were deficient in this important ingredient, the odor of which is quite characteristic, and very perceptible, in genuine Hoffmann's anodyne.

Notwithstanding these deficiencies in the commercial article, this medicine has a great and wide-spread reputation, and indeed there is no medicine of its class so much used; it is prescribed for internal use almost to the exclusion of ether, being adapted to admixture with aqueous solutions.

Some of its favorite combinations will be found under the head of extemporaneous pharmacy. Its dose is from 20 drops to f℥j.

Spiritus Ætheris Nitrici, U. S. (*Sweet Spirit of Nitre.*)

This is directed to be made by the action of nitric acid, evolved spontaneously from nitrate of potassa by sulphuric acid, on alcohol. It is collected by distillation, and purified by redistilling from an alkaline carbonate; although found among the pharmaceutical preparations along with the other ethers in the *Pharmacopœia*, like them, it is almost invariably made by the manufacturing chemist. That of Dr. E. R. Squibb, of Brooklyn, N. Y., is considered the best in the market.

Sweet spirit of nitre is a solution of nitrous ether (hyponitrite of oxide of ethyl, C_4H_5O,NO_3) in alcohol. It is a transparent, volatile, bright liquid, of a greenish-yellow tint, fragrant fruity odor, without pungency; it boils at 156° to 158°, sp. gr. .840 to .841, mixing in all proportions with water, alcohol, and ether. By being kept a long time it becomes acid, and may have a crystal of bicarbonate of potassa kept in the bottle. Aldehyde is an impurity which gives it a tendency to turn brown with strong solution of potassa. According to Dr. Squibb, the article made strictly by the officinal process, gives a deep straw color with a dilute solution of potassa within half an hour. Much of the sweet spirit of nitre is of very deficient strength as regards its ethereal ingredient, being mixed with water and alcohol to suit the price charged. It is said that the term spirit. nitri dulc. is applied by some of the wholesale dealers to the weak article, and spirit. æther. nit. to the strong. If skilfully adulterated, its specific gravity would be preserved at about the normal standard, but to an experienced observer it would be deficient in the proper odor, and the sweet and rather pleasant taste. In view of its use as a very mild diaphoretic and sedative, especially for children, its admixture with alcohol is highly injurious as it is criminal.[1]

Uses.—Spirit of nitric ether is very extensively used as a mild refrigerant and diaphoretic; in febrile complaints, it is much combined with antimonial wine, citrate of potassa, &c.; as a diuretic it is much used in connection with the preparations of digitalis and squill. Its dose is from ten drops, for a child, to two fluidrachms for an adult.

CHLOROFORMUM, *U. S.*

This compound, the vapor of which is so largely employed for anæsthetic purposes in surgical and obstetric practice, while in the liquid form it is one of the most useful of chemical solvents, is peculiarly an American remedy; it was first prepared in 1831, by Samuel Guthrie, of Sackett's Harbor, New York, and was first introduced prominently as an anæsthetic agent by Dr. Simpson, of Edinburgh; it is prepared according to the *Pharmacopœia* by distilling alcohol from chlorinated lime, but is made exclusively by manufacturing chemists, and probably by processes very much modified from that given in the books.

It is a heavy colorless liquid, very clear and bright, sp. gr. 1.49, sp. gr. of its vapor 4.2. Its odor is fragrant, fruity; its taste very sweet and pungent. It is very soluble in alcohol and ether, but not in water.

When equal volumes of chloroform and pure concentrated sulphuric acid are shaken together, and then allowed to separate, there should be but a faint tinge of color imparted to the acid, and only a very slight, almost imperceptible elevation of temperature should occur. Pure chloroform is liable to undergo decomposition by age, shown by the evolution of chlorine gas; in order to preserve it from this deterioration when commenced, the addition of eight drops of alcohol to each fluidounce is recommended. Alcohol is, however, a common adulteration of chloroform, and may be detected as follows: Potassium does not decompose pure chloroform, the surface of the metal being only covered with small gas bubbles; if much alcohol be present the entire mixture becomes quite colored, attended with the liberation of acid fumes. Chloroform, on being shaken with the nearly pure orange-colored mixture of bichromate of potassa, sulphuric acid and water, and allowed to remain quietly for a time, assumes a light-green color; if 5 per cent. of alcohol is present the mixture separates into two sharply-divided layers, the lowest having a green color. The same occurs when ether is present. If water is present, potassium immersed in it will be rapidly oxidized.

The chief impurities, however, are products of the reaction, which, in properly rectified chloroform, or chloroform made from pure alcohol, are never present; these subtle carbohydrogen compounds are frequently perceptible as oily-looking globules, floating through the liquid, and are always shown by the color imparted by admixture with sulphuric acids as above.

It is a powerful solvent of camphor, caoutchouc, gutta percha, wax, resins, iodine, and of the vegetable alkaloids and neutral crystalline principles generally. Its property of dissolving camphor in so large

[1] For a full history of the preparation of this important medicine on a scale adapted pharmaceutists, see *American Journal of Pharmacy*, vol. xxviii. p. 289.

proportion, is one of its most remarkable peculiarities, and adapts it as a vehicle for that medicine.

A solution of gutta percha in chloroform in the proportion of one drachm to the fluidounce forms a very mild and pleasant application to abraded surfaces and cuts, which is less adhesive than collodion, and does not contract in drying. Chemically, chloroform is the terchloride of formyle, having the composition C_2H,Cl_3.

Under the very incorrect name of chloric ether, a mixture of chloroform and ether, in the proportion of one part of the former to three of the latter, by measure, is much used as an anæsthetic agent, being considered by some surgeons less stimulating than ether, while its depressing effects are less marked than those of chloroform.

One of the chief uses of chloroform and ether in medicine, is for the purpose of producing an anæsthetic or benumbing effect during surgical operations and parturition. This effect is produced by the inhalation of their vapors, which appear to be absorbed by the blood, and, by acting on the nervous centres, suspend their functions. One of the chief causes of fatal effects of chloroform given by inhalation has undoubtedly been its imperfect quality as found in commerce. Though the increase of its use of latter years is well known, the number of deaths reported has been greatly diminished in the last three years, and the explanation is undoubtedly found in the improved quality of the article of commerce, as well as in the greater care and judgment with which it is now administered.[1] The quantity necessary to be inhaled varies in different individuals, though perhaps the most usual dose by the lungs is of chloroform f℥j to f℥iij—of ether, f℥ss to f℥ij. Both these liquids are also given by the stomach, and used externally in anodyne liniments.

Professor Landerer, after many observations, has repeatedly recommended the use of chloroform against sea-sickness, which, in doses of from five to ten drops, given in a little syrup or cognac, alleviates the nausea and resuscitates the patient from his extreme prostration. I have tried this in my own case, and, as I confidently believe, with advantage, though not with complete relief.

The dose of chloroform by the stomach is from 20 to 60 drops, taken on sugar, or appropriately suspended and combined. (See *Extemporaneous Preparations.*)

Iodoform, $C_2 HI_3$.—Dissolve 5 parts carbonate of potassa, placed in a long-necked flask, in 12 parts water; in this solution 6 parts of iodine are dissolved, 6 parts alcohol added, and the whole gently heated until all color has disappeared. On cooling, the greater part of iodoform crystallizes out, and the mother liquor yields but little more on the addition of water, but contains iodide of potassium. Six parts of iodine yield ⅔ parts, or about 11 per cent. of iodoform.

Iodoform appears in yellow, rhombohedral crystals, of pearly lustre, a peculiar saffron odor, and a faintly sweet peculiar taste. It evaporates entirely when exposed to the air.

[1] See paper read before the N. Y. Academy of Medicine, by Dr. E. R. Squibb, *American Medical Monthly*, July, 1857.

This compound acts as an antiseptic and anti-miasmatic. Taken internally, it produces all the effects of iodine, without any irritation, and has been given in doses ranging from 1 to 7 grains. It has likewise been employed with asserted beneficial effect as an inhalation in diseases of the lungs, and externally in the form of suppositories and ointments.

Amylic alcohol, fusel oil, $C_{10}H_{12}O_2$.—This alcohol, which has been referred to as an impurity of alcohol, is contained in the products of fermentation of potatoes, grain, and grape husks. To obtain it in a state of purity from the ordinary grain fusel oil, which may be obtained at distilleries, the crude fusel oil is agitated with an equal bulk of water, the water removed and the oil distilled with about its own weight of dry carbonate of potassa; the potato fusel oil, distilling at first, still contains some alcohol, and the receiver is therefore changed as soon as the temperature in the retort has risen to 268°, when it remains stationary. This part of the distillate is the pure amylic alcohol.

It may also be obtained sufficiently pure for all purposes if the crude oil is at once distilled over a slow fire, and the receiver changed when the temperature has attained 268°; a rectification of this product is necessary, and the first portion of all the distillates may be preserved for future use, when it may be added to other portions of crude fusel oil.

Fusel oil, thus purified, is a thin, oily liquid, crystallizing at —4° F. It has a penetrating disagreeable odor, and a hot, acrid taste. The inhalation of its vapor and its internal administration are poisonous, producing coughing, nausea, vomiting, vertigo, fainting, prostration of the lower extremities, convulsions, asphyxia, and death. Ammonia has been recommended to counteract these deleterious effects.

It is not used in medicine, but has attained considerable importance in the arts, chiefly for the artificial production of perfumes and fruit essences, and for the preparation of valerianic acid by the use of oxidizing agents. (See *Valerianic Acid.*)

Artificial Fruit Essences.

The artificial fruit essences now so largely employed for making artificial fruit syrups and flavoring extracts for culinary purposes, belong to the class of ethers; they are solutions of compounds of organic acids with ordinary ether and amylic ether, in deodorized alcohol. The World's Exhibition in London has particularly stimulated the inquiry into these compounds, and the examination of samples on exhibition proved their real character; but little practical information has been published with reference to their preparation, the manufacturers keeping their processes secret, in consequence of which the quality and adaptability of the essences, as they occur in commerce, vary exceedingly.

The following gives the results of the various scientific investigations on some of the most prominent of these essences:—

Jargonelle pear oil is an alcoholic solution of acetate of oxide of amyle, which may be obtained by digesting fusel oil with strong acetic acid for several days, but more satisfactorily by the following process: 1 part of fusel oil, 2 parts of acetate of potassa, and 1 part of sulphuric acid, are mixed and distilled. The distillate is washed with a weak solution of potassa, then dried by chloride of calcium, and rectified over oxide of lead to abstract the last quantities of free acetic acid. This ether is a light volatile liquid, boiling at about 270°. Its constitution is expressed by $C_{10}H_{11}O$, $C_4H_3O_3$.

Bergamot pear oil is similar to the former: 5 parts of acetate of oxide of amyle, mixed with 1½ part of acetic ether, are dissolved in from 100 to 120 parts of alcohol.

Apple Oil.—In the preparation of valerianic acid from fusel oil, the distillate separates into two layers, the upper stratum, of which is an oily liquid, consisting principally of valerianate of oxide of amyle. It is washed with a weak solution of carbonate of soda, then with water, afterwards dried with chloride of calcium and distilled, preserving that portion which comes over at 270° to 274°; it consists of $C_{10}H_{11}O$, $C_{10}H_9O_3$. One part of this ether, dissolved in 6 or 8 parts of alcohol, furnishes apple oil.

Oil of Pineapples.—For the preparation of this essence, the making of butyric acid is necessary. As obtained by the saponification of butter, some difficulties are presented in freeing it of caprylic, caprinic, and vaccinic acids, it is therefore best to prepare it artificially by butyric fermentation, for which purpose 100 parts of starch sugar, or cane or milk sugar, are dissolved in water, and set aside in a warm place, with 10 parts of old cheese; or a mixture of 100 parts of sugar, 150 parts milk, and 50 parts of powdered chalk, are allowed to ferment in a warm place; if diluted with water, fermentation takes place quicker. After the cessation of the evolution of gas, the liquid, on evaporation, furnishes butyrate of lime, 10 parts of which are to be dissolved in 40 parts of water, and distilled with 3 or 4 parts of muriatic acid; from the distillate the acid is separated by saturating it with chloride of calcium, the oily liquid is rectified, and that portion coming over at 327° is preserved as pure concentrated butyric acid.

Two parts of this acid are mixed in a tubulated retort with 2 parts by weight of alcohol and 1 part of sulphuric acid; after the reaction has taken place, the mixture separates into two strata, the upper of which is washed with water, dried with chloride of calcium, and rectified; it is then butyric ether, has a specific gravity of .9, and boils above 230°; it is composed of C_4H_5O, $C_8H_7O_3$.

To avoid the preparation of free butyric acid, the ether may be prepared by heating the powdered butyrate of lime with a mixture of alcohol and sulphuric acid, skimming off the ether and treating it as above. The essence of pineapples is made by dissolving 1 part of this ether in 8 or 10 parts of alcohol.

Banana essence is prepared from a mixture of acetate of oxide of amyle and some butyric ether, by dissolving it in alcohol.

Essence of raspberries is usually made by mixing acetic ether with an alcoholic essence of orris root.

Quince Essence.—In making this essence pelargonic acid has to be prepared as a first step. This acid is contained in the oil of pelargonium roseum, from which it may be obtained by combining it with potassa, but more advantageously it is made from oil of rue, by heating it in a retort with nitric acid previously diluted with an equal measure of water, removing from the fire as soon as the reaction commences, afterwards boiling with cohobation until nitrous acid vapors cease to be evolved, the oily acid is then removed, washed with water, combined with potassa, and a neutral strong smelling oil separated, after which the solution of pelargonate of potassa is decomposed by sulphuric acid.

Pelargonic acid is now sufficiently pure for the preparation of the ether; it still contains a resinous substance, from which it may be purified by rectification, combining with caustic baryta, and decomposing the crystallized salt with diluted sulphuric acid. Pelargonic acid, by a continued digestion with alcohol, is converted into pelargonic ether, which is obtained purer and in a shorter time, by saturating an alcoholic solution of pelargonic acid with muriatic acid gas, washing the separated ether with water, and drying it over chloride of calcium. If the pure ether is sought this may be rectified; it consists of C_4H_5O, $C_{18}H_{17}O_3$.

The pelargonic, also called œnanthic, ether, dissolved in alcohol constitutes the essence of quince.

Fusel Oil of Wine.—Though pelargonic ether is generally called œnanthic ether, many chemists apply the latter name to the pure fusel oil of wine, which, though closely analogous to the former, they assert to be a different compound. This fusel oil is the cause of the persistent smell of all or most wines, and is quite distinct from their *bouquet*, which in some wines is wanting altogether. It is obtained by careful distillation of the ferment of wines mixed with half its measure of water, a little œnanthic acid may be removed by agitation of the distillate with some carbonate of soda, the liquid is then heated, the ether rises to the surface, and is obtained free of water by standing over chloride of calcium.

The fusel oil of grain spirits contains a small portion of the same ether.

CHAPTER V.

FIXED OILS AND FATS.

THE fixed oils and fats form so natural a group that they may be conveniently classed together, though both of vegetable and animal production.

They resemble the preceding groups of ternary organic principles in being nutritious in the sense in which that term applies to non-nitrogenized principles. The very large proportion of carbon they contain peculiarly adapts them to maintain, by combustion in the lungs and capillaries, the heat required in the various processes of the economy. In medicine, they are used for this in connection with certain demulcent, alterative, and cathartic properties, pertaining to the particular individuals of the group. They constitute the chief vehicles for medicines to be applied externally, whether in ointments in which the oil is usually not decomposed, or in liniments and plasters, in some of which a decomposition of the oil is effected, as will appear in the sequel. The fixed oils enter largely into the food of animals, and of the human race; they are accumulated particularly in the fruit and seeds of plants, and they exist in the straw and stalks as well as the seed of the cereal grasses, where they are associated with other nutritive materials.

Rancid oils are directed to be purified by boiling with water in which calcined magnesia is suspended, or by filtration through charcoal, though neither of these processes is very effectual.

A great many processes are resorted to for the purification and bleaching of oils for use in the arts, but no chemical agents should be used in the case of those oils designed for use in medicine.

The following proportions of fixed oils have been ascertained to exist in the several substances named: in Indian corn, 8.8 per cent.; oats, 6.9; fine wheat flour, 1.4; bran from wheat, 4.6; rice, 0.25; hay and straw, from 3 to 5; olive seeds, 54; flaxseed, 22; almonds, 46; walnuts, 50; cocoa-nut, 47; yelk of eggs, 28; cow's milk, 3.13 per cent.

Adulterations.—The chief adulterations to which the fixed oils are subject, are mixtures of the finer and more expensive kinds with the cheaper. These may frequently be detected by variations of the specific gravity from the normal standard, though as the several oils only vary from .865 to .970 sp. gr., detection by this means becomes a matter of considerable delicacy. It has been proposed to apply this test at the temperature of boiling water, but we have too little data to make this generally available. The sp. gr. of each of the fixed oils mentioned in this work, as far as known, is given in the table on pages 326 and 327.

The odor of oils, if carefully observed, will be found a good means of detecting their adulterations, especially if heat is applied. A known pure sample being obtained may be heated in a spoon and compared with a quantity of the suspected oil similarly heated.

The presence of fish oil in the vegetable oils is detected by passing a stream of chlorine through them. The pure vegetable oils are not materially altered, but a mixture of the two turns dark brown or black.

Solubility in alcohol is another fact which is useful in determining the genuineness of oils. Castor oil is soluble in its own weight of alcohol of .820 sp. gr. Croton oil dissolves in the same proportion in alcohol of .796 sp. gr. Olive oil is nearly insoluble. Oil of almonds dissolves in 25 parts of cold and 6 parts of boiling alcohol.

The boiling point of fixed oils varies from 500° to 600° F., so that we might detect the admixture of the volatile oils, hydro-carbons from coal, &c., by raising the temperature and noticing the point at which ebullition commences, and the nature of the distillate.

Chemical History.—The fixed oils and fats differ from the foregoing ternary principles in being separable into several proximate principles, which have been pretty well studied. These are *olein*, *stearin*, and *margarin*. When a fixed oil is heated with a caustic alkali, it is decomposed into glycerin with an organic acid which unites with the alkali and forms a soap. Thus olein is resolved into oleic acid and glycerin; stearin into stearic acid and glycerin, and margarin into margaric acid and glycerin.

M. Fremy has also shown that the oils, and neutral fatty bodies in general, are converted into fatty acids by concentrated sulphuric acid, and the use of sulphuric acid as a test for the several oils has been extensively studied, and the reaction tabulated. (See *Cooley's Cyclopædia of Practical Receipts*, article Oils.)

Olein, oleate of glycerin, forms the fluid portion of fats and oils, and exists in nearly all of them. It remains liquid at a low temperature. Oleic acid, $C_{36}H_{34}O_4$, is obtained by saponifying olein, and afterwards decomposing the soap by an acid, when it is set free as an oily, almost colorless liquid, lighter than water, with an acid reaction; it unites with bases, forming salts; those with alkalies are soluble in water, those with other metallic oxides and with the earths are insoluble; oleate of lead is the basis of lead plaster.

Stearin, stearate of glycerin, forms the solid part of mutton suet and beef fat; and *stearic acid*, $C_{36}H_{36}O_4$, forms salts similar to those of oleic acid.

Margarin, margarate of glycerin, enters into human fat, and into that of the carnivora; it is also present in most vegetable fixed oils. *Margaric acid* is prepared from margarin, or by the action of nitric acid on stearic acid; it is represented by the formula $C_{34}H_{34}O_4$, containing C_2H_2 less than stearic, which it resembles in most of its properties. Margarate of lead is also present in lead plaster.

Besides these principles, found in the most common oils and fats, there are others which may be mentioned, though of little practical utility to the physician or pharmaceutist. In palm oil, palmitic acid, $C_{32}H_{32}O_4$; in cocoa-nut oil, coco-stearic acid, $HO,C_{26}H_{25}O_3$; in the butter of nutmegs or oil of mace, myristic acid, $HO,C_{28}H_{27}O_3$, are all found combined with glycerin.

Wax and spermaceti are complex products of the animal kingdom, somewhat resembling solid oils or fats, but destitute of glycerin.

This subject brings into view the preparation of lead plaster, which is highly important to the pharmaceutist as the basis of most of the class of plasters which are for convenience introduced in this work among the extemporaneous preparations.

Emplastrum Plumbi, U. S. *Lead Plaster.* (*Oleo-Margarate of Lead.*)

This is made usually on a large scale by manufacturing pharmaceutists, some of whom make it, with its kindred preparations, their leading or exclusive articles of manufacture.

The process for the preparation of lead plaster requires that olive oil (lard oil does not produce a nice product) should be boiled with finely-powdered semivitrified oxide of lead (litharge) and water (the proportions are given in the *Pharmacopœia*) for a long time, until they unite into a mass of a soft solid consistence, which is tenacious, and readily rolled upon a wet marble slab into rolls of suitable size, which are allowed to harden by maceration in a trough of cold water and subsequent exposure for a long time to the air; one gallon of oil yields about twelve pounds of plaster. The process is a tedious one, and requires to be pursued with strict reference to many precautions suggested by experience, which seem scarcely appropriate to a work of the scope and design of the present.

Lead plaster is usually found in commerce, in rolls of various sizes, from half an ounce to half a pound in weight, called diachylon, simple diachylon, or lead plaster; sometimes, though rarely, it is spread upon cotton cloth by machinery, and sold by the yard like adhesive plaster cloth. It is milder and less irritating in its action upon highly inflamed surfaces, though less adhesive than that well-known and useful application. Postponing to another chapter the practical details in regard to these, and the numerous compounds into which they enter, I need only refer here to the utility of glycerin as a constituent of emollient plasters, and to the fact that much of the lead plaster now made is deprived of this ingredient by long washing and kneading with water, and is hence peculiarly apt to become dry and crisp by age.

Glycerin, U. S.

Glycerin, $C_6H_7O_5+HO$, is a colorless, odorless, sweet liquid, resembling syrup, having a sp. gr. of 1.26; it may be classified among sugars, see page 291; it is generally stated to be a hydrate of the oxide of a hypothetical radical glyceryle, C_6H_7. Glycerin is separated from oils in the process of their saponification, and is directed to be obtained by evaporation from the water in which lead plaster has been made, care being taken to precipitate any lead held in solution, by sulphuretted hydrogen; it is, of recent time, much employed as a substitute for oils, having a remarkable property of soothing irritable conditions of the mucus surfaces, and at the same time mixing in all proportions with water and alcohol, though not with ether.

It is a most useful application in the dry and parched condition of the mouth so often present in disease, to which it may be applied either by painting it over the dry surface with a brush, or by swallowing it diluted with water. For a certain form of deafness resulting from dryness of the tympanic membrane it is one of the best of remedies. It is used in certain scaly skin diseases, as lepra. It is a useful application to sore nipples, also to burns and excoriated surfaces, and is added to poultices to keep them moist. Its substitution for almond and olive oil, in the preparation of delicate ointments, is seldom productive of advantage; it must be remembered that it is not miscible with the fixed oils. It is not liable to become rancid as oils are, and it imbibes the essential oils from plants digested in it with remarkable avidity, so that it is well adapted to the preparation of liniments and lotions; it is also miscible with soaps. From its remarkable solvent power over chemical agents it is much used in Pharmacy, and the name glyceroles is applied to solutions containing it.

The idea has occurred to me of using it as a vehicle for subacetate of lead, which, on admixture with common oils as in Goulard's cerate, is always converted into a compound of the oil-acid with oxide of lead; and, on admixture with water, as in lead-water, immediately commences to be decomposed, and to deposit carbonate of lead so that the solution in a short time becomes inert. By experiment, I find glycerin miscible in all proportions with liquor plumbi subacetatis, and have inserted, under the name of *linimentum plumbi subacetatis*, a formula which I think an improvement on any of the old preparations of lead.

There are several qualities of glycerin in our markets, the cheapest, which is made from the waters from which soap has been separated, that which is collected as a residuary product from the plaster manufacture, and that which is distilled from fats by the highly heated steam. Of the latter, which is the best variety, that imported from Price's Candle Co., London, is to be preferred; it is destitute of odor and has the requisite specific gravity. This article is made from palm oil, while that obtained from the refuse of the manufacture of stearin candles from lard is seldom destitute of an odor when heated, which is fatal to its use for a large number of the purposes to which it is applied.

When made by distillation, glycerin is often contaminated with *acroleine*, a peculiar volatile principle to which it owes its acridity. Some specimens have a saline taste, evincing important impurities in view of the uses to which it is applied. The following recipe for the preparation of glycerin is given by Dorvault in *L'Officine*, and is translated for the use of any who are disposed to experiment upon the production of this useful article, premising that the proportion of glycerin is so small that one gallon of oil only yields half a pound of the product: Take of a fixed oil or fat a convenient quantity, saponify it by milk of lime, then separate the liquid from the insoluble lime soap; add to the liquid sufficient diluted sulphuric acid to precipitate as sulphate the excess of lime held in solution. Evaporate by a water bath, and treat the residue with strong alcohol, which, on evaporation, will leave the glycerin.

The lime soap which is here a residuary product, is, as far as I know, quite useless, and unless this can be made available for some purpose as yet unknown, this recipe will be deficient in the element of economy.

List of the Principal Fixed Oils and Fats used in Medicine.

1. Vegetable Oils.

Oleum olivæ, *U. S.* (sweet oil or olive oil). From the fruit of olea Europea, by expression, sp. gr. .9109 to .9192.

" amygdalæ, *U. S.* From kernels of fruit of A. communis by expression, sp. gr. .917.

" sesami (benne oil). From the seeds of sesamum indicum and orientale.

" lini, *U. S.* (flaxseed oil). From the seed of linum usitatissimum, sp. gr. .9347.

" arachadis (groundnut oil). From kernels of fruit of arachis hypogæa by expression, sp. gr. .874. ?

" bertholetiæ (Brazil nut oil). From kernels of fruit of B. excelsa, sp. gr. .917.

" cacao (butter of cocoa). From roasted seeds of theobroma cacao, sp. gr. .892.

Oleum cocois (cocoanut oil). From the kernel of the cocos nucifera.
" macidis (solid). From the arillus of the fruit of myristica fragrans.
Myristicæ adeps, expressed from the nutmeg of myristica fragrans.
Oleum palmæ (solid), obtained from the fruit of elais guineensis.
" papaveris (poppy oil). From the seeds of papaver somniferum, sp. gr. .9243.
" ricini, *U. S.* (castor oil). From seeds of ricinus communis, sp. gr. .9612.
" tiglii, *U. S.* (croton oil). From the seeds of croton tiglium, sp. gr. .947 to .953.

2. Animal Oils.

Adeps, *U. S.* (lard). Prepared fat of sus scrofa, the hog.
Butyrum (butter). See page 304. From cream by mechanical agitation.
Sevum, *U. S.* (mutton suet). The prepared suet or fat, from ovis aries.
Oleum adipis (lard oil). The olein separated from lard by expression, sp. gr. .9003.
" bubulum, *U. S.* (neat's-foot oil.) From the bones of bos domesticus, the ox.
" cetacei (spermaceti oil). From the cavity in the upper jaw of physeter macrocephalus.
" morrhuæ, *U. S.* (cod-liver oil). From the livers of gadus morrhua, sp. gr. .9230 to .9315.

Of the foregoing list several are quite bland, agreeable, and destitute of active properties; of these oleum olivæ, oleum amygdalæ, oleum sesami, oleum papaveris, oleum arachadis, may be substituted for each other for internal use.

Olive oil, of the finest quality met with in commerce, virgin oil, salad oil, has a pale yellow or greenish color, and a very faint and agreeable odor; its taste is bland and pleasant, though sometimes a little acrid; its specific gravity, at 77° F., is stated at .9109, .9176 at 59° F. It is soluble in one and a half times its weight of ether, but almost insoluble in alcohol; it generally contains a solid deposit of oleo-margarin in cold weather, which is readily fused by a slight elevation of temperature. The best generally comes in bottles which hold from f℥xij to f℥xxiv, or in small flasks covered by wicker work, which, after they are emptied, come in play for small chemical operations. The common impure oil, is generally rancid, acid, and disagreeable, and often abounds in green coloring matter.

The detection of adulterations in olive oil is a matter of no great difficulty to the connoisseur, as any admixture of inferior oils affects the taste perceptibly. The following are, however, more generally applicable.

Pure olive oil, when shaken in a vial half filled, gives a "*bead*" which rapidly disappears, but if adulterated the bubbles continue longer before they burst. Pure olive oil completely solidifies if immersed in ice, but if one-third of poppy oil is present it does not freeze at all at the temperature of ice. When carefully mixed with one-twelfth part of its volume of a solution of four ounces of mercury, in eight fluidounces and six drachms of nitric acid, sp. gr. 1.5 it becomes a firm fat in three or four hours, without any separation of liquid oil. The other edible oils do not solidify with acid nitrate of mercury, and the hardness of this mass is dependent on the purity of the oil. Animal oils solidify with this nitrate, but if olive oil is mixed with them it floats on the surface of the coagulum and may be decanted. And when heated this coagulum exhales the well-known odor of rancid fats.

Pelouze has investigated the subject of the acidification of fixed oils, and confirms the fact already known, that foreign substances with which fatty bodies are contaminated exert a similar action upon them that a ferment does upon saccharine fluids, setting free the fatty acids. He has also found that when oleaginous seeds are crushed so as to break up their cells and bring their contents into close contact, the neutral fatty bodies contained in them are spontaneously converted into fatty acids and glycerin. This phenomenon is analogous to what takes place in the grape, the apple and other fruits, the sugar contained in which is converted into alcohol and carbonic acid as soon as the cells which separate it from the ferment are destroyed. When extracted immediately, these oils are perfectly free from any traces of acid. The difference in quality between good and bad olive oil is thus explained, the former being extracted before the lapse of time has allowed of this peculiar fermentative action.

Almond oil is procured from the kernels by expression, the best being imported from England. It has about the specific gravity of olive oil, and is without its green tinge of color, so that it generally makes a whiter ointment. It is generally imported in jugs. Almond oil is soluble in 25 parts of cold and 6 parts of boiling alcohol. In selling and prescribing it, care should be taken that it be not confounded with the essential oil of bitter almond.

It is well known that some wholesale drug houses fraudulently substitute for this valuable oil, oil of poppy seed, which is little over half its value; the fraud may be detected by mixing upon a glass or porcelain slab a few drops of the suspected oil with about an equal number of drops of nitric acid; the oil of poppies, being a drying oil, soon becomes hard, while the almond oil retains its fluidity.

Oil of Benne Seed.—Sesamum orientale has been produced in this country, and is recommended as a desirable production to add to our agricultural resources. The plant grows well, particularly in the South, and has been estimated to yield twenty bushels of the seed to the acre; the yield of oil approaches two and a half gallons to the bushel. The seeds should be planted as soon as the frost is out of the ground in drills three feet apart, and six inches distance along the drills.

Poppy seed oil is imported in casks in considerable quantity from Germany, where it is frequently employed as a substitute for sweet oil for table use, and by some practitioners is preferred to oil of almonds. In this country it is made use of for the same purposes, and is besides often fraudulently substituted for, or mixed with olive and almond oil, which see.

Oleum macidis, oleum myristicæ expressum, oleum adipis, oleum lini, oleum bertholetiæ, oleum cocoa, oleum bubulum, oleum cetacei, and oleum palmæ, are seldom used for any internal form of administration, but in common with olive and almond oil have their special adaptations and uses in the arts, and for topical applications in medicine.

Expressed oil of nutmegs as it occurs in commerce is of the consistence of suet, and has a mixed white and yellow color, and a strong odor of nutmegs; it is prepared in the East India Islands by exposing the bruised nutmegs contained in a bag to the vapors of boiling water and subjecting it to pressure between heated plates. It is entirely soluble in boiling ether; leaves nearly one-half behind on being treated with cold ether; the residue is white, pulverulent, inodorous. It is chiefly used for external applications where a mild stimulant is required.

Expressed oil of mace is now met with very seldom in commerce; it is prepared in a manner similar to the above, has the consistency of butter, a reddish color, and an agreeable strong odor and taste of mace.

Lard oil, which is a tolerably pure form of olein, when freshly and skilfully prepared, is seldom met with in commerce free from a very disagreeable rancid odor; on this account it is rarely employed in medicine. It is said to be largely exported for admixture with olive oil.

Linseed or flaxseed oil is chiefly used to mix with the carbonates of lead and zinc in the manufacture of the pigments known as white lead and white zinc; it is sometimes substituted for this use by a variety of inferior oils, which possess the same drying or oxidizing property. Boiled linseed oil, particularly if litharge or acetate of lead is mixed with it in boiling, is remarkable for the rapidity with which it dries into a hard varnish-like material. It is sometimes used as a cathartic in doses of one or two ounces.

Oil of Groundnuts.—A fine oil is now extensively made both in France and in this country, by expressing groundnuts between hot plates in the same way that linseed oil is prepared. Its chief use, as far as I can learn, is to adulterate almond and olive oils. It is remarkably free from unpleasant properties, and if thrown into commerce under its own proper name, would no doubt answer many purposes both in the arts and in medicine. Oil of groundnuts has been employed in place of neat's-foot oil for citrine ointment, which, however, is apt to be too soft when thus prepared.

Cocoanut oil is obtained by expression from the kernel of the cocoanut; it is of the consistency of suet between 40° and 50°, and semifluid between 75° and 85°; it has a peculiar odor which is owing to the presence of caprylic and capronic acids in small quantities, which for the greater part may be removed by digesting the oil for several hours with coarsely-powdered charcoal, and filtering through paper in a warm place. It has been proposed by M. Pettenkofer, as a substitute for lard, especially in ointments which contain much vegetable matter, or aqueous solutions, of which it is able by trituration to take up one-third more than lard. Its keeping well without getting rancid admirably adapts it for such purposes, and also for hair oil; it is readily absorbed by the skin and, therefore, is not so apt to stain the garments and bedclothes.

Oil of brazil-nuts, oleum bertholetiæ, when properly made, is of a bright amber color, has the peculiar smell and taste of the nut, and congeals at 24° F. Dr. Donnelly, of Philadelphia, has used it as a substitute for olive oil in plasters and ointments, and found it to be well adapted for such purposes. One gallon of oil requires six pounds of litharge to saponify, and yields a good plaster of a rich cream color, and 12 oz. of a superior glycerin.

Neat's-foot oil, as usually met with, is so offensive [illegible] in one officinal preparation, in which it is often substituted [illegible] lard oil—unguentum hydrargyri nitratis. It may be [illegible] good enough for internal use, and in England it is said to [illegible] for frying fritters; it does not thicken by age.

Spermaceti oil is the clearest and thinnest of the whale [illegible] remarkably adapted for greasing heavy machinery, for which [illegible] it is in great demand; it is also a fine oil for burning, but [illegible] used in medicine or pharmacy, except by those few practitioners who believe it fully equal to cod-liver oil.

Palm oil is consumed largely in the manufacture of soap, to which it imparts its peculiar odor and yellow color; of this, however, it is deprived by exposure to air and light. It is a very extensive article of commerce in England, entering into many of the cheaper varieties of soap, and in pharmacy being used in the manufacture of plasters, certain pomades and ointments. It is a soft solid, melts at [illegible] F., sp. gr. .968.

Oleum ricini, oleum tiglii, oleum morrhuæ, oleum maydis, and oleum cocois, are medicinal, and used as internal remedies.

Castor oil is a viscid, transparent, light yellow-colored oil, specific gravity .9575, at 77°. Its taste and smell, when of fine quality, are very slight, though its extreme viscidity renders it disagreeable. It is peculiar in being miscible with absolute alcohol, in all proportions, and in rendering other oils, mixed with it in certain proportions, also soluble; it also dissolves some alcohol, but this property diminishes with the strength of the alcohol. The two principal kinds are, the American oil, which is produced principally in our Western States and comes in casks, and the East India oil, which is imported in tin cans from Bombay and Calcutta. The latter article is, I think, the best, either from the constant agitation to which it is subjected in the hold of the vessel during a long voyage, a great part of the time in the tropics, producing a separation of its albuminous ingredient and thus clarifying it, or from some peculiarity in its preparation. A can of this oil is often found cloudy near the bottom, while the upper portion may sometimes be racked off remarkably clear and free from odor and taste.

The English castor oil so much esteemed here is selected from the best East India oil and submitted to filtration, and afterwards bleached by exposure to the sun. The blue tinge of color of bottles in which it is sold, by neutralizing the yellow rays reflected from the oil, give it the appearance of great freedom from color. (See Pharmaceutical Notes of Travel, by the author, *Am. Journ. Pharm.*, vol. xxx. p. [illegible].)

The *Palma Christi*, which produces the valuable seed yielding this oil, is a beautiful annual plant, readily cultivated in our climate from the seed. It grows to the height of from six to ten feet with us, and is one of the most ornamental of annuals for garden or lawn.

The seeds are powerfully acrid and cathartic. The activity of these and the oil depends upon a principle, said to be resinoid, which is invariably present in it, and is modified by its bland demulcent properties, rendering it one of the most useful of cathartics.

Great quantities of castor oil are consumed in the preparation of applications for the hair, it being now generally preferred to bear's oil, which was formerly much in vogue for this purpose. For greasing the hair, it should have a small admixture of alcohol to diminish its viscid properties, while for hair restoratives, such as are called katharion, tricopherous, &c., the alcohol is in larger proportion, the oil being added to diminish the drying and crisping properties of the spirits used. Two good recipes for these preparations are given below—

Perfumed Hair Oil.

Take of Castor oil . . . . f℥x.
Very strong alcohol . . . . . f℥ij.
Ess. of jessamine . . . . . . fʒij.
Mix.

Any other essential oil may be substituted for the essence of jessamine, and we usually label the vials according to their perfume, and color the rose oil red.

Hair Restorative.

Take of Castor oil . . . . f℥vj.
Alcohol . . . . f℥xxvj.
Dissolve, then add—
Tinct. of cantharides (made with strong alcohol) . . . . f℥j.
Ess. of jessamine (or other perfume) . fʒiss
Mix.

This preparation has the property of rendering the hair soft and glossy, at the same time that, by its tonic and stimulant properties, it tends to arrest its premature decay. To accomplish this it should be rubbed thoroughly into the roots at least once a day.

Croton oil, like the foregoing, is the product of the seeds of one of the family euphorbiaceæ. It is imported in bottles holding about twenty ounces. Its powerful irritant and drastic cathartic properties, in doses of from one to two drops, are well known. In applying it as a local irritant for producing a pustular eruption, it is usually diluted with twice the quantity of olive oil; it should then be carefully and conspicuously marked *for external use.*

The use of croton oil mixed with castor oil, in the so-called castor oil capsules, is frequently the cause of violent purging, when a mild and pleasant effect was anticipated. The substitution in this way of a powerful for a mild and wholesome remedy in a popular form of medicine should be corrected by the interference of the physician and pharmaceutist.

Pure croton oil is soluble in about its own bulk of very strong alcohol, but in two or three days nearly all the oil separates. One of the most ready ways of testing its quality is to try its effect upon the skin; if pure, the speedy appearance of the eruption may be anticipated.

Cod-liver oil is largely prepared upon our New England coast, and that of Newfoundland, in connection with the cod fisheries. Three different commercial varieties are produced, which vary in quality according to the skill and care expended in their preparation. *Pale* cod-liver oil is prepared in New England by cutting up the fresh livers and throwing them into water in a large tank arranged for the application of heat. A fire being kindled, the oil rises to the surface and is skimmed off; by standing, even after being barrelled, a deposit separates which allows of the clear oil being racked off. It is abundant in our markets within a few years, being used exclusively in medicine, and commanding a price, by the gallon, of from $2 to $3.

The other most common variety is the *dark brown* oil. The livers being thrown into a heap exposed to the sun, are thus allowed to become decomposed, and the oil is collected as it flows out from the corrupting mass. The dark brown oil is rancid, having a disagreeable empyreumatic odor, and a taste which is bitter, besides being acrid, as in the other case. It is used extensively by curriers. Its price is usually about $1 per gallon.

The *pale brown cod-liver oil* is intermediate in its properties between the foregoing; it is by some preferred to either, and by several customers with whom I have met is said to disagree less with the stomach. This variety is not so common in commerce. Many dealers do not procure it at all. I have obtained it by the gallon at from $1 25 to $1 75 per gallon. There are all grades of quality between the finest and commonest oils.

The large admixture of other fish than the cod in the produce of the New England fisheries and the consequent admixture of the livers, has induced a very general opinion that the Newfoundland oil, as representing the oil of the livers of the cod exclusively, is to be preferred. This is the kind of oil sold chiefly in England, and upon which the reputation of the oil was mainly founded in the first instance. Excellent cod-liver oil is made in London from the livers of the fresh fish brought to that market. The firm of Allen and Hanburys supply their extensive demand from this source. The livers are placed in a large iron pan over a coal fire, and heated to about 180° F., stirring constantly; the oil which exudes is then strained, and is ready for use.

The following description of the *Newfoundland* manufacture, it will be seen, differs from that of New England, though the three varieties produced are here differently named; it is compiled from an article by Dr. Edward H. Robinson, *Am. Journ. Pharm.*, vol. xxvi. p. 1.

On the Banks of Newfoundland, the fish are obtained within from one to five miles from shore, and if the day be favorable, the fisherman fills his boat (which is small) at least twice during the day. As soon as the boat is filled, they are taken on shore and handed over to women and children, who split the fish for drying, carefully putting the livers into a clean tub or some other article used for the purpose. All the fish being thus prepared, and spread on sheds to dry, the livers are carried to a cool place where they are kept until evening, by which time another boat load of fish has generally been obtained.

Treating this second lot as the first, the livers are now all put together in a large shallow vessel of iron, usually about five feet square, and three in depth; which vessel is again inserted into another and larger, which is set into masonry and partly filled with water. A fire is then kindled under the outer vessel and kept burning until the greater part of the oil has been separated from the livers. The fire is then extinguished, and, when cool, the oil is dipped out and introduced into new or clean casks. What oil remains in the livers is now pressed out, but not being of as good quality as that made without pressure, it is put into a separate cask, constituting an inferior quality.

The casks containing the oil are now put in a cool place, and undisturbed for five or six days, at the end of which time a considerable sediment has fallen, leaving a pure oil on top, which is carefully drawn off and put into other casks; the oil is now fit to be sent into the market. This constitutes the best quality of cod-liver oil. The color of this variety is a pale yellow, having a specific gravity, at 63° F., of .9240; has a slight fishy taste, though not very disagreeable to most persons, leaving an impression of acridity on the fauces. In some parts, where the fishermen are too poor to purchase the water bath, the fresh livers are put into a common iron pot used for domestic purposes; moderate heat is then applied. As soon as the livers are somewhat broken down and softened, they are taken from the pot and introduced into a coarse canvas bag, and, by pressure, the greater part of the oil is forced out. This variety is not of quite as fine quality as that made with the steam bath; the color is rather darker, has a slight empyreumatic taste, and is apt to leave a peculiar burning sensation in the fauces when swallowed, which is perceptible some time after.

Another variety, of an inferior quality, is made in larger vessels which remain at sea for weeks together without going to the shore. The method of obtaining this variety is as follows: As fast as the fish are caught and dressed, the livers are thrown into barrels placed on deck, the tops of which remain uncovered. The livers are exposed to the action of the sun's rays, decomposition soon ensues, and the oily matter separates. That part which first rises to the top is skimmed off and put into a separate cask. The color of this variety is yellow approaching to a brown. It is commonly known as *straits* oil. The commonest variety of all is made from the remnants of the casks from which the straits oil has been drawn. In this variety complete putrefaction has taken place. It is of a very dark color, has an extremely offensive smell, and is more disagreeable than the other varieties. This is known as *banks oil.*

The following particulars of the process, as conducted by Charles Fox & Co., of Newfoundland, show the application of more extended arrangements to the same branch of manufacture.

The boats go out early in the morning and return about four o'clock in the afternoon. The fish, on landing, are handed over to the "fish-room keeper," whose duty it is to split and open the fish, and to deposit their livers in small tubs, holding 17 or 18 gallons each. These tubs are soon afterwards collected from the different fish-rooms, and conveyed to the manufactory. The livers here are thrown into tubs containing pure cold water, and, after being well washed and jerked over, are placed on galvanized iron-wire sieves to drain. They are next put into covered steam jacket-pans and submitted to a gentle heat for about three-quarters of an hour, after which the steam is turned off, cold air admitted, and the whole allowed to repose for a short time, during which the livers subside, and the oil separates and floats on the top; the oil is then skimmed off into tin vessels and passed through flannel strainers into tubs, where it is left to subside for about 24 hours. From these the purer upper portion of oil is run into a very deep galvanized iron cistern, and again left to clarify itself by defecation for a few days.

The *London Pharmaceutical Journal*, October, 1853, announced that a patent has been recently obtained by Sir James Murray for a process by which cod-liver oil may be completely deodorized. This is accomplished by agitating it in high pressure cylinders with carbonic acid gas. None of the deodorized oil having yet found its way to this country, it is probable that some practical difficulty has prevented the success of the process.

The composition of cod-liver oil, as inferred from the analysis of Dr. De Jongh, is similar to that of other fatty oils, with the exception of a peculiar organic substance, called by him *gaduin*, and also some of the constituents of bile, with traces of iodine, bromine, &c.

More recently, Dr. F. L. Winckler has investigated its chemical nature, and regards this oil as an organic whole of a peculiar chemical composition, differing from that of all other fatty oils hitherto employed as medicines. According to this eminent chemist, it contains no glycerin, but by saponification yields oleic and margaric acids, and the hydrated oxide of the organic radical, *propyle* (C_6H_7); existing also in ergot and in the liquor of pickled herring. From this, Dr. Winckler infers that cod-liver oil cannot be substituted by any other officinal oil. Propylamine ($NH_2C_6H_7$), a product of the reaction of ammonia on cod-liver oil, is also found by Winckler in normal urine and sweat; and, viewing its formation as probable by the reaction in the system by which cod-liver oil is assimilated and burnt up in the lungs, he founds upon this his theory of the utility of cod-liver oil in medicine.

CHAPTER VI.

ON VOLATILE OILS, CAMPHORS, AND RESINS.

VOLATILE OR ESSENTIAL OILS.

THIS highly important and interesting class of proximate principles contains an immense number of individuals which are distinguished from each other by striking sensible, as well as chemical and physical peculiarities. By far the largest number are derived from plants, in which they exist ready formed, although some are the products of a sort of spontaneous fermentative action set up among principles contained in the plants in the presence of water; others are products of the destructive distillation of organic substances.

The natural volatile oils are mostly prepared by mixing plants or parts of plants containing them, with water, and, after maceration for a certain length of time, subjecting the mixture to distillation. The distillate is usually milky, and on standing separates, most of the oil rising to the top, or, in a few instances, subsiding, while the water continues charged to saturation with the oil. Although the boiling point of these oils is much above that of water, many of them are readily volatilized in contact with steam at 212°, and are hence conveniently prepared in the way above described.

The unpleasant odor at first perceived in the distillate was formerly believed to be empyreumatic, but is now said to be due to portions of tin dissolved from the neck of the still or the condensing worm, and to disappear with the subsequent oxidation and separation of this metal, and its separation as a flocculent precipitate which is often mistaken for an algaeric vegetation.

Some highly odoriferous plants which yield by this process very sparse and unsatisfactory results, are found to impart their volatile oils better by digesting with fixed fatty bodies, which, when treated with strong alcohol, yield the volatile oils to that solvent, forming essences. Numerous oils or essences used in perfumery are prepared in this way. Others are prepared by direct expression from the vessels containing them, as the oils obtained from the rind of the lemon and bergamot fruits; while others are obtained, associated with their resins and camphors, by the use of ether.

The volatile oils are mostly soluble in water to a very limited extent; and in turn dissolve a small proportion of water, which separates at low temperatures. They are mostly soluble to an unlimited extent in anhydrous alcohol, ether, and the fixed oils.

By the destructive distillation of most organic substances, liquids are obtained which possess the general physical characters of volatile oils, and may be classed as empyreumatic oils, though many of them are designated as peculiar chemical compounds. Creasote, which is treated of at page 286, is an illustration of this. These are more properly treated of under the heads of the several sources from which derived, than in this connection.

The perfume of most plants is due to the gradual elimination, diffusion, and oxidation, in very minute qualities, of their volatile oils. Every one must have noticed that in the moist morning and evening atmosphere, the odor of flowers is greatly enhanced, a phenomenon which is partly due to the power of vapor of water to aid in the diffusion of the volatilized oils, and probably partly to an increased tendency to oxidization in contact with aqueous vapor. According to Liebig, the perfume of essential oils is strong in proportion to their tendency to oxidize in the air, though their degree of volatility has an important bearing on this property. Their odor is generally strong in proportion to the oxygen in their composition. Certain oils containing no oxygen may be temporarily deprived of their characteristic odors by distillation from freshly-burnt lime in an apparatus exhausted of air or filled with carbonic acid gas. The odor of essential oils is apt to be less delicate or grateful after they have been isolated than when spontaneously exhaled by the plant, and by time and exposure many of them not only lose their delicacy of flavor, but become less limpid, assuming a darker color and more resinoid consistence. In the process of drying certain plants at a moderate heat, the oil seems to improve in flavor, while very little of it is dissipated, so that the aromatic seeds, as of fennel and caraway, the unexpanded flowers of clove, &c., as found in commerce, yield full proportions of essential oils, and of finer quality than the imported oils obtained from them when fresh. Valerian is an instance of the smell being greatly increased by age, owing to the oxidation of the oil.

Carbo-Hydrogen Essential Oils.

The most simple group of essential oils is that which consists of carbon and hydrogen alone. Some of these have been already referred to as frequently associated with the oxygenated essential oils. There are a number produced by plants and obtained by distillation. The coniferæ, aurantiaciæ, and piperaceæ yield nearly all that are known. Although these are so similar in composition, they are, as usually obtained, as dissimilar in many of their properties as they are unlike the members of the oxygenated group. As already stated, when absolutely pure and exposed to no oxidizing influences, they are quite inodorous, and it is impossible in this state to distinguish oil of lemon from oil of turpentine, or oil of juniper from oil of neroli. As soon as they are exposed to ordinary external influences, however, they develop their characteristic odors and become less limpid and colorless. As a class, they are the least soluble in alcohol and in water. Several of them are among the most useful of vegetable stimulants. The composition of the carbo-hydrogen essential oils is $C_{20}H_{16}$, or $C_{10}H_8$, or some multiple of C_5H_4.

1. *List of Plants yielding Binary Volatile Oils.*

They are all dicotyledons, and with the exception of Dippel's animal oil, the oils of this series are carbo-hydrogens of the formula $C_{20}H_{16}$; they are therefore called terebenes or camphenes.

Dipteraceæ.

Dryobalanops camphora, Borneo camphor tree.[1]

Terebinthaceæ.

Amyris elemifera, Elemi tree—resin.
Boswellia serrata, East India Olibanum tree—resin.

Leguminosæ.

Copaifera (various species)—oleo-resin.

Piperaceæ.

Piper cubeba, cubeb—fruit.
" nigra, black pepper—fruit.

Coniferæ.

Abies canadensis, hemlock spruce fir—resin.
Juniperus communis, juniper—fruit tops and wood.
Juniperus sabina, savin—leaves.
" Virginiaca, red cedar—leaves.
Pinus pumilio, mountain pine—oleo-resin.
" palustris, &c., various species of pine—oleo-resin.

Empyreumatic Products.

From asphaltum—oil of asphaltum.
" amber—oil of amber.
" tar—oil of tar.
Natural product—petroleum.
From animal matter—Dippel's animal oil. Consists of organic alkaloids, has an alkaline reaction, is poisonous; is darkened by light and air; used as an antispasmodic in doses of 5 to 25 drops.

---

[1] Camphor oil or Borneen exists in the cavities of the trunk.

Oxygenated Oils.

A very large number of oxygenated oils are known to exist, although, according to the views of some, many of this class consist of members of the former class combined with peculiar camphors. Others have regarded the members of this series as oxides of oils of the carbohydrogen series. Many important members of this class are obtained from the natural families Umbelliferæ, Labiatæ, Lauraceæ, and Compositæ, but they are very widely diffused in other divisions of the vegetable kingdom. The oils from the leaves, bark and fruit of several species of Rosaceæ, when obtained by distillation with water, contain hydrocyanic acid, and possess decidedly sedative and even poisonous properties, while the flowers of the same plants and all parts of the herbaceous Rosaceæ are destitute of any nitrogenized element.

Of the complex series derived chiefly from the Cruciferæ, and containing sulphur, one only, that of garlic, numbers oxygen among its elements. Only three of the oxygenated oils, those of cinnamon, gaultheria, and bitter almond, have as yet been produced by chemical processes from other vegetable principles. This extraordinary attainment of modern chemistry leads to the inference that many others of this class are capable of artificial production.

The oxygenated volatile oils, though heavier than the carbohydrogens, are, with a few exceptions, lighter than water; their specific gravity ranges from .82 to 1.09. See *Chemical History*, &c., p. 342.

The oxygenated oils, like the carbo-hydrogens, are mostly local and general stimulants: some of them are of the kind called carminatives, used to expel wind in colic; others are stomachics, promoters of digestion; a few, from their influence upon the brain, rank as antispasmodics. Not a few of both classes are chiefly valued as perfumes, whether for the toilet or in pharmacy.

Most of the spices, as nutmeg, mace, pimento, cloves, contain oxygenated oils, which, in connection with peculiar camphoraceous or resinous ingredients, give them their value as condiments or seasoners.

The herbs used in soups and stuffings, and rendering savory many otherwise tasteless dishes, all contain essential oils, and most of them of this series. It will be observed that none of the essential oils rank as narcotics, except in overdoses, though those of camphor, valerian, serpentaria, &c., as before stated, are used as cerebro-spinal stimulants and antispasmodics.

As a class of essential oils, the oxygenated are the most soluble in water, and enter into the *Aquæ Medicatæ* introduced among the Galenical preparations.

2. *List of Plants Yielding Oxygenated Oils.*

(Mostly dicotyledons, but few monocotyledons.)

DICOTYLEDONS.		
Ranunculaceæ.		
Nigella sativa—small fennel flower	seed	16 oz. yield 4 scr.; pure oil is opalescent; dissolves in 30 p. alc.
Magnoliaceæ.		
Drimys Winteri—Winter's bark	bark	16 oz. yield 10 to 20 grs.
Illicium anisatum—Star anise	seed	$C_{20}H_{16}$ and $C_{20}H_{12}O_2$; the latter solid below 50°, melts at 62°, boils at 430°. (See umbelliferæ.)
Violareæ.		
Viola odorata—Sweet violet	flowers	blue; delightful fragrance, yield very small.
Tiliaceæ.		
Tilia Europæa—European linden	flowers	yield exceedingly small; oil thin, colorless, very fragrant.
Aurantiaceæ.		
Citrus aurantium—Sweet orange " limetta—Bergamot lemon " limonum—Lemon " medica—Citron " vulgaris—Seville orange	leaves flowers and peel of fruit	The oil obtained from orange leaves is called *essence de petit grain;* that from the flowers of citrus vulgaris is the real *oil of neroli*, though probably the flowers of other species are mixed with them before distillation; oil from the peel is mostly $C_{20}H_{16}$; all contain $C_{20}H_{18}O_2$.
Guttiferæ.		
Canella alba—White cinnamon	bark	16 oz. yield 40 grs. aromatic.
Rutaceæ.		
Diosma crenata—Buchu	leaves	16 oz. yield 51 to 68 grains; yellowish-brown, diuretic.
" odorata, serratifolia	leaves	
Gallipea cusparia—Angustura	bark	16 oz. yield 7 to 23 grs.
Ruta graveolens—Rue	herb	Is principally $C_{20}H_{20}O_2$; stim. antispasmod. emmenagogue.
Leguminosæ.		
Genista Canariensis—Canary rosewood	wood	80 lbs. yield from 9 to 16 drachms of oil. Oil of rhodium.
Rosaceæ.		
Cydonia vulgaris—Quince	peel	16 oz. yielded by expression 4 grs.
Rosa centifolia—Hundred-leaved rose	petals	100℔ rose leaves yield less than 3 dr.; below 86° it assumes the consistence of butter.
Rosa sempervirens — Evergreen rose, and other species.	"	
Sanguisorba officinalis—Common burnet	root	color blue; cordial.
Spiræa ulmaria—Meadow sweet	herb	Is hydruret of salicyle $C_{14}H_6O_4$; boiling point 350°; sp. grav. 1.173.
Myrtaceæ.		
Caryophyllus aromaticus—Cloves	flower-buds	$C_{20}H_{16}$ and caryophyllic acid $C_{20}H_{12}O_5$; boils at 470° F.
Eugenia pimenta—Allspice	fruit	yield as much as 6 per cent.; compos. like oil cloves $C_{20}H_{16}$ and $C_{20}H_{12}O_5$.
Melaleuca cajeputi—Cajeput	leaves	$C_{20}H_{16} + 2HO$, green; stimul. antispasm.
Myrtus communis—Common myrtle	leaves & flowers	Very fragrant; 100℔ fresh leaves yield 2½ to 4½ oz.
Crassulaceæ.		
Rhodiola rosea—Rose-root	root	1℔ yields 1 dr., substitute for oil of rhodium.
Umbelliferæ.		
Anethum graveolens—Dill.	seed	Carminative; soluble in 1440 parts of water.

Angelica Archangelica—Angelica	root	16 oz. yield ½ to 1 drachm.
Apium petroselinum—Parsley	herb	$C_{20}H_{16}$ and $C_{12}H_8O_2$. Occasionally used in medicine.
Carum carui—Caraway	fruit	$C_{20}H_{16}$ and carvol $C_{20}H_{14}O_2$, carminat.
Cicuta virosa—Water hemlock	"	Identical with oil of cumin seed.
Coriandrum sativum—Coriander	"	16 oz. yield ½ to 1 dr., sp. gr. .85 ; $C_{20}H_{16}$ and $C_{20}H_{18}O_2$.
Cuminum cyminum—Cumin	"	Cymol $C_{20}H_{14}$ and cuminol $C_{20}H_{14}O_2$; acrid.
Daucus carota—Carrot	"	16 oz. yield 30 grs. ; diuretic, stimulant.
Fœniculum vulgare—Fennel	"	Composition like oil of anise ; but $C_{20}H_{12}O_2$ still liquid at 14°, boils at 440°.
Galbanum officinale—Galbanum	resin	Taste and smell like resin, camphorous ; sp. gr. .912.
Imperatoria ostruthium—Masterwort	root	$C_{20}H_{16}$ and hydrur. angelyle $C_{10}H_8O_2$; boiling commence at 335°.
Phellandrium aquaticum—Water dropwort	fruit	16 oz. yield from 2 scr. to 2 dr. ; golden yellow ; taste sweetish, afterw'ds burn'g.
Pimpinella anisum—Anise	"	Like oil of star anise ; see magnoliaceæ, also compositæ.
Caprifoliaceæ.		
Sambucus nigra—Common elder	flowers	Yield small ; mild stimulant.
Valerianeæ.		
Valeriana officinalis—Valerian	root	Borneen $C_{20}H_{16}$ and valerol $C_{12}H_{10}O_2$.
Compositæ.		
Achillea millefolium—Yarrow	herb and flowers	16 oz. yield 5 to 13 grs. ; sp. gr. .9 ; color blue or deep green.
Anthemis nobilis—English chamomile	flowers	16 oz. yield 22 to 55 grs. ; spec. gr. .908 ; hydrur. angelyle $C_{10}H_8O_2$, angelicic acid $C_{10}H_8O_4$ and $C_{20}H_{16}$. Color blue or green.
Arnica montana—Arnica	root and flowers	1℔ flowers yields about 3 grs. ; of root ½ dr. : both lighter than water.
Artemisia absinthium—Wormwood	herb and flowers	Comp. $C_{20}H_{16}O_2$; crude oil brownish-green.
Artemisia dracunculus—Tarragon	herb	Composition like oil anise, $C_{20}H_{12}O_2$ liquid ; boils at 400°.
" contra, Judaica and santonica (Semen contra, S. cynæ)	flower buds	Spec. grav. .91 to .97 ; dissolve in an equal part of alcohol.
Erigeron Canadense—Canadian fleabane	herb	Spec. grav. .845. Anti-hæmorrhagic.
Erigeron Philadelphicum—Philadelphia fleabane	"	Yield very small. "
Inula helenium—Elecampane	root	16 oz. yield from ¼ to 1 dr.
Matricaria chamomilla—German chamomile	flowers	Resembles oil of anthemis ; color blue.
Tanacetum vulgare—Tansy	herb	Yellow or greenish ; taste warm, bitter.
Ericaceæ.		
Gaultheria procumbens—Wintergreen	herb	Comp. $C_{20}H_{16}$ and Methylsalycic acid $C_{16}H_8O_6$; boiling point 412°.
Jasmineæ.		
Jasminum grandiflorum and fragrans—Jessamine	flowers	Yield very small ; extracted by a fixed oil, from which alcohol takes it up ; very fragrant.
Labiatæ.		
Hedeoma pulegioides—Pennyroyal	herb	Carminative, emmenag., spec. grav. .948.
Hyssopus officinalis—Hyssop	"	Odor persist. arom. ; taste hot, camphor's.
Lavandula spica—Spike lavender	herb and flowers	Oleum spicæ, similar to and sold for cheap oil of lavender ; that usually kept is fictitious, princ. turpentine.

Lavandula vera—True lavender	herb and flowers	$C_{20}H_{16}O_2$ and $C_{16}H_{14}O_2$; the lightest oil from selected flowers is most fragrant.
Marrubium vulgare—Horehound	herb	Very small quantity.
Melissa officinalis—Lemon balm	"	Used for flavoring medicines, also in perfumery.
Mentha aquatica—Watermint	"	This and other species of mentha are often mixed with peppermint in distilling the oil; yields nearly 1 scr. to the pound.
" crispa—Curled-leaved mint	"	Not so cooling as peppermint; freezing in the cold.
Mentha piperita—Peppermint	"	$C_2H_{20}O_2$ and alsoopter; boiling point 365°; best distilled by steam.
" pulegium—Europ. pennyroyal	"	$C_{20}H_{16}$ and $C_{20}H_{16}O_2$; 100℔ fresh herb yield rather less than 1℔; spec. gr. .927; boils at 395°.
Mentha viridis—Spearmint	"	Spec. grav. .91; $C_{35}H_{28}O$? (Kane); boiling point 320°; 100℔ fresh herb yield 3 oz.
Monarda punctata—Horsemint	"	$C_{30}H_{21}O$ and thymol $C_{20}H_{14}O_2$; solid at 40° F.; rubefac.
Nepeta cataria—Catnep	"	16 oz. fresh herb yield 9 grs.; carminative.
" citriodorata—Lemon catmint	"	16 oz. yield 7½ grs.; odor pleasant; fulminates with iodine.
Origanum majorana—Sweet marjoram	"	Pale yellow; tonic, stimulant; its camphor is $C_{14}H_{15}O_6$.
Origanum vulgare—Origanum	"	$C_{50}H_{40}O$,? boils at 354°; rubefac.; oil of commerce often adulter.
Rosmarinus officinalis—Rosemary	"	$C_{45}H_{38}O_2$? boiling point 365°.
Salvia officinalis—Sage	"	$C_{12}H_{10}O$ and $C_{18}H_{15}O_2$.
Thymus serpyllum—Lemon thyme	"	Used like other aromatics; also for scenting soaps.
Thymus vulgaris—Garden thyme	"	Comp. thymen $C_{20}H_{16}$ and thymol $C_{20}H_{14}O_2$.
Chenopodeæ.		
Chenopodium ambrosioides—Mexican tea	"	16 oz. yield 26 grs.; burning aromatic taste and smell.
Chenopodium anthelminticum—wormseed	seed	$C_{20}H_{16}$ and $C_{20}H_{16}O_2$; anthelmintic.
Laurineæ.		
Cinnamomum aromaticum—Chinese cinnamon	bark	Comp. $C_{20}H_{16}$, hydrur. cinnamyle, $=C_{18}H_8O_2$, cinnamic acid $C_{18}H_8O_4$ and resin.
Cinnamomum Zeylanicum—Ceylon cinnamon	"	(same as above)
Cinnamomum Loureirii—(Cassia buds)	flower buds	Agreeably aromatic, hot.
Laurus nobilis—Bay tree	berries	16 oz. yield ½ to 1 dr.; sp. grav. .914; comp. $C_{20}H_{16}O$, contains two isomeric oils.
Sassafras officinale—Sassafras	wood and bark	$C_{20}H_{16}$ and $C_{20}H_{10}O_4$; boils at 440°.
Myristiceæ.		
Myristica moschata—Nutmeg	kernel	Ol. nuc. moschat.; yield 6 per cent.; sp. gr. .92 to .95.
" " "	arillus	Oleum macidis is oftener met with in commerce; the stearopter is $C_{16}H_{15}O_6$.
Santalaceæ.		
Santalum myrtifolium—White saunders	wood	16 oz. yield ½ to 2 dr.; used in perfumery.
Aristolochiaceæ.		
Asarum Canadense—Canada snakeroot	root	Light colored, fragrant.
Asarum Europæum—Asarabacca	"	Yield 12 grs. pr. 16 oz.; spec. grav. 1.018, comp. C_8H_4O; camphor C_8H[illegible]O_2.
Serpentaria Virginiana—Virginia snakeroot	"	Yield about ½ per cent.; color green.

Euphorbiaceæ.		
Croton eleuteria—Cascarilla	bark	16 oz. yield 27 to 68 grs.; spec. grav. .92: used for fumigation; $C_{14}H_{10}O$ and another oil.
Urticeæ.		
Humulus lupulus—Hop	strobiles	Spec. grav. .91; $C_{20}H_{16}$ and $C_{20}H_{18}O_2$.
MONOCOTYLEDONS.		
Zingiberaceæ.		
Alpinia galanga—Galangle	root	16 oz. yield 1 to 3 scr.; taste sim. cardam.
Curcuma zedoaria—Zedoary	root	16 oz. yield 1 dr.; thick, yellowish white.
Elettaria cardamomum—Cardamom	seed	Odor penetrating; aromatic; taste hot, camphorous.
Zingiber officinale—Ginger	root	16 oz. yield ½ to 2 dr.; compos. $C_{20}H_{16}$ + variable prop. HO.
Irideæ.		
Crocus sativus—Saffron	pistils	16 oz. yield 1½ dr., yellow, heavier than water, acrid; by keeping it turns white and lighter; probably the active princ.
Aroideæ.		
Acorus calamus—Calamus	root	100℔ fr. rt. y'ld 16 oz.; $C_{13}H_{10}O$ & oth. oils.

3. *List of Plants yielding Volatile Oils containing Hydrocyanic Acid.*

(All belong to the family of rosaceæ, most to the sub-family amygdaleæ, and a few to pomaceæ.)

Amygdalus communis, var. amara—Bitter almond	kernels	These oils are very similar in their sensible properties: the oil of almond is hydruret of benzyle $C_{14}H_6O_2$, in which hydrocyanic acid HC_2N is dissolved. All are poisonous.
Cerasus (various species)—Cherry	bark	
Persica vulgaris—Peach	leaves & kernels	
Prunus domestica and others—Plum		25℔ of bitter almond cake after the expression of the fixed oil yield about 2 oz.
Pyrus communis and malus—Pear and apple	leaves & kernels	

4. *List of Plants yielding Sulphuretted Oils.*

(Mostly cruciferæ.)

DICOTYLEDONS.		
Cruciferæ.		
Alliaria officinalis—Jack by the hedge	leaves and root	C_6H_5S, if distilled from fresh spring root it is $C_8H_5NS_2$
Capsella bursa pastoris—Shepherd's purse	seed	C_6H_5S and $C_8H_5NS_2$.
Cochlearia armoracia—Horse-radish	root	$C_8H_5NS_2$; 100℔ fresh root yield nearly 7 oz.
Cochlearia officinalis—Common scurvy grass	herb	Same comp.
Iberis amara—Bitter candytuft	herb and	Same comp.
Lepidium sativum, campestre, &c.—Cress	seed	C_6H_5S; is decomposed on rectification.
Raphanus raphanistrum—Wild mustard	seed	C_6H_5S and $C_8H_5NS_2$.
Sinapis nigra—Black mustard	seed	$C_8H_5NS_2$; yield 5 per cent.
Sisymbrium nasturtium—Water-radish	seed	Same and C_6H_5S.
Thlapsi arvense—Treacle mustard	herb and seed	C_6H_5S.
Umbelliferæ.		
Ferula assafœtida—Assafœtida	gum-resin	C_6H_5S with other compounds of sulphur and C_6H_5.
" persica (?)—Sagapenum	"	Contains C_6H_5S.
MONOCOTYLEDONS.		
Liliaceæ.		
Allium sativum—Garlic	bulb	C_6H_5S and C_6H_5O.

Oils that may be obtained artificially.

1. *Oxygenated.*

Oil of cinnamon from styrone $C_{18}H_{10}O_2$, by platina black $= C_{18}H_8O_2$ hydruret of cinnamyle.

Oil of gaultheria from 2 parts crystal. salicylic acid $C_{14}H_6O_6$. 2 anhydrous methylic alcohol $C_2H_4O_2$ and 1 $SO_3 = C_{14}H_5(C_2H_3)O_6$.

2. *Nitrogenated.*

Oil of bitter almonds, from styracine $C_{36}H_{16}O_4$ by NO_5, besides benzoic and nitro-benzoic acids also $= C_{14}H_6O_2$ and $H_{11}C_2N$.

3. *Sulphuretted.*

Oil of mustard, from iodide of propylene, C_6H_5I, by sulpho-cyanuret of potassium $K,C_2NS_2 = C_6H_5(C_2N)S_2$.

Chemical History.—Notwithstanding the admitted crude and imperfect preparation of the volatile oils of commerce, and the fact that they consist of different proximate principles varying in their relative proportions to each other, and therefore in the results of their analyses; yet much light has been thrown upon their chemical history by the labors of chemists.

Volatile oils are classed as in the foregoing tables: 1. Carbo-hydrogens or camphenes; 2. Oxygenated oils; and 3. Oils of a more complex nature, generally containing sulphur or nitrogen, and being the products of fermentation. The natural volatile oils belonging to the first class all have the composition $C_{20}H_{16}$, and from nearly all of the second class by fractional distillation a liquid of the same composition may be obtained, having a lower boiling point and being thinner, and of less specific gravity than that portion distilling at a higher temperature; the former is called *elæopten;* the latter, *stearopten*, contains oxygen and frequently has the composition of ordinary camphor $C_{20}H_{16}O_2$, oxide of camphene, or its composition corresponds with a hydrate of camphene $C_{20}H_{18}O_2$ (Borneo camphor), $C_{20}H_{20}O_4$ (juniper camphor), $C_{20}H_{22}O_6$ (lemon camphor). A similar hydrate may be obtained from turpentine, and most other camphenes by treating them with a mixture of nitric acid and alcohol, when *terpin* $C_{20}H_{16}+6HO$ crystallizes, which in vacuo loses 2HO.

By the action of hydrochloric acid gas on the camphenes, a combination of the two is effected, which may be liquid or solid; if the latter, it is crystalline, and from its resemblance to camphor has been called artificial camphor. The behavior of a number of the camphenes towards polarized light has been observed; most of them deviate its plane to the left side; the carbo-hydrogen of oil of lemon is an exception, it turning the polarized light towards the right.

All *pure* volatile oils are believed to be colorless, though a few have not as yet been obtained entirely destitute of color, while a few are so readily influenced by air and light, as, after rectification, to assume coloration in a short time (oil of cinnamon and cassia). There are very few colored oils which cannot be freed from color by rectification or fractional distillation; oleum matricariæ and anthemidis have a blue color; oleum millefolii a green, sometimes a blue; oleum absinthii a deep brown color; oleum sem. nigellæ which is of a brownish color, has the property of fluorescence the blue color, being also observable in its solutions in alcohol and ether.

The volatile oils, by absorbing oxygen from the atmosphere, assume a deeper color, which passes through yellow, reddish or greenish, to brown, those to which a color naturally belongs, also undergo this change, generally passing through green to brown. This change, as a general rule, takes place very slowly with the natural carbo-hydrogens; oxygenated oils change more quickly, usually the more so, the more oxygen they contain. With the deepening of the color, the fluidity of the volatile oils is lessened owing to a resinification taking place, some gradually assuming the consistence of resins; at the same time the odor is altered and rendered more or less unpleasant.

The less stearopten oils contain, the less are they influenced by change of temperature, while from all a few crystals may be obtained in the cold, unless they have been entirely deprived of the water, they have dissolved in minute quantities. As the carbo-hydrogens are not solidified by a low temperature, a change in the amount of the stearopten must necessarily alter the freezing and melting point of the volatile oils, the latter of which is always several degrees above the former. G. H. Zeller, from his own observations with oils prepared by himself, gives the following :—

Oleum anisi	solidifies at	43° to 66° F.,	liquefies at	68° to 72° F.
" " stellati	" "	54° to 59° "	" "	63.5° "
" arnicæ flor.	" "		" "	100° "
" fœniculi (mostly elæopt.)	"	bel. + 5° "	" "	21° "
" " (rich in stearopt.)	" "	41° to 45° "		
" matricariæ	" at	10° to 5° "	" "	21° "
" petroselini	" "	36° to 50° "		
" rosæ German	" "	88° "	" "	100° "

The boiling point is variable from the same cause; volatile oils commence to boil at comparatively low temperatures, when elæopten with little stearopten distils over; gradually the boiling point rises and the distillates contain more of the stearopten; the boiling point of any pure compound of the volatile oils is stationary.

The relations between certain essential oils, organic acids and neutral principles found in plants, constituting regular series of chemical compounds, though not as yet discovered to extend to any great number of them, are among the most curious and interesting developments of modern chemistry. The following syllabus embraces most of these :—

Benzyle Bz	$C_{14}H_5O_2$.
Hydruret of Bz, oil of bitter almond . . .	$C_{14}H_5O_2+H$.
Oxide of Bz, anhydrous benzoic acid . . .	$C_{14}H_5O_2+O$.
" crystallized " . . .	$C_{14}H_5O_2+O+HO$.
Cynamyle, Ci	$C_{18}H_7O_2$.
Hydruret of Ci, oil of cinnamon . . .	$C_{18}H_7O_2+H$.
Oxide of Ci, cinnamic acid	$C_{18}H_7O_2+O$.
Cumyle	$C_{20}H_{11}O_2$.
Hydruret of cumyle, oil of cumin . . .	$C_{20}H_{11}O_2+H$.
Oxide " cuminic acid . . .	$C_{20}H_{11}O_2+O$.
Thymyle, Th	$C_{20}H_{13}$.
Hydruret of Th, "cymale, cymin," . . .	$C_{20}H_{13}+H$.
Oxide of Th, oil of thyme	$C_{20}H_{13}+O_2+HO$.
"Carvol," oil of caraway	$C_{20}H_{14}O_2$.
"Carvacrol," creasote of camphor . . .	$C_{20}H_{14}O_2$.
Rutyle, Rut	$C_{20}H_{19}O_2$.
Hydruret of Rut, oil of rue	$C_{20}H_{19}O_2+H$.[1]
Salicyle, Sal	$C_{14}H_5O_4$.
Hydruret of Sal (spirous acid)[2] . . .	$C_{14}H_5O_4+H$.
Helicin+2 aq.	$C_{14}H_6O_4+C_{12}H_{12}O_{12}$ (sugar)
Saligenin	$C_{14}H_6O_4+H_2$.
Salicin+2 aq.	$C_{14}H_8O_4+C_{12}H_{12}O_{12}$.
Salicylic acid	$C_{14}H_5O_4+O+HO$.
Salicilate of oxide of methyle, oil of gaultheria .	$C_{14}H_5O_5+C_2H_3O$.

[1] The aldehyde of caprinic acid.

[2] Oil of spiræa (*see* Acids).

ADULTERATIONS.

Essential oils are liable to be adulterated with fixed oils, with alcohol, and with other and cheaper essential oils. The mode of detecting these adulterations is as follows:—

With Fixed Oils.—Oils thus adulterated leave upon bibulous paper a greasy spot, which remains even after long-continued heating over the flame of a lamp. Sometimes, owing to the essential oil being partially resinified, it leaves a mark which is devoid of transparency and possesses a peculiar gloss, while the stain from a fixed oil is transparent, and, when completely absorbed by the paper, devoid of a distinct gloss—besides, when soaked in alcohol and heated, the resinous stain can be wiped off, while the fatty stain cannot be removed. When the mixture is distilled with water, the volatile oil passes over while the fixed oil remains, and may be saponified with alkali. On dissolving the volatile oil in strong alcohol, in the proportion indicated in the Table of Solubilities, page 346, the greater part of the fixed oil remains undissolved. Small proportions of fixed oils may escape detection, if soluble to any extent in alcohol, and this difficulty is increased by the increased solubility of the fixed oils from admixture with essential oils.

With Alcohol.—When the proportion of alcohol is considerable, the greater part of it may be extracted by water, the liquid becoming turbid, and the oil finally separating. When the quantity of the adulteration is small, it is better to shake it with olive oil, which dissolves the essential oil, and separates the alcohol in a layer floating on the surface. The quantity of alcohol is shown *approximately* by shaking the adulterated oil with an equal bulk of water in a minim measure or test-tube graduated for the purpose, and observing the diminution of its volume. Into a graduated tube, two-thirds filled with the oil, some pieces of chloride of calcium may be introduced, and a gentle heat applied for a few minutes with agitation. If no alcohol is present, the lumps of chloride of calcium appear unaltered on cooling; if it contains alcohol, they will show a disposition to coalesce, and if it is in considerable proportion, a fluid layer will separate at the bottom, on which the oil will float. This is especially applicable to oil of lemon, of which 480 grains, mixed with 15 of alcohol, liquefies 3 grains of chloride of calcium. The suspected oil being agitated with dry acetate of potassa, if dissolved. on mixture with sulphuric acid, and heating, the odor of acetic ether is evolved, recognizable by its odor. Nitric acid added to oil of bitter almonds, will only give off nitrous fumes in case of its adulteration with alcohol.

With other Essential Oils.—One means of detecting these common adulterations is by triturating a small quantity on the hand and noticing the odor after it is dried, or in setting fire to a small portion and blowing it out again, when the foreign odor may generally be perceived. If, on agitating the suspected oil with its own bulk of strong alcohol, it is not completely dissolved, probably oil of turpentine, or some other rather insoluble oil, is present. Most carbohydrogens require over 10 parts of alcohol, of .85 sp. gr., to dissolve them.

Oil of savine is soluble in 2 parts of alcohol of this strength, which affords a means of detecting its adulteration by oil of turpentine.

Oils of copaiba, cubebs, and the empyreumatic oils, are recognized by the absence of a violent fulminating reaction with iodine.

The carbohydrogens prevent the reaction of the oxygenated oils with nitroprusside of copper.[1] See page 348.

The behavior of nitric acid, as shown in the table appended, is also useful in detecting adulterations in those cases where the pure oils are little affected by it; in the case of sulphuric acid no advantage results from a comparison. The carbohydrogens are not characteristically affected by this agent.

The variable composition of the volatile oils, owing to the different conditions of the plants and the circumstances of their growth, renders the task of testing them very delicate and uncertain, and all the properties and reactions of an oil should therefore be carefully noted before forming a conclusion.

The following tabulated statement of the principal properties and reactions of the essential oils are designed to furnish, with the foregoing remarks on their chemical history and adulterations, a more complete series of tests for their purity than any heretofore published. They are prepared with the aid of John M. Maisch, of Philadelphia, to whose remarks on this class of bodies, published in the Proceedings of the American Pharmaceutical Association for 1858, the reader is referred.

1. *Carbohydrogens or Camphenes.*

As already stated, most of the volatile oils contain an elæopten composed of carbon and hydrogen, usually in the same proportion as oil of turpentine, and accordingly the number of carbohydrogens might be increased to probably the entire number of the volatile oils. We will class in this group only those which are obtained directly from their plants, or after a simple rectification, their number will then be small and confined to the families of coniferæ, leguminosæ, and piperaceæ, and to some empyreumatic oils. Although their composition is so much alike, there is a marked difference in the odor, the boiling point and their optical behavior. Berthelot's researches have proved the existence of different oils of turpentine, which, though otherwise alike, deviate the polarized light in a different degree, and enter into somewhat differing combinations with hydrochloric acid. Their composition being $C_{20}H_{16}$, or some multiple of C_5H_4, they may be regarded as the radical of camphor, as the following table shows:—

Camphene . . .	$C_{20}H_{16}$.	Lemon camphor . .	$C_{20}H_{16} + 6HO$.
Borneo camphor . .	$C_{20}H_{16} + 2HO$.	Camphor, from camphora officinarum . .	$C_{20}H_{16}O_2$.
Terpin (Juniper camphor) . . .	$C_{20}H_{16} + 4HO$.	Camphoric acid . .	$C_{20}H_{16}O_3$.

So far as examined, these carbohydrogens are not altered in appearance on being boiled with nitroprusside of copper, a reagent of much interest in

[1] Preparation of nitroprusside of copper by Wittstein's process: 10 ounces nitric acid, sp. gr. 1.20 is stirred into 4 ounces powdered ferrocyanuret of potassium, afterwards digested on a water bath until the filtered solution is precipitated with a slate color by a protosalt of iron; the liquid is then diluted with twice its measure of water, neutralized with carbonate of soda, heated to the boiling point, filtered, and precipitated with sulphate of copper; the precipitate is well washed and dried at a moderate heat.

connection with the essential oils; they even have the power to prevent a certain quantity of this body from acting on the oxygenated oils. The following table will exhibit their qualities:—

	Yield from 16 oz. of raw material.[1] Smallest.		Largest.		Specific gravity between	Solubility in — parts alcohol of .85 sp. gr.	Compound with HCl are:	Action of alcohol and NO_5.	Behavior to iodine.	NO_5 sp. gr. 1.28.	SO_3 sp. gr. 1.727.
	℥	gr.	℥	gr.							
Oleum terebinthinæ					.86 & .90	10 to 12 clear	Solid and liquid	Terpin	Very fulminating	Hard resin	
Oleum camphoræ (from dryobalanops camphora)							Solid	Terpin			
Oleum copaibæ					.87 & .91	20 to 30 turbid	Bihydrochloride is solid	Terpin after some time	Faintly fulminating	Hard resin	
Oleum cubebæ	6	48	20	—	.92 & .93	27 opalescent	Solid $C_{20}H_{32}+2HCl$	Terpin	Yellow and gray vapors	Hard resin	Carmine red.
Oleum elemi (from resina elemi)					.852		Liquid and solid	Terpin			
Oleum juniperi (from juniperus communis)	—	23	3	—	.85 & .91	10 to 12 turbid	Liquid $3C_{20}H_{32}+2HCl$	Terpin after considerable time	Very fulminating	Hard resin	Balsam.
Oleum piperis nigri	1	—	3	12	.86 & .99		Not solid				
Oleum pini semin; S. oleum templinum (from pinus picea)	9	54	11	—	.84 & .856	10 turbid	"	Terpin after several months	Very fulminating	Brittle resin	
Oleum sabinæ (from juniperus sabina)	1	12	6	—	.89 & .94	2, with more opalescent	"		Very fulminating	Thin balsam	
The empyreumatic oils											
Oleum asphalti					.86 & .92	30 clear	"	No terpin	Dissolv. quietly	Thin balsam	Blood red.
Oleum petræ					.75 & .80	18 clear	"		Insoluble	No evolut. of NO_4; unaltered	Not colored.
Oleum succini					.80 & .89		"		Dissolves slowly	Thick balsam	

2. *Oxygenated Oils.*

As oxygenated oils are composed of two or more different liquids, the analysis of them should give the composition of these compounds, though many are little known. The empirical formulæ will never convey a correct idea of the composition of these oils, inasmuch as each individual oil varies much when obtained from fresh or dried plants, from plants grown in a rich or poor soil, and even collected in different seasons; the stearopten, the oxygenated part varies so much in quantity or proportion as to sensibly affect the specific gravity, the boiling point, as well as the freezing and melting point; all these characters, when given of an oil, belong to a particular one, and may be modified in another oil of like purity.

With the action of reagents, for the same reasons, there are certain final results, nearly alike for the same pure oil, differing though it may in the proportion of its components, or in the degree of its oxidation, the intermediate changes by a reagent from the pure rectified oil to the final result, which are sometimes interesting and characteristic, may be lost on account of the resinification.

[1] The yield is here inserted as of interest, though not pertinent to the special object of the table.

	Yield from 16 oz. dry material.				Specific gravity observed.		Solubility of 1 part oil in alcohol of sp. gr. 0.85.	REACTION WITH			
	Smallest.		Largest.		Low-est.	High-est.		Iodine.	NO_4 specific gravity 1.28.	SO_3 specific gravity 1.727	Color of SO_3 after reaction.
	℥	gr.	℥	gr.							
Ol. absinthii	3	30	1	20	.88	.97	āā and more	No vapors	Hard resin	Blue, violet	
" anethi	2		8		.88	.95	In all prop.	Quick sol. few vapors	Brown resin		
" anisi	1	30	3	48	.97	1—	5 parts	Few yellow vapors	Soft resin	Solid	Purple
" " stellati	1	48	4	30	.97	.98	5 parts	Few vapors	Thick balsam.	Solid blood red	Blood red.
" aurantii flor.[1]		14		31	.82	.90	1 to 3, more opalescent		Soft resin	Balsam	
" " fruit[1]	3	6	3	12	.83	.88	7 to 10, slightly turbid	Fulminating (for aurantii flor., fruit, and bergami)	Brittle resin		
" bergami[1]	2	48	3	18	.856	.89	½, more opalescent		Soft resin		
" cajeputi					.91	.97	āā and more	Slow sol.	Thin balsam		
" calami		35	2	25	.89	.99	"	Little heat	Brittle resin	Soft resin	Blood red.
" cardamomi min.	5		6		.93	.94	"	Yellow vapors	Soft resin	Yellowish brown	
" cari	3	30	11	30	.90	.97	"	Few or no vapors	Brittle resin	Balsam	
" caryophylli	10		32		1.03	1.06	"	Slow sol. little heat	Evolves NO_4 brittle resin	Solid; prussian blue	
" cassiæ		16	2	40	1.04	1.09	"	Slow sol. little heat	"	Soft resin olive green	Purple
" chenopodii sem.			1	15		.908					
" cinnamomi ver.	1		3		1.006	1.09	"	Heat, no vapors	Thick balsam	Solid, brown, green, purple	
" cumini	1	24	5		.90	.97	3 parts	Gray vapors	No evolution of NO_4 consist. butter	Carmine	
" fœniculi	2	10	6	48	.89	1—	2 to 4.	Few vapors	Soft resin	Solid carmine	Carmine to blood.
" hyssopi	1	12	2		.89	.98	1 to 4, more opalescent	Few yellow vapors	Soft resin	Balsam	
" lavandulæ flor.	4		6		.87	.95	āā and more	Fulminating	Soft resin	Balsam	
" limonis	2		2	30	.84	.88	10, turbid	Fulminating	Soft resin		
" macidis	2		12		.92	.95	6 parts	Very fulminating	Soft resin	Brownish	Br'n to blood.
" majoranæ	1		3		.89	.90	1, more slightly opalescent	Yellow vapors	Thick balsam	Bluish red	
" matricariæ		3		30	.92	.94	8 to 10 parts	Few yellow vapors	Brittle resin	Soft resin	
" melissæ		3		21	.85	.97	5 to 6	Yellow vapors	Soft resin		
" menthæ crispæ	1	20	3		.87	.97	āā and more	Quick sol. few yellow vapors	Hard resin	Balsam	
" " piperitæ	1		2	40	.84	.97	1, 2, or 3 parts; more opalescent	Solution, no reaction	Thin balsam	Balsam	
" origani vulgaris		9	3		.87	.90	12 to 16, turbid	Fulminating	Hard resin	Dark-blood red	

[1] The yield has reference to the undried or recent plants.

	Yield from 16 oz. dry material. Smallest.	Yield from 16 oz. dry material. Largest.	Specific gravity observed. Lowest.	Specific gravity observed. Highest.	Solubility of 1 part oil in alcohol of sp. gr. 0.85.	REACTION WITH Iodine.	REACTION WITH NO_5 specific gravity 1.28.	REACTION WITH SO_3 specific gravity 1.727.	Color of SO_3 after reaction.
Ol petroselini	ʒ gr. 1[1]	ʒ gr. 4[2]	1.015	1.14	2½ to 3	Fulminating	Evolves NO_4, hard resin	Violet, deep-blood red	
" rosæ German	2.4[5] 1.2[4]	4 6 3.	} .814		100, turbid	No reaction	Little thicker	Very light reddish brown	
" rosmarini	1	3	.88	.93	āā and more	Few yellow vapors	Thin balsam	Light reddish brown	
" rutæ	2[3]	28.7[3]	.84	.91	1, more floc.	Slow sol.	Thin balsam		
" salviæ	30	1 40	.86	.92	āā and more	Few yellow vapors	Thin balsam	Carmine	
" sassafras cort.	3	5 47	1.07	1.09	4 to 5 parts	Quick sol.	Evolves NO_4		Green to red.
" serpylli	.5	30	.89	.95	āā and more	Few yellow vapors	Soft resin	Balsam, brown carmine	
" spicæ	1	2	.88	.98	"	Fulminating	Thin balsam		
" tanaceti	38	52	.91	.95	"	Quiet sol.	Soft resin		
" thymi	30	3	.87	.90	"	Few yellow vapors	Thick balsam	Brown carmine	
" valerianæ	26	2 20	.87	.97	"	Little heat	Hard resin	Red brown, deep violet	

In the above table, where no coloration is given for the action of SO_3 on the oils, it is brown, more or less associated with yellow and red; the few marked brown are but very lightly colored. The coloration of SO_3 by the oils is only mentioned where it is characteristic, all others impart to SO_3 a red color more or less combined with yellow and brown.

The Nitroprusside of Copper Test.—The color imparted to oxygenated oils, so far as examined, is characteristic and striking: For ol. cajeputi viride, olive green; ol. caryoph., pink, violet, cherry red, reddish brown, opaque; ol. cassiæ, hyacinthine, deep brown, red; ol. chenopodii, instantly brown, red; ol. millefolii, pale blue, dark green; ol. monardæ, colorless, green, brown, black. The others are yellow or brown, combined with yellow and red. (See *Proceed. Am. Pharm. Association*, 1858, p. 344.)

The presence of any of the pure carbohydrogens prevents the reaction of a certain portion of the nitroprusside of copper, which must be used as a test in very small quantity. For the preparation of this salt see foot-note on page 345.

3. *Nitrogenated Oils.*

The only few known contain prussic acid, from which they may be freed without materially altering their odor. They are not pre-existent in the plant from which they are derived, but are the results of a reaction in the presence of water, between amygdalin with emulsin or similar compounds.

[1] From the herb. [2] From the seed.
[3] This yield has reference to the undried or recent drugs.
[4] From salted petals. [5] From dried herb.

	Yield from 1lb.	
Oleum amygdal. am.	16 grs. to 1 dr. 20 grs.	Sp. gr. 1.04–1.07. Boiling point, 320° to 390° F.; reacts acid on litmus paper. Iodine is dissolved in small quantity. No reaction. Nitric acid, no reaction in cold; on boiling very little nitrous acid is evolved. Sulphuric acid dissolves an equal quantity of oil, by water separated, little thickened. Alcohol of .85 miscible in all proportion. Nitroprusside copper, no reaction. Product of boiling with caustic potassa in excess dissolves in water.
" cerasi sem.	25 grs.	
" lauro-cerasi fol.	40.5 grs.	

4. *Sulphuretted Oils.*

The sulphuretted oils are compounds of allyle, as the following table will show:—

Allyle	C_6H_5	Sulphuret of allyle (oil of garlic)	$C_6H_5 + S$.
Oxide of allyle,	$C_6H_5 + O$	Sulphocyanuret of allyle (oil of mustard)	$C_6H_5S + C_2NS$.

Of the oils belonging to this group, only oil of mustard has been used medicinally, particularly in alcoholic solution, under the name of spiritus sinapis, as a powerful rubefacient. But the activity of all the plants yielding these oils is due to them, at least principally so. The following have been employed: mustard seed, garlic, horseradish, assafœtida, sagapenum. Some of the plants are valued for culinary purposes, owing to the presence of the compounds of allyle. It is worthy of note that, with the exception of assafœtida, sagapenum, and garlic, all belong to the family of cruciferæ, many of whose plants likewise yield an abundance of fixed oils, for which, in many parts of Europe, they are extensively cultivated (Brassica, &c.).

Camphors.

This class of solid crystalline substances has already been shown to have a close relation to the essential oils. Common camphor, $C_{20}H_{16}O_2$, is obtained from an evergreen-tree growing in China and Japan, the roots and twigs of which are cut into chips and placed with water in large iron vessels, surmounted by earthen capitals furnished with a lining of rice straw. A moderate heat being applied, and the camphor volatilized by the steam, it collects upon the straw in a crude and impure condition, and is collected and packed for exportation as crude camphor. It is refined by resublimation, and then constitutes the valuable and characteristic drug so familiar to almost every one. As already stated, camphor is an oxide of the radical $C_{20}H_{16}$, and one of the so-called camphene series.

Some of the essential oils can be converted into camphors by solution in water and long exposure. The carbohydrogen constituents of these combine with the elements of water to form hydrates, which appear to be true camphors. These are solid, colorless, crystalline, fusible bodies, less volatile than the essential oils, soluble in alcohol and ether, and partially in water.

Some of the substances usually treated of as neutral crystalline principles are classified by the German chemists as camphors; of this number cantharidin, the active principle of Spanish flies, and nicotianin, one of the constituents of tobacco, may be instanced. There is much obscurity now connected with the precise habitudes and relations of these and other crystalline principles associated with oils and otherwise distributed in plants.

Three different kinds of camphor have been distinguished by their behavior in the polariscope, one turning the ray of polarized light to the left, one to the right, and one being inactive. The camphor deviating to the right is stated to be that from laurus camphora.

Camphor deviating to the right.—The vapor conducted over red hot iron gives an oily liquid containing naphthalin and a hydrocarbon of the composition of benzole. Under the influence of heat and nitric acid, 6 eq. of oxygen combine with camphor to form camphoric acid, $C_{20}H_{16}O_8$, which deviates light to the right. Anhydrous phosphoric acid and fused chloride of zinc produce water and cymol $C_{20}H_{14}$.

Camphor deviating to the left.—From the oil of matricaria parthenium, that portion distilling between 200° and 220° C. With nitric acid this furnishes camphoric acid which deviates light to the left.

Inactive Camphor, from the volatile oils of many of the labiatiæ, lavender, marjoram, sage, &c. These are without effect upon polarized light.

The camphors from oil of tansy and valerian, and that from sage by nitric acid, have not been tested by the polariscope.

Borneo camphor, obtained from dryobalanops camphora, is a hydrate of borneen, and has the composition $C_{20}H_{18}O_2$. It is said to be deposited by moist oil of valerian. Its alcoholic solution deviates polarized light toward the right. By the action of nitric acid it loses two of hydrogen, and is converted into common camphor.

Ordinary camphor exists in solution in the crude oils of lavender, rosemary, spearmint, and origanum; it is also produced by the action of nitric acid on oil of sage. Löwig also describes numerous camphors, of which the following are illustrations: Lemon camphor, a compound of oil of lemon and water, has the composition $C_{20}H_{22}O_6$; but, by being heated, loses two atoms of water. Juniper-berry water, treated with caustic potassa, yields a camphor$=C_{20}H_{20}O_4$. The crude oil distilled from parsley seed, dissolved in water, after a few days, deposits a camphor$=C_{12}H_7O_4$.

Resins.

The resins are very extensively diffused in the vegetable kingdom, being generally present in every plant containing an essential oil, as also in many which do not. The definition of a resin is rather vague, but we may, in a general way, describe among this class substances which are solid at ordinary temperatures, inflammable, fuse readily in boiling water, do not volatilize unchanged, become negatively electric by rubbing; are insoluble in water, soluble in alcohol, and partially so in ether and oil of turpentine. They are mostly inodorous, and are readily incorporated with fatty bodies by fusion. They are not, as a class, disposed to crystalline forms, being mostly amorphous; their ultimate composition is carbon, hydrogen, and oxygen.

The origin of resins is mostly in the action of the air on essential oils, which lose part of their hydrogen and absorb oxygen; this may occur, as in the case of turpentine and copaiva, in the plants producing them, or after the extraction of the essential oils. To this fact may be traced their mixed character. The volatile oils being usually mixtures of two or more oils, the resins are apt to be constituted of several similar though not identical resins. By treatment with alcohol, ether, oil of turpentine, &c., the different constituents can generally be separated. Many of the resins—those containing most oxygen—play the part of acids, and are, in fact, designated as such; these form with alkalies compounds, some of which are soluble and others insoluble in alcohol, while some are quite indifferent to the action of alkalies. Some so-called soft resins possess strong odors; these are usually imperfectly oxidized, and contain portions of essential oil.

Resins generally resemble the corresponding essential oils in their stimulating effects, though some of them, which may be termed acrid resins, including the cathartics, appear to bear no relation to the essential oils. A few of the gum resins are adapted, by their control over the nervous system, to use as antispasmodics.

Syllabus of Resins.

I. *Resins Proper.*

Name, Origin, &c.	Composition and Properties.	Uses.
Cistineæ. Ladanum, labdanum. From Cistus Creticus & Cyprious.	Volatile oil. 86 per cent. resin, $C_{40}H_{30}O_4$. 7 per cent. wax.	Obsolete.
Zygophylleæ. Guaiaci resina, *U. S.* From Guaiacum officinale.	80 per cent. resin. Guaiacic acid. Gum extractive.	Alterative stimulant.
Terebinthaceæ. Elemi. From Amyris elemifera and zeylanica.	60 per cent. acid resin sol. in alcohol, indifferent resin crystallizing from sol. in hot alcohol. 10 to 13 per cent. volatile oil.	Stim. in Ointments.
Mastich. From Pistacia lentiscus.	Acid resin sol. in cold alcohol, $C_{40}H_{31}O_4$. Resin soluble in hot alcohol, $C_{40}H_{31}O_2$. Trace of volatile oil.	Adjunct in pills and in varnish.
Leguminosæ. Copaiva resin. From Copaiba, *U.S.*	Soft indifferent resin. Copaivic acid $C_{40}H_{30}O_4$. Crystallizable from solution in petroleum.	
Anime. From Hymenæa courbaril.	Acid resin soluble in cold alcohol. Indifferent resin $C_{40}H_{33}O$, cryst. from hot alcohol sol. 2 per cent. volatile oil.	
Copal. From Hymenæa verrucosa and other trees?	1. Resin, soft, fusible in water-bath, sol. in alcohol, 72 per cent. and oil of turpentine. 2. Resin, soft, fusible below 212° F., sol. in alcohol, ether, & oil of turpentine. 3. Resin, white, not so readily fusible, soluble in alcohol and ether. 4. Resin, white, still less fusible, sol. in alcohol. solution of potassa, insol. in alcohol and ether. 5. Resin, gelatinous, insol. in all menstrua.	Used in varnishes.
Resin of Peruvian balsam. From Balsamum Peruvianum, *U.S.*	Acid $C_{40}H_{28}O_6$, crystallizes in rhombic prisms.	

NAME, ORIGIN, &c.	COMPOSITION AND PROPERTIES.	USES.
Convolvulaceæ. Resinæ jalapa. From Ipomœa jalapa, *U. S.*	Convolvulin, rhodeoretin, $C_{42}H_{36}O_{8}$.	See *Jalapin*, page 189.
Urticeæ. Extractum cannabis. From cannabis Indica.	Neutral resin soluble in alkalies associated with chlorophylle.	Narcotic. See *Extracts*.
Euphorbiaceæ. Lac (shellac and seedlac). From Croton lacciferum by the puncture of Coccus lacca, and from ficus religiosa and indica.—(*Urticeæ.*)	Different resins, wax, gluten, coloring matter.	In varnishes, cements, &c.
Euphorbium. From various species of Euphorbia.	One resin dissolving easily, and another with difficulty in cold alcohol—a third insoluble in cold alcohol, but crystallizes from hot alc. solut. ($C_{40}H_{30}O_{6}$.)	Acrid, cathart., vesicant, &c. Obsolete.
Coniferæ. Dammar. From Dammara Australis.	Dammaryl $C_{45}H_{36}$ (polymeric with oil of turpentine). Dammaric acid, $C_{40}H_{30}O_{8}$.	
Sandarac. From Juniperus communis in warmer climates, and from Thuja articulata.	$C_{40}H_{31}O_{6}$, easily soluble in alcohol. $C_{40}H_{31}O_{5}$, not easily soluble in alcohol. $C_{40}H_{30}O_{6}$, soluble in boiling alcohol.	In varnishes.
Resina, *U.S.*[1] From Terebinthina, *U.S.*	Colopholic acid, taken up by cold alcohol 70 per cent. Pinic, amorphous silvic acid, taken up by cold alcohol 70 per cent. Silvic acid, $C_{40}H_{30}O_{4}$, crystallizes from hot alcohol.	
Fossil Resins. Succinum, *U.S.* Amber.	2 Resins, volatile oil, succinic acid, and bitumen, by action of NO_{5} artificial musk.	
Asphaltum.	Most probably the product of oxidation of oleum petræ. Many bituminous resins are mixtures of asphaltum and petroleum.	

II. *Natural Oleo-Resins.*

NAME, ORIGIN, &c.	COMPOSITION AND PROPERTIES.	USES.
Leguminosæ. Copaiba, *U. S.* Sp. gr. .916 to 1. From various species of Copaifera.	31 to 80 per cent. volatile oil. 1.6 per cent. soft brown resin. Copaivic acid, see *Resins Proper*.	Diuretic, Stimulant
Coniferæ. Terebinthina, *U. S.* From Pinus palustris, and other species of Pinus.	About 17 per cent. volatile oil. Resina, *U.S.*	Stim. emmenagogue.
Terebinthina Veneta. From Larix Europæa, Venice turpentine.	About 20 per cent. volatile oil. Resin.	In stimulating external remedies.
Terebinthina Canadensis. From Abies balsamea, balsam of fir.	40 per cent. resin sol. in alcohol. 33.4 sub resin sol. in alcohol with difficulty. 18.6 per cent. volatile oil.	do.

III. *Gum Resins.*

NAME, ORIGIN, &c.	COMPOSITION AND PROPERTIES.	USES.
Guttiferæ. Gambogia, *U. S.* From Stalagmitis cambogioides and several species of Garcinia.	19.5 per cent. gum. 80 per cent. gambogic acid.	Powerful cathartic.

[1] Resin from pinus maritima contains pimaric acid $C_{40}H_{30}O_{4}$, which, by being heated for some time, is converted into silvic acid.

NAME, ORIGIN, &c.	COMPOSITION AND PROPERTIES.	USES.
Terebinthaceæ. Myrrha, *U.S.* From Balsamodendron myrrha.	40.81 per cent., 40 per cent. Arabin. 44.76 per cent. resin. 2.18 per cent. volatile oil.	Astringent and emmenagogue.
Bdellium. From Balsamodendron Africanum.	59 resin, 9.2 gum, 30.6 bassorin and volatile oil.	Obsolete.
Olibanum. From Boswellia serrata and an Amyris (?)	4 per ct. (Stenhouse) volatile oil, gum, at least 2 resins, one of which = $C_{40}H_{30}O_6$.	For fumigation.
Umbelliferæ. Galbanum, *U.S.* From Bubon galbanum, Ferula ferulago, and Galbanum.	66.86 per cent. resin. 19.28 per cent. gum. 6.34 per cent. volatile oil.	Stim., antispasmodic.
Assafœtida, *U. S.* From Ferula assafœtida.	26 per cent. gum, 4.6 per cent. sulphuretted volatile oil, 47.2 per cent. resin, malates, acetates, sulphates, and phosphates.	Antispasmodic.
Sagapenum. From Ferula Persica.	54 per cent. resin, 32 per cent. gum, Sulphuretted volatile oil.	Stim. like assafœt.
Ammoniacum, *U. S.* From Heracleum gummiferum.	22 per cent. gum. 72 per cent. resin.	Stim. expectorant.
Opopanax. From Pastinaca opopanax.	42 per cent. resin. 33 per cent. gum. Sulphuretted vol. oil.	Antispasmodic. Obsolete.
Asclepiadeæ. Scammonium Smyrna. From Periploca secamone?	An adulterated resin of Convolvulus scammonia?	Cathartic?
Convolvulaceæ. Scammonium, Aleppo. From Convolvulus scammonia.	Convolvulin, resin, wax, extractive, gum, sugar, starch. Commercial article from 5 to 80 per cent. resin.	Cathartic.

IV. *Balsams.*

NAME, ORIGIN, &c.	COMPOSITION AND PROPERTIES.	USES.
Styraceæ. Benzoinum, *U.S.* Sp. gr. 1.063. From Styrax benzoin.	Benzoic acid, average 15 per cent. *a.* Resin, $C_{70}H_{42}O_{14}$, soluble in ether, not in KO,CO_2. *b.* Resin, $C_{30}H_{20}O_5$, soluble in KO,CO_2, not in ether. *c.* Resin, $C_{40}H_{22}O_9$, soluble in alcohol, not in ether.	
Leguminosæ. Balsamum Peruvianum, *U.S.* Sp. gr. 1.14 to 1.16.	Cinnamic acid, 6.94 per cent. Oil or cinnameine, 69 per cent. 23.1 per cent. resin, $C_{40}H_{28}O_8$.	Stimulating expectorant.
Balsamum tolutatum, *U. S.*	Resin, 88 per cent. Cinnamic acid, 12 per cent. Volatile oil, 0.2 per cent.	do.
Balsamineæ. Styrax, *U.S.* Semifluid juice of liquidambar orientale[1]	Benzoic acid. Styracine. Cinnameine. (?) 2 resins.	do.
Gum wax, semifluid juice of Liquidambar styraciflua.	Cinnamic acid. (?) Styracine. (?) Resin. (?)	Little used as yet. See *Syrups*.

REMARKS ON THE RESINS, OLEO RESINS AND BALSAMS.

As shown in the syllabus, most of the resins proper are used exclusively in varnishes, and in the various modifications of stimulating and rubefacient applications.

Amber is employed exclusively for the products of its decomposition. Oil of amber produced from it by distillation is a powerful

[1] According to Hanbury, *London Pharm. Journ.*, 1857.

rubefacient, with antispasmodic effects, which adapt it to the treatment of hysteria and other nervous affections; artificial musk is obtained by treating f℥j of oil of amber with f℥iiiss of strong nitric acid, a peculiar resinoid substance is the result, which after washing may be dissolved in alcohol, and the tincture made in the proportion of ℥j to f℥x of alcohol, is given in teaspoonful doses; it is esteemed a good substitute for musk.

Guaiacum, formerly considered a gum resin, is now classed among resins proper, though the presence of a peculiar acid somewhat resembling benzoic and cinnamic, may entitle it to a place among balsams, should that group be extended to embrace a wider range of resinous substances.

Burgundy pitch and the so called hemlock gum (pix Canadensis) are well known ingredients of strengthening and rubefacient plasters, which will be considered under the appropriate head. Elemi is a popular substitute for common resins in an unofficinal ointment much prescribed by surgeons.

Of the *oleo* resins, the three turpentines differ in their proportion of resin to oil and their consequent consistence. White turpentine of commerce though exuding from the tree in a liquid form, is always found nearly or quite solid, while balsam of fir, and Venice turpentine continue more or less fluid at ordinary temperature. The former of these is much used for mounting objects for the microscope, and for cementing ambrotypes upon glass, its perfect transparency and great adhesiveness adapting it to these uses. The latter is perhaps rarely met with in our commerce, being substituted by a factitious article, said to be composed of about 24 lbs. of resin to the gallon of oil of turpentine. It is esteemed as a useful ingredient in the finest qualities of sealing-wax.

Copaiva, which is very commonly called balsam copaiva, is highly esteemed for its stimulating effects on the mucous surfaces; it is variously combined with mucilage or with alkali in prescriptions mentioned under the appropriate head, and is prescribed in the *Pharmacopœia* in the form of pill mass to be made with magnesia. (See *Pilulæ*.)

The chemical distinction between gum resins and balsams is observed in the foregoing syllabus, though in commerce it has no significance. Strictly speaking, the balsams are those resinous bodies which are known to contain either benzoic or cinnamic acid.

Most of these drugs are possessed of decided medicinal effects; ammoniac, benzoin and tolu, are chiefly used as stimulating expectorants. Assafœtida, galbanum and sagapenum (the latter almost obsolete), are distinguished by powerful effects on the nervous system. Myrrh is peculiarly adapted to the relaxed conditions of the system, consequent on pulmonary and uterine affections; it is well suited to combinations with iron, and is directed in several emmenagogue pills, and in the officinal mistura ferri composita.

Among the gum resins we have two drastic cathartics, gamboge and scammony; and among the resins proper, jalapin and euphorbium; to these might be added several cathartic resins, prepared by similar processes to that for jalapin from podophyllum and other resinous roots, but which have been omitted from this syllabus, as it was designed chiefly to display at one view the characteristic vegetable products produced by exudation from the several trees. Olibanum is almost exclusively used for fumigation, being employed alone and combined with cascarilla, and benzoin, as incense, in the ceremonies of the Roman Catholic churches.

The balsams vary in their consistence. Benzoin is solid, hard and brittle; Peruvian balsam (formerly called myroxylon) is fluid; Tolu is intermediate, being a very soft and readily fusible solid. The best storax is liquid, but an article is also met with in a granular condition, which is very impure. This balsam is little used, though directed in some of the old recipes. Our native "gum wax," as it has been called, has a very strong resemblance to storax, its consistence being semi-fluid and its color and odor almost identical.

Several products of scientific interest have been discovered by the decomposition of the balsams. *Styracin*, the resin of styrax, is obtained by treating the balsam with caustic soda in solution, dissolving the residue in alcohol and ether, and crystallizing; when acted on with nitric acid this yields the same products of decomposition with cinnamic acid. By distillation of the soda solution left in its preparation, *styrole* is obtained, while cinnamic acid is left in the residue. Styrol has the composition $C_{16}H_8$, and styracin is a compound of cinnamic acid with a peculiar alcohol, bearing the same relation to hydrated cinnamic alcohol as common alcohol does to acetic acid. Several similar compounds have been discovered, and it is probable that chemists will hereafter find all the acids of the benzoic and cinnamic series, to form such oxides or ethers, and hydrated oxides or alcohols. (See *Gregory's Chemistry.*)

Tests for Purity.

Guaiacum.—Entirely soluble in 85 per cent. alcohol and less so in ether, gives a blue color to mucilage of gum Arabic and milk.

Mastich.—Softens by chewing, not entirely soluble in alcohol, wholly taken up by ether, chloroform and oil of turpentine, not by fixed oils.

Copal.—Readily fusible, soluble in rectified oil of turpentine. See syllabus for behavior to alcohol and ether.

Jalap Resin and Scammonium.—By the action of alkalies under the influence of heat, it is converted into convolvulic (rhodeoretinic) acid, which is soluble in water. The solution of the resins in alkalies may be rendered slightly opalescent by sulphuric acid, but is not precipitated.

Copaiva.—If adulterated with fixed oil, this may be detected by the stain produced on paper; pure copaiba, after the evaporation of the volatile oil by the application of a little heat, leaves a *resinous* stain, which has a *greasy* margin if balsam was adulterated with fixed oil.

Or, the balsam is boiled for several hours in an open vessel with water to drive off the volatile oil; pure balsam leaves a brittle resin, which is soft from an adulteration of fixed oil.

Fixed oils, except castor oil, may be detected by their insolubility in 90 per cent. alcohol, pure balsam furnishes a clear solution.

An adulteration with turpentine (oleo-resin) is easily detected by the odor produced by the evaporation of the oils, on dropping the suspected balsam upon a hot brick.

Balsamum Peruvianum.—The surest way to find an adulteration with castor oil, is to distil about 20 grammes until about 10 grammes have passed over,

and the residue begins to become charred. The distillate which separates into an aqueous and oily stratum, is agitated with caustic baryta, the oil removed, and agitated with a concentrated solution of bisulphide of soda. Genuine balsam Peru on dry distillation furnishes products, which with bisulphite of soda do not form a crystalline combination. The crystals obtained by this process from its admixture with castor oil, on being recrystallized from alcohol, have the odor of œnanthol, and the composition $C_{14}H_{13}O,SO_2+NaO,SO_2$.

CHAPTER VII.

ON ORGANIC ACIDS.

ORGANIC ACIDS are distinguished as a class by characteristic properties. They combine with inorganic and organic alkalies, some of them in several different proportions, according to the number of equivalents of basic water combined with them. Thus, citric is a tribasic acid, containing three equivalents of water; tartaric bibasic, containing only two; and benzoic containing but one equivalent of water, besides the water of crystallization, is monobasic. These acids are found in nature both free and combined with organic and inorganic bases. Some are very commonly diffused throughout the vegetable kingdom, as tannic; others exist exclusively in one family of plants, as meconic acid in the papaveraceæ. Some, although existing naturally, are capable of artificial production from other organic material, as oxalic and valerianic. This whole class, and that of organic alkalies, have a much closer relation to inorganic compounds, than the neutral crystalline and uncrystallizable principles. They all contain oxygen, and are destitute of nitrogen in their composition; an exception, however, is hydrocyanic acid, which in all its chemical relations bears a close resemblance to the inorganic hydre-acids.

The organic acids are capable of numerous changes during the process of life of the organisms by which they are produced, or after their introduction into the circulation of living animal or vegetable beings. These changes are the result of obscure processes of nature, and of conditions and functions of the organs, which we are unable to imitate by art. Chemistry, however, has in some instances arrived by artificial means, at close imitations of nature, and has produced changes which furnish connecting links between compounds, having, apparently no relation to each other.

Of the organic acids, those occurring in plants are by far the most important as medicines, and of the very few animal acids employed most, though formerly regarded as exclusively belonging to the animal kingdom, have subsequently been discovered to be direct products of decomposition of vegetable principles, and are even generated by certain plants in their normal processes of growth and assimilation.

In the present chapter the numerous acids are thrown together in groups, either from their diffusion in certain classes of vegetables, from the harmony of some of their physical or chemical relations, from their associations with other organic principles, or from the value attached to them as medicinal agents.

First Group.—Fruit Acids.

These acids occur in the fruits of many plants of the families aurantiaceæ, rosaceæ, grossularieæ, in grapes, tamarinds, in short, in all succulent acidulous fruits, and at certain periods of their maturity, in a free state, with the exception of oxalic acid, which is comparatively seldom met with in an uncombined state, though widely diffused, wholly or partly neutralized by certain vegetable alkaloids, or inorganic bases. They are all agreeable refrigerants, and, as such, have a very extensive use; combined with alkalies or magnesia, they act in large doses as laxatives; oxalic acid and its compounds are poisonous, unless in minute doses.

Acetic acid, $HO,C_4H_3O_3$. Occasionally in plants, product of fermentation.
Oxalic " $2HO,C_4O_6+4$ aq. In rhubarb, sorrel, many officinal roots, herbs and barks.
Tartaric " $2HO,C_8H_4O_{10}$. In grapes, tamarinds, &c., obtained from wine deposits.
Uvic " $2HO,C_8H_4O_{10}+2$ aq. In the deposit of some grape juices.
Malic " $2HO,C_8H_4O_8$. In apples, sumach berries, the berries of mountain-ash, &c.
Citric " $3HO,C_{12}H_5O_{11}+2$ aq. In lemons, oranges, currants, gooseberries, tomatoes.

Acetic acid has been already referred to as produced in the destructive distillation of wood, and also as a product of the spontaneous change which takes place in articles of the saccharine and amylaceous group by the catalytic action of ferments. (See p. 284.)

Oxalic acid is an instance of an important vegetable acid existing ready formed in plants, and also capable of artificial production. Most of the oxalic acid of commerce is obtained by the action of nitric acid on sugar or starch, the organic principle being oxidized at the expense of the acid. Nitrous acid fumes and carbonic acid gas are evolved, and oxalic acid is formed, which is collected and crystallized, and most extensively used as a bleaching agent. If nitric acid has been employed in sufficient quantity, no saccharic acid is formed; the nitrous acid evolved is employed in the manufacture of sulphuric acid or for other purposes where oxidation is required. It is not officinal.

The alkaline oxalates are soluble, but the other salts are mostly insoluble in water. Oxalic acid and its salts are decomposed by a red heat, into carbonic acid and carbonic oxide, without leaving any charcoal. If heated with sulphuric acid the same decomposition takes place. Carbonic oxide CO is inflammable. If mixed with sand and heated, dry oxalic acid yields formic acid, and but little carbonic acid is given off if the temperature is well regulated. The precipitate formed by chloride of barium and lime-water is soluble in nitric and muriatic acids. The silver precipitate dissolves in nitric acid and ammonia. Insoluble oxalates, boiled in concentrated solution of carbonate of soda, are decomposed, oxalate of soda being held in solution.

Acidum Tartaricum, U. S.

This valuable acid is prepared from bitartrate of potassa or cream of tartar, by the addition of carbonate of lime, whereby insoluble tartrate of lime is formed with the excess of acid of the bitartrate and neutral tartrate of potassa left in solution. This is decomposed with chloride of calcium, which forms an additional quantity of tartrate of lime. Lastly, the insoluble tartrate of lime is purified by washing, and decomposed by sulphuric acid, which liberates the tartaric acid. This, on evaporation, crystallizes in colorless crystals, with a tendency to the form of oblique rhombic prisms (citric acid is more in right rhombic prisms). It has a sour taste, resembling, though not identical with, that of citric acid. It is soluble in an equal weight of water, from which solution alcohol throws down no precipitate. This is rather a stronger acid than citric, 100 grains saturating 133.5 grains of bicarbonate of potassa. It is most usually sold in powder. Its principal use is in preparing effervescing and refrigerant drinks, and as a substitute for citric acid.

The salts used medicinally are the tartrates of potassa, soda, ammonia and iron, the bitartrates of potassa, soda and ammonia, and the double salts of potassa and soda, potassa and ammonia, potassa and boracic acid, potassa and borate of soda, potassa and iron, ammonia and iron.

Tartaric acid may be recognized by the copious white crystalline precipitate it furnishes on adding it in excess to any neutral salt of potassa. The precipitate formed by both this and citric acid with acetate of lead should be soluble in nitric acid.

Neutral tartrates are precipitated on the addition of acetate of potassa and free acetic acid; the precipitate by chloride of calcium is soluble in cold caustic potassa, separates on boiling, and redissolves on cooling; the precipitate by lime-water dissolves in free tartaric acid, and in chloride of ammonium, and tartrate of lime crystallizes out after some time.

If not carefully prepared, the following impurities may be present: heavy metals, detected by sulphuretted hydrogen, sulphuric acid by chloride of barium, muriatic acid by nitrate of silver, oxalic acid by a solution of sulphate of lime.

Solution of tartaric acid and its salts are decomposed by oxygen like citric acid; by oxide of manganese it is converted into formic and carbonic acids.

The following well-marked varieties of tartaric acid have been distinguished:—

1. *Dextrotartaric acid*, the ordinary tartaric acid, which in the free state and combined with certain inactive bases turns polarized light to the right. If its salt with cinchonia is heated to 338° F., in five or six hours it has been changed for the greatest part into

2. *Paratartaric, uvic or racemic acid*, which occurs naturally in cream of tartar from certain localities. It and its salts have a neutral behavior towards polarized light. Its double salt with ammonia and soda is obtained in crystals, one-half of which show a hemiedric form to the right, the other half the same form to the left; the former contain dextrotartaric, the latter the lævotartaric acid. From a solution of paratartrate of cinchonicine crystals of the lævotartrate, and from a solution of paratartrate of quinicine, the dextrotartrate is deposited first, leaving the greatest part of the salts with the opposite acid in solution.

3. *Lævotartaric acid* may be obtained, like the preceding, from its lime salt; it deflects polarized light to the left.

4. *Inactive tartaric acid* is obtained with the paratartaric acid as above, or by heating paratartrate of cinchonicine to 338° F. It has no action on polarized light, and cannot be resolved into the right and left tartrate.

5. *Metatartaric acid.* By melting dry powdered dextrotartaric acid in an oil bath; the change takes place in a few seconds at 340° to 356° F. The acid is hygroscopic; its lime salt is soluble.

6. *Isotartaric or tartralic acid.* If the heat in the last process has been applied too long, the product contains this acid also. The lime salt is syrupy, uncrystallizable, and by boiling is resolved into metatartaric acid and metatartrate of lime.

All of these acids are of the same composition, $C_8H_6O_{12}$, and, excepting the last, are bibasic.

Pyrotartaric Acid, $2HO,C_{10}H_8O_6$.—Tartaric acid yields by dry distillation at between 350° F. and 370° F. water, carbonic and pyrotartaric acids, scarcely any secondary products. This acid is very soluble, fusible, and not precipitated by neutral lead salts.

Malic Acid.

Malic acid is difficult to purify if prepared from the juice of tart apples; the juice of the fruit of Sorbus aucuparia, Rhus glabrum, and typhinum contains a considerable quantity, which may be obtained by precipitating with sugar of lead, recrystallizing, and decomposing by hydrosulphuric acid. The juice of the rhubarb plant, after being clarified by isinglass, and evaporated to the consistence of syrup, yields about 3½ per cent. of crystallized bimalate of potassa. The acid crystallizes in four and six sided needles and prisms, is deliquescent, and dissolves in water and alcohol.

The acid and its salts are not precipitated by lime-water; chloride of calcium occasions a precipitate soluble in acids; the precipitate by acetate of lead melts in boiling water, assuming the appearance of resin fused in water.

Though malic acid is present in many pharmaceutical preparations, none of its salts have been used in medicine with the exception of an impure malate of iron, which, in Europe, is still largely employed as a mild chalybeate, under the name of Extractum ferri pomatum; malate of manganese has likewise been somewhat used.

Malic acid has acquired some importance as a material for the preparation of succinic acid.

Menispermic or coccalinic, solanic, and probably also *nicotic, igasuric* (in nux vomica and Ignatia beans), *fungic* (in boletus, helvella, &c.), and others are identical with malic acid.

The decomposition of malic acid by various influences is as follows:—

1. If heated with an excess of potassa to 300° F., it is converted into oxalic and acetic acids.

2. By quick dry distillation it is converted into equisetic or pyromalic acid, $C_8H_6O_{10} = C_8H_4O_8 + 2HO$.

3. If heated in an oil bath to 300° F., until vapors cease to be emitted, it has been converted into *fumaric* or *paramalic acid.*

4. Neutral malate of lime, $C_8H_4Ca_2O_{10}$, if kept under water, particularly by the action, as ferment, of beer yeast or old cheese, is converted into succinic, acetic, and carbonic acids, $3C_8H_6O_{10} = 2C_8H_6O_8 + C_4H_4O_4 + 4CO_2 + 2HO$.

5. If by this fermentation hydrogen is evolved with the carbonic acid gas, another change takes place, butyric acid being formed, $2C_8H_6O_{10} = C_8H_8O_4 + 8CO_2 + 4HO$.

6. By long contact, no butyric, acetic, or succinic acid is obtained, but another product of decomposition; lactic and carbonic acids—$2C_8H_6O_{10} = C_{12}H_{12}O_{12} + 4CO_2$.

Acidum Citricum, U. S.

This is procured from lime or lemon-juice by neutralizing the acid with chalk, and from the citrate of lime thus formed liberating the citric acid by means of sulphuric acid.

It is in large transparent crystals without color, with a strong, but agreeable acid taste, decomposed by heat, very soluble in water and in weak alcohol, deliquescing in moist weather. Specific gravity 1.6. As usually obtained in crystals, it consists of one equivalent of the tribasic acid + one (sometimes two) equivalent of water of crystallization. It is not sold in the form of powder. According to the *U. S. Pharmacopœia*, 100 grains of crystallized citric acid will saturate 150 grains of bicarb-potassa, which is on the supposition of one equivalent of water of crystallization being present. Its principal consumption is in the preparation of so-called lemon syrup, and solution of citrate of magnesia. This latter preparation has increased the quantity of the acid used immensely, so that the price had, at one time, advanced to more than double its former average. The subsequent reduction to near its former rate has probably arisen from an increased supply. To make artificial lemon-juice, add citric acid ℥ixss to water Oj; fresh oil of lemon ♏j; and sugar ʒj. This solution is much employed in making effervescing draughts. (See *Potassæ citras.*)

There are not many salts of citric acid used in medicine, but most of them very extensively; they are the citrates of potassa, magnesia, iron, quinia and morphia, and the double salts of ammonia and iron, of potassa and iron, and strychnia and iron.

Citric acid and its salts are precipitated on being boiled with a large excess of lime-water; the greater part of the precipitate redissolves on cooling; neutral citrates are precipitated by chloride of calcium.

Citric acid is scarcely ever adulterated or impure; if tartaric acid should be present, it may be detected by a concentrated solution of citrate of potassa; oxalic acid by a solution of sulphate of lime, and sulphuric by a diluted solution of chloride of barium; in both the last cases the appearance of a precipitate is promoted by nearly neutralizing the acid with an alkali.

The solution of citric acid and of its salts is decomposed by the influence of oxygen, with the formation of mould, and a slimy precipitate of apparently organic structure. On fusing the acid with hydrate of potassa, it is converted into oxalic and acetic acids, $C_{12}H_8O_{14}+2HO=C_4H_2O_8+2C_4H_4O_4$.

SECOND GROUP.—*Derivatives of the Fruit Acids.*

The acids placed in this group may be artificially obtained from the fruit acids; they are also found in a number of vegetables and vegetable products, and two of them are productions of animal organisms. Of their number, three have been more or less used in medicine, the others, as yet, are not employed either in medicine or in the arts.

Formic acid,	HO,C_2HO_3.	In ants, nettles, ergot, the leaves of some pines, old turpentine, &c.
Succinic "	$2HO,C_8H_4O_6$.	In amber, wormwood, melampyrum nemorosum, &c.
Aconitic "	$2HO,C_8H_2O_6$.	In various species of aconitum, delphinium, yarrow, &c.
Fumaric "	$2HO,C_8H_2O_6$.	In fumaria (fumitory), Iceland moss, &c.
Equisetic "	$2HO,C_8H_2O_6$.	In equisetum fluviatile, and limosum.
Lactic "	$2HO,C_{12}H_{10}O_{10}$.	In dulcamara, bellis perennis, primula veris, from milk, &c.

Formic Acid.

Chloroform and iodoform are compounds of the same radical formyle, C_2H, of which formic acid is the hydrated oxide; it is prepared artificially from tartaric acid, starch, lignin, fibrin, grape sugar, sugar of milk, &c., by distilling them with the black oxide of manganese and sulphuric acid.

The following proportions are recommended: 1 part of sugar, 2 water, 3 manganese, and 3 sulphuric acid diluted with 3 water; or, 1 starch, 4 water, 4 manganese, and 4 sulphuric acid. The acid is to be gradually added in a large retort, capable of holding fifteen times the quantity of the whole mixture; after the violent reaction has subsided, heat is applied, and distilled to near dryness; the distillate is saturated with carbonate of lead, the solution evaporated to crystallize, so as to leave acetate of lead in the mother liquor; the crystals are distilled with sulphuric acid and water, equal parts.

It is a colorless, volatile liquid, of a peculiar penetrating odor, and producing inflammation if applied to the skin. All its salts are soluble in water; from the salts of silver, mercury, gold, &c., formic acid reduces the metals. The formates are decomposed into carbonic oxide and water by concentrated sulphuric acid.

A solution of formic acid in alcohol is still occasionally employed abroad as a rubefacient under the name of spiritus formicarum, prepared by distilling 4 pounds of alcohol from 2 pounds of ants.

Succinic Acid.

Spermaceti, tallow, or margaric acid, if for several days digested, without boiling, with nitric acid of medium strength, yields, on evaporation, succinic acid. It is also prepared by fermentation of impure malate of lime as follows: Rub old cheese, 1 part, into an emulsion, and digest with the lime salt, 12 parts, and 40 parts of water, at a temperature below 112° F., for four to six days, until gas ceases to be emitted; the precipitate is now washed, dilute sulphuric acid added to neutralize the carbonate of lime, the same quantity of acid added and boiled until the precipitate has lost its sandy nature; the liquid is filtered off and evaporated until a pellicle is formed, when the lime is precipitated with sulphuric acid, and the filtrate further evaporated; the crystals may be recrystallized and purified with animal charcoal. It may also be obtained from amber by distillation.

The crystals are colorless, without odor; they have an empyreumatic smell if prepared from amber. They dissolve in 5 parts of water, and are not dissolved by cold nitric or chromic acid, or chlorine; heated upon platina foil, they leave but little charcoal; and if adulterated with benzoic acid, their hot aqueous solution will separate crystals on cooling.

A solution of succinate of ammonia is the only preparation medicinally employed, and it is questionable whether its invigorating action in low states of the nervous system is not mostly due to the oils with which it is associated. The Prussian *Pharmacopœia* gives the following directions for preparing it.

Liquor Ammonii Succinatis.—Rub to 1 ounce succinic acid, 1 scruple rectified oil of amber, dissolve in 8 ounces distilled water, and add 1 ounce (containing 15 grains of Dippel's animal oil), or a sufficient quantity, of pyro-oleous carbonate of ammonia.

Aconite Acid.

It is obtained by heating citric acid for several hours with muriatic acid, evaporating and extracting by ether. It is in colorless, granular crystals; its lime salt is at first soluble in water, but once crystallized it dissolves with great difficulty.

By distillation, the following three new acids may be obtained, all of which have the composition $2HO,C_{10}H_4O_6$: itaconic, citraconic, and mesaconic or citracantic acids.

Fumaric or Paramaleic Acid.—By precipitating the clarified juice of fumaria officinalis with acetate of lead, decomposing the washed precipitate by sulphuretted hydrogen, and recrystallizing the acid from hot water. Crystalline scales, soluble in 200 parts cold water; soluble in alcohol and ether; not precipitated by the salts of lime, baryta, and strontia; silver salts are entirely precipitated by this as by muriatic acid. The fumerate of lead is taken up by boiling water, but without previously melting (difference from malic acid).

Equisetic or Maleic Acid.—By distillation of malic acid, or by heating fumaric to 400° F.

Oblique rhombic prisms; taste acid, acrid; easily soluble in water and alcohol, and in ether; melts at 320°, distils at 350°. If heated for some time to 265° F., is again converted into fumaric acid. Its salts resemble those of fumaric acid; silver salts are not precipitated by it; its lead salt is not soluble in water.

By fermentation, fumaric and maleic acids are converted into succinic acid.

Lactic Acid.

Lactic acid is contained in many old officinal extracts as a product of fermentation of their saccharine constituents, or of malic acid. For medicinal use it is prepared by the so-called lactic fermentation. The following process of Wackenroder is one of the most simple: 25 parts sugar of milk, 20 parts finely powdered chalk, 100 parts skimmed milk, and 200 parts water are digested at about 75°; in six weeks the chalk will be dissolved, the whole is then heated, but not to boiling; the cheese is strained off, pressed, the decanted liquid is clarified by albumen and evaporated to let the lactate of lime crystallize; the recrystallized salt is decomposed either by sulphuric or by the exact quantity of oxalic acid.

It is a colorless, uncrystallizable syrup of strong acid taste; the concentrated has a specific gravity of 1.215; by oxidizing agents it is converted into oxalic acid.

Its salts are insoluble in ether, most of them slightly soluble in cold water and alcohol. The iron salt has been of late much used in medicine as a mild chalybeate.

The diluted acid must not be precipitated by chloride of barium—absence of sulphuric acid, by sulphate of lime—absence of oxalic acid, by sulphuretted hydrogen—absence of metallic oxides, or after neutralization with ammonia, by oxalate of ammonia—absence of lime.

THIRD GROUP.—*Acids representing wholly or in part the Medicinal Virtues of Plants.*

The acids arranged in this group have very few chemical properties in common; they are interesting because they are wholly or in part the active principles of the plants in which they have been generated. If those grouped in division *a*, be excepted, the acid properties of most of these acids are not very decided; some of them are unable to decompose the carbonates, and quite a number have been long taken for neutral principles. Of the whole number, phloridzic and santonic acids only have been employed in medicine in their isolated condition; chrysophanic acid is attracting considerable attention as the active principle of our most popular cathartics.

(a) *Connected with Volatile Oils and Resins.*

Angelicic acid, $HO,C_{10}H_7O_3$. In the root of angelica, masterwort, &c.
Guaiacic " $C_{12}H_8O_6$. In the resin and wood of guaiacum.
(See also Group V., Division *a*.)

Angelicic acid may be obtained by the action of potassa on oil of chamomile, imperatorin and peucedanin; it is more advantageously prepared by exhausting 12 parts of angelica root with 1 part hydrate of lime and sufficient water, evaporating, distilling with the addition of sulphuric acid, and redistilling the distillate after saturation with potassa and decomposing with sulphuric acid; large crystals appear after some time, valerianic and acetic acids remain in solution. Long colorless prisms, without water of crystallization, odor aromatic, boiling point 374°. They are little soluble in cold water, easily in boiling water, alcohol, ether, oil of turpentine and fixed oils. Its salts are crystallizable, and its compound with ether has the odor of rotten apples. It is decomposed by excess of caustic potassa into acetic and propionic acids.

Guaiacic Acid.—To obtain it the resin or wood is exhausted with warm alcohol, and after distilling off the greater part and separating the resin, is neutralized with carbonate of baryta, evaporated to a syrupy consistence, decomposed by sulphuric acid and purified by dissolving in ether.

The resin of guaiacum yields by dry distillation guaiacene, a light volatile oil which is the oxide of a camphene, and has the composition of guaiacic acid minus $2CO_2 = C_{10}H_8O_2$.

(b) *Mostly Bitter Acids, some Poisonous.*

Hederic acid, $C_{15}H_{12}O_4$. In the seed of common ivy.
Picrotoxic " $C_{20}H_{12}O_8$. In cocculus indicus.
Phloridzic " $C_{24}H_{16}O_{14}+12$ aq. In the bark of many fruit trees, especially the apple tree.
Chrysophanic acid, $C_{20}H_{10}O_8$. In rhubarb root, senna, doçk root, parmelia parietina, &c.
Santonic " $C_{30}H_{18}O_6$. In levant, wormseed, from artemisia santonica, &c.
Cahincic " $2HO,C_{32}H_{24}O_{13}+3$ aq. In cahinca root.
Polygalic " $C_{36}H_{24}O_{20}$. In the root of polygala amara and senega.
Cetraric " $2HO,C_{36}H_{14}O_{14}$? In Iceland moss.
Anacardic " $C_{44}H_{32}O_7$. In cashew nuts.
Digitalic and digitoleic. In the herb of digitalis.

Hederic Acid.—The seeds are freed of fat by ether, afterwards exhausted by boiling alcohol; on cooling, the acid separates in colorless needles or tablets. It is insoluble in water and ether; without odor, of acrid taste; colored purple by concentrated sulphuric acid. The salts are mostly gelatinous. It is sometimes difficult to free the acid of a tannin adhering to it.

Picrotoxic Acid, Picrotoxin.—After the fixed oil of cocculus indicus is expressed, the acid crystallizes from the decoction of the residue with diluted muriatic acid, in colorless prisms, of an extremely bitter taste; they are very poisonous. (See *Detection of Poisonous Alkaloids.*)

Phloridzic Acid, Phloridzin.

It crystallizes from the tincture of apple-tree bark, prepared with warm diluted alcohol. The crystals are yellowish needles of a silky lustre, easily soluble in alcohol, ether and boiling water; it is destitute of odor, and has a bitter, somewhat astringent taste; it fuses at 220°, is solid again at 266°, and liquid at 320°.

It yields formic acid on being treated with sulphuric acid and oxide of manganese; phloridzein$=NC_{21}H_9O$, by ammonia; by diluted acids phloretin and sugar, $C_{24}H_{16}O_{14}+2HO=C_{12}H_6O_4+C_{12}H_{12}O_{12}$.

It has been used with asserted success as a substitute for quinia in the treatment of intermittent fevers.

Chrysophanic Acid.—Synonyms of this acid in various states of purity, are parietinic acid, rhein, rhabarbarin, rheumin, rhabarbaric acid, rhaponticin, rumicin, lapathin. It is prepared by extracting parmelia parietina or rhubarb with weak alkaline alcohol, precipitating by carbonic acid, dissolving in 50 per cent. alcohol containing a little caustic potassa, precipitating by acetic acid, dissolving in boiling alcohol, mixing the filtrate with water and recrystallizing from alcohol. It crystallizes in golden yellow needles of metallic lustre, inodorous, nearly tasteless, nearly insoluble in cold water, soluble in alcohol and ether, and in sulphuric acid without decomposition, in alkalies with a dark red color; its salts are very changeable.

Investigations performed by Professor Schroff, tend to show that the cathartic principle of rhubarb is chrysophanic acid, which is modified in its action by the other constituents of the root, so that while powdered rhubarb acted within twelve hours, Geiger's rhabarbarin purged in nineteen, Brandes' rhein in twenty, pure chrysophanic acid in twenty-four hours; on the other hand he found the duration of the activity of rhubarb to be about twenty-four hours, that of rhein and rhabarbarin three, and of chrysophanic acid five days; during this time eight grains of the latter produced twelve thin yellow evacuations, without the least griping. The acid prepared from parmelia parietina shows no difference from that prepared from rhubarb. The quickness of action of rhubarb, in pharmaceutical preparations must be due to excipients or adjuvants which render the chrysophanic acid soluble.

The active vegetable principle of senna, likewise appears to be chrysophanic acid, combined in such a way as to be easily soluble in water, nearly insoluble in strong alcohol, and supported in its action by a large amount of saline constituents, viz: sulphates, phosphates and tartrates of alkalies and alkaline earths; the senna extract prepared with strong alcohol has no cathartic properties. Dr. Martius has not succeeded in completely isolating chrysophanic acid from senna, but the reactions indicate its presence as well as the presence of two or three other bodies first discovered in rhubarb, namely, aporetin, phæoretin, and probably erythroretin.

Winkler's cathartin, found in the ripe fruit of rhamnus catharticus, is also believed to be this acid in an impure state.

Chrysophanic acid, when taken internally, passes into the urine, where it may be easily recognized by its striking a characteristic red color with alkalies. The same reaction takes place after the administration of rhubarb and senna; with the latter given in the form of infusion or aqueous extract, this reaction would often take place after fifteen minutes and last until twelve hours after the evacuations had taken place.

The root of rumex obtusifolius, and probably other species, owe their laxative properties likewise to chrysophanic acid. (See *American Journal of Pharmacy*, xxxi. 153.)

Santonic Acid (*Santonin*).

Preparation: 4 parts of Levant wormseed are digested with 1½ hydrated lime, and 20 alcohol of 56 per cent.; the alcohol is distilled off, and the filtrate now contains santonic acid and a brown amorphous resin; it is boiled and decomposed by acetic acid. The impure crystals are washed with a little alcohol, dissolved in 8 or 10 parts of 80 per cent. alcohol, digested with animal charcoal, filtered and crystallized.

Flat hexagonal or feathery prisms, little soluble in cold water, more in ether; at 176° F. 27 parts of alcohol dissolve 10 parts santonic acid. The ethereal solution is intensely bitter. Exposed to the light the crystals change their color to a golden yellow and burst to pieces; adulteration with other white substances may thus be easily detected. The alcoholic solution is colored carmine red by caustic alkalies and their carbonates, that which has been colored yellow by the light furnishes a yellow solution, from which white santonic acid crystallizes.

The santonates are decomposed by being boiled with water. The potassa salt is uncrystallizable. The soda salt, which on account of its solubility has been proposed as a substitute for the acid, is obtained by digesting its alcoholic solution with carbonate of soda, evaporating, redissolving in strong alcohol and crystallizing. Large crystals are obtained by evaporating spontaneously a concentrated aqueous solution. Its composition is NaO,HO, $C_{30}H_{18}O_6+7HO$, and it therefore contains 74 per cent. santonic acid. Santonic acid is much employed as a very reliable vermifuge, and often exhibited to children in the form of confections or troches. Dose for children, ½ to 1 grain 2 or 3 times daily.

Cahincic acid on which the strong diuretic virtues of cahinca root depends, is obtained by distilling the alcohol from the tincture, treating the extract with water, filtering, adding milk of lime gradually until all bitterness has disappeared, and treating the cahincate of lime with alcoholic oxalic acid; on cooling fine needles of the acid are obtained, which have a silky lustre, odorless, at first tasteless, afterwards an astringent feeling in the throat. Little soluble in ether and water, easily in alcohol. Alkalies and diluted mineral acids decompose cahincic acid into glucose and kinovic acid. The cahincates are not crystallizable.

Polygalic Acid, Senegin, Polygalin.—The root is extracted with alcohol evaporated to syrupy consistence, and this treated with ether to separate fat; after some time a precipitate forms which is collected on a filter, dissolved in boiling alcohol, treated with animal charcoal and filtered. White amorphous powder, without odor, at first tasteless, afterwards very acrid, astringent in the throat, sternutatory, little soluble in cold water, the solution foams like soap-water; it is easily soluble in alcohol, insoluble in ether. With concentrated sulphuric acid in contact with air it undergoes the following changes: yellow, red, it dissolves, then blue, grayish, colorless. It is poisonous, producing difficulty of breathing, vomiting, &c. The salts are uncrystallizable.

Cetraric Acid.—Iceland moss is extracted by boiling alcohol and carbonate of potassa, the liquid acidulated with muriatic acid and mixed with four or five volumes of water. The precipitate consists principally of cetraric and lichenstearic acids. It is dissolved in eight or ten times its quantity of boiling weak alcohol and filtered, on cooling the lichenstearic acid crystallizes in quadrangular plates, afterwards the cetraric acid in needles; the needles are separated from an amorphous body, and several times recrystallized. Very thin needles, intensely and purely bitter taste, nearly insoluble in water, soluble in boiling alcohol, little in ether. The acid is destroyed by mineral acids, and by boiling its solution in alcohol or its alkaline salts. The soluble salts have an intensely bitter taste, but cannot be evaporated without losing their bitterness.

Anacardic acid is obtained from the pericarp of cashew-nuts by treating the residue of the ethereal tincture with water, to separate tannic acid, dissolving in alcohol, and digesting with hydrated oxide of lead; the anacardate of lead is decomposed by sulphuret of ammonium, and the anacardate of ammonia decomposed by sulphuric acid. The impure acid is purified by washing, recombining with lead, and decomposing by diluted sulphuric acid. Crystalline masses, without odor, of a faint aromatic, afterwards burning taste, liquefies in contact with air, and assumes a rancid smell. Metallic salts are precipitated by it.

Digitalic Acid.—The alcoholic extract of the aqueous extract of digitalis, is treated with ether, which dissolves the acid and digitalin; caustic baryta precipitates digitalate of baryta, which by decomposition with sulphuric acid yields the acid. It crystallizes with difficulty in needles, has a peculiar odor, is not volatilizable; soluble in water, alcohol, less in ether; the alcoholic solution keeps unaltered. Many salts are soluble, but prone to change when kept in solution.

Digitaleic Acid.—The precipitate of the aqueous extract by acetate of lead is washed, decomposed by carbonate of soda, the filtrate precipitated by muriatic acid, recrystallized from hot alcohol. Green needles in star-like groups, bitter acrid taste, agreeably aromatic odor; little soluble in water, soluble in alcohol and ether. Its salts are yellow or green, and insoluble, except those with alkalies, whose solutions foam like soap-water.

FOURTH GROUP.—*Acids combined with Alkaloids.*

It has not been ascertained yet of all alkaloids in which combinations they occur naturally. The large number of vegetable acids in existence, and the difficulties often attending their complete isolation, make the recognition of an acid in its natural association a matter of no ordinary difficulty, and have led to the proposal of many new names for acids long before known, before their identity with those newly discovered had been established beyond a doubt. The greater the difficulty in isolating an acid, or the more widely diffused it is throughout organic nature, the more will be its liability to receive constantly new names from plants hitherto not subjected to a complete analysis. It is necessary only to refer for the illustration of this subject to malic acid, which has been named at various times after quite a number of plants; under its head, attention has been drawn to various acids, mostly connected with alkaloids, which, by later investigations, have been proved to be malic acid. Of acids treated of in the second group, the following would likewise belong to this fourth group: fumaric acid, in glaucium luteum combined with glaucina; aconitic acid in aconitum napellus combined with aconitia. Meconic and kinic acids are interesting on account of some of their reactions.

Chelidonic	acid,	$3HO,C_{14}HO_9$ 2 aq.	In celandine with lime, sanguinarina and chererythrina.
Meconic	"	$3HO,C_{14}HO_{11}+6$ aq.	In opium, with morphia.
Veratric	"	$HO,C_{18}H_9O_7$.	In cevadilla seed, with veratria.
Columbic	"	$C_{42}H_{22}O_{14}$.	In colombo root, with bebeerine.
Kinic	"	$2HO,C_{28}H_{20}O_{20}+2$ aq.	In Peruvian bark, with quinia, cinchonia.
Kinovic	"	$HO,C_{48}H_{34}O_{10}$.	In quinquina nova, and true Peruvian bark.

Chelidonic Acid.—Celandine contains, while young, chiefly malic acid; when in flowers, malic acid has disappeared, and the juice contains chelidonic acid.

To prepare it, the juice is coagulated by heat, the filtrate, after being acidulated with nitric acid, is precipitated by nitrate of lead, which must not be added in excess; the precipitate is decomposed by hydrosulphuric acid, the free acid combined with lime, the salt recrystallized, decomposed by carbonate of ammonia, and afterwards by muriatic acid.

Chelidonic acid crystallizes in colorless needles, soluble in water and alcohol. Most of the salts are colorless; the tribasic salts are, with the exception of those containing colored bases, of a lemon color.

Meconic Acid.—The meconate of lime obtained on the manufacture of morphia is dissolved in dilute muriatic acid, and heated to boiling, when, on cooling, acid meconate of lime crystallizes, which is treated again in the same way; meconic acid now crystallizes, is purified by repeated crystallizations, combined with ammonia or potassa, and lastly precipitated by muriatic acid.

Colorless scales or prisms of a pearly lustre, taste faintly acid and astringent; little soluble in cold water and ether, soluble in hot water and alcohol. Sesquisalts of iron are colored deep red by a trace of acid, the coloration is not affected by boiling, dilute acids, or chloride of gold (difference from sulphocyanurets); this test is characteristic for the presence of opium.

Komenic acid, $C_{12}H_4O_{10}=C_{14}H_4O_{14}—2CO_2$, by heating meconic acid to 390°, or by boiling its solution, particularly with dilute muriatic acid.

Hard warty crystals, colorless, insoluble in absolute alcohol, slight acid taste; bibasic.

Parakomenic acid, $C_{12}H_4O_{10}$, in small quantity, on the dry distillation of the former. Feathery needles, very acid taste; bibasic.

Pyromeconic acid, $C_{10}H_4O_6=C_{12}H_4O_{10}—2CO_2$, by the dry distillation of meconic or komenic acid. Crystallizes in colorless, lustrous needles, scales, or octahedrons; fuses at about 250°; sublimes, is easily soluble in alcohol and water; taste very acid, afterwards bitter; monobasic, a weak acid.

All these derivatives of meconic acid show that characteristic coloration with sesquisalts of iron.

Veratric Acid.—The alcoholic tincture of cevadilla seed is acidulated with sulphuric acid and precipitated by lime, the filtrate is distilled and decomposed by an acid.

It crystallizes in four-sided needles; sublimable, soluble in alcohol and boiling water. The veratrates of the alkalies are crystallizable and soluble in water and alcohol.

Columbic Acid.—The alcoholic extract of columbo root is treated with lime, and the lime salt decomposed by muriatic acid. White crystalline floccules, nearly insoluble in water, little in ether, easily in alcohol. The latter solution is precipitated by neutral acetate of lead, but not by acetate of copper.

Kinic Acid.—The bark is exhausted by cold water, the alkalies precipitated by a little lime, more lime precipitates the cinchotannic acid and coloring matter, the filtrate is evaporated, the crystals of kinate of lime decolorized with animal charcoal, and decomposed by oxalic acid.

Oblique rhombic prisms, acid taste, soluble slowly in 2½ parts cold water, little in alcohol, scarcely in ether. Most salts are soluble. Heated over its melting point, it is decomposed into benzoic and phenylic acids, salicylous acid, hydrokinone and benzol. With oxide of manganese and sulphuric acid it is converted into kinone, carbonic and formic acids.

Kinone, $C_{12}H_4O_4$, long yellow prisms, fusible, volatilizable, little soluble in cold water, soluble in alcohol and ether. With sulphuretted hydrogen it turns immediately red, precipitates floccules, which, after drying, are olive green.

Hydrokinone, $C_{12}H_6O_4$, by dry distillation of kinic acid, or from kinone by the action of sulphurous or hydriodic acids. Colorless prisms, inodorous, fusible, volatile; easily soluble in water and alcohol. Oxidizing agents precipitate needles of

Green hydrokinone, $C_{12}H_6O_4+C_{12}H_4O_4$, of a beautiful green metallic lustre; fusible, but decomposed on volatilizing, little soluble in water, more in alcohol.

Kinovic Acid.—If the bark which comes in commerce under the name of quinquina nova is boiled with milk of lime, and the solution decomposed with muriatic acid, kinovic acid is separated, which is purified by dissolving in alcohol and treating with animal charcoal.

It is a resin-like mass of a bitter taste, little soluble in water, more in alcohol, ether, and alkalies; concentrated sulphuric acid dissolves it with a red color; with sulphate of copper a dirty green precipitate of kinovate of copper is produced.

Fifth Group.—*Acids derived from Essential Oils.*

But few of the numerous essential oils naturally contain acids, and have, in consequence thereof, an acid reaction; most oils, however, on exposure to the atmosphere, become oxidized, and while they assume a thicker consistence, their chemical nature is partly changed, and they now, in alcoholic solution, impart a red color, more or less decidedly, to blue litmus paper—they have become resinified. A similar change takes place by subjecting the essential oils to the influence of nitric or chromic acid, or other strong oxidizing agents. Thus the essential oils yield a large number of acids, mostly of a nature which may be termed resinous. The following embrace those only that are important in a medicinal point of view, or interesting on account of their relation to other bodies. We class them in four divisions:—

(a) *Acids occurring in the freshly-distilled Crude Oils.*

Hydrocyanic acid,	HC_2N.	In the oils of amygdaleæ and pomaceæ. See *Nitrogenated Oils.*
Salicylous "	$HO,C_{14}H_5O_3$.	The oil of herbaceous plants of the genus spiræa.
Methyl-salicylic acid,	$HO,C_{16}H_7O_5$.	The oxygenated part of oil of wintergreen.
Caryophyllic "	$HO,C_{20}H_{11}O_3$.	The oxygenated part of oil of cloves.

Hydrocyanic Acid.

Hydrocyanic or prussic acid, as formed by a reaction between amygdalin and emulsin, and as an ingredient in the volatile oils distilled from many plants belonging to the natural family of rosaceæ, has already been referred to (see *amygdalin and nitrogenated volatile oils*), but for pharmaceutical use, the acid is prepared artificially, and the *U. S. Pharmacopœia* gives two processes, the starting-point for each being the decomposition of ferrocyanuret of potassium by sulphuric acid.

Potassii ferrocyanuretum, U. S., *yellow prussiate of potassa*, is only made on a large scale from animal matter free of bones. They are either first subjected to dry distillation in order to gain part of the nitrogen as ammonia, and the remaining charcoal, which is highly charged with nitrogen, is fused together with small fragments of iron and potash; or the first part of the process being omitted, the animal matter is at once subjected to a red heat in conjunction with potash and iron. After long-continued heating and stirring, a combination has been effected, the fused mass now containing cyanide of potassium, which, when dissolved in water, combines with finely-divided iron, and crystallizes into large yellow tabular prisms, which have a sweetish bitter taste, are soluble in four parts of cold water, and insoluble in alcohol.

They are composed of two equivalents of cyanide of potassium, one of cyanide of iron, and three of water $=2KCy+FeCy+3HO$. The water of crystallization is given off in a dry, warm atmosphere, and the crystals become white and pulverulent. This salt has an extensive use in the arts, and is employed for the preparation of ferrocyanuret of iron, hydrocyanic acid, and all its compounds.

This salt is little used in medicine; it is not poisonous, but in very large doses is apt to produce vertigo, coldness, and fainting; it has been recommended as an alterative, antiphlogistic, and tonic astringent in the dose of from ten to twenty grains internally, and externally, in an eye-salve, composed of from five to twenty grains to one drachm of cocoa-butter.

The commercial salt, though not chemically pure, is sufficiently pure, if it is well crystallized and dissolves in two parts of boiling water.

Argenti Cyanuretum, U. S.; *Cyanide of Silver*.—According to the *Pharmacopœia*, the hydrocyanic acid, produced from two ounces of ferrocyanuret of potassium, is conducted into a solution of two ounces of nitrate of silver.

The cyanide of silver is precipitated as a white, tasteless, inodorous powder, which is darkened by the light, is insoluble in diluted nitric acid, but decomposed by it at a boiling temperature. It is soluble in ammonia, and in cyanide of potassium, and consists of one equiv. of cyanogen, and one of silver $=AgCy$. It is little used, sometimes externally in ointments as an antisyphilitic.

Acidum Hydrocyanicum Dilutum, U. S.—From the above two preparations, the *Pharmacopœia* gives two distinct processes, the first of which is intended for making hydrocyanic acid in larger quantities, while the second process is given for its extemporaneous preparation, and is particularly applicable for the use of the physician.

First Process.—Take of ferrocyanuret of potassium ℥ij, sulphuric acid ℥iss, distilled water q. s. Mix the acid with distilled water f℥iv, and pour the mixture when cool into a glass retort. To this add the ferrocyanuret of potassium, previously dissolved in distilled water, f℥x. Pour of the distilled water f℥viij into a cooled receiver; and, having attached this to the retort, distil by means of a sand bath, with a moderate heat, f℥vj. Lastly, add to the product, distilled water f℥v, or q. s. to render the diluted hydrocyanic acid of such strength that 12.7 grains of nitrate of silver dissolved in distilled water may be accurately saturated by 100 grains of the acid, and give 10 grains of the cyanuret of silver, which, corresponding with 20 per cent. of its own weight of anhydrous hydrocyanic acid, indicates 2 grains, or 2 per cent. of it in 100 grains of the officinal acid.

The difficulties in this process are twofold: 1st. It is difficult to conduct the distillation in an ordinary uncovered retort on account of the excessive bumping occasioned by the escape of the acid vapor through the mixed liquid and precipitate; and 2d. It is exceedingly troublesome to adjust the strength of the distillate to the officinal

24

standard. The first of these difficulties may be overcome, but the precision necessary to be observed in regard to the strength of so powerful a medicine as this, and the impossibility of regulating by the proportions employed the amount of the acid generated and absorbed by the water in the receiver, make it necessary to determine its strength by experiment at each operation. This may be accomplished by testing, say 100 grains of the acid distillate with nitrate of silver before diluting it, carefully washing the resulting cyanide of silver, drying and weighing it, then calculating the degree of dilution required by the weight of this precipitate. If of proper strength, this would be 10 grains, as above, but in this experiment of course a larger yield would be obtained. The equation would then be as follows: As the known weight of the precipitate from acid of standard strength, is to the weight of cyanide obtained from the distillate, so is the quantity of the acid weighed to the quantity to be obtained by dilution. Suppose the precipitate to have weighed 11.5 grains—then 10 : 11.5 : : 100 : 115; or to every 100 grains of the distillate 15 grains of water must be added to make the officinal diluted hydrocyanic acid.

The plan that I would recommend to the inexperienced is to saturate the acid which comes over by the officinal process without special reference to the quantity of water in the receiver, with nitrate of silver, as stated above, to form the officinal cyanide of silver, and further proceed, after carefully washing and drying the product, by the second process of the *Pharmacopœia*.

Second Process.—

Take of Cyanuret of silver . .	Fifty grains and a half.
Muriatic acid . . .	Forty-one grains.
Distilled water . .	One fluidounce.

Mix the muriatic acid with the distilled water, add the cyanuret of silver, and shake the whole in a well-stoppered vial; when the insoluble matter has subsided, pour off the clear liquid and keep it for use. Diluted hydrocyanic acid should be kept in closely-stoppered vials excluded from the light. In preparing this medicine, a slight excess of muriatic acid is not objectionable, giving it greater stability, and as the commercial acid is nearly always weaker than that of the *Pharmacopœia*, it should be added as long as any precipitate is produced. It is usually put up in f℥j ground-stoppered vials, the imported kind called Saxony is the best; each vial being inclosed in a tin can. The only apparent objection to this process is its expensiveness; this is, however, less than would at first appear. The reaction between muriatic acid and the cyanide results in the production of hydrocyanic acid and chloride of silver, thus—$AgCy + HCl = H,Cy + AgCl$. Now, the chloride of silver is convertible into pure metallic silver by the introduction into it while in the condition of a moist powder, of a strip of zinc, which abstracts the chlorine, the chloride of zinc becoming dissolved, and the pure silver remaining as a gray-colored spongy mass or powder, which, on being washed and treated with nitric acid, yields the soluble nitrate ready for any further use.

The country practitioner, who wishes to be prepared for every emergency in his practice, may, with advantage, supply himself with a suitable f℥j vial, containing 50½ grains cyanide of silver, to which the mixed muriatic acid and water may be added when the occasion arises.

The diluted acid prepared as above is a colorless liquid, frequently having, from the presence of iron, a slight blue tint, of a peculiar odor and taste; it is entirely volatilized by heat. It contains two per cent. of anhydrous acid (HCy). Its use in medicine has been very much avoided by practitioners, on account of the violent poisonous character of the anhydrous or concentrated acid; but in the diluted form, in which it is officinal, it is no more dangerous than many other remedies constantly prescribed, and, notwithstanding the alleged variable strength of the commercial article, I believe it will be found as nearly uniform as most other pharmaceutical preparations.

As a sedative and antispasmodic, it is a favorite with some practitioners, who employ it simply mixed with mucilage, or with the galenical preparations of digitalis, valerian, &c. It should not be prescribed with strong alkaline, ferruginous, or other metallic salts.

In this country, no stronger hydrocyanic acid is used than the officinal; in other countries, however, its strength varies materially. The acid of the London, Dublin, and Prussian *Pharmacopœias* is of about the same strength as our own, that of the Edinburgh *Pharmacopœia* contains about 3¼ per cent., Scheele's acid 5 per cent., and some European pharmacopœias even a much larger proportion of anhydrous acid. The dose of our officinal acid being ♏ij to ♏v, is so small that there is no necessity for employing a stronger acid in formulas, which would be liable to lead to dangerous mistakes; besides, it must be remarked that strong acids are very prone to spontaneous decomposition, while that of the officinal strength, if not exposed to the light, or to a continued high temperature, keeps well for a considerable time. Of course the vials are to be well-stoppered on account of the volatility of the acid.

Potassii Cyanuretum, U. S.; *Cyanide of Potassium.*—This salt may be mentioned in this place, as having all the medicinal properties of hydrocyanic acid; it is given as a substitute for it. It is prepared by fusing ferrocyanuret of potassium with carbonate of potassa until effervescence ceases, when the clear liquid is poured off the precipitated oxide of iron, and, immediately after cooling, put into well-stoppered bottles. It is then in white fused masses of a powerful caustic taste, and a composition which is expressed by the formula KCy, though it is usually contaminated by carbonate and cyanate of potassa.

The pure cyanide is equal to ⅖ of its weight of hydrocyanic acid, the officinal to somewhat less. The dose is $\frac{1}{16}$ grain, which, with proper care, may be gradually increased to ½ grain; it is given dissolved in alcohol or water.

It is a useful chemical agent for removing the stains of nitrate of silver and durable ink, and its utility as a solvent for metallic oxides is well known in electro-metallurgy and photography.

Salicylous or Spirous Acid.—It is artificially obtained by oxidation of salicin or populin and by fermentation of helicin. 3 parts salicin are mixed with 3 parts bichromate of potassa, and 24 parts water; to this 4½ parts sulphuric acid in 12 parts water are added, and after the reaction has ceased, heat is applied, and distilled as long as with the water an oily liquid comes over, which is taken up by ether and left after its evaporation.

It is an oily liquid, colorless or reddish, of an agreeable aromatic odor and burning taste; specific gravity 1.17; it freezes at 5° F., and boils at 340° F.

The salicylites, when kept moist, are decomposed, acquiring a rose odor; this reaction has been proposed for the formation of an artificial rose-water.

If salicylous acid is heated with potassa, it is converted into *salicylic or spiric acid*, $2HO,C_{14}H_4O_4$, which is of importance as the acid contained in the following.

Methyl-salicylic acid, or oil of wintergreen, $HO,C_2H_3O,C_{14}H_4O_4 = C_{16}H_8O_6$, is the oil obtained by distillation with water from gaultheria procumbens. It is a colorless or reddish-yellow oil, of a well-known characteristic odor. By distillation with an excess of baryta it is converted into carbolate of oxide of methyle, while by the dry distillation of an alkaline or earthy salicylate, a carbonate and carbolic acid is formed, $C_{14}H_6O_6 = 2CO_2 + C_{12}H_6O_2$ (carbolic acid).

Caryophyllic or Eugenic Acid.—If oil of cloves is treated with solution of potassa or soda, and the light carbohydrogen distilled off, the acid may be easily separated by a mineral acid.

It is a colorless oil, of 1.079 specific gravity, the odor and taste of cloves; it resinifies in contact with the air. The caryophyllates of alkalies and alkaline earths are crystallizable; metallic salts are either precipitated or colored blue, violet, or green.

(b) *Products of Oxidation by the Atmosphere.*

Valerianic acid, $HO,C_{10}H_9O_3$.	From valerol in oil of valerian and valerian root.
Benzoic " $HO,C_{14}H_5O_3$.	In old oil of bitter almonds, benzoin, from cinnamic acid by NO_5.
Cinnamic " $HO,C_{18}H_7O_3$.	In old oil of cinnamon, storax, Tolu, Peru balsam, &c.

Valerianic Acid.

This important acid which is developed spontaneously by the oxidation of valerol, one of the ingredients of oil of valerian, is also met with in the root of angelica archangelica, in the inner bark of sambucus niger, in assafœtida, &c., and is artificially obtained by the oxidation of protein compounds, some fatty acids, but particularly of amylic alcohol or fusel oil. Of the various processes recommended, the following by Wittstein is one of the most satisfactory. To 10 lbs. bicarbonate of potassa, and 10 quarts of water, is gradually added a mixture of 10 lbs. of sulphuric acid, and 2 lbs. of rectified fusel oil; of this mixture 8 quarts are distilled, the residue is mixed with 6 lbs. sulphuric acid, and again distilled. The mixed distillates are saturated with carbonate of soda, the separating oil is removed, the remaining solution boiled to drive off all oil, and then decomposed by sulphuric or phosphoric acid; the distillate requires to be once more rectified, and furnishes then, if the operation has been properly conducted, 1 lb. of concentrated valerianic acid.

It is a colorless liquid, of a disagreeable odor of valerian, and old cheese, and a similar acid taste; its sp. gr. is .937, its boiling point 347° F.; it is inflammable, dissolves in 30 parts cold water, and in all proportions of alcohol and ether; it dissolves camphor and some resins.

The salts have an unctuous touch, and are inodorous when perfectly dry, but mostly have the odor of the acid; they revolve when thrown upon the water in a crystallized state, like the butyrates. Most of them are soluble in water or alcohol, or in both liquids.

The following salts have been used medicinally: the valerianate of ammonia, zinc, iron, bismuth, morphia, quinia and atropia.

Acidum Benzoicum, U. S.

This, with cinnamic acid is considered characteristic of the class of medicines called balsams. The two acids are closely allied in their chemical nature, as has been already shown; they are also related to salicylic and allied acids.

For medicinal use it is readily obtained from benzoin by sublimation. For this experiment, which is an interesting one to the pharmaceutical student, the following simple directions are to be observed. Select an iron or tinned iron pan or cup—a common pint cup, without a handle, will answer—and, having covered the bottom with some powdered benzoin mixed with sand, stretch over the top of it a piece of porous paper, which may be secured at the edge by a string, but preferably by glue or some firm paste. Now fold a tall conical or straight-sided cap of the diameter of the pan, and tie it, or cement it securely round the upper edge, and set the whole in a sand bath, or over a slow and well-regulated source of heat, leaving it for several hours. On removing the cap, it will be found to contain brilliant white feathery crystals of benzoic acid. The residue in the cup, by being again powdered, mixed with sand, and heated, will yield another, though a less abundant and less beautiful crop of crystals. As thus obtained, benzoic acid has a faint and agreeable balsamic odor, with very little taste, being nearly insoluble.

The process of Scheele consists in boiling the balsam with hydrate of lime, and treating the benzoate of lime thus formed with muriatic acid. Thus procured, benzoic acid has but little odor, and is ill adapted to the uses to which it is usually applied in medicine and pharmacy. Sometimes the process of sublimation is resorted to at first, and from the residue the remaining acid is extracted by Scheele's process, after which the whole is mixed.

The virtues of the acid are, partly at least, dependent on the odorous principle with which it is associated. Its salts have no smell if prepared from the chemically pure acid, but they retain some of the odor of the officinal acid if prepared from it. Of the salts only the benzoates of ammonia and of soda have been occasionally employed.

Benzoic acid if distilled with caustic potassa in excess, is converted into carbonic acid and benzol, $C_{14}H_6O_4=2CO_2+C_{12}H_6$; in the animal organism it is changed into hippuric acid, from which it may be reproduced on boiling with muriatic acid; hippuric acid occurs naturally in the urine of herbivorous animals, and from this source the German article, occasionally met with in our commerce, is derived; it has a peculiar urinous odor, and quite a different appearance from the sublimed article, having been crystallized from an aqueous solution.

Detection of Impurities.—All fixed impurities are left behind on volatilizing some of the acid; hippuric acid is detected by its odor, by leaving charcoal on heating, and by evolving ammonia on heating it with lime; cinnamic acid imparts the odor of bitter almonds to the distillate, with bichromate of potassa and sulphuric acids.

Cinnamic Acid.—To prepare this acid, liquid storax is first distilled with water, to obtain styrol, afterwards treated with carbonate of soda (residue is styracin); the solution is evaporated, decomposed by muriatic acid, the cinnamic acid after washing, distilled and the last impure portions are treated again with soda. In a similar way it is obtained from Tolu balsam (here the residue is Tolu ol.). Colorless prismatic and scaly crystals, melting at 264°. F., boiling and distilling at 655° F.; little soluble in cold water (less than benzoic acid), easily soluble in alcohol. With excess of baryta or lime it is converted into carbonic acid and cinnamen ($C_{16}H_8$); with bichromate of potassa and sulphuric acid into oil of bitter almonds (principal distinction from benzoic acid), and by distillation with hypochlorite of soda into a chlorinated volatile oil of agreeable odor. When fused with hydrate of potassa it is decomposed into acetic and benzoic acids.

(c) *Acids obtainable by artificial oxidation of Volatile Oils.*

Anisic acid, $HO,C_{16}H_7O_5$. From oil of anise and fennel by oxidation.
Pelargonic acid, $HO,C_{18}H_{17}O_3$. From oil of rue by diluted NO_5, and in oil of geranium.
Rutinic " $HO,C_{20}H_{19}O_3$. From oil of rue by NO_5, and in various animal fats.
Angelicic " $HO,C_{10}H_7O_3$. From oil of chamomile by KO. (See *Third Group.*)

Anisic Acid.—To prepare it, 6 parts of bichromate of potassa are dissolved in 9 parts water, and heated with 7 parts concentrated sulphuric acid and 1 part oil of anise, diluting with cold water and recrystallizing from alcohol; the yield is half a part.

Large colorless prisms, nearly tasteless, nearly insoluble in cold water, easily in boiling water, in alcohol, and ether. Melts at 347° F., sublimes at higher temperature in white needles; distilled over baryta, is decomposed into carbonic acid and anisol, $C_{16}H_8O_6=2CO_2+C_{14}H_8O_2$. Its salts are crystallizable.

Pelargonic acid is contained in oil of rose geranium as distilled from the leaves of pelargonium roseum.

The pure acid is a colorless oil, of a peculiar odor; crystallizes in cold weather and boils at 500°; its compound with ether is interesting for its agreeable odor of quinces. (See *Pelargonic Ether.*)

Rutinic or caprinic acid is contained in the butter of cows and goats, but only with difficulty separated from the other fatty acids. Cod-liver oil, cocoanut oil, and the fusel oil of alcohol prepared from beetroot-molasses likewise contain it. From the latter it is separated by first washing it with carbonate of soda, saponifying it with potassa, decomposing with tartaric acid, and crystallizing from alcohol.

It appears in white crystalline masses, of a peculiar "buck's" odor, easily soluble in alcohol and ether.

(d) *Acids obtained from Empyreumatic Oils.*

Phenylic acid, $HO,C_{12}H_5O$. In coal tar; from salicylic and kinic acids, and some resins.
Carbazotic " $HO,C_{12}H_2(NO_4)_3O_2$. By NO_5 from salicin and its derivatives, from coumarin, phloridzic and phenylic acids, silk, indigo, &c.

Carbolic or Phenylic Acid, Spirol, Salicon.—It occurs in castor, and the urine of many domestic animals.

Coal tar is distilled, the product between 300° and 400° is saturated with strong solution of potassa, the oil is removed, the salt decomposed by muriatic acid; the carbolic acid washed with water, dried with chloride of calcium, rectified, cooled to about 12° F., the liquid decanted, and the crystals quickly dried. Long colorless needles, melting at 95°, boiling at 369° F., but with little water liquid; not very soluble in water, in all proportions in alcohol and ether, soluble in concentrated acetic acid. By nitric acid it is converted into picric acid; it crystallizes with solid potassa, and distilled with it is not decomposed. The test recommended for it on page 286 is unreliable, as many resinous woods, by moistening with muriatic acid, and subsequent exposure to light, acquire a blue, violet, or green color (R. Wagner).

As before stated, carbolic acid is generally sold for *creasote*, which, it appears, is a name applied by chemists to various empyreumatic liquids; the following is given as the principal differences of wood creasote from phenylic acid: it remains liquid at 17° F., boils at 397° F., remains colorless if pure. Strong ammonia dissolves it in the cold; with solid potassa it forms a liquid compound, and probably some crystalline scales; if distilled with it it is decomposed, and an aromatic oil is obtained; its formula has been given as $C_{24}H_{14}O_5$ (Völckel), $C_{26}H_{16}O_4$ (Gorup), $C_{14}H_8O_2$ (Williams).

Picric Acid, Carbazotic Acid, Welter's Bitters.—The cheapest method of preparing it is from coal tar, but from indigo it is better obtained in a pure state.—1 part indigo is boiled with 10 to 12 parts of nitric acid, specific gravity 1.43, gradually added until nitrous acid ceases to be evolved; the picric acid crystallizes on cooling, and is purified by combining with an alkaloid, and precipitating by nitric acid.

Yellow scales or octahedrons, soluble in 86 parts water of 60°, easily soluble in alcohol and ether, explosive when suddenly heated; it colors the skin yellow, is very bitter, and is a dye for silk and wool, but not for cotton. Its salts are yellow, crystallizable, very bitter, soluble, and explosive by heating. It has been occasionally used in medicine, and is said to be employed in France in making beer, in place of hops.

SIXTH GROUP.—*Astringent and Allied Acids.*

These acids are widely diffused throughout the vegetable kingdom, and have many properties in common. They are all with two exceptions uncrystallizable, inodorous, of an astringent taste, and soluble in water and alcohol. The solutions are precipitated by gelatin and albumen, most metallic oxides and the vegetable alkaloids; iron salts are generally rendered dark green, blue, or black. They are weak acids, and if kept in a moist state, are rapidly changed in contact with the air; their salts are quickly darkened while in solution, or, if insoluble, while being washed upon a filter. Owing to this property, their composition and the nature of their changes are, in many cases, still a matter of controversy. The following syllabus contains not only the astringent acids, properly so called, but also some allied acids and some of their derivatives:—

Gallotannic acid, $C_{54}H_{22}O_{34}$. Acidum tannicum, *U. S. P.* } In galls from quercus infectoria, Chinese galls from distylium racemosum.
Gallic acid, $3HO,C_{14}H_3O_7$. In uva ursi, sumach, &c., the seed of mangoes (mangifera Indica) contain 7 per cent.
Pyrogallic acid, $HO,C_{12}H_5O_5$. By destructive distillation of the former.
Quercotannic " ? In oak-bark, black tea, &c.
Catechutannic " ? In catechu, probably by oxidation of catechuic acid.
Catechuic acid, $C_{17}H_9O_7+3$ aq. In catechu.
Coffeotannic " $C_{28}H_{16}O_{14}$. In coffee, cahinca root, the leaves of ilex Paraguayensis.
Viridinic " $C_{28}H_{14}O_{16}$. In coffee, product of oxidation of the tannin.
Boheatannic " $C_{28}H_{16}O_{20}$. In small quantity in tea, besides gallotannic acid.
Moritannic " $C_{36}H_{14}O_{18}+2$ aq. Crystallizable; in fustic, wood of morus tinctoria (fustic)
Moric " $C_{36}H_{14}O_{18}+2$ aq. In fustic; is the yellow dye stuff.
Kinotannic " ? In kino.
Cephaëlic " $HO,C_{14}H_8O_6$. In the root of ipecacuanha.
Cissotannic " $C_{20}H_{12}O_{16}$. The red coloring matter of leaves in fall.
Xanthotannic " $C_{23}H_{15}O_4$. The yellow coloring matter of autumnal leaves.

Acidum Tannicum, U. S.

Gallotannic acid is conveniently prepared by treating powdered galls in a narrow covered displacer, with hydrated or washed ether. The ethereal tincture which passes separates, upon standing, into two layers; the lower one is aqueous, thick, and of a light buff or straw color; it contains the tannic acid, which, by the action of the small portion of water in the washed ether, has been dissolved out from the galls. The upper layer or stratum of liquid is limpid and specifically much lighter than the other; it has a greenish color, and contains very little tannin, but a small amount of coloring matter from the galls. To obtain the dry product, the light layer is poured off and purified by distillation, and combined with water for another operation, while the thick heavier layer is evaporated in a capsule by a carefully regulated heat till dry. If a white and very porous product is desired, the capsule should be inverted towards the end of the evaporation, so as to expose the thick syrupy liquid to the radiated heat. It is swelled up and whitened as the liquid is disengaged. The whole of the liquid which comes through may be evaporated without the precaution of pouring off the top layer, but the tannin is then apt to have a greenish tinge. In large manufacturing establishments, apparatus is, of course, constructed for saving all the ether for future use. Fig. 191 represents a suitable apparatus for small operations. *A* is an adapter, such as is used for coupling retorts and receivers; *B* is a wide-mouth receiving bottle; *C* is a glass tube passed through the cork, and drawn out to a capillary orifice for the escape of air as the liquid drops in. The adapter is designed to be stopped at bottom with a cork notched, as shown in Fig. *E;* and, as the lower orifice would be too small to allow a free passage of the liquid if the powder were tightly compacted into it, a portion of sand, either alone or mixed with powdered galls, is filled in to the lower part. Fig. *F* represents the broken beak of a retort cut round at its broken end, and adapted to a similar use. I have usually employed for this purpose, in teaching the student the process on a small scale, a Farina Cologne bottle cracked off evenly near the bottom, thus forming a still better shaped tube for the purpose. To prevent undue evaporation of ether, a stout, though loosely-fitting cork, may be introduced into the upper end, or it may be covered with a piece of bladder perforated with a few pin-holes. The yield of tannic acid by this process is from 30 to 60 per cent. of the galls employed.

Fig. 191.

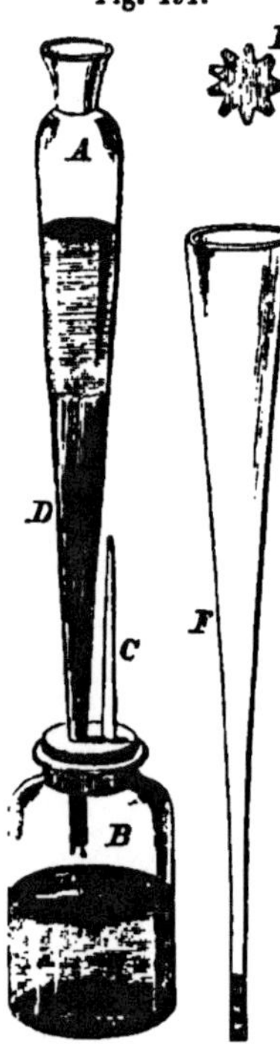

Displacers for making tannic acid.

Mohr, Sandrock, and others assert the syrupy liquid to be a concentrated solution of tannin in ether, which is not miscible with ether, except by the intervention of a little alcohol; they therefore reject the employment of aqueous ether, which has a tendency to swell up the powdered galls, and retard percolation, and recommend a mixture of 90 per cent. alcohol and ether (one to twenty parts, Guibourt).

Tannin is soluble in fixed and volatile oils; it readily dissolves in water, glycerin, alcohol, and absolute ether. The concentrated ethereal solution contains 46.5 to 56.2 per cent. of tannic acid (Mohr), and is insoluble in ether. Could this be a chemical compound between oxide of ethyle and tannic acid? 18 equivalents of the former =481 to 1 equivalent of the latter =618, require exactly 56.2 per cent. of tannin and 43.8 per cent. of ether.

Acidum Gallicum, U. S.

Gallic acid is made by subjecting a portion of powdered galls to long-continued action of air and moisture. This may be accomplished in an evaporating capsule loosely covered with paper. The powder is first made into a paste with water, and water repeatedly added to this as it dries, until after the lapse of thirty days (*U. S. P.*), when the whole of the tannic has passed spontaneously into gallic acid. In extracting this from the moist mass, advantage is taken of the solubility of gallic acid in hot water, and its ready precipitation on cooling; all that is necessary is to press out from the pasty mass its water, and, rejecting this, to digest the remaining paste in hot water, and filter the solution while hot through animal charcoal to decolorize it, and a nearly white crystalline powder of gallic acid is obtained.

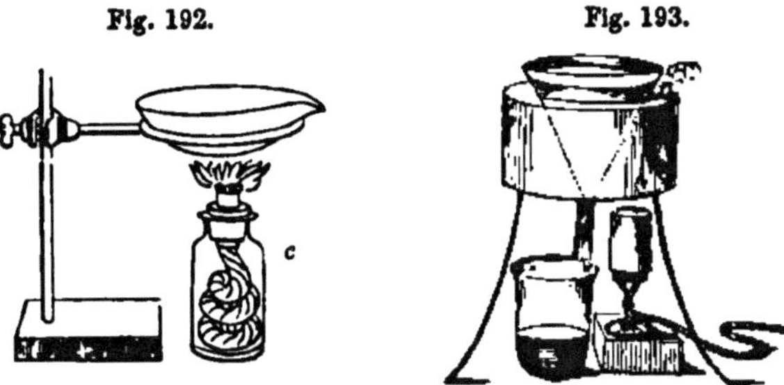

Fig. 192. Evaporating dish and lamp. Fig. 193. Water-bath funnel.

Fig. 180 represents the use of the evaporating dish for the hot solution, and Fig. 181 the arrangement usually adopted for filtering the solution while hot. Care must be taken in these processes not to employ vessels of tinned iron, which, by the exposure of a small surface of iron, may blacken the whole product.

The amount of gallic acid obtained from galls is about 20 per cent.; the ferment inducing the change of tannic into gallic acid, is identical with pectase; emulsin, yeast, albumen, and legumin are without action, on the contrary they retard the influence of pectase. Tannin, according to Strecker, is decomposed into 3 equivalents of gallic acid and 1 of grape sugar: $C_{54}H_{22}O_{34}+8HO=3C_{14}H_{6}O_{10}+C_{12}H_{12}O_{12}$.

The same decomposition of tannic acid is induced by the influence of diluted sulphuric acid, and the process for obtaining gallic acid can be materially shortened if, instead of exposure to the atmosphere, galls or tannin are treated with sulphuric acid at the boiling point. Otherwise the process remains the same as above given.

Gallic acid is soluble in cold water in about the proportion of 4 grains to the ounce. Its salts with the alkalies and alkaline earths are crystallizable; at a boiling temperature, sesquisalts of iron are decomposed by being reduced to protosalts, carbonic acid being given off at the same time.

In common with tannin, it is usually given in pills, and used externally in ointments or solution. It is likewise used in hair dyes, an ammonical solution of nitrate of silver being afterwards employed to produce the color.

Paraellagic or rufigallic acid, $=C_{14}H_4O_8+2HO$, is formed by the action of 5 parts sulphuric acid on 1 part dry gallic acid, until sulphurous acid is given off; by cooling it and throwing it gradually in cold water, it is separated into the crystalline, and amorphous paraellagic acid, both insoluble in water, subliming to vermilion-red prismatic crystals, soluble with difficulty in alcohol and ether, and not furnishing pyrogallic acid.

Ellagic or bezoaric acid is a product of decomposition of gallotannic along with gallic acid. An infusion of galls deposits the acid as a grayish powder, which is washed with boiling water, dissolved by an alkali, and precipitated by an acid. The oriental bezoars, certain animal concretions, consist of the greater part of this acid. It is a light yellowish crystalline powder, tasteless, nearly insoluble in water.

Tannoxylic acid is formed by the action of caustic potassa on gallotannic or gallic acid at ordinary temperatures. Composition $C_{14}H_6O_{12}$, that is gallic acid, $C_{14}H_6O_{10}+2O$. The lead salt is a brick-red precipitate.

Tannomelanic acid by the action of potassa at the boiling heat, with evolution of carbonic acid; the lead salt is dark brown. Composition $C_{12}H_4O_6$, that is tannoxylic acid, $C_{14}H_6O_{12}—2HO—2CO_2$.

Pyrogallic Acid, $C_{12}H_6O_6$=gallic acid $C_{14}H_6O_{10}—2CO_2$.—The best and cheapest method for preparing it is from the dry aqueous extract of galls in Mohr's benzoic acid apparatus in a bath of sand or chloride of zinc, heated as accurately as possible to 400° F., and towards the end of the process a little higher. 100 parts of dry extract yield about 5 parts perfectly pure pyrogallic acid, and the same amount of impure, to be purified by another sublimation. By dry distillation of Chinese galls in small retorts, Liebig obtained a liquid, yielding, on evaporation, 15 per cent. brown crystallized pyrogallic acid.

White laminæ or needles of a pearly lustre, soluble in 2¼ parts water at 55° F., less in alcohol and ether; the solutions do not affect litmus paper; its taste is very bitter; fusible at 240° F., boiling at about 400°, at 480° it is blackened and converted into metagallic acid. Solution of pyrogallic acid, if dropped into milk of lime, produces a characteristic red coloration, changing to brown. Protosulphate of iron produces a bluish black color, a trace of sesquisalt changes it to a dark green. Sesquisalts of iron color a solution of the acid red; hydrated sesquioxide of iron and a pyrogallate give a dark blue liquid and precipitate.

It is much employed in photography on account of its great sensitiveness to light in combination with silver, and for dyeing hair brown and black. The salts are more soluble than the gallates.

Metagallic, Gallhuminic Acid, $C_{12}H_4O_4$,= pyrogallic $C_{12}H_6O_6—2HO$.—By decomposition of pyrogallic acid at 480°, also from gallic and tannic acids. It is black, tasteless, insoluble in water, soluble in caustic alkalies.

Medical Properties.—The relative utility of tannic and gallic acids, which are too apt to be confounded by physicians, depends upon the fact that the former acts directly upon the mucous membranes with which it comes in contact, arresting hemorrhage or other excessive discharge by its direct effect on the gelatin frequent in them. It is hence a direct and powerful styptic, while gallic acid, by entering the circulation, produces an astringent and tonic impression upon the more remote organs which cannot be directly impressed. The dose of tannic acid is from two to ten grains, that of gallic acid from five to twenty, several times a day. The former is much used in ointments as a substitute for powdered galls, in about one-fourth the quantity, and is also well adapted to astringent injections instead of the less soluble vegetable astringents. Its action is considered somewhat different (harsher) than that of the modified forms of tannic acid contained in kino, krameria, cinchona, &c.

The list which follows contains the names of different vegetable astringents owing their activity wholly or in part to gallic or a tannic acid, and below are found, in a condensed form, the results of the chemical investigation of the tannins, contained in our officinal and otherwise important plants.

List of Vegetable or Tannic Acid Astringents.

Catechu, *U. S.*; extract of wood of acacia catechu. Gum catechu.
Chimaphila, *U. S.*; leaves of C. umbellata. Pipsissewa.
Cinchona, *U. S.*; bark of different species cinchona. Peruvian bark.
Diospyros, *U. S.*; unripe fruit of D. Virginiana. Persimmon.
Galla, *U. S.*; morbid excrescence in quercus infectoria. Galls.
Geranium, *U. S.*; rhizoma of G. maculatum. Cranesbill.
Geum, *U. S.*; root of G. rivale. Water avens
Granatum fructus cortex, *U. S.*; from punica granatum. Pomegranate.
" radicis cortex, *U. S.*; " " "
Hæmatoxylon, *U. S.*; wood of H. Campechianum. Logwood.
Heuchera, *U. S.*; root of H. Americana. Alum root.
Kino, *U. S.*; inspissated juice of various plants. Kino.
Krameria, *U. S.*; root of K. triandra. Rhatany.
Quercus alba, *U. S.*; the bark. White oak bark.
Quercus tinctoria, *U. S.*; the bark. Black oak bark.
Rosa gallica, *U. S.*; the petals. Red roses.
Rubus villosus, *U. S.*; the root. Blackberry-root.
" trivialis, *U. S.*; " Dewberry-root.
Spiræa, *U. S.*; root of spiræa tomentosa. Hardhack.
Statice, *U. S.*; the root of S. Caroliniana. Marsh rosemary.
Tormentilla, *U. S*; the root of potentilla, T. Tormentil.
Uva ursi, *U. S.*; leaves of arctostaphylos, U. U. Bearberry leaves.

Quercotannic Acid.—Similar to gallotannic, but yields no gallic or pyrogallic acid.

Catechu, or mimotannic acid, precipitates gelatine, protosalts of iron grayish-green; sesquisalts are colored brownish-green; tartar emetic is not precipitated; yields no sugar with SO_3.

Catechuic Acid, Catechin.—White crystals scarcely soluble in cold water, and not precipitated by starch, gelatine, tartar emetic or vegetable alkaloids; by acetate of lead white, by sesquichloride of iron dark-green; by oxidation catechutannin is formed. (See *American Journal of Pharmacy*, xxviii. 326.)

Rufocatechuic, rubinic acid, in the oxidized alkaline solution of the former. The tannin in *krameria* yields a similar red acid by spontaneous oxidation.

Kino, or coccotannic acid, precipitates sesquisalts of iron, but not tartar emetic; by oxidation red.

Coffeotannic Acid.—Colorless needles; yields kinone with SO_3 and MnO_2 (see *Kinic*

Acid); sesquisalts of iron are colored green; protosalts, tartar emetic and gelatine not precipitated.

Viridinic Acid.—From the former by alkalies; its solutions are green, the lead salt blue.

Boheatannic acid is precipitated with sugar of lead by ammonia.

Cinchotannic Acid.—Precipitated by sesquisalts of iron green, by tartar emetic, starch, gelatine and albumen, is soluble in diluted acids.

Cinchona Red.—A product of oxidation of the former; various ingredients of bark have received this name; that of H. Heasiwetz is of a chocolate or black color, soluble in alcohol, ether and alkalies.

Moritannic Acid.—Yellow prisms; precipitated by gelatine, sesquisulphate of iron (greenish-black), sugar of lead (yellow), and partly by tartar emetic, with BO_3 a gelatinous mass.

Rufimoric Acid.—$C_{16}H_6O_5+HO$, brick-red floccules, with alkalies carmine-red solution, with alum, baryta and tin, dark-red lakes.

Moric Acid, Morin.—White, crystalline, with alkalies yellow, with sesquichloride of iron garnet-red; olive-green precipitate with protosalts of iron.

Oxyphenic, Pyromoric, Pyrocatechuic Acid.—By dry distillation of all tannins, imparting a green-color to iron salts.

Cephaëlic, Ipecacuanhic Acid.—Very bitter; colors sesquichloride of iron green, violet, black.

Cissotannic Acid.—A weak acid, its nature discovered by Wittstein.

Xanthotannic Acid.—Similar to the former, discovered by Ferrein.

SEVENTH GROUP.—*Acids of Animal Origin.*

Two acids have been described in the second group, which for a long time had been supposed to be exclusively of animal origin, though likewise formed by the decomposition of certain organic compounds of vegetable products; modern chemistry, however, has established the fact that formic and lactic acids are both produced during the natural healthful life of some vegetable organisms, and that the nettles, for instance, owe their powerful irritant effect to the same acid that nature has provided for the defence of ants, wasps and bees.

Vegetable acids, to the exclusion of but a few compounds, which from their chemical behavior may be classed with the acids, are destitute of nitrogen; the acids arranged in this group all contain nitrogen, one also sulphur, and are produced by the functions of some of the most important organs of animal economy; they comprise the acids found in the muscles, occurring in urine, and being the active constituents of bile. None of them have been used in medicine in a free state; the impure soda salt of one of the biliary acids, however, has been somewhat employed as a substitute for inspissated bile, and others may probably be found useful if attention is drawn to them.

Inosinic acid, $HO,C_{10}H_6N_2O_{10}$. In the juice of the meat of most animals.
Uric " $2HO,C_{10}H_2N_2O_4+4$ aq. Free and combined in the urine of birds, reptiles, some molluscs and insects; in the urinary sediment and calculi of man and quadrupeds.
Hippuric " $HO,C_{18}H_8NO_6$. In the urine of man and herbivorous animals.
Choleic " $HO,C_{52}H_{42}N_{12}$. As soda salt in the bile of most animals.
Hyocholeic acid, $HO,C_{54}H_{42}NO_9$. Combined with soda, potassa and ammonia in the bile of the hog.
Sulphocholeic " $C_{52}H_{45}NS_2O_{14}$. In small quantity in the bile of the ox, and other animals.

Inosinic Acid.—The mother liquor of the preparation of creatine is precipitated by alcohol, the crystals in hot solution are decomposed by chloride of barium; the crystallizing inosinate of baryta decomposed by sulphuric acid, and the concentrated solution of inosinic acid precipitated by alcohol.

Inosinic acid has an agreeable taste of broth; its alkaline salts are easily soluble in water, and crystallize from a concentrated solution on the addition of alcohol; all other salts are sparingly soluble.

This acid is important as an ingredient of the various culinary and dietetic preparations of meat, which likewise contain the following:—

Creatine $C_8H_9N_3O_4 + 2$ aq.—Though creatine is a neutral substance, it may be well to refer to it in this place. It is prepared by expressing fresh meat, macerating it several times with water, and subjecting it each time to strong pressure. From the mixed liquids, albumen and fibrin are removed by coagulating with heat, and solution of baryta is added as long as a precipitate occurs; the filtrate is evaporated at a moderate heat to a syrupy liquid, and set aside to crystallize.

The flesh of chickens and game is easy to clarify; the former contains the largest, fishes the least quantity of creatine. It is in colorless pearly crystals without taste or action on litmus; it is soluble in 75 parts of cool water, and 100 parts of absolute alcohol. By boiling with baryta it is decomposed into an organic alkaloid, sarkosina and urea; by boiling with strong acids, it loses 2HO and is converted into kreatinine. (See *Organic Alkaloids.*)

Uric Acid.—The following is the method recommended by Arppe. The solution of 9½ oz. of borax in 8¼ gall. water is heated to boiling, with two linen bags immersed in it, each of which contains 3¼ lbs. of pigeon's excrements; after one hour the bags are withdrawn, ¼ lb. sal ammonia is added and the liquid allowed to cool. The liquor is decanted, the precipitate washed with cold water, and boiled with a diluted solution of borax; the filtrate while warm is decomposed by a warm mixture of 5 drachms of sulphuric acid and 1 oz. of water; the crystalline acid is combined with potassa, repeatedly recrystallized and decomposed by sulphuric acid. Yield =.33 per cent. It is obtained by a similar process from guano.

Dry uric acid is a white crystalline powder of silky lustre; scarcely soluble in cold water, insoluble in alcohol and ether; is decomposed by concentrated nitric acid into alloxan and urea; the solution of urea in diluted nitric acid, evaporated until it has assumed a red color, yields on the addition of very diluted ammonia *murexide* or purpurate of ammonia.

The quantity of uric acid in urine is determined by precipitating this liquid with an acid; if no albumen is present, muriatic acid will answer, otherwise acetic, or, better, phosphoric acid is to be used; the liquid retains of uric acid only .009 per cent. of its weight, which loss is usually made up by the precipitation of coloring matter. Uric acid has a tendency to form acid salts; nearly all the urates are little soluble or insoluble in water.

Hippuric Acid.—The quantity of hippuric acid in urine is increased by taking benzoic or cinnamic acid, benzoic ether and other compounds relating thereto.

Gregory's process for obtaining it is as follows: the fresh urine of cows or horses is mixed with milk of lime in excess, boiled, strained and evaporated to ⅛ its original measure; it is then supersaturated with muriatic acid, and the crystallized acid purified by again combining it with lime and decomposing with muriatic acid.

The urine of cows contains 1.3, of horses .38 per cent. of hippuric acid; in putrefied urine it is changed to benzoic acid.

It crystallizes in prisms or needles of a very acid taste, which are easily soluble in alcohol and boiling water, nearly insoluble in ether. By destructive distillation it yields hydrocyanic acid, benzoic acid, benzoate of ammonia and similar compounds; by boiling with diluted mineral acids it is converted into benzoic acid and glycocoll: boiling alkalies produce the same change. It is extensively used in Europe for preparing benzoic acid artificially.

The hippurates are mostly soluble in boiling alcohol, and with the exception of the sesquisalt of iron, also soluble in boiling water; the alkaline salts are easily soluble in the cold.

The Biliary Acids.

On this subject, Dr. Strecker has published valuable investigations, which have thrown some light on the constituents of bile, hitherto but very imperfectly understood.

Choleic, or glycocholeic acid is the intrinsic ingredient of bile of most animals in the form of choleinate of soda. To prepare the pure acid, fresh bile is precipitated by acetate of lead, the precipitate extracted with boiling 85 per cent. alcohol, the solution decomposed by sulphuretted hydrogen and the filtrate allowed to cool with the addition of the wash water of the precipitate. Another method consists in evaporating fresh beef gall, exhausting with cold absolute alcohol, adding a little ether, decanting after several hours from the plaster-like mass, and treating with more ether. Thus prepared it contains paracholeic acid, which is left behind on treating it with boiling water.

It crystallizes in very thin white needles, is easily soluble in alcohol, little in water and ether; the aqueous solution has a sweet, slightly bitter taste. If boiled with alkalies it is converted into cholalic acid $=C_{48}H_{40}O_{10}$, and glycocoll.

Paracholeic acid is left behind as stated above, in pearly scales, has precisely the same composition, and appears to be merely a modification of choleic acid.

Impure *choleinate of soda, bilin* of Berzelius, has been proposed as a substitute for ox-gall in doses varying from 5 to 15 grains 3 or 4 times daily. An easy mode of preparation is by evaporating fresh ox-gall to one-half, precipitating slimy and coloring matter by alcohol, treating the filtrate with animal charcoal, evaporating and washing with ether.

Hyocholeic acid is prepared by dissolving in fresh hog's gall sulphate of soda, which precipitates the hyocholeinates with some coloring matter; this is dissolved in strong alcohol, decolorized and precipitated with ether; dilute sulphuric acid gradually separates the acid. It is a white resinous mass, which fuses immersed in hot water and dissolves easily in alcohol.

Sulphocholeic, taurocholeic acid is obtained by precipitating fresh ox-gall with sugar of lead; the filtrate is repeatedly precipitated by a little subacetate of lead, and filtered until the precipitate has a white color, when subacetate of lead with some ammonia is added, the white precipitate decomposed by sulphuretted hydrogen, and the filtrate evaporated in vacuo to a thick syrup.

EIGHTH GROUP.—*Acids connected with Coloring Matters.*

The organic coloring matters are chemical compounds, the character of which is not clearly ascertained, except in a few instances. All those substances which in their dry state or in solution are remarkable for decided coloration, may be called coloring principles; sanguinarina and hydrastia have been thus classified; they are, however, alkaloids, and will be treated of in their proper place. Of the coloring matters in the following lists, many of those placed in division *a*, have acid properties so decided as to decompose the salts of carbonic acid; the properties of others are not so easily recognized, as they frequently dissolve in acids and alkalies with different colors, and in such solutions are readily affected by atmospheric oxygen, particularly at high temperatures. But as far as the latter property is concerned, they are not the only acids changed in this way, the whole group of tannins and their derivatives are equally unstable, and probably even more so, than many coloring acids.

Most of those which follow are precipitated by acetate or subacetate of lead, and may be obtained in a free state by decomposing such precipitates, diffused in alcohol, by sulphuric acid or sulphuretted hydrogen. Compounds may be formed with alumina, if their mixture with a solution of alum is precipitated by ammonia; such colored precipitates are called *lakes*.

(a) *Acids from Phanerogamic Plants.*

Carthamic acid, $C_{14}H_8O_7$, *carthamin*. In carthamus. Amorphous, green, metallic lustre; little soluble in water; soluble in alcohol; purple, alkalies, red.

Crocic " $C_{20}H_{13}O_{11}$, *polychroite*. In saffron. Brilliantly red; by NO_5 green, by SO_3 indigo blue (tests for saffron); slightly soluble in water.

Rottleric " $C_{22}H_{10}O_6$, *rottlerin*. In the hairy covering of the fruit of rottlera tinctoria. In India used for dyeing silk. Brilliant yellow crystals.

Chrysophanic " $C_{28}H_{10}O_6$. In senna, rhubarb, &c. (See also *Rhamnin*.)

Gentisic " $C_{28}H_{10}O_{10}$. In gentian root. Yellow needles, not bitter; soluble in alcohol.

Santalic " $C_{30}H_{14}O_{10}$, *santalin*. Microscopic red crystals; insoluble in water.

Ruberythrynic " $C_{32}H_{18}O_{19}$. In madder, the root of rubia tinctorum. Yellow prisms; soluble in hot water, alcohol, and ether; by a ferment in madder, alkalies, and dilute acids, it is decomposed into glucose and

Alizarin, $C_{20}H_6O_6$. Sublimed in orange-colored, anhydrous prisms; from solutions, in brownish yellow prisms with 4HO; with alkalies purple, with lime and baryta, blue.

Purpurin, $C_{18}H_6O_6+HO$. By decomposition of madder by yeast under water; red or orange needles; with alkalies yellowish red, with lime and baryta purple.

Anchusic " $C_{35}H_{20}O_8$. In anchusa, alkanet root. Deep red; insoluble in water; the salts purple or blue.

Brazilic " $C_{36}H_{14}O_{14}$, *brazilin*. In Brazil wood. Yellowish-red prisms; soluble in alcohol and water.

Quercitric " $C_{36}H_{19}O_{21}$. In quercitron bark. Crystalline, chrome yellow, bitterish; soluble in alcohol. By dilute SO_3 into glucose and

Quercetin, $C_{24}H_8O_9$, crystalline, yellow; by SO_3 and MnO_2 yields formic acid.

Luteolic " $C_{40}H_{14}O_6$, *luteolin*. In French weld from reseda luteola. Yellow needles by sublimation; nearly insoluble in water.

Hæmatoxylic " $C_{40}H_{17}O_{15}$, *hæmatoxylin*. In logwood, from hæmatoxylon campechianum. Yellow prisms; little soluble in water; lose 8HO by heat.

Curcumic " ? *curcumin*. In turmeric, curcuma longa; yellow powder; slightly soluble in water; soluble in alcohol and ether, brown by alkalies.

(b) *Acids from Cryptogamic Plants.*

They are generally nearly colorless, or of a light red color, but, by various treatments, they yield some of the much esteemed pigments of commerce, of which litmus is employed as an important test in chemistry.

Orsellic, $C_{16}H_8O_8$. From lecanoric acid by boiling with milk of lime.

Parellic, $C_{18}H_6O_8$
Lecanoric, $C_{3}H_{14}O_{14}$
Erythric, $C_{44}H_{16}O_{16}$
} In various species of lecanora, variolaria, roccella, &c. Heat and alkalies change it to orceine, $C_{14}H_8O_4+2$ aq, which, by ammonia, is converted into orcine, $C_{14}H_7NO_6$, the principal coloring matter of *archil* and *cudbear*.

Litmus is probably obtained from the same lichens by a different process; its coloring principles are derivatives of orcine. The following have been distinguished; all are amorphous and little soluble in water:—

Azolitmin, $C_{14}H_7NO_8$; that is orcine, $C_{14}H_8O_4+NH_3+O_8=C_{14}H_7NO_8+2HO$.—Deep brown red, amorphous, soluble in alkalies with blue color. Its lakes are blue and purple.

Spaniolitmin, light red, insoluble in alcohol and ether, soluble in alkalies blue, lakes blue and purple.

Erythrolitmin, light red, easily soluble in alcohol. The hot solution deposits it in soft deep-red granules. Its lakes are purple.

Erythrolein, semiliquid; easily soluble in alcohol and ether with dark-red color, in ammonia purple. Its lakes are purple.

(c) *Azotized Vegetable Coloring matters.*

There are but two of this division, which have not the least relation to each other; moreover, one is a complex body never obtained in a state of purity.

Indigogen $C_{16}H_6NO_2$. In the juice of various plants yielding indigo.
Chlorophyll $C_{18}H_9NO_8$. The green coloring matter of leaves and herbs.

Indigogen, or Indigo white, is contained in the juice of plants yielding indigo in a state of combination with alkalies; owing to its proneness to oxidation, it is difficult to be obtained in a state of purity. During the process of fermentation of the leaves, it is oxidized and converted into indigo blue, other matters being separated at the same time, the whole constituting commercial indigo.

Chlorophyll is the name given to the green coloring matter of leaves; it is contained in globules or granules composed of a green membrane and semiliquid matter, enveloping a granule of amylum (Böhm), or it is a transparent colorless membrane, containing a green liquid with some minute granules. The different parts have not been separated, and consequently its chemical relation is as yet uncertain. It furnishes a green lake.

It has been asserted, that *xanthein* and *cyanin*, a yellow and a blue principle, furnish all the innumerable shades of the yellow, blue, green and red colors, which we admire in the petals of flowers; they are then in combination with one another, with various alkalies and acids.

(d) *Coloring Matters from Animal Sources.*

Carmic' acid, $C_{28}H_{14}O_{16}$. In cochineal.
Euxanthic " $2HO,C_{42}H_{16}O_{20}$. In Purree, an East Indian pigment.
Hæmatin $C_{44}H_{22}N_3O_6Fe$. In the blood of all vertebrate animals.

Carminic acid, obtained by precipitating a decoction with acetate of lead and separating the lead by sulph. hydrogen, is a friable brownish purple mass, easily soluble in alcohol and water; yields by dry distillation oxyphenic acid. On account of this last-mentioned property, some chemists think it identical with rufimoric acid, probably combined with a minute quantity of ammonia. This is the basis of carmine.

It is asserted that the flowers of monarda didyma contain the same coloring matter.

Euxanthic Acid.—Purree,[1] is chiefly euxanthate of magnesia, used for dyeing silk. The free acid appears in yellow prisms of a high lustre, is

[1] A yellow Chinese dyestuff of doubtful origin.

scarcely soluble in water, but soluble in alcohol and ether; its salts are yellow and crystallizable.

Hæmatin, Hæmatosin.—To prepare it, blood is liberated of its fibrin by beating, the liquid mixed with six measures of a concentrated solution of sulphate of soda, the filtered hæmatocrystallin is boiled with alcohol acidulated with sulphuric acid, the filtrate precipitated by carbonate of magnesia or ammonia, and the clear liquor evaporated.

It is a brownish-red powder, without taste or smell, insoluble in water, alcohol, and ether, but soluble in alkaline or acidulated liquids, producing a crimson-colored solution which carbonic and sulphuric acids blacken, oxygen brightens, and protoxide of nitrogen turns purple. With concentrated sulphuric acid, hydrogen is disengaged, and hæmatin is obtained free of iron, which is less soluble; by aqueous hypochlorous acid, it is colored black; all other coloring matters are destroyed by the same agent.

The *detection of blood* is sometimes very important in chemico-legal analysis. A solution of the blood stains is made and evaporated at a very low temperature; advantage is taken of the solubility of hæmatin in caustic potassa, which likewise separates iron rust or earthy matters that may be present.

The following are the characteristic tests for blood:—

1. The dry extract, on being heated in a glass tube, becomes black, at the same time giving off white vapors with the odor of burning feathers, which produce a brown color on curcuma paper.

2. By heating to redness with a little sodium, dissolving in water, mixing the filtrate with a mixed proto and per salt of iron, and supersaturating with muriatic acid; a precipitate of Prussian blue occurs.

3. An aqueous solution coagulates on boiling, the coagulum dissolves in caustic potassa and the liquid has a greenish color.

4. Chlorine water produces a decolorization and a white flocculent precipitate.

5. Nitric acid precipitates fine grayish floccules.

6. Tannin causes a grayish violet precipitate.

(See observations of Prof. Wittstein in *American Journal of Pharmacy*, xxix. page 30.)

CHAPTER VIII.

ON THE ALKALOIDS.

The whole subject of organic chemistry is comparatively new, the discovery of the existence of the vegetable alkaloids, the most important class of organic principles, dating back only to 1817, when Sertürner, a German apothecary, announced the existence of morphia.

The study of all classes of organic bodies has since progressed rapidly, many discoveries have been announced, which have been subjected to revision and been superseded by others, and this process is still going on; all that the pharmacologist can expect to do, is to present the actual state of knowledge upon the several subjects under examination, awaiting the progress of analytical and synthetical investigations to confirm existing views, or to present others more in accordance with the requirements of exact science.

In the present uncertain state of chemical knowledge in regard to the alkaloids, we shall follow the classification indicated by nature in her morphological developments, and arrange the natural alkaloids as the other classes of organic chemical principles upon a botanical basis; those of animal origin and those produced by artificial processes being grouped separately.

The alkaloids as a class, are the most powerful of organic principles, displaying their effects especially on the nervous system, which they so forcibly impress as to constitute many of them virulent poisons; a few, however, seem nearly destitute of active properties. They all contain nitrogen, and by destructive distillation, or by heating with alkalies, evolve ammonia; they evince their alkalinity by restoring the color to reddened litmus, and though not always crystalline or even solid, they combine with acids to form definite salts which are crystalline; they also, like the alkalies proper, form double salts with bichloride of platinum.

Most of the alkaloids are sparingly soluble in water, but dissolve freely in alcohol, especially with heat; some dissolve in ether, fixed and essential oils, and almost all in benzine, bisulphuret of carbon and chloroform, which may hence be used for their extraction. They are all precipitated from solution, whether alone or combined as salts, by tannic acid, which is hence, when taken immediately, one of the best chemical antidotes for them; they are precipitated by alkalies.

Alkaloids do not exist free in plants, but are generally combined with peculiar vegetable acids. Certain natural families of plants are distinguished by containing the same or similar alkaloids in their several species, while in other instances the same plant contains two or more different alkaloids. Opium contains nine, St. Ignatius bean three, sabadilla and veratrum three, while the different species of cinchona are known to contain at least four.

It is believed that all really poisonous plants contain an alkaloid or neutral characteristic principle, except, perhaps, those few acrid poisons which owe their activity to resins. It is remarkable that the development of the active principle is frequently only in one organ of the plant, and only at a certain period of its growth.

There is no convenient and scientific classification of the natural alkaloids, and their composition which is known, at least empirically, affords no clue to their properties and relations; indeed, their separation from some of the class of peculiar neutral principles, though sanctioned by a single well-known chemical distinction, seems forced and unnatural when we compare their physical and therapeutic properties, and is constantly lost sight of by writers.

Considering the recent discovery of most of this class, it might be expected that a uniform system of nomenclature would obtain in regard to them. This, however, is only measurably the case; they are most usually named from the generic title of the plants from which first derived, or from some distinguishing property; but by many they are indiscriminately terminated by *in* or *ia*. This practice is contrary to the rule adopted by common consent in this country, appropriating to the neutral principles the former, and to the alkaloids the latter, termination. Even the officinal alkaloids are constantly misnamed from a disregard to this rule. In converting the foreign names into our own Latinized form, some discrepancies arise, as aconitina and aconitia, quinidina and quinidia, applied to the same substances.

The mode of preparation of the alkaloids varies with their habitudes, and particularly according to their solubility and that of their native combinations. When the native salt is soluble, as meconate of morphia, and the alkaloid is itself insoluble, there is no difficulty in its extraction, the simple addition of a strong alkali to the infusion of the vegetable substance neutralizes the organic acid with which the alkaloid was associated, and it is thrown down in a more or less pure form. It more frequently happens that the native alkaloid salt is not so freely soluble in water, and then a diluted acid is employed for its extraction; so that its salt with an inorganic acid is obtained, and, this being decomposed by an alkali, yields the pure precipitated alkaloid. In a large number of cases, however, these simple methods of extraction are quite useless, and complex processes are necessarily resorted to. Some of these are founded upon the alkaloid being separated from its associated principles by subacetate of lead. Some processes direct ether, benzine or chloroform as the solvent, which separates the alkaloids from the other proximate principles present, and deposits them upon evaporation. The volatile alkaloids are, of course, prepared by appropriate modifications of the process of distillation.

It is not intended to go into detail on these processes except in a few cases, as many of the alkaloids are seldom called for, and those in use are prepared almost exclusively on a large scale by chemical manufacturers.

. The use of animal charcoal for its powerful absorbent properties, and the subsequent extraction of the alkaloid by appropriate solvents, is a process sometimes resorted to with success.

Chemical History.—The study of the native alkaloids has not as yet revealed their actual composition, the empirical formulas only being ascertained by our present means of analysis. From their behavior to tests we know that they have a certain relation to ammonia, and it is by the study of the artificial alkaloids that we are able to form an idea of the real chemical nature of the whole class.

By the destructive distillation of many nitrogenated substances, compounds are obtained containing nitrogen, and having the behavior of alkaloids; they are closely allied to ammonia, this base, though generally classed amongst the inorganic compounds, is, in fact, merely the last stage of decomposition of organic nitrogenated bodies, containing only two elements, nitrogen and hydrogen. Like it, the compounds referred to have strong alkaline properties, in some instances even stronger than ammonia, and, as already stated, like the strong inorganic alkalies, readily form crystallizable double salts with bichloride of platinum.

The organic alkalies, chiefly on account of their strong affinity for acids, and of their property for evolving ammonia when heated with caustic potassa, have long been viewed by some chemists, especially Berzelius, as compounds of ammonia with another complex body; since the discovery of the artificial alkaloids, and the investigations into their constitution, this view has been somewhat modified so as to consider them as ammonia, in the composition of which one or more equivalents of hydrogen have been substituted by a radical, and since this view of their composition has obtained the number of the artificial alkaloids has been largely increased, and the probability has been shown of its further increasing to a surprising extent.

Among the inorganic compounds, even some metals are capable of replacing one or more equivalents of hydrogen to form bases, as in the well-known instances of cuprum ammoniatum and hydrargyrum ammoniatum of the *Pharmacopœia;* it now remains to be shown how the elements are grouped in compounds of this nature, and which of the atomic elements or groups may be substituted for the hydrogen in ammonia to form alkaloids.

Such substituting compounds we find among the carbohydrogens, such as methyle C_2H_3, ethyle C_4H_5, propyle C_6H_7, butyle C_8H_9, amyle $C_{10}H_{11}$, capryle $C_{16}H_{17}$, phenyle (benzid) $C_{12}H_5$; oxygenated radicals like benzoyle $C_{14}H_5O_2$, cumyle $C_{20}H_{11}O_2$, &c.; the elements forming hydracids, bromine, iodine, chlorine, cyanogen; hyponitric acid NO_4, and a great variety of other elements and groups.

The newly-formed compounds have an alkaline character as long as they correspond with the composition of ammonia. As a general rule, the compounds with the radicals of the hydracids have a weaker basic character, which becomes less decided as the number of equivalents of these radicals is increased in the alkaloid; when they assume the composition of four equivalents of the element of the hydracid group, all alkalinity is lost; such compounds, however, do not correspond with ammonia or the oxide of ammonium in composition. The artificial alkaloids, after combining with acids, correspond closely in composition with the ammonia salts.

Series of Alkaloids containing Phenyle, $C_{12}H_5$, illustrating the foregoing.

Phenylamin (anilina)	$N(C_{12}H_5)H_2$.
Methylanilina	$N(C_2H_3)(C_{12}H_5)H$.
Ethylanilina	$N(C_4H_5)(C_{12}H_5)H$.
Diethylanilina	$N(C_4H_5)_2(C_{12}H_5)$.
Methyl-ethylanilina	$N(C_2H_3)(C_4H_5)(C_{12}H_5)$.[1]
Chloranilina	$N(C_{12}H_5)ClH$.
Bichloranilina	$N(C_{12}H_5)Cl_2$.
Trichloranilina	$N(C_{12}H_5)Cl_3$ (not a base).
Bromanilina	$N(C_{12}H_5)BrH$.
Iodinanilina	$N(C_{12}H_5)IH$.
Cyananilina	$N(C_{12}H_5)CyH$.
Nitranilina	$N(C_{12}H_5)(NO_4)H$(void).[2]

The chemical behavior of all the organic bases is closely allied to ammonia; there are particularly three reactions characteristic of this class:—

1. The residue of the treatment of uric acid with nitric acid is of a reddish color, and dissolves in ammonia with a beautiful purple, forming murexid. Precisely similar is the behavior of the organic alkaloids, though from their different composition, this color is somewhat altered; nicotia produces the purest purple, anilina a more violet color (Schwarzenberg).

2. Their behavior to Sonnenschein's test is alike. Whether free or combined with an acid, all alkaloids of the combination of ammonia are precipitated by phosphor-molybdic acid with various shades of yellow, some pulverulent, some flocculent, some voluminous. The following exhibits his results:—

[1] Similar combinations are formed with amyle, butyle, and other carbohydrogens.

[2] Chlorine, bromine, iodine, &c., in the proportion of two atoms, are less basic, and where three atoms enter into the compound, it ceases to have basic properties.

The precipitate is:—

Light yellow and flocculent with morphia, veratria, jervia, aconitia, emetia, atropia, daturia, ethylamin, diethylamin, triethylamin, methylamin, dimethylamin, trimethylamin, and anilin.
Light yellow and voluminous with caffeina, theobromina, conia, nicotia.
" " " *pulverulent* " mercuramin.
Yellowish-white and flocculent with quinia and cinchonia.
" " " *voluminous* " strychnia.
Brownish-yellow and flocculent " narcotina and piperina.
" " " *voluminous* " codeia.
Ochre-yellow and flocculent with brucia.
Dirty-yellow and flocculent with berberina.
Orange-yellow and flocculent with colchicia.
Sulphur-yellow and flocculent with sinamin.
Lemon-yellow and flocculent with quinolina.
" " " *pulverulent* with solania.

3. Another very important test for the discovery of the alkaloids is Scheibler's *phosphor-tungstate of soda*, which precipitates the organic alkaloids; a solution containing only $\frac{1}{200000}$ part of strychnia is rendered opalescent.

The reagent is prepared by adding phosphoric acid to tungstate of soda, and has been, as far as experiments performed on dogs are reliable, recommended as an antidote to poisonous alkaloids, with which an insoluble compound is formed, that cannot be assimilated.

These precipitates are all insoluble or nearly so in water, alcohol, ether and in dilute mineral acids, with the exception of phosphoric. Concentrated nitric acid, acetic, tartaric, citric, oxalic acids dissolve them on boiling, separating them again on cooling; citric acid, however, easily reduces the phosphor-molybdic acid. Caustic alkalies, their carbonates, borates, phosphates, tartrates, and acetates, dissolve the precipitates, some separating again the organic alkaloid. The oxides of the earthy metals, silver and lead, and their carbonates gradually decompose them liberating the base. .000071 gramme of strychnia in one cubic centimetre of solution is very plainly precipitated.

Asparagin, sinapolin, urea, hydrocyanic, hippuric, uric, and similar acids, and nitrogenous bodies, digitalin, meconin, and similar organic neutral principles are not precipitated.

For chemico-legal analyses Sonnenschein proposes the following easy way of detecting the alkaloids. The substances are several times exhausted with water strongly acidulated with muriatic acid, evaporated at about 90° F., to a thin syrupy consistence, diluted with water, after standing, filtered; precipitated by phosphor-molybdic acid in excess, the precipitate washed with water on a filter, acidulated with nitric and phosphor-molybdic acid, mixed with hydrate of baryta to alkaline reaction, and heated in a flask with a tube attached to gain ammonia and other volatile bases in muriatic acid. The residue is treated with carbonic acid, evaporated, exhausted with alcohol and evaporated; if necessary, recrystallized to purify the bases.

The phosphor-molybdic acid is prepared by precipitating molybdate of ammonia with phosphate of lime, the yellow precipitate is well washed with water, suspended in water, and dissolved by carbonate of soda, evaporated and heated to expel ammonia; if reduction should take place, it is moistened with NO_5, and again heated to redness; the mass is then dissolved in warm water and mixed with NO_5 to strong acid reaction, and diluted to ten times the weight of the dry salt; after filtering it has a golden yellow color; must be preserved against ammoniacal vapors.

Besides the method by phosphor-molybdic acid as above, the following older method of testing for the alkaloids, first proposed by Stas, has been more frequently tried and found successful.

The substance is mixed with twice its weight of pure strong alcohol and a little tartaric or oxalic acid, and heated to 160° to 165° F., after cooling, filtered, washed with strong alcohol, and the liquors evaporated below 95° over sulphuric acid or in a current of air; the remaining aqueous liquid is passed through a wetted filter, to separate fats, and again evaporated to near dryness; the product is exhausted with cold 95 per cent. alcohol, evaporated, dissolved in very little water, bicarb. soda or potassa added until carbonic acid ceases to be evolved, and agitated with four or six times its measure of rectified ether free from oil of wine. The residue, after evaporation of some of the ethereal solution, shows the presence of either a liquid or solid alkaloid. If the former, the ether is shaken with a little of a strong solution of caustic soda or potassa, decanted, the residue washed with ether, the liquids mixed with a little diluted SO_3. This ether then contains the animal substances, the water, the salts of nicotia, conia, and ammonia; sulphate of conia is slightly soluble in ether. The aqueous solution is decomposed by potassa and agitated with ether, the ether evaporated spontaneously; to get rid of all traces of ammonia, the residue is placed for a moment in vacuo over SO_3. Conia and nicotia may be easily distinguished by their odor; conia is insoluble, nicotia soluble, in water. In water mixed with conia, a few drops of chlorine water produce white precipitate.

If the alkaloid be solid, the ethereal solution is treated with soda or potassa, decanted, washed with much ether, evaporated, dissolved in little alcohol, evaporated, dissolved in water acidulated with SO_3, evaporated in vacuo or above sulphuric acid, treated with pure carbonate of potassa, then with absolute alcohol, which, on evaporation, yields the alkaloid crystallized. If, after the decomposition by an alkali, the addition of ether is delayed, morphia, which immediately after precipitation is more soluble, becomes crystalline, and ether then takes up but traces of it; alcoholic ether, however, takes up larger quantities of morphia. Otto therefore advises to add more soda to the washed (with ether) solution to prevent crystallization of morphia, then add muriate of ammonia, when, on evaporation, all morphia will crystallize out.

The volatile alkaloids, besides being obtained by means of ether, are obtained by distilling the aqueous acid solution with soda.

Meconic Acid.—For the detection of opium, it is not necessary to isolate the alkalies, since the reaction of meconic acid with sesquichloride of iron is unmistakable evidence of its presence. The substance is treated with alcohol and a few drops of muriatic acid, evaporated, dissolved in water, filtered, boiled with excess of magnesia, filtered, acidulated with muriatic acid, and a solution of sesquichloride of iron added; a deep brown red coloration indicates the presence of meconic acid.

1. *Syllabus of Natural Quaternary Alkaloids.*

	Ranunculaceæ.	
Aconitum Napellus.	Aconiti folia, *U.S.* " radix, "	Aconitia, $C_{60}H_{47}NO_{14}$. Napellina, ?
Delphinium staphisagria.	Staphisagria.	Delphinia, $C_{27}H_{19}NO_2$.
" consolida.	Delphinium, *U. S.*	Staphisaina, $C_{22}H_{23}NO_2$.
Hydrastis Canadensis.	Yellow root.	Hydrastia ?
Helleborus niger.	Helleborus, *U. S.*	Helleboria, ?
	Menispermaceæ.	
Cissampelos pareira.	Pareira, *U. S.*	Cissampelina, $C_{36}H_{21}NO_6$.

Anamirta cocculus.	Cocculus Indicus.	Menispermina, $C_{18}H_{12}NO_2$.
Cocculus palmatus.	Colomba, *U. S.*	Berberina, $C_{42}H_{18}NO_9$.
Cœscinium fenestratum.	Columbo wood.	
Berberideæ.		
Berberis vulgaris.	Barberry root.	Berberina, $C_{42}H_{18}NO_9$. Berbina. ?
Papaveraceæ.		
Papaver somniferum.	Opium, *U. S.*	Morphia, $C_{34}H_{19}NO_6$. Narcotina, $C_{42}H_{21}NO_{14}$. Codeia, $C_{36}H_{21}NO_6$. Thebaia, $C_{38}H_{21}NO_6$. Narceina, $C_{46}H_{29}NO_{18}$. Opiania, $C_{66}H_{37}NO_{21}$. Papaverina, $C_{40}H_{21}NO_8$. Phormia, $C_{30}H_{18}NO_{14}$. Opina, ?
Sanguinaria Canadensis.	Sanguinaria, *U. S.*	Sanguinarina, $C_{36}H_{16}NO_8$.
Chelidonium majus.	Celandine.	Chelidina, $C_{40}H_{20}N_3O_6$.
Glaucium luteum.		Glaucina, ? Gaucina, ?
Fumariaceæ.		
Corydalis fabacea, bulbosa, tuberosa, and formosa.	Turkey corn, &c.	Corydalina, $C_{50}H_{30}NO_{20}$.
Fumaria officinalis.	Fumatory.	Fumarina, ?
Violareæ.		
Viola odorata.	Viola, *U. S.*	Violia, ?
Anchieta salutaris.		Anchietia, ?
Byttneraceæ.		
Theobroma cacao.	Chocolate nut.	Theobromia, $C_{14}H_8N_4O_4$.
Camellieæ.		
Thea Bohea.	Chinese tea.	Theina identical with caffeina. (See *Celastrineæ* and *Cinchonaceæ.*)
Sapindaceæ.		
Paullinia sorbilis.	Guarana.	
Rutaceæ.		
Peganum harmala.	Harmel rue.	Harmalina, $C_{26}H_{14}N_2O_2$. Harmina, $C_{26}H_{12}N_2O_2$.
Celastrineæ.		
Ilex Paraguayensis.	Paraguay tea.	Caffeina. (See *Cinchonaceæ.*)
Leguminosæ.		
Geoffroya Jamaicensis.	Jamaica cabbage-tree bark.	Jamaicina ?
" Surinamensis.	Surinam " "	Surinamina ?
Umbelliferæ.		
Conium maculatum.	Conium, *U. S.*	Conhydrina, $C_{16}H_{17}NO_2$. (See *Conia* among the ternary alkaloids.)
Cinchonaceæ.		
Various Peruvian barks of the genus cinchona.	Cinchona, *U. S.*	Quinia, $C_{40}H_{24}N_2O_4$. Quinidia, $C_{40}H_{24}N_2O_4$. Cinchonia, $C_{40}H_{24}N_2O_2$. Cinchonidia, $C_{40}H_{24}N_2O_2$.
Jaen and Cusco bark. **Para bark.** **Pitaya bark.** **Carthagena bark.**	Unofficinal barks.	Aricia, $C_{40}H_{21}N_2O_6$. Paricia, ? Pitayia, ? Carthagia, ?
Cephaëlis ipecacuanha.	Ipecacuanha, *U. S.*	Emetia, $C_{30}H_{24}NO_8$?
Coffea Arabica.	Coffee.	Caffeina, Theina, $C_{16}H_{10}N_4O_4+2$ aq.
Compositæ.		
Arnica montana.	Arnica, *U. S.*	Arnicina, ?
Apocynaceæ.		
Strychnos nux vomica.	Nux vomica, *U. S.*	Strychnia, $C_{42}H_{22}N_2O_4$. Brucia, $C_{46}H_{26}N_2O_8$.
" Ignatia.	St. Ignatius bean.	Igasuria, $C_{44}H_{26}N_2O_8$.
Cerbera, unknown species.	Pao pereira.	Pereirina ?
Solanaceæ.		
Solanum dulcamara and other species.	Dulcamara, *U. S.*	Solania, $C_{42}H_{35}NO_{14}$.

Atropa belladonna.	Belladonna, *U. S.*	Atropia, $H_{34}H_{23}NO_6$. Belladonnia, "
Datura stramonium.	Stramonium, *U. S.*	Daturia, identical with atropia?
Hyoscyamus niger and albus.	Hyoscyamus, *U. S.*	Hyoscyamia, $C_{34}H_{23}NO_6$.
Laurineæ.		
Nectandra rodiei.	Bebeeru bark.	Bebeerina, $C_{38}H_{21}NO_6$. Sepeerina, ?
Piperaceæ.		
Piper longum, nigrum and album.	Piper, *U. S.*	Piperina, $C_{70}H_{37}N_2O_{10}+2$ aq.
Piper caudatum.	Cubeba clusii.	
Melanthaceæ.		
Veratrum album, sabadilla viride.	Veratrum, *U. S.*	Veratria, $C_{64}H_{52}N_2O_{16}$. Sabadillia, $C_{40}H_{26}N_2O_{10}$? Jervia, $C_{60}H_{45}N_2O_5$.
Colchicum autumnale.	Colchicum, *U. S.*	Colchicia. ?

2. *Syllabus of Artificial Quaternary Alkaloids.*

Quinicia, $C_{40}H_{24}N_2O_4$.	From quinia and quinidia.	(See *Cinchona Alkaloids.*)
Cinchonicia, $C_{40}H_{24}N_2O_2$.	From cinchonia and cinchonidia.	
Tropia, ?	From atropia.	
Porphyrharmina ?	From harmalina and harmina.	

3. *Native Ternary Alkaloids.*

Leguminosæ.		
Spartium scoparium.	Scoparius, *U.S.*, Broom.	Sparteina, $NC_{15}H_{14}$.
Umbelliferæ.		
Conium maculatum.	Conium, *U.S.*, Hemlock.	Conia, $NC_{16}H_{15}$.
Lobeliaceæ.		
Lobelia inflata.	Lobelia, *U. S.*	Lobelina, ?
Solanaceæ.		
Nicotiana tabacum.	Tabacum, *U.S.*, Tobacco.	Nicotia, $N_2C_{20}H_{14}$.
Rosaceæ.		
Pyrus communis.	Flowers Sorbus aucuparia, Cratægus monogyna and oxycantha.	Secalina, or Propylamin. } NC_6H_9.
Chenopodeæ.		
Chenopodium vulvaria.	Herb.	
Fungi.		
Secale cornutum.	Ergota, *U. S.*	

4. *Artificial Ternary Alkaloids.*

(a) *By Decomposition of Native Alkaloids, mostly with Potassa or other Alkalies.*

Conia, $NC_{16}H_{15}$. From conhydrina by anhydrous phosphoric acid.

Ethylamin, NC_4H_7. From narcotina; thin colorless liquid, boiling at 66° F.; strong ammoniacal odor; burning with a yellow flame; miscible with water; strong base.

Propylamin, NC_6H_9. From narcotina and codeia. (See *Secalina.*)

Methylamin, NC_2H_5. From narcotina, codeia, morphia, caffeina by potassa; a liquefiable gas, ammoniacal odor; very soluble in water; burns with a yellow flame; strong base.

Piperidina, $NC_{10}H_{11}$. From piperina by a mixture of soda and lime.

(b) *From Alkaloids, and in Coal Tar.*

Lepidina, $NC_{20}H_9$. From cinchonia by potassa; colorless oil; distils at 500°.

Pyridina, $NC_{10}H_5$. Like former; distils at 242°; soluble in water.

Lutidina, $NC_{14}H_9$. Like former; distils at 310°; aromatic oil separated from its aqueous solution by heating.

Pyrrolina, NH_8O_5. Like former: distils at 271°; agreeable ethereal odor; colors pinewood moistened with HCl carmine red; turns red with NO_5.

Quinolina or **Leucolina**, $NC_{18}H_7$. From quinia, cinchonia, strychnia, berberina by potassa; oily; disagreeable bitter almond odor; distils at 462°; dissolves much water, in which it is little soluble.

Picolina, $NC_{12}H_7$. From piperina and cinchonia by potassa; distils at 275°; pine wood is colored yellow.

(c) *From other Sources.*

Toluidina, $NC_{14}H_9$. From nitrotoluol by NH_3 and HS; from oil of turpentine by NO_5 and KO; little soluble in water, easily in other solvents; liquid at 104°; boiling at 388°; intensely yellow with pine wood.

Anilina, $NC_{12}H_7$. From coal-tar; from indigo by KO, from nitrobenzol by HS and NH_4S, &c.; vinous odor; aromatic taste; boiling point 360°; by NO_5 deep blue, yields picric acid. Synonyms crystallin, benzidamin, phenylamin.

Aconitia, U.S.

This alkaloid is directed to be prepared from the root by extracting with boiling alcohol, evaporating, treating the alcoholic extract with a mixture of water and dilute sulphuric acid. The sulphate being decomposed by ammonia, yields a precipitate of aconitia, which requires to be purified, and is then in the condition of a white or yellowish powder, containing water. It is, when anhydrous, in the form of a brittle mass, usually of a yellowish brown color; with difficulty it may be obtained in crystalline grains. It imparts a sensation of numbness to the tongue, which is extremely powerful and characteristic. It is sparingly soluble in water, though forming soluble salts on the addition of acids; it dissolves freely in ether, alcohol, and chloroform. Being a very small product of the root, it is extremely expensive and liable to adulteration; probably very little that is sold as such is reasonably pure.

Aconitia is one of the most virulent of poisons, and extreme caution is necessary if used internally. Externally applied, it produces on the skin a prickling sensation followed by numbness and a feeling of constriction. Its principal use is in cases of neuralgia, in ointment made by triturating the alkaloid first with a little alcohol or oil, and then with an unctuous vehicle. From a half to two grains are added to one drachm of the ointment. The galenical preparations of aconite will answer every useful purpose to which aconitia can be applied. The salts of aconitia are uncrystallizable, or with difficulty obtained in a crystalline state; they are as poisonous as the pure alkaloid.

Concentrated nitric acid dissolves the alkaloid without coloration; concentrated sulphuric acid imparts a yellow, afterwards a reddish violet color.

Napellina occurs in the genus aconitum, with aconitia in very small proportion. It may be obtained from the crude aconitia, which is dissolved with as little ether as possible; the residue is dissolved in absolute alcohol, precipitated by acetate of lead, treated with sulphuretted hydrogen, then with carbonate of potassa, evaporated, exhausted by absolute alcohol, and decolorized by animal charcoal. It is a white electrical powder, of a bitter, afterwards burning taste; pure ether dissolves it with some difficulty. It is distinguished from aconitia by not being precipitated by ammonia, from its diluted solution in muriatic acid, and by being more soluble in dilute alcohol.

Delphinia.—The alcoholic extract of the seed of delphinium staphisagria is treated with dilute sulphuric acid, precipitated with an alkali, again dissolved in dilute sulphuric acid, the coloring matter precipitated by a few drops of nitric acid, the alkaloïd by potassa; it is then obtained by evaporation of its solution in absolute alcohol, one pound yields about one drachm.

It is a light yellowish or white powder; its taste is burning, acrid, very persistent in the throat; it is soluble in alcohol and ether; the salts are bitter and acrid, some deliquescent.

Staphisaina.—If delphinia is dissolved in ether, this alkaloid remains behind as a yellowish, uncrystallizable mass, of an acrid taste, which forms acid salts.

Hydrastia is prepared by treating the aqueous extract of yellow root with magnesia, and extracting the precipitate with boiling alcohol.

Brilliant yellow crystals, insoluble in water, sparingly soluble in cold alcohol and ether, soluble in chloroform and boiling alcohol, fusible in heated turpentine; it has an alkaline reaction on litmus; by concentrated nitric acid it is colored deep red. Concentrated sulphuric acid has little action in cold; when heated a purple color is produced; concentrated muriatic acid dissolves it.

The salts, which are intensely bitter, have not been obtained in crystals yet.

Hydrastin is much employed by the eclectics as a valuable tonic, which has an especial action on diseased mucous tissues. It is given in doses of from three to five grains several times a day.

Helleboria is obtained by treating the root with alcohol containing one-fiftieth sulphuric acid; the tincture is treated with magnesia, the filtrate acidulated with sulphuric acid, water is added, the alcohol distilled off, filtered, decomposed with carbonate of potassa, and by shaking with ether, the alkaloid obtained in solution. It is white, crystalline, easily soluble in water, alcohol, and ether; taste bitter and acrid; not volatile; as it evolves ammonia when treated with potassa, its proper place appears to be among the alkaloids, though its chemical nature is not known.

Cissampelina or Pelosina.—It is prepared by carefully precipitating an infusion of the root made with sulphuric acid water, washing, drying at 212°, and dissolving in absolute ether, which is free from alcohol and water.

The yellowish hard semitransparent mass is colored yellow by sunlight; without smell; taste disagreeably sweetish bitter; soluble in alcohol and ether; insoluble in water, but swelling up and combining with it; in this state it has an alkaline reaction.

The alkaloid and its salts are rapidly oxidized.

Menispermina is contained in the shell of cocculus Indicus. To prepare it, the alcoholic extract is first extracted by cold water, then by hot water, from which solution mineral acids precipitate picrotoxic acid in crystals; the filtrate is precipitated by an alkali, the precipitate extracted with acetic acid, again precipitated, washed with cold alcohol, and the alkaloid extracted by ether.

It crystallizes in needles or prisms, which are very bitter.

Berberina is one of the active principles of barberry and colombo root. It is prepared from the aqueous extract by treating it with 82 per cent. alcohol, distilling it off, crystallizing the alkaloid in a cool place, and purifying it by recrystallization.

It is best extracted from colombo wood, the wood of coscinium fenestratum, a tree growing in Ceylon. The decoction of the wood is evaporated, the extract treated with boiling alcohol, filtered while hot, distilled to an oily residue, which, after twenty-four hours, is filled with crystals of berberina; the mother liquor is removed, and the crystals purified by a recrystallization from alcohol, and treating with animal charcoal.

It crystallizes in fine yellow needles, containing 12 HO, of a strongly bitter taste, insoluble in ether, easily soluble in boiling water and alcohol. By concentrated sulphuric acid it is dissolved with an olive-green color; by concentrated nitric acid, red with nitrous acid fumes; by distillation with lime it yields quinolina.

It is a dye for silk, cotton, wool, and linen. Its salts have a yellow color, and are crystallizable.

Berbina (*Oxyacanthin*).—The bark of barberry root is extracted with alcohol, mixed with one-eighth water, the alcohol distilled off, the filtrate evaporated, berberina crystallized out, the mother liquor precipitated by carbonate of soda, and the precipitate treated with sulphuric acid and animal charcoal.

White powder, colored brown by sunlight, bitter; nearly insoluble in water, soluble in alcohol, ether, fixed and volatile oils.

The salts are crystallizable, colorless, bitter.

The Opium Alkaloids and their Salts.

The various kinds of opium, as produced in different localities, always contain morphia, on which the activity of opium depends in a large degree; narcotina and some other alkaloids are likewise always present, but some species contain, besides them, one or two alkaloids which have not been found in opium as generally produced. Besides the acid and neutral principle, there have been discovered nine distinct alkaloids, many of which, however, are still little known.

Morphia.

Morphia, which is the only one commonly used in medicine, was first discovered, and is the most abundant. It is the best and most familiar of the alkaloids.

There are various processes for its preparation, of which that of the *Pharmacopœia*, already adverted to, is the simplest and best for the student who may be disposed to attempt this, by no means difficult experiment. Reduced in quantity to suit the purpose, it is nearly as follows:—

Take of	Opium, sliced	℥j.
	Solution of ammonia . . .	f℥ss.
	Water,	
	Alcohol,	
	Animal charcoal, of each . .	sufficient.

Macerate the opium with f℥vj of water, working it with the hands or a pestle, as described under the head of *Tincture of Opium*, into a paste (if powdered opium is used, this is unnecessary); then digest it for twenty-four hours, and strain. Macerate or digest the residue in the same way, successively, with similar portions of water, and strain; then mix the infusions, evaporate to f℥viij, and filter. To the concentrated aqueous solution thus obtained add first f℥vj of alcohol, and then fʒij of solution of ammonia, previously mixed with about f℥ss of alcohol; cover the vessel and set it aside. After twenty-four hours pour in the remaining fʒij of solution of ammonia, mixed, as before, with alcohol, and again set aside that the morphia may crystallize out. The only remaining process is to purify the crystals which are formed in the bottom of the vessel. This is done by dissolving them in boiling alcohol, and filtering, while hot, through animal charcoal. A common flask will serve for the solution, and, for small operations, the application of heat to the funnel will be unnecessary. It may be conveniently arranged over an evaporating dish. The filtered liquid, as it falls, will be immediately cooled by contact with the dish, and the extended surface will favor the spontaneous evaporation of the alcohol, so that a small crop of crystals (40 to 60 grains) of morphia may be expected.

This is an excellent method of testing the value of specimens of opium, except that, for approximate results, it is not necessary to carry out the last part of the directions, but is as well to take the weight of the crystallized morphia as at first thrown down. The animal charcoal deprives the product of color, but is apt to absorb a portion of alkaloid also; so that, to get the entire yield, the charcoal should be digested in a further portion of alcohol, which should be added to the filtrate. The motive for using alcohol with the ammonia added to the concentrated liquid in the first instance, is to take up the resinous coloring matters, which would otherwise contaminate the precipitate.

Morphia, as thus obtained, is in small but brilliant prismatic crystals, containing 2HO, or nearly six per cent., which are transparent and colorless, intensely bitter when dissolved, but nearly insoluble in water, also insoluble in ether. It dissolves in about thirty parts of boiling alcohol, in fixed alkaline solutions, and with great facility in dilute acids, which it neutralizes, forming salts. One hundred parts of chloroform dissolve .57 of morphia; if heated with caustic potassa, methylamin is evolved. Of course, it is entirely dissipated by heat.

In powder, it strikes a deep blue color with neutral salts of sesquioxide, or with sesquichloride of iron, decomposes iodic acid with liberation of iodine, and forms, with nitric acid added to it in powder, a red compound passing into yellow; with nitric containing some sulphuric acid, it strikes a green color; chlorine colors morphia diffused in water orange, then red, and after solution yellow, and ultimately causes a flocculent precipitate.

Morphia may be considered pure, if ether takes nothing up, if it is wholly soluble in alcohol, and when its solution in diluted nitric acid is not precipitated by nitrate of silver, nitrate of baryta, phosphate and oxalate of ammonia.

Officinal Salts.—These are three in number, as follows: sulphate, muriate, and acetate. They are made by forming solutions of the alkaloids in the appropriate acids and evaporating.

Morphiæ Sulphas, U. S.—This is in white feathery crystals, very soluble in water, of an intensely bitter taste. It is by far the most common of the morphia salts. DOSE, one-eighth to one-fourth grain.

Morphiæ Murias, U. S.—This is most used in England, where it is officinal as morphiæ hydrochloras. It is somewhat less soluble in water, though sufficiently so for use in medicine. DOSE, the same as of the sulphate.

Morphiæ Acetas, U. S.—This is a white powder, seldom crystalline in appearance. It is apt to be deficient in the proportion of the acid ingredient, and to be comparatively insoluble, in which case a few drops of acetic acid to the liquid will make a clear solution. This is much used for external application, though adapted also to the form of powder or pill. DOSE, the same as of the foregoing.

Morphiæ Citras.—In some parts of the United States a solution of this salt is employed. It is prepared by dissolving 16 grains of morphia with 8 grains citric acid and ½ grain cochineal in one ounce of water. It is considered 2½ times stronger than laudanum; its dose is 10 drops.

Valerianate of morphia is an unofficinal salt, made by neutralizing the alkaloid with valerianic acid. Its dose is from one eighth to one-half grain.

Narcotina is a brilliant crystalline principle, which is easily obtained by extracting aqueous extract of opium with ether, which leaves it, on evaporation, nearly pure. It is nearly insoluble in water; its alcoholic solution is very bitter, but has no alkaline reaction; it is insoluble in alkalies and lime-water; 100 parts of chloroform dissolve 37.17 parts, and 1 ounce of olive oil 1.2 grain of narcotina; it is not acted on by sesquisalt of iron or pure nitric acid, but sulphuric, with but a trace of nitric acid, colors it blood red. Its salts are generally acid and crystallize with difficulty. Narcotina is not narcotic. It has been given as a tonic and antiperiodic, in doses as high as half a drachm, without the production of narcotic symptoms. The following four homologous varieties of narcotina have been distinguished, which, by treatment with caustic potassa, yield homologous volatile bases:—

Normal narcotina, $C_{42}H_{91}NO_{14}$, yields ammonia.
Methylic narcotina, $C_{44}H_{23}NO_{14}$, yields methylamin.
Ethylic narcotina, $C_{46}H_{25}NO_{14}$, yields ethylamin.
Propylic narcotina, $C_{48}H_{27}NO_{14}$, yields propylamin.

Narcotina, by the influence of dilute SO_3 and hyperoxide of manganese, is decomposed into water, opianic acid, and the following stronger alkaloid.

Cotarnina.—Crystallizing in colorless prisms, easily soluble in boiling water, intensely bitter, alkaline reaction. The various homologous kinds of narcotina appear to furnish also homologous kinds of cotarnina:—

Normal cotarnina, $C_{22}H_{9}NO_{6}$. Methylic cotarnina, $C_{24}H_{11}NO_{6}$.
Ethylic cotarnina, $C_{26}H_{12}NO_{6}$. Propylic cotarnina, $C_{28}H_{13}NO_{6}$.

Codeia crystallizes in octohedral or prismatic crystals, with two equivalents of water, soluble in alcohol, ether, and in boiling water. It is not precipitated by ammonia, and is insoluble in fixed alkalies; it is colored yellow by nitric acid. Its salts are neutral, and have a bitter taste.

In doses from one-fifth to one-half grain, it is said to produce a tranquillizing effect, while over two grains produce sleep, with stupefaction, and sometimes with nausea and vomiting.

Thebaia, or paramorphia, is contained in the precipitate produced by lime in an infusion of opium, from which it is obtained by extracting with muriatic acid, precipitating by ammonia, and crystallizing from ether.

The small alkaline crystals have an acrid taste, are little soluble in water, and colored red by sulphuric acid.

Narceina occurs in very thin prisms, of a bitter taste, which are fusible at 197.5°, and easily soluble in hot water. Its combinations with acids are obtained with some difficulty; they are rendered blue by a little water, colorless by more water, blue again by fused chloride of calcium.

Opiania is contained in Egyptian opium; it crystallizes in long prisms, which are insoluble in water, but dissolve in hot alcohol. It has an alkaline reaction, a bitter taste, and is narcotic. Nitric acid renders it yellow, if added to its solution in sulphuric acid, blood-red changing to light yellow.

Papaverina is an alkaloid in small acicular crystals, which turn blue with sulphuric acid; with muriatic acid in excess it forms very insoluble colorless prisms, which possess a high refractive power. It is insoluble in water, little soluble in alcohol and ether.

Phormia, or pseudomorphia, has been obtained by Pelletier only from a few lots of opium, after precipitating the sulphate of morphia by ammonia, and evaporating the mother liquid, white micaceous scales are separated, containing about one-tenth per cent. of SO_3; after removing the acid by ammonia, the crystals of phormia are not so lustrous as before, and it is not so soluble in water, it is insoluble in absolute alcohol and ether, somewhat soluble in alcohol of .833 sp. gr., soluble in caustic soda and potassa. Nitric acid colors it red, oxidizing it ultimately to oxalic acid. Neutral salts of sesquioxide of iron render it blue; the blue solution, in sesquichloride of iron, turns green on boiling; on the addition of ammonia, wine-red. It is not poisonous.

Opina or Porphyroxin.—Powdered opium is exhausted by cold ether, then by a weak solution of carbonate of potassa, again by ether, codeia, thebaia, and opina are dissolved; the extract of the last tincture is dissolved in muriatic acid, precipitated by ammonia (codeia remains in solution), the precipitate is treated with alcohol, which, leaving thebaia behind, dissolves opina. It crystallizes in fine needles, soluble in alcohol, ether, and dilute acids; solutions in mineral acids turn purplish red on boiling.

The following is Merck's TEST FOR OPIUM:—

The concentrated solution is treated with caustic potassa, and shaken with ether; a strip of paper having been dipped several times in the ethereal solution, is moistened with muriatic acid, and exposed to the vapors of boiling water; on account of the opina, the paper will acquire a red color, if opium had been present in the liquid. (See also *Meconic Acid.*)

Sanguinarina, or Chelerythrina.

This alkaloid is derived from the root of one of our most familiar indigenous plants, by exhausting it with weak sulphuric acid, precipitating by ammonia, dissolving it out by ether, and precipitating by sulphuric acid. It is a white, pearly substance, of an acrid taste, very soluble in alcohol, also soluble in ether, in fixed and volatile oils. With acids it forms soluble salts, which are remarkable for their beautiful red, crimson, and scarlet colors. From this it is inferred that a native salt of this alkaloid is the occasion of the brilliant color of the fresh juice of the plant. The alkaloid is poisonous.

Chelidina.—The precipitate, as above, which is insoluble in ether, is exhausted with dilute sulphuric acid, the solution precipitated by ammonia, and the precipitate crystallized from acetic acid, when colorless flat crystals remain, which are free of acetic acid, have a bitter taste, and dissolve in alcohol, fixed and volatile oils.

It forms colorless, acidulous salts, of a purely bitter taste, which are not poisonous.

Another alkaloid has been discovered by Prof. E. S. Wayne, in the ethereal solution of sanguinarina; its sulphate remains dissolved in ether after sanguinarina is precipitated; its salts are of a deep red color. (See *Am. Journ. of Pharm.*, vol. xxviii. p. 520.)

Glaucina is prepared from the juice of the herb of glaucium luteum, by precipitating it with sugar of lead, treating the filtrate with sulphuretted hydrogen, precipitating it with tannin, decomposing the precipitate by lime, and crystallizing from alcohol.

It is in pearly scales, of a burning, acrid taste, soluble in boiling water, ether, and alcohol. It assumes a red color in the light, dissolves in sulphuric acid, with a greenish-blue color, rendered reddish by dilution, and precipitated by ammonia, with a blue color. Its salts are acrid.

Picroglaucina, gaucina, is prepared from the root in a similar way. It is in white crystalline scales, of a bitter, nauseous taste, soluble in water, alcohol, and ether, and colored deep green by sulphuric acid. The salts are crystallizable, and of a bitter, nauseous taste.

Corydalina.—The juice of the root is precipitated by acetate of lead, dilute sulphuric acid and ammonia; the last precipitate yields the alkaloids to alcohol. It has also been obtained from the American species, though by a different process.

Soft grayish white lumps or powder, colorless prisms or scales, without odor, nearly tasteless, insoluble in water, soluble in ether and alcohol, alkaline reaction, the solutions are greenish-yellow; it melts in boiling water, is soluble in caustic alkalies; the salts are soluble, very bitter, somewhat crystallizable; nitric acid, even in dilute solutions, colors corydalina red or blood-red, destroying it at the same time. (See *Am. Journ. of Pharm.*, vol xxvii. p. 205.)

Fumarina is similar to the foregoing, but soluble in water and insoluble in ether.

Violia.—The alcoholic extract is treated with ether, then boiled with sulphuric acid and water, precipitated with oxide of lead, the precipitate treated with alcohol. Similar in its action to emetia; but differing chemically from it by rendering reddened litmus paper green, and being more soluble in water, less in alcohol. Some violets, however, contain *emetia.*

Anchietia.—In the root of anchieta salutaris, which is successfully used in Brazil, for the treatment of various skin diseases.

The bark of the root is mashed and allowed to ferment, extracted with muriatic acid and water, evaporated and precipitated by ammonia; by treatment with animal charcoal and repeated crystallization from alcoholic solution it is obtained pure. Yield about .42 per cent.

Straw-yellow needles, insoluble in ether and water, easily soluble in alcohol, no smell, taste sharp, nauseous; nitric acid colors it orange-yellow to chrome-yellow; sulphuric acid violet to blackish.

The salts are soluble, crystallizable; the muriate is colorless, crystallizing from hot water in star-like needles, after which it is insoluble in water.

Theobromina.—It is prepared from the chocolate nut, by a process similar to that for obtaining caffeina. It dissolves with difficulty in boiling water, alcohol and ether; boiling solution of caustic baryta dissolves it, and it separates again on cooling. It has a slightly bitter taste, is unalterable in contact with the air, is rendered brown on exposure to a heat of 480°, and sublimes at between 554° and 563°, leaving but little charcoal.

Its salts resemble those of caffeina. The tannate is soluble in an excess of tannic acid in alcohol and boiling water. With chlorine it is converted into methylamin.

Caffeina, Thein, Guaranin, Psoralein.—It is prepared from the hot infusion of tea or coffee by precipitating the tannic acid with subacetate of lead, boiling the mixture, filtering, removing the excess of lead by hydrosulphuric or sulphuric acid, evaporating the clear liquor and recrystallizing the product.

A. Vogel, Jun.'s, method is as follows: Powdered coffee is extracted by commercial benzol, this is distilled off, leaves an oil and caffeina behind; the oil is removed by a little ether or by water, from which latter liquid the alkaloid crystallizes on cooling.

Coffee contains about ½ per cent., tea (gun-powder) 1 to 4 per cent., ilex Paraguayensis (psoralea glandulosa), .13 per cent. of *caffeina.* **Black tea contains more caffeina than green tea.**

It crystallizes in needles, losing 2HO water of crystallization at 302° F.; it melts at 352° and sublimes at 725° without decomposition; it is soluble in alcohol, ether, chloroform and hot water, cold water dissolves but little. If boiled with nitric acid, the yellow liquid assumes a purple color.

Its salts and double salts are well defined and crystallizable, some are decomposed by water. It produces a crystalline precipitate with nitrate of silver, and with iodide of potassium and mercury. Tannate of caffeina is obtained as a white precipitate, soluble in boiling water.

Caffeina is not an alimentary, but a poisonous substance, producing death in various animals, by palsying the nervous system. (*Dr. Stuhlmann.*) Its citric acid salt, with excess of the acid, has been used with considerable success in the treatment of sick-headache. (See *Extemporaneous Pharmacy.*)

Harmalina.—The seeds of peganum harmala (ruta sylvestris), a plant of Southern Russia, are used there as a dye, and are said to be inebriating and soporific.

The neutralized infusion with acidulated water is saturated with table salt, in which solution the chlorides are insoluble; the purified salts are precipitated by excess of ammonia, when harmina crystallizes first in needles, afterwards harmalina in scales. Colorless scales or octohedrons, nearly tasteless, with difficulty soluble in water and ether.

The salts are of a sulphur yellow color, not dyeing; of a purely bitter taste; precipitated by excess of acids or inorganic salts. By digestion with alcohol another alkaloid,

Porphyrharmina, harmala of Goebel, is obtained of a red color, yielding red salts and dyeing.

Harmina is a product of oxidation of harmalina; it crystallizes in colorless prisms; its salts are colorless, but otherwise resemble those of harmalina. Harmina and harmalina are splendid red dyes, if previously converted into porphyrharmina.

Jamaicina is obtained from the cabbage-tree bark, Geoffroya jamaicensis, also called andira inermis.

The aqueous infusion is precipitated by basic acetate of lead, treated with sulphuretted hydrogen and evaporated. It crystallizes in yellow quadrangular tables, bitter, soluble in water, little in alcohol, melting below the boiling point of water. The salts are yellow, bitter, some crystallizable; in small doses they produce restlessness, in larger purging. It is said to be vermifuge.

Surinamina.—From the bark of andira retusa (Geoffroya surinamensis), is prepared similarly to the above. It crystallizes in fine white microscopic needles, without taste or smell, nearly insoluble in cold water and ether, soluble in boiling alcohol and boiling water.

The Cinchona Alkaloids and their Salts.

Quinia.

This alkaloid is prepared from various species of cinchona bark, which contain it in combination with kinic acid and the astringent principle called cincho-tannic acid. These combinations being only partially soluble in water, resort is had to an acid which liberates the alkaloid in a soluble form. That used in our officinal process for preparing the sulphate of quinia is muriatic, which is mixed with water in which the powdered bark is boiled. The very soluble muriate of quinia contained in this decoction is decomposed, giving up its acid to the lime, while the quinia is liberated, and, being insoluble, is precipitated with the excess of lime added, the water retaining the chloride of calcium resulting from the reaction, and most of the impurities, in solution. The precipitated quinia and excess of lime being now digested in alcohol, the former is dissolved, and the impure quinia is obtained by evaporating this alcoholic solution. The remaining part of the process consists in converting this into the officinal sulphate, at the same time rendering it pure. To accomplish this, the amorphous mass is dissolved in diluted sulphuric acid, and filtered through bone black, which contains sufficient carbonate of lime to neutralize the excess of sulphuric acid, and thus facilitate the crystallization of the sulphate as the solution cools. This process requires to be repeated, with the addition of acid, if the charcoal is too alkaline, till a white and pure product is the result.

The desire has been often expressed for a method to prepare this alkaloid without alcohol: the following is the process of Herring, who substitutes in place of it, oil of turpentine or benzole:—

Powdered bark is boiled with caustic soda, to remove extractive, gum and coloring matter, exhausted with dilute sulphuric acid, evaporated at about 120°, filtered, precipitated by caustic soda, washed, redissolved in SO_3, recrystallized, treated with animal charcoal, and by fractional crystallizations purified from the other alkaloids.

The soda liquor is supersaturated with muriatic acid, evaporated, filtered, treated with hydrate of lime, from which precipitate the alkaloids may be extracted by oil of turpentine or benzole. On adding dilute SO_3, a solution of the alkaloid is obtained to be purified as above.

Quinia occurs in silky needles, or in a crystalline powder, fusible at 194° to an electrical mass, soluble in about 400 parts of water, 60 parts ether, 2 parts alcohol or chloroform, 24 parts of olive oil, also in alkalies, carbonate of ammonia, chloride of calcium, &c. Its solution in concentrated nitric acid turns yellow by heat, the solution in sulphuric acid is colored only at a high temperature.

Its salts are mostly crystallizable; their solution shows a blue fluorescence, which is rendered green on the addition of chlorine water, and subsequently ammonia—too much chlorine causes a brown color. A solution of quinia in diluted sulphuric acid, mixed with some acetic acid and alcohol, and heated to 130°, yields, after the addition of tincture of iodine, beautiful emerald green crystals of iodosulphate of quinia, which are nearly colorless by transmitted light. The solution of its salts is precipitated by alkalies, their carbonates and bicarbonates; but if they had been previously sufficiently acidulated with tartaric acid, bicarbonate of soda produces no precipitate. If their solution is treated first with chlorine water, free from hydrochloric acid, and subsequently with finely-powdered ferrocyanide of potassium, a red coloration is produced. Quinia salts are precipitated by ferrocyanide of potassium, the precipitate is dissolved on boiling and by an excess of the precipitant. (Differences from cinchonia.)

Quiniæ Sulphas, U.S.—Of the salts, the neutral sulphate (formerly called disulphate) is mostly employed. Its mode of preparation has been given above. It is in feathery white crystals, much interlaced; of its eight equivalents of water, six are given off by exposure to dry air, while the remaining two are driven off at 248°. It dissolves in 740 parts of cold and 30 parts hot water, in 60 parts of alcohol, but scarcely in ether. The addition of a mineral or of certain organic acids renders it easily soluble.

The salts of quinia are all used as tonics; the sulphate, especially, is a well-known antiperiodic and febrifuge. The dose varies from one to twenty grains. It is given in powder, pill, mixture, and solution. (See *Extemporaneous Pharmacy.*)

The following unofficinal salts are occasionally prescribed:[1]—

Quiniæ Murias.—The Dublin *Pharmacopœia* orders 437 grains of crystallized sulphate of quinia (equivalent to 382 grains of the salt dried at 212°) dissolved in 30 ounces of boiling water, to be precipitated by 123 grains of chloride of barium, and the filtrate evaporated until a pellicle forms. It crystallizes with 3HO in needles of a pearly lustre, more soluble than the sulphate. Baryta is detected by sulphuric acid, sulphate of quinia by chloride of barium.

Quiniæ Hydriodas.—5 parts of effloresced sulphate of quinia dissolved in alcohol and decomposed by an alcoholic solution of 3 parts of iodide of potassium, precipitates sulphate of potassa, and yields, on cooling and evaporating, hydriodate of quinia in fine crystalline needles.

Quiniæ antimonias is precipitated by double decomposition of antimoniate of potassa and sulphate of quinia, and crystallized from hot water or alcohol. It has been administered in periodical diseases in doses of from six to ten grains during apyrexia, and it is stated to be rarely necessary to give it a second time.

Quiniæ Arsenis.—Quinia is precipitated from 100 parts of its sulphate, dissolved in 600 parts alcohol, and boiled with 14 parts arsenious acid, the filtrate, on cooling, separates needles of this poisonous salt. It may be given with caution in doses from one-quarter to one-half grain several times a day.

Quiniæ lactas is obtained by saturating lactic acid with quinia, or by double decomposition of the baryta salt of the former with the sulphate of the latter, and crystallizes in soluble needles.

Quiniæ tartras is crystallized in needles from the hot solution of quinia in tartaric acid.

Quiniæ citras is separated in needles from the hot mixture of citrate of soda added to sulphate of quinia until an acid reaction is shown to test paper.

Quiniæ et Ferri Citras.—Dr. Squibb saturates 330 grains of citric acid with freshly-precipitated sesquioxide of iron in a warm place; to this is added in the cold the quinia from 78 grains of effloresced sulphate, and, after solution, dried by spontaneous evaporation (*Am. Jour. Ph.*, xxvii. 294). It is stated to crystallize in greenish scales by saturating a hot solution of citrate of the sesquioxide of iron with quinia. As usually met with, it differs little in appearance from the garnet-colored scales of citrate of iron, and varies very much in composition. The usual dose is from 2 to 5 grains, in pill.

Quiniæ Acetas.—Seventeen parts of the effloresced sulphate of quinia is dissolved in boiling water and mixed with six parts of crystallized acetate of

[1] See Phosphorous Compounds for Quiniæ Phosphas and Quiniæ Hypophosphas.

soda; acetate of quinia crystallizes in white feathery needles, nearly insoluble in cold water. (See remarks in *Am. Jour. Ph.*, xxx. 385.)

Quiniæ valerianas is officinal in the Dublin *Pharmacopœia*, which prepares it by double decomposition between muriate of quinia and valerianate of soda. It is also obtained by dissolving freshly-precipitated quinia in diluted valerianic acid, heating to near the boiling point, and crystallizing by cooling; the mother liquors are evaporated below 125°. It combines the tonic properties of quinia with the antispasmodic effects of the valerianates.

Quiniæ Tannas.—Tannic acid precipitates tannate of quinia from all solutions which have not been too much acidulated; it has little taste on account of its little solubility in neutral liquids.

Quiniæ gallas is obtained by double decomposition between a hot solution of sulphate of quinia and gallate of potassa. It is in crystalline granules, or a white powder, almost insoluble in water, soluble in alcohol and dilute acids.

Quiniæ Kinas.—To obtain this natural salt directly from the bark, the following process is given by Henry and Plisson. The extract is dissolved in 8 parts of water, nearly neutralized by carbonate of lime, then cautiously neutralized by hydrated oxide of lead; from the filtrate the lead is removed by sulphuretted hydrogen, after which the evaporated liquid is treated with alcohol of .842, the alcohol distilled off and the residue repeatedly treated with water and alcohol until nothing is separated by these liquids. It is obtained in white crystalline warts, soluble in 4 parts of water, and 8 parts of alcohol.

Quiniæ Hydroferrocyanas.—1 part sulphate of quinia, 1½ parts ferrocyanuret of potassium, and 7 parts of boiling water yield the salt on cooling, which is to be recrystallized from alcohol. It appears in greenish-yellow needles, which are insoluble in water. Pelouze asserts it to be quinia mixed with some Prussian blue. Dollfuss found it to be $C_{40}H_{24}N_2O_4+2(FeCy+2HCy)+6HO$.

Quinidia.

This name is now generally applied to an alkaloid which is isomeric with quinia, but differs from it in turning polarized light to the right. It occurs, in company with the other alkaloids, in many cinchona barks, particularly those imported from New Grenada.

It is obtained from its sulphate by decomposition with ammonia, and crystallizes in shining colorless efflorescing crystals, which are readily reduced to a white powder; they melt without decomposition, and, on cooling, concrete into a grayish white crystalline mass. When ignited, they burn with the odor of kinole and the volatile oil of bitter almonds; they have a less intensely bitter taste than quinia. This alkaloid is nearly insoluble in water, soluble in 12 parts of alcohol and 143 of ether, and its solution turns to a green color like quinia when successively treated with chlorine water and ammonia; a solution of either alkaloid even in 700,000 parts of water, according to Herapath, shows a dispersion of light with a bluish milky coloration. Quinidia, treated with tincture of iodine under the same circumstances as quinia, yields crystals which appear garnet red by transmitted light, and bluish red in reflected light. Quinidia is the only cinchona alkaloid yielding, with the solution of an iodide, a nearly insoluble precipitate, hydriodate of quinidia.

Quinidiæ sulphas is more soluble than sulphate of quinia, and remains in the mother liquor after the quinia salt has been crystallized. When the cheaper barks above referred to are manipulated with, this salt is an important product; it is largely produced, and by some used as a substitute for quinia. As generally found in commerce, it contains cinchonidia, and comes in long, shining white crystals, interlaced, and resembling those of sulphate of quinia. It is soluble in 130 parts of cold water, freely soluble in alcohol, and almost insoluble in ether. It contains six equivalents of water of crystallization.

Cinchonia.—This is another unofficinal alkaloid usually accompanying quinia. Huanuco bark contains almost exclusively cinchonia, which, when first isolated from this bark, was called huanucina, under the supposition of its being a distinct alkaloid. It may be obtained from this bark by a process similar to that for the preparation of quinia. It is in white needles, insoluble in alkalies, ether, and cold water, but soluble in 13 parts of boiling alcohol; chloroform dissolves 4.3; olive oil, 1 per cent. of cinchonia. It is less bitter than quinia and quinidia, fuses at 330° to an amorphous mass, and at a higher temperature partly sublimes without decomposition; polarized light is deviated to the right.

Its salts are generally more soluble than the corresponding salts of quinia; they are precipitated by the caustic alkalies and their carbonates; and in not too diluted solutions the bicarbonates likewise cause a precipitate after the previous addition of tartaric acid. Under similar circumstances cinchonia does not produce the reaction of quinia with chlorine and ferrocyanuret of potassium. The precipitate of ferrocyanide of potassium in cinchonia salts is insoluble in an excess of the precipitant, but crystallizes from its hot solution; its composition corresponds with the quinia salts. The cinchonia sulphate, if treated with iodine similarly to sulphate of quinia, yields a brick-red deposit.

Cinchoniæ Sulphas.—If cinchonia occurs in barks with quinia and quinidia, this salt remains behind in the mother liquor after the crystallization of the other sulphates.

It crystallizes in white pearly oblique prisms, containing 2HO, soluble in 54 parts of cold water, in 7 parts alcohol, not in ether. On the addition of sulphuric acid it passes into the very soluble acid sulphate. The other salts of cinchonia may be prepared like the corresponding quinia salts; the following have been occasionally used:—

Cinchoniæ murias is in silky prisms, easily soluble in water and alcohol.

Cinchoniæ hydroiadas crystallizes in needles.

Cinchoniæ tannas is a yellowish powder, soluble in alcohol.

Chinchoniæ Acetas.—If acetic acid is saturated with cinchonia, on evaporation granular or scaly crystals of the acetate are left, which are easily soluble in water.

Cinchonidia often constitutes the greatest part of commercial quinidia; as it contains no water of crystallization, it is not efflorescent in the air.

Its principal peculiarities are: solubility in ether, deviation of polarized light to the left, and no reaction with chlorine water and ammonia. By Dr. Herapath's test, viz: treating with iodine like quinia, the resulting iodosulphate of cinchonidia is so similar in appearance to the corresponding quinia salt, that it can only be distinguished from it by a little difference in the tint caused by transmitted light.

The base discovered by Wittstein, and called by him cinchonidia, is a mixture of various alkaloids, but principally of cinchonia and Pasteur's cinchonidia.

Quinicia and Cinchonicia.—The acid sulphates of quinia or cinchonia, if heated for three or four hours to about 250° or 266°, are converted into alkaloids, isomeric with the original bases, the former into quinicia, and the latter into cinchonicia, and but very little coloring matter; the neutral salts suffer partial decomposition at that temperature after melting. Both are nearly insoluble in water, soluble in alcohol, easily combine with carbonic acid, deplace ammonia from its salts, and deviate the polarized light a little to the right. The optical behavior of the different alkaloids, therefore, is as follows:—

Quinia, considerably to	left.	Cinchonia, considerably to	right.
Quinidia, "	right.	Cinchonidia, "	left.
Quinicia, feebly	right.	Cinchonicia, feebly	right.

Chinoidina or Quinoidina.—Is a product of alteration of the cinchona alkaloids. Drying of the barks, or exposure of solution of alkaloids to the sun, and the influence of a high temperature appear to favor this alteration. It is prepared by precipitating the mother liquor, from which the sulphates of the other alkaloids have been crystallized, by carbonate of soda, and extracting with alcohol.

It is a reddish-brown, resin-like mass, entering into combination with acids like the unaltered alkaloids. The salts are resinous, uncrystallizable, very bitter. It is isomeric with quinia, and has, therefore, been also called amorphous quinia. Pasteur supposes it to be uncrystallizable quinicia and cinchonicia.

It has strong febrifuge properties, and is very efficient in doses double of that of the sulphate of quinia, either in pills or dissolved with a little sulphuric acid. It may be considered pure if it is entirely soluble in alcohol, and in diluted sulphuric acid.

Precipitated extract of bark is the same preparation as the above. It differs from the extractum calisayacum, referred to on page 186 by not containing the crystallizable alkaloids.

Of the remarkable principles above described as existing in cinchona barks, cinchonia was the first discovered, having been isolated in an impure state as early as 1803, and fully described as an alkaloid by Pelletier and Caventou in 1820. Quinia was discovered soon after by the same chemists. Not until 1833 was the existence of quinidia announced. In that year, Henry and Delondre announced its discovery, but afterwards abandoned the idea of its being a distinct principle; so that no further attention was bestowed upon it until, about the year 1844, the celebrated German chemist, Winkler, investigated its properties, and conferred upon it the name quinidine, which, to correspond with our nomenclature, is changed to quinidia. Pasteur has since proved that quinidia as it occurs in commerce is generally composed chiefly of another alkaloid to which he gave the name cinchonidia; he likewise discovered the artificial isomeric alkaloids quinicia and cinchonicia.

On page 407 will be found an account of other similar alkaloids, discovered in particular barks, and most of them not fully investigated.

The former scarcity and high price of sulphate of quinia, occasioned in part by the restrictions placed upon the trade in genuine Calisaya bark by the Bolivian government, had the effect to direct the attention of physicians to other and similar remedial agents; but, notwithstanding the frequent announcement of favorable results from the trial of such, there seems a general disposition to withhold confidence from any but the products of that remarkable family of South American trees whose history has been so long connected with the cure of periodical diseases. The introduction into commerce of large quantities of cheap cinchona barks from new sources, has been another result of the long-continued scarcity of the older and officinal kinds. Notwithstanding these have been regarded by many with jealousy, and doubts have been entertained of their therapeutic value, the study of their chemical history has shown that some of them are not less rich in alkaloids than the finest monopoly barks, and experiments in regard to the therapeutic value of their characteristic alkaloids have shown a close resemblance in physiological effects to quinia itself. Some Bogota barks are now extensively employed for the manufacture of quinia, the price of which has, in consequence thereof, considerably decreased; these barks, beside the other alkaloids, abound in quinia.

Dr. Pepper and other practitioners connected with hospital practice, have used sulphate of quinidia in the same or less doses than the quinia salt, and with equal success; and its value and efficacy are confirmed by the experience of others in private practice.

Sulphate of cinchonia, which had been generally overlooked, has also been much used of latter time as a substitute for the quinia salt; and, although some physicians assert that larger doses of it are required, I am told by Dr. Conrad, the Apothecary of Pennsylvania Hospital, that in that Institution the three cinchona alkaloids are used indiscriminately and in the same doses. Through Dr. R. P. Thomas I am informed that the cinchonia salt has been used with satisfaction as a substitue for that of quinia in the Philadelphia and Northern Dispensaries, in the Western Clinical Infirmary, and Philadelphia Hospital, Blockley, where many intermittents are daily under treatment.

Quinoïdine is sold at a still lower price than either of the crystallized products. I am told that the demand for it has not justified manufacturers in preparing all that is produced for sale.

Detection of Adulterations and Impurities in Sulphate of Quinia.—The behavior of the cinchona alkaloids and their salts has been mentioned under their respective heads, and, with the aid of these tests, it is not very difficult to distinguish the alkaloids, when pure, from each other. There is more difficulty experienced in detecting the presence of one alkaloid in another, or in finding out foreign substances sometimes fraudulently mixed with them. The following are the various tests proposed for these purposes.

1. *Zimmer's test.*—Sixty drops of ether, twenty of aqua ammonia, and ten grains of the sulphate, previously dissolved in fifteen drops of water and ten drops of dilute sulphuric acid, made of one part, by weight, of sulphuric acid, to five of water, are mixed in a test tube; the quinia, being soluble in the ether, will not appear, but any admixture of cinchonia, or above ten per cent. of quinidia, will separate as a layer of a white powder, between the aqueous liquid and the supernatant ether. If quinidia be present, it will be dissolved by a large addition of ether, while cinchonia will not. If less that ten per cent. of quinidia is present, the mixture will be clear, but the quinidia will soon crystallize, while quinia will, after a while, gelatinize the ethereal solution.

2. *Rump's test* is said to be even more delicate than the former. Six grains of the sulphate, one-half drachm of ether, two or three drops of aqua ammonia, are well agitated in a test tube; pure sulphate

of quinia will yield a perfectly transparent solution; if five per cent. of sulphate of quinidia is present, the solution will likewise be clear, but, after a while will become turbid; ten per cent. of quinidia will leave a portion undissolved; with less than five per cent., the solution is to be evaporated spontaneously, quinidia will then be left in crystals, but quinia as a gummy mass.

3. *Liebig's test.*—Fifteen grains of the salt are rubbed with two ounces of aqua ammonia, this is heated until nearly all odor of ammonia has disappeared, and agitated with two ounces of ether. If a turbidness remains on the margin of the two liquids, cinchonia is present.

The ethereal solution may, besides quinia, also contain quinidia, which, like the above, will be left in crystals on spontaneous evaporation.

4. The presence in the sulphates of cinchona alkaloids of common adulterations may be detected as follows:—

The sulphates are entirely soluble in cold dilute sulphuric acid, and entirely dissipated by heat. *Sulphate of lime* may be detected by its insolubility in alcohol, and by remaining, after ignition, on a piece of platina foil. *Starch* would remain insoluble in dilute acid and in alcohol, and would be recognized by the well-known iodine test. *Stearic* and *margaric acids* and *resins* would float in the acid solution, and be dissolved by ether. *Salicine*, if more than ten per cent. were present, would show, with concentrated sulphuric acid, a red color. *Phloridzin* would be detected as yielding a yellow color with the same reagent, or by the yellow, red, and blue color imparted to it by gaseous ammonia under a bell glass. *Sugar* or *mannite* would be blackened by concentrated sulphuric acid. *Oxalate of ammonia* would be detected by giving off ammoniacal vapors with caustic potassa. Solution of caustic baryta dissolves *salicine*, *phloridzin*, *gum*, *mannite*, &c., but leaves the alkaloids and sulphate of baryta; in the solution, after it has been freed from baryta by carbonic acid, these substances may be detected.

Besides the above, the following alkaloids have been discovered in various barks.

Aricina, derived from Arica, the port from whence the bark is sent, is prepared like the other cinchona alkaloids, and crystallizes in white, transparent needles, which gradually develop a bitter, warming, sharp taste, melt between 356° and 374°, are insoluble in water, soluble in ether, alcohol, and ammonia. It is colored green by concentrated nitric acid

The salts are crystallizable, bitter, easily soluble in water and alcohol, insoluble in ether.

Paricina has been discovered in Para bark, by Winckler.

It is a white mass, uncrystallizable, electric when rubbed to powder, little soluble in water, easily soluble in ether and alcohol, and is left, after evaporation, as a golden-yellow, resinous mass. Its salts are amorphous, resinous.

It appears to bear to aricina the same relation as chinoidina to quinia.

Pitayia, discovered by Peretti, is prepared from the aqueous extract, which is exhausted by alcohol, evaporated, dissolved in water, and precipitated by ammonia, washed with ether, and crystallized from boiling water.

It is in colorless prisms, volatile, not bitter. Its salts are bitter and crystallizable.

Carthagia, discovered by Gruner, in Carthagena bark, crystallizes in needles, is tasteless, insoluble in water, soluble in alcohol.

Its salts are bitter, crystallizable, resembling the quinia salts, but are said to be destitute of febrifuge qualities.

Emetia.

Emetia is the active principle of ipecacuanha, and is also present in the roots of several species of viola.

The root is extracted by acidulated water, and precipitated by ammonia; to obtain it pure and white, according to Merck, it is dissolved in dilute muriatic acid, precipitated by corrosive sublimate, dissolved in alcohol, decomposed by sulphuret of barium to precipitate mercury, and sulphuric acid to precipitate baryta, diluted with water, the alcohol evaporated, and the sulphate of emetia precipitated by ammonia.

It is a white, inodorous powder, not crystalline, of a bitter taste, soluble in alcohol, sparingly so in water, nearly insoluble in ether and fixed oils, fusible at about 120° F. Its native salt existing in the root is taken up by water, wine, and diluted alcohol. It assumes a dirty green color by sulphuric acid, is converted first into a yellow, bitter, resinous substance, afterwards into oxalic acid. In minute doses it acts as a powerful emetic; in larger doses it is poisonous. Nearly all its salts are easily soluble in water; the acid salts, according to Liebig, are crystallizable. The commercial *emetia* is very impure, and not preferable for ordinary use to the various Galenical preparations of ipecac, in which the peculiar astringent and acid principles are associated with the alkaloid.

The *emetinum impurum* of some *pharmacopœias*, which is the French *emetin colorée*, is obtained by exhausting the alcoholic extract of ipecacuanha with water, neutralizing with carbonate of magnesia, and evaporating the filtrate.

Arnicina is prepared by exhausting the flowers with alcohol mixed with some sulphuric acid, treating the tincture with lime, and the filtrate with sulphuric acid, an excess of carbonate of potassa and ether, which dissolves it.

It is solid, slightly bitter, not acrid; its odor resembles that of castor; it is slightly soluble in water, more in alcohol and ether. It is little known.

The Alkaloids of Strychnos and their Salts.

Strychnia, U. S.

The *pharmacopœia* directs the rasped seed of nux vomica; but, as their comminution in the dry state is a work of no little difficulty, it is best to first heat them with some water, or expose them to hot steam; they will become thoroughly softened, and, while still warm, may be easily bruised in a warm mortar, or between two iron cylinders; then they are treated with water acidulated with muriatic acid; after concentration, the muriate thus formed is decomposed by lime, which precipitates the strychnia along with the excess of lime employed, and some impurities. The alkaloid is now dissolved out from the precipitate by boiling alcohol, and deposited, on evaporating and cooling. To purify it still further, it is next converted into a sulphate, boiled with animal charcoal, and precipitated by ammonia. St. Ignatius' bean contains a large proportion of strychnia and less brucia than nux vomica, but is not so abundant and cheap.

Strychnia, as thus prepared, is a white or grayish white powder which may be crystallized by the slow evaporation of an alcoholic solution. It is distinguished by extraordinary bitterness. It is soluble in boiling ordinary alcohol, but to a limited extent only in water, and nearly insoluble in absolute alcohol and ether. Its best solvents are 70 per cent. alcohol, and volatile oils. Chloroform dissolves 20 per cent., and olive oil one per cent. of strychnia. Perfectly pure strychnia is not affected by nitric acid. The following are its most reliable tests: Rub a very little of the powder with a few drops of sulphuric acid on a slab, and add a minute quantity of solution of chromate of potassa. A splendid violet color will be produced if it contain strychnia. Or thus: add a little of the powder to a few drops of sulphuric acid containing $\frac{1}{100}$ of nitric; it will form a colorless solution; but, on the addition of a little peroxide of lead, a bright blue color will be developed, which will pass rapidly into violet, then gradually into red, and ultimately to yellow. Its solution in sulphuric acid is colored red by chlorous and chloric acids, and by chlorates; a solution of the rose-colored sulphate of manganese causes a violet color, the same color is produced by ferridcyanide of potassium, and this reaction is not affected by the presence of other organic substances.

The salts which strychnia forms are mostly crystallizable and soluble. Their solutions are precipitated by fixed alkalies and their carbonates, and the precipitate is insoluble in an excess of the precipitant; the precipitate caused by ammonia dissolves, but afterwards crystallizes from an excess of it. Sulphocyanide of potassium produces a white crystalline deposit; the precipitate with gaseous chlorine is soluble in ether and alcohol. If acidulated with tartaric acid, a white precipitate occurs by bicarbonate of soda.

Adulterations with mineral substances are discovered by the residue left after ignition or after solution in boiling alcohol. Brucia is detected by the red color on the addition of sulphuric acid.

The following salts have been occasionally used in medicine, chiefly on account of their solubility. They are mostly prepared by neutralizing the acid with strychnia, and evaporating:—

Strychniæ sulphas contains 7HO; it crystallizes in prisms and cubes, is efflorescent, and contains 75 per cent. strychnia. It is used, on account of its solubility, in preference to the alkaloid.

Strychniæ nitras crystallizes in needles of a pearly lustre, which are insoluble in alcohol.

Strychniæ murias is in silky needles, easily soluble in alcohol.

Strychniæ hydriodas is obtained by double decomposition as a white crystalline powder, little soluble in water, more in alcohol, and containing nearly 73 per cent. strychnia.

Strychniæ iodas is likewise obtained by double decomposition, and crystallizes in flat pearly needles, soluble in alcohol, but little in cold water.

Strychniæ acetas crystallizes with difficulty in white silky needles, very soluble in alcohol and water.

Strychniæ tannas is a white precipitate, scarcely soluble in water.

The medicinal uses of strychnia are those of a tonic, with a special action upon the nerves of motion. It is much employed in a variety of diseases. Dose, one-twelfth to one-sixth of a grain.

In doses of two or three grains, strychnia is one of the most powerful and fatal of poisons. Immense quantities are sold for the purpose of killing animals, particularly dogs, on whom the most certain and rapidly fatal effect is produced by its use. In cases of poisoning by strychnia, the most prompt and vigorous efforts are necessary to arrest its effects. The jaws must be prevented from becoming permanently closed, as in tetanus. Emetics should be tried, but will seldom act. Tannic acid or other astringents will precipitate the alkaloid in an insoluble form. Chloroform has been found to arrest the effects of the poison. In one memorable case I saw the life of an individual saved by the application of the poles of a magnetic battery over the stomach, which aroused that organ, and, by excessive vomiting, produced the relaxation of the spasm.

Brucia.

If strychnia is crystallized from a hot alcoholic solution, the mother liquor contains nearly all the brucia; but it may be entirely freed from strychnia by nitric acid. From the neutral solution, the strychnia salt crystallizes first, leaving bruçia in the mother liquor; the acid solution, however, separates the brucia salt first in hard, four-sided prisms, while the strychnia salt crystallizes afterwards in fine needles.

It crystallizes in oblique four-sided prisms, dissolves in 850 parts cold, 500 parts boiling water, is easily soluble in alcohol, insoluble in ether; volatile oils dissolve a small quantity. Chloroform dissolves 56 per cent., and olive oil nearly 2 per cent. It contains 8HO.

The salts are bitter, crystallizable, precipitated by alkalies and alkaline earths, by morphia and strychnia; an excess of ammonia dissolves its precipitate; if acidulated with tartaric acid, no precipitate occurs on the addition of bicarbonate of soda; concentrated nitric acid dissolves brucia and its salts to an intensely red fluid, which subsequently acquires a yellowish red, and by heat a yellow tint; if now protochloride of tin or sulphuret of ammonium is added, an intense violet color is produced.

Of the salts used medicinally, the neutral sulphate crystallizes in needles with 4HO; the neutral nitrate is a gum-like mass, but the acid nitrate is crystallizable in four-sided prisms. Brucia is a less powerful therapeutic agent than strychnia, being safely employed in doses of from two to four grains.

Igasuria.

The mother liquors of the former two, after their precipitation by lime, contain this alkaloid.

It crystallizes, is very bitter, dissolves in 200 parts of boiling water, in weak alcohol, in acids and alkalies. Sulphuric acid imparts a rose color, which turns yellowish and greenish.

The salts are soluble, crystallizable, and poisonous. They are precipitated in presence of tartaric acid by alkaline bicarbonates.

Schutzenberger has found that what has been called Igasuria is a mixture of various alkaloids, which he purified by fractional crystallization. They are all colorless, intensely bitter, poisonous like strychnia, soluble in boiling water and alcohol, little in ether; they crystallize in transparent needles or pearly scales, are colored red by nitric acid, lose their water of crystallization at 212°. Their salts are easily crystallizable. They are distinguished by affixing the letters of the alphabet:—

Igasuria, *a*, $C_{34}H_{26}N_2O_3+6HO$. Very little soluble.
" *b*, $C_{36}H_{26}N_2O_{14}+6HO$. Little soluble.
" *c*, $C_{36}H_{24}N_2O_8+6HO$. Moderately soluble.
" *d*, $C_{34}H_{26}N_2O_6+6HO$. " "
" *e*, $C_{36}H_{26}N_2O_8+6HO$. Soluble.
" *f*, $C_{42}H_{30}N_2O_8+6HO$ or 8HO. Moderately soluble.
" *g*, $C_{42}H_{28}N_2O_{12}+6HO$. Very little soluble.
" *h*, $C_{42}H_{26}N_2O_{12}+6HO$. Moderately soluble.
" *i*, $C_{40}H_{26}N_2O_{14}+6HO$. " "

Schutzenberger thinks they are products of brucia, altered by the process of life in the organs of the plant.

Pereirina is obtained from the bark of an unknown tree, probably of the genus cerbera, called in Brazil, pao pereira. It is prepared like the cinchona alkaloids, and lastly dissolved by ether. It is a yellowish-white amorphous, bitter mass, on melting, blood-red, has an alkaline reaction, is little soluble in water, soluble in alcohol and ether. Concentrated sulphuric acid dissolves it with violet color, which afterwards turns brown, on diluting with water, olive-green and grass-green. Nitric acid dissolves it with a blood-red color, changing to grayish-brown. The salts are little known, they are precipitated by the oxalates, and are said to have febrifuge properties.

Alkaloids of the Solanaceæ.

Solania occurs in the berries of solanum nigrum, and verbascifolium, the berries and germs of solanum tuberosum, and in the whole herb of solanum dulcamara.

It is prepared from the potato germs by maceration with water, acidulated with sulphuric acid, mixing with hydrate of lime, and exhausting the precipitate with boiling alcohol; on cooling the greater part is separated. It crystallizes in colorless prisms, without odor; its taste is faintly bitter, nauseous, causes a persistent acrid feeling in the throat. It has an alkaline reaction, is little soluble in cold water, ether, alcohol and fixed oil. It is a weak base, its salts are soluble, few crystallizable, and have a bitter taste, with lasting acrimony.

Solania, as obtained from the various species of solanum, according to Moitessier, differs to a considerable extent in its physical properties. Various different alkaloids have probably been confounded under this name. Prepared from solanum dulcamara, it has the composition $C_{42}H_{35}NO_{14}$, and all its salts are amorphous.

Atropia.—The infusion of belladonna is precipitated by a solution of iodine in iodide of potassium, the precipitate decomposed by zinc and water; precipitated by carbonate of potassa, the alkaloid is crystallized from alcohol.

It is in needles of a silky lustre, without odor, and of a bitter, acrid, almost metallic taste; it dilates the pupil more than any other alkaloid; to act on the pupil, atropia must have entered the circulation (Harley). It melts at 212°, is soluble in 200 parts of cold, 50 parts of boiling water, without crystallizing on cooling, by continued boiling it dissolves in 30 parts of water, from which the greater part crystallizes; it dissolves in 1½ parts cold alcohol; the solution in 6 parts of boiling ether gelatinizes on cooling into a transparent jelly. Chloroform dissolves 50, olive oil 2.3 per cent. atropia. The salts are crystallizable, without odor, and with the taste of atropia, they are mostly soluble in water, alcohol and alcoholic ether, not in pure ether; all are very poisonous. Sulphuric acid dissolves the alkaloid without color, after some time the solution turns red and black. It is colored yellow by chlorine. Nitric acid dissolves it with a pale yellow color, afterwards orange, then colorless. The solution is then still precipitated by tannin, but does not contain any atropia, as the pupil is not dilated.

In contact with air it is easily converted into another alkaloid, which Berzelius has called *tropia*. It is very soluble in water, yellowish, not crystallizable, of a disagreeable odor, and strong alkaline reaction.

Belladonnia is the yellow resin adhering to atropia and preventing it from crystallizing.

Crude atropia is dissolved in a weak acid, neutralized by carbonate potassa to separate a body opalescing in blue, an alkali is added, taking care not to produce a pulverulent precipitate, as long as the precipitate appears oily and resin-like, this is collected on linen, dissolved in an acid, treated with animal charcoal, if necessary again fractionally precipitated, and dissolved in absolute ether.

A gum-like mass remains behind, of little bitterness, and a burning, sharp taste; it melts on heating and decomposes with the smell of hippuric acid; it is easily soluble in pure and officinal ether, in absolute and dilute alcohol, scarcely soluble in water; though strongly alkaline, it is less so than atropia; from the sulphate it is precipitated by ammonia as a white powder, which soon becomes resin-like. It was discovered by Hübschmann.

Daturia.—From the seed of stramonium by extracting with alcohol, treating with a little lime, acidulating with sulphuric acid, distilling off the alcohol, removing the oil, precipitating by carbonate potassa, expressing, treating with alcohol, sulphuric acid, and animal charcoal, and crystallizing from alcohol.

Daturia has been proved to be chemically identical with atropia. Its pharmacodynamical properties have been studied by Professor Schroff, and carefully compared with atropia. His conclusions are, that their qualitative action is alike, but that there exists a vast difference in their intensity, daturia being nearly twice as strong and powerful, as atropia.

Here the question arises: Is there no doubt at all about the chemical identity of both alkaloids? May they not be only very similar in their composition and chemical behavior?

Hyoscyamia is obtained from the juice of hyoscyamus, after coagulation of the albumen by neutralizing it with lime, adding carbonate of potassa, and extracting with ether.

It crystallizes in needles of silky lustre, when pure without odor; its taste is acrid, tobacco-like. With a carefully regulated heat it may be distilled. It has a strong alkaline reaction, dissolves in water, alcohol and ether; and is easily decomposed when in solution. Of the salts, some few are crystallizable; they must be evaporated in vacuo to prevent them from becoming oxidized; they are soluble in water and alcohol, without smell, and have the taste of the base.

Bebeerina is best prepared from the commercial so-called sulphate of bebeerina by precipitating it with ammonia, removing the tannin with oxide of lead or lime, and boiling with alcohol; the evaporated mass is repeatedly treated with absolute ether, and evaporated.

It is amorphous, lemon yellow, bitter, of an alkaline reaction, scarcely soluble in water, soluble in 13 parts ether, and 5 parts absolute alcohol. The salts are yellow, bitter, amorphous, precipitated and decomposed by nitric acid.

The commercial sulphate of bebeerina is in dark brown glittering slabs, readily soluble in water by the aid of acids. It is esteemed as a tonic and antiperiodic, and is given in doses of three to ten grains, to the amount of a scruple or a drachm, between the paroxysms in intermittents.

Sepeerina (from the Dutch name sepeeri for bebeeru), remains behind after the exhaustion of bebeerina by ether.

Amorphous, reddish-brown, little soluble in water, soluble in alcohol. The salts are amorphous, of a brown color, and generally obtained in very shining laminæ, almost resembling crystalline scales.

Piperina.—Powdered white pepper is exhausted by alcohol; this is distilled off, the extract mixed with a solution of potassa, which dissolves resinous and coloring matter; the precipitated greenish powder is piperina, which is purified by repeated crystallizations.

It crystallizes in four sided prisms, colorless when pure, when chewed for some time developing a hot peppery taste, scarcely soluble in water, easily in alcohol, the solution is neutral to litmus, and has a burning pepper taste. It melts at 212°, losing 2 equivalents of water. It dissolves in cold sulphuric acid with a deep red color, and is a weak base.

Distilled with potassa at 320° picolina is obtained leaving a body of the following combination: $C_{70}H_{37}N_2O_{10}+(C_{58}H_{30}NO_{10}+KO)$ and piperina may be regarded as a combination of picolina, with another body not isolated yet, viz: $C_{58}H_{30}NO_{10}+C_{12}H_7N$.

Piperidina $= C_{10}H_{11}N$ is probably ethyl-allyl-amin $N(C_4H_5+C_6H_5)+H$. By distillation of piperina with 2½ to 3 parts of soda-lime, Cahours obtained two alkaloids and a neutral liquid of benzoin odor. One of the bases, called piperidina, is obtained by saturating the distillate with fused potassa, and saving by fractional distillation of the separated oil, that part coming over at 212°, which amounts to about $\frac{9}{10}$ of the distillate.

It is a colorless liquid, strongly alkaline, of an ammoniacal odor and taste, lighter than water, in which it dissolves in all proportions; it precipitates the salts of the metallic oxides. Its salts are crystallizable.

Veratria, U. S.

Veratria is procured from cevadilla seeds by treating them with alcohol, evaporating the tincture to an extract, and treating this with water acidulated with sulphuric acid; this solution, containing sulphate of veratria, is next decomposed by magnesia, which is added in excess; the precipitated veratria thrown down is now washed and separated from the excess of magnesia by alcohol, from which it is obtained by evaporation, but requires still further purifying with animal charcoal, &c. A pound of the seeds yields about a drachm of veratria.

This product is a white, uncrystallizable powder, extremely acrid when diffused in the air, producing excessive irritation of the nostrils. It is freely soluble in alcohol, less so in ether, and almost insoluble in water, but soluble in diluted acids, from which ammonia and solution of tannin throw down white precipitates. Among its most striking peculiarities are the intense red color it assumes on the addition of sulphuric acid, and the yellow solution it forms with nitric. Veratria, as procured by the officinal process, is a complex body, and contains two alkaloids, *sabadillia* and *jervia*, with some resinous matter.

The medical uses of veratria are confined chiefly to gouty and neuralgic affections, in the treatment of which it is used internally in doses of one-twelfth to one-sixth grain, repeated, or externally, in ointment, of about ℈j to the ounce.

The following is the process for obtaining the alkaloids pure, and ascertaining their properties.

Veratria.—Commercial veratria, if dissolved in much alcohol, and mixed with water until a precipitate just commences to appear, this yields, on evaporation, a white, crystalline powder, mixed with a brown, resinous mass, which can be removed by washing with cold alcohol. The powder, if dissolved in strong alcohol, and evaporated spontaneously, leaves large, rhombic, colorless prisms, which effloresce in the air, become porcellanous and pulverulent, are insoluble in boiling water, but rendered opaque, readily soluble in alcohol and ether. Sulphuric acid colors it yellow, then carmine red; muriatic acid produces a deep violet solution, forming oily drops on the surface. The acids are completely neutralized, but the solutions do not crystallize on evaporation.

Sabadillia crystallizes in colorless prisms, which are soluble in boiling water, melt at 390° F., and have a very acrid taste. It is easily soluble in alcohol, but does not crystallize from this solution; it is insoluble in ether, and, from its solution in dilute sulphuric acid, is not precipitated by ammonia. It is not sternutatory. (Hübschmann.)

Jervia.—The precipitate by soda, containing the alkaloids, is boiled with dilute sulphuric acid; on cooling, the sulphate of jervia is precipitated. The precipitate may be decomposed by carbonate of soda, and recrystallized from alcohol.

It is nearly insoluble in water, soluble in alcohol, crystallizes in colorless prisms with 3HO, loses its water of crystallization on heating, then melts, and above 375° is decomposed.

Jervia and its soluble salts are precipitated from their solutions by muriatic, sulphuric, and nitric acids, forming therewith nearly insoluble salts; they, however, dissolve in alcohol.

Colchicia.—According to Aschoff, the root is to be exhausted by cold water, precipitated by basic acetate of lead, the filtrate neutralized by carbonate of soda, the filtrate precipitated by tannin, this precipitate washed, expressed, dissolved in eight parts alcohol, and digested with freshly precipitated oxide of iron; the filtrate is evaporated, the residue dissolved in a mixture of equal parts of alcohol and ether, evaporated, and again dissolved in water.

The corns gathered in spring yielded but .75 grains, in the fall as high as 6.5 grains from the pound; the seed 16 grains to the pound.

It is a white, amorphous mass, of a bitter, not acrid taste, without odor, when moist of a feeble narcotic odor. It is easily decomposed in aqueous solution, is not sternutatory or hygroscopic, is fusible and inflammable, easily soluble in water and alcohol, less in absolute ether. It has no reaction on vegetable colors. The following is its behavior to reagents:—

It is soluble in SO_3, with a clear yellow color; in NO_5, yellow; the undissolved colchicia is brownish-red, then violet, brownish-green, brown-red;

fuming NO_5 (containing nitrous acid) impart to it a violet or indigo-blue, afterwards yellow, color. The solution of $\frac{1}{1000}$ colchicia is colored lemon yellow by muriatic acid. Bichromate of potassa and sulphuric acid impart a green color. Iodine causes a kermes-colored, gelatinous precipitate, soluble in alcohol and water. Chlorine-water a yellow precipitate, soluble with orange color in ammonia. No crystallizable compounds have been obtained with acids, except that J. E. Carter thinks he obtained a crystalline sulphate.

Hübschmann was unable to saturate two drops of dilute sulphuric acid with colchicia, though he and Carter both found it to act slowly on reddened litmus paper, and on paper colored with rhubarb.

By external applications, several painful cases of rheumatism have been relieved by it. If given internally, one-sixtieth ($\frac{1}{60}$) grain three times daily, continued, if necessary, for several weeks, has a most salutary effect in rheumatic complaints. It opens the bowels even of those who have been suffering from constipation. (See *Thesis* of J. E. Carter, of Philadelphia, *Am. Journ. Pharm.*, vol. xxx. p. 205.)

Colchiceine, $C_{35}H_{20}NO_{11}$.—Oberlin obtained no colchicia by Geiger and Hesse's process, but, on dissolving the product in water, acidulating with muriatic acid, evaporating until of an intense yellow color, by water a white precipitate was thrown down, crystallizing from alcohol and ether in pearly lamellæ, nearly insoluble in water, soluble in alcohol, ether, woodspirit, chloroform, ammonia, potassa; in sulphuric acid with yellow, in muriatic acid with pale yellow, in nitric acid with intense yellow color, changing to violet, deep red, light red and yellow. It is very poisonous.

It is neutral to test paper. It remains to be investigated whether or not it is a product of decomposition of colchicia by the influence of muriatic acid.

Tests for Distinguishing the Alkaloids.

The following, taken from Dr. A. T. Thompson, conveys, in a compact form, the leading facts applicable to distinguishing the alkaloids. Some *general* characteristics are noticed at the beginning of this chapter, and some *particular* ones under the several heads.

Method of Distinguishing the following Vegetable Alkaloids—Atropia, Brucia, Delphia, Emetia, Morphia, Solania, Strychnia, Veratria—when they are in powder.

Treat the powder first with nitric acid, which is colored red by *brucia*, *delphia*, *morphia*, and the *strychnia* of commerce, but not by pure strychnia. If the reddened acid become of a violet hue on the addition of protochloride of tin, after the nitric solution has cooled, the alkaline powder is *brucia;* if the reddened acid gradually become black and carbonaceous, it is *delphia*. If the powder be soluble without decomposition, and decompose iodic acid, evolving free iodine, it is *morphia;* if it is not fusible, and does not decompose iodic acid, it is *strychnia*. If the powder greens, instead of reddening nitric acid, it is *solania*; if it is insoluble in ether, and does not redden nitric acid, it is *emetia;* if it be soluble in ether, and does not redden nitric acid, but melts when heated, and volatilizes, it is *atropia;* if it is thus affected by ether and nitric acid, but is not volatilized, it is *veratria*.

The Ternary Alkaloids.

Sparteina.

A concentrated decoction of broom is distilled with soda, and several times rectified.

It is a colorless oil, which, in contact with water, soon becomes opalescent, and is colored brown by the air; it smells faintly like anilina, has a very bitter taste, and is narcotic; its boiling point is 550° F. Acids are perfectly neutralized; the salts are soluble, the muriate and nitrate not crystallizable.

Conia

Is most abundant in the fresh plants gathered before flowering, and in the seed, from which it is obtained by distillation with caustic potassa, purifying the sulphate by dissolving it in alcoholic ether, and again distilling with potassa.

Conia is a volatile yellow, oily fluid (specific gravity .89), with a very characteristic odor resembling that of the urine of the mouse. It is neutral to test paper when anhydrous, but decidedly alkaline when containing some water. It is soluble in 100 parts of water, floating on its surface when distilled with it. Alcohol dissolves it readily, as also ether, the fixed and volatile oils. It does not dilate the pupil.

Like other volatile alkaloids of the composition of substituted ammonia, it occasions white clouds when approached with a rod moistened with muriatic acid. This test, when applied to the extract of conium, after adding to it on a tile a few drops of solution of potassa, is much resorted to, in connection with the odor, in judging of the quality of that extract.

When exposed to the air, conia undergoes oxidation, being converted into a brown resinous matter, ammonia, and butyric acid. By concentrated muriatic acid it is colored purple changing to blue; chlorine produces thick white vapors of a lemon odor.

It neutralizes the acids, forming soluble salts, some of which are crystallizable, while those with oxygenated acids are mostly decomposed on evaporation and leave a gummy residue.

Conia, $=NC_{16}H_{15}$, often contains variable proportions of methylic conia, $=NC_{18}H_{17}$, and æthylic conia, $NC_{20}H_{19}$, which appear to be as poisonous as the normal alkaloid.

In this connection it is proper to mention the quaternary alkaloid, discovered by Wertheim, accompanying conia.

Conhydrina

Occurs chiefly in the flowers and seed of conium; to prepare it, the crude conia is neutralized with sulphuric acid, the salt extracted with alcohol to separate ammonia, evaporated, treated with concentrated caustic potassa, then with ether; this is distilled off, and by very slow fractional distillation in an oil bath, the conia is separated; between 300° and 400° crystals of conhydrina are sublimed.

It is in colorless, pearly crystalline lamellæ, sublimes slowly below 212°, is soluble in water, alcohol, and ether; by distillation with anhydrous phosphoric acid, conia is obtained, 2HO being abstracted: $NC_{16}H_{17}O_2 - 2HO = NC_{16}H_{15}$.

Its action on animals is similar to conia, but weaker. The salts have not been studied yet.

Lobelina

Was discovered by the late Professor S. Calhoun, of Philadelphia, in 1834, and first isolated in a state of purity by Professor Procter, in 1842. It is most conveniently obtained by extracting the seed with alcohol acidulated with acetic acid, which forms a fixed salt with the alkaloid, evaporating and treating with magnesia, and then with ether, from which it may be obtained by evaporation.

It is a liquid lighter than water, and when dropped into that fluid rises to its surface and spreads out like a drop of oil, then gradually dissolves without agitation, forming a transparent solution. It is very soluble in alcohol and ether, the latter readily removing it from an aqueous solution; it also dissolves in fixed and volatile oils. It forms crystallizable salts, with numerous acids.

It is not obtained on an economical scale for use in medicine. Lobelina, as it exists in the plant combined with lobelic acid, is decomposable by a moderate heat, as also by the action of strong acids.

Nicotia, or Nicotina,

Is prepared in the following manner: The acid infusion of tobacco is evaporated to about one-half, distilled with caustic potassa, the distillate neutralized by oxalic acid, treated with anhydrous alcohol, decomposed by potassa, and the alkaloid dissolved by ether. By rectification in a current of hydrogen, it may be obtained colorless.

It is a colorless, oily liquid, of strong tobacco odor, a burning sharp taste, heavier than water, specific gravity 1.048. It is inflammable, has an alkaline reaction, is soluble in water, and water is soluble in it to some extent; miscible with alcohol, ether, and olive oil, scarcely soluble in oil turpentine. It becomes yellow by keeping, absorbing oxygen from the air, which gradually turns it thick and brown. It boils at 482° F., but volatilizes at a much lower temperature. The vapor which rises is so powerful in its smell and irritating properties that one drop of it diffused in a room renders the atmosphere insupportable. The volatility of this principle insures its diffusion, along with empyreumatic products, in tobacco smoke, so that it is inhaled to a certain extent by smokers. It exists in the different commercial varieties of tobacco in about the following proportions: Havana 2 per cent., Maryland 2.3, Virginia 6.87, Kentucky 6.09.

Orfila has lately investigated the properties of nicotia, and ascertained with precision its chemical habitudes. These are detailed in a paper copied in the *American Journal of Pharmacy*, vol. xxiv., p. 142, from the *London Pharmaceutical Journal.* See also a paper by Professor Procter in *Proceedings of the American Pharmaceutical Association*, 1858, p. 295.

Its salts have a burning taste of tobacco, are very soluble in water, deliquescent, and difficult to crystallize.

Secalina

Has the composition of propylamin, methylæthylamin, and trimethylamin, and is identical with one of them, probably the former, as it may be obtained from propylic narcotina[1] by distillation with potassa. Besides the plants mentioned in the *Syllabus*, it has been obtained

[1] See page 397.

from herring-pickle, crabs, the spirits in which anatomical preparations have been kept, and the urine of man. When artificially prepared, it is best known as *Propylamin.*

Propylamin is most economically prepared from herring-pickle by distillation with caustic potassa, neutralizing the distillate with muriatic acid, purifying the salt by dissolving it in strong alcohol or alcoholic ether, and again distilling with potassa.

It is a colorless liquid of a strong odor of herrings, and a sweetish astringent taste; it is soluble in water, has an alkaline reaction, produces white vapors with muriatic acid. Its salts are mostly soluble in water and alcohol, and crystallizable.

According to Dr. Awenarius, of St. Petersburg, it appears to be a true specific for rheumatic affections, the acute as well as the chronic. He administered it in mixtures, containing 24 drops of propylamin to 6 ounces of mint-water sweetened with 2 drachms of sugar, and gave it in doses of a tablespoonful every two hours.

See papers on this subject by Professor Procter in *Proceedings of the American Pharmaceutical Association*, 1857, and *American Journal of Pharmacy*, xxxi. 125 and 222.

Alkaloids of Animal Origin.

Some animal tissues and liquids contain alkaline substances or are decomposed into such by the influence of various chemical agents. These animal alkaloids, however, are as yet of little importance in a medicinal point of view; and it remains here merely to draw attention to a few of them which are either contained in culinary and dietatic articles, or are of importance from their presence in various secretions.

Syllabus of Animal Alkaloids and the Products of their Decomposition.[1]

Sarkosina, $C_6H_7NO_4$. From creatine by boiling with BaO; rhombic prisms or scales, easily soluble in water.

Glycina, $C_4H_5NO_4$ or *Glycocoll.* In the bile; by treating glue or similar substances with boiling alkalies or acids; sweet rhombic crystals, easily soluble in water and ordinary alcohol.

Leucina, $C_{12}H_{13}NO_4$. By putrefaction of casein, from glue like glycina. Shining scales, easily soluble in water, alkalies, and muriatic acid, little in alcohol; fused with KO yields valerianic acid.

Tyrosina, $C_{18}H_{11}NO_6$. By acids or alkalies upon casein, glue, albumen, &c., silky needles, soluble in acids and alkalies, little in water, insoluble in alcohol and ether.

Guanina, $C_{10}H_5N_5O_5$. In the excrements of spiders and in small quantity in guano; white powder, insoluble in water, somewhat soluble in lime and baryta water; its salts crystallizable.

Taurina, $C_4H_7NS_2O_6$. In bile after decomposition by acids or by fermentation; six-sided prisms, easily soluble in water, little in alcohol; taste cooling.

Urea, $C_2H_4N_2O_2$. In the urine of the mammalia, particularly the carnivorous.

As urea has been proposed as a remedial agent, it may be well to give its mode of preparation.

Urine is evaporated to a syrupy consistence, mixed with an equal volume of nitric acid, and set aside for twenty-four hours in a cool place; the crystals are redissolved in boiling diluted nitric acid to destroy coloring matter, if necessary digested with animal charcoal, and subsequently decomposed by carbonate of baryta. After evaporation, the mass is exhausted by alcohol.

[1] See Inosinic Acid and Creatine, p. 381.

For its artificial preparation Liebig gives the following directions: A mixture of four parts finely powdered anhydrous ferrocyanuret of potassium, and two parts black oxide of manganese is heated to redness, and constantly stirred until it has ignited; it is extracted with cold water, the solution mixed with a solution of three parts sulphate of ammonia, evaporated, the sulphate of potassa removed as much as possible, and the residue exhausted with boiling ordinary alcohol.

Urea crystallizes in long, colorless prisms, easily soluble in water and alcohol, containing no water of crystallization, and fusing at 248° F.

It has been recommended as a good and reliable diuretic, in doses of from five to ten grains, several times a day, in diabetes, albuminuria, and dropsy.

Ureæ nitras is precipitated from a concentrated solution of urea by strong nitric acid in anhydrous white shining scales, soluble in 8 parts of water, little in nitric acid and alcohol. Its action is said to be similar to urea, and it has been recommended as a solvent for vesical calculi composed of ammonio-phosphate of magnesia.

CHAPTER IX.

ON NEUTRAL ORGANIC PRINCIPLES MOSTLY PECULIAR TO A LIMITED NUMBER OF PLANTS, AND POSSESSED OF MEDICINAL PROPERTIES.

FORMERLY, the virtues of most medical plants were attributed to *extractive* matter, though this as obtained from various sources and by different analytical processes, was known to vary somewhat in its properties.

In the progress of investigation many of these plants have been found to possess certain well-defined proximate principles, sometimes crystalline and sometimes amorphous, to which appropriate names have been given. If *alkaline*, these names should terminate in *ia*; if *neutral* or *subacid*, in *in* or *ine*. This arrangement, which would conduce to accuracy, if invariably observed, is, however, not adhered to universally, and in Europe is repudiated by some high authorities.

The *neutral organic principles* are conveniently considered together, and will be separately presented with reference to their leading characteristics. Some of these are amorphous, some liquid or pulverulent, and others distinctly crystalline.

The neutral principles are in some instances active, and in others appear to possess little power of affecting the system. Some of them contain nitrogen, while most others consist of merely carbon, hydrogen, and oxygen. These principles occasionally unite with acids, forming crystalline compounds, which are, however, acid in their properties; others combine with alkalies, forming crystallizable salts. They are generally precipitated by tannic acid, and many of them by subacetate of lead. The modes of obtaining these principles are various, and sometimes difficult to follow, though the solubilities and chemical peculiarities of each, when ascertained, indicate approximately its mode of extraction.

In a work of the design and scope of the present, it will suffice to display the more striking peculiarities of these principles, none of which are officinal, in a syllabus, and to give the processes of extraction and the leading chemical and medicinal characteristics, only in a few cases including the more important and familiar.

There are here, as in the case of the alkaloids, no known chemical relations upon which we would be justified in founding a scientific classification of these principles, and here, as in treating of the other proximate principles of plants, we will find the botanical arrangement of the plants themselves to afford the best grouping. The natural families of plants, though arranged upon a purely botanical basis, are found to exhibit remarkable chemical and physiological relations among the products of their individual members; this agreement, as yet but imperfectly recognized owing to our limited knowledge of the actual composition of organic proximate principles, is probably one of the great universal harmonies of nature which in the progress of science must be more fully developed and made known.

Syllabus of Plants and their Neutral Characteristic Principles.

1. *Ternary Compounds.*

Ranunculaceæ. Pulsatilla pratensis. (Anemone pretensis.)	*Anemonin*, associated with anemonic acid, rhombic crystals, nearly insoluble in ether; product of the decomposition of the acrid oil of ranunculus scleratus. Poisonous.
Magnoliaceæ. Liriodendron, *U. S.* Magnolia, *U. S.*	*Liriodendrin*, crystallizable, white, soluble in alcohol and ether, bitter, pungent.
Menispermaceæ. Colomba, *U. S.* Root of Cocculus palmatus.	*Columbin*, $C_{42}H_{22}O_{14}$, colorless, rhombic prisms, very bitter, soluble in 30 per cent. alcohol, in alkalies, precipitated by acids. Associated with *berberina*.
Papaveraceæ. Opium, *U. S.* From Papaver somniferum.	*Meconin*, $C_{20}H_{10}O_8$, white acicular crystals, soluble in 265 parts cold, 18 boiling water, ether, alcohol and volatile oils; acrid.
Caryophylleæ. Saponaria officinalis, *U. S.* Gypsophylla struthium. Agrostemma githago.	*Saponin* $C_{36}H_{22}O_{24}$, *Struthiin*, *Githagin*, identical; soluble in hot water and alcohol, insoluble in ether; taste sweetish, afterwards acrid and bitter, frothing in solution, sternutatory; identical with polygalic acid, which see; with SO_3, produces *sapogenin*.
Aurantiaceæ. Limonis cortex, *U. S.* Citrus limonum and citrus aurantium, the seed.	*Hesperidin*, in the spongy portion of lemon peel, bitter. *Limonin*, $C_{42}H_{25}O_{13}$. From the seed by alcohol, crystalline, bitter, soluble in alkalies; red color with SO_3.
Guttiferæ. Garcinia mangostana,[1] bark of the fruit.	*Mangostin*, $C_{40}H_{22}O_{10}$, golden yellow scales, without smell or taste, insoluble in water, soluble in alcohol and ether, dilute acids and alkalies.
Erythroxyleæ. Erythroxylon cocoa, leaves.	*Erythroxylin*, volatile needle shaped crystals, very bitter, probably identical with caffein.
Hyppocastaneæ. Æsculus hippocastanum. (Horse chestnut), the bark.	*Æsculin*, $C_{60}H_{33}O_{37}$ or $C_{48}H_{24}O_{26}$, *polychrom*, colorless powder, without smell, bitter, nearly insoluble in cold water and ether, soluble in alkali. (See page 425.)

[1] Used in the East India islands as a remedy for intermittents.

Plant	Principle
Various species of Æsculus and barks of the genus *Pavia*.	*Paviin*, similar to æsculin, though not identical. (See page 425.)
Rutaceæ. Angustura, *U. S.* Bark of Gallipea Cusparia.	*Cusparin*, tetrahedral crystals, soluble in acids and alkalies, and in 200 parts water; precipitated by tannic acid.
Xanthoxylum piperitum, the fruit.	*Xanthoxylin*, volatile, insoluble in water, soluble in alcohol, ether; aromatic resinous taste; stearoptene from the oil.
Xanthoxylum, *U. S.* The bark of X. fraxineum.	*Xanthoxylin* of Dr. Staples, not investigated, probably identical with xanthopicrite (Dr. Wood).
Xanthoxylum corribæum,[1] or X. clava herculis, the bark.	Xanthopicrite of Chevalier & Pelletan; crystallizable, bitter.
Simarubaceæ. Quassia, *U. S.*, and Simaruba, *U. S.*	*Quassin*, $C_{20}H_{12}O_6$, white opaque granules, inodorous, intensely bitter, very soluble in alcohol, less so in ether, slightly in water which is increased by mixture with alcohol. (See page 425.)
Celastrineæ. Ilex opaca. (The American holly,) the fruit.	*Ilicin*,[2] acicular crystals, intensely bitter, slightly acrid, soluble in water and alcohol, freely in ether; precipitated by tannin.
Rhamneæ. Rhamnus frangula and cathartica. The unripe berries (buckthorn).	*Rhamnin*, volatile, tasteless, yellowish crystals; soluble in alkalies with yellow color (Fleury). *Cathartin* of Winkler, from the ripe fruit. Cathartic dose 1 to 3 grs. (See *Crysophanic Acid.*)
Leguminosæ. Dipterix odorata, fruit (Tonka beans). Melilotus officinalis, flowers.	*Coumarin*, $C_{18}H_6O_4$.[3] Colorless, quadrangular prisms; odor and taste aromatic; destroyed by SO_3, by NO_5 converted into nitro-coumarin and picric acid, by boiling with alkalies, coumaric acid $C_{18}H_8O_6$, 1 lb. tonka yields 108 grs.
Scoparius, *U. S.* (Broom.)	*Scoparin*, $C_{21}H_{11}O_{10}$, soluble in alkalies; precipitated by acids; little soluble in water, more soluble in alcohol, without odor or taste; oxidized by NO_5 to picric acid, appears to be the diuretic principle. (Stenhouse.)
Ononis spinosa, the root.	*Ononin*, $C_{62}H_{34}O_{27}$, colorless needles; little soluble in water, insoluble in ether, slowly soluble in boiling alcohol; red with SO_3; with caustic baryta into formic acid and *onospin*, which with diluted SO_3 or HCl, into sugar and *ononetin*. *Onocerin*, $C_{12}H_{10}O$, another crystallizable principle, not altered by boiling, as above.
Granateæ. Granat radix, cort, *U. S.*	*Punicin*, acrid, uncrystallizable, oily, powerful errhine.
Myrtaceæ. Caryophyllus, *U. S.*	*Caryophyllin*, $C_{20}H_{16}O_2$, yellow prisms, without taste or smell; soluble in ether and boiling alcohol. *Eugenin*, $C_{24}H_{15}O_5$, yellow pearly scales, becomes red with NO_5; isomeric with caryophyllic acid.

---

[1] Used in the Antilles as a febrifuge.

[2] In the first edition of this work, this principle as obtained from the leaves of the European species was classified among the uncrystallizable principles, but the crystalline principle has been discovered as above, by Dr. P. Pancoast, a graduate of the Philadelphia College of Pharmacy, as announced in his inaugural thesis. (See *American Journal of Pharmacy*, vol. xxviii. p. 312.)

[3] Coumarin also exists in Asperula odorata, *Rubiaceæ*, Anthoxanthum odoratum, *Gramineæ*, and some other herbs.

Cucurbitaceæ. Bryonia alba.	*Bryonin*, $C_{48}H_{80}O_{38}$, very bitter, soluble in water and alcohol, and insoluble in ether. *Bryonitin*, crystals, soluble in alcohol 95 per cent., and ether.
Colocynthis, *U. S.* The fruit of Cucumis colocynthis.	*Colocynthin*, $C_{56}H_{42}O_{23}$, amorphous? (See page 425.) *Colocynthitin*, obtained in white prisms from the part of the alcoholic extract insoluble in water and cold alcohol; soluble in hot alcohol and ether.
Elaterium, *U. S.*, from the fruit of Momordica elaterium (spirting cucumber).	*Elaterin*, $C_{20}H_{14}O_5$, colorless prisms, very bitter, acrid; insoluble in alkalies and in water; soluble in alcohol and ether.
Umbelliferæ. Petroselinum sativum. The herb.	*Apiin*, $C_{24}H_{14}O_{13}$, white powder, tasteless; nearly insoluble in cold water; gelatinizing from hot solution; blood red with FeO,SO_3. *Apiol*, yellowish, oily, non-volatile, acrid, pungent, heavier than water; soluble in alcohol, ether, chloroform. (See page 219.)
Daucus carota.	*Carotin*, $C_{10}H_{16}$? copper red, microscopic crystals, no odor or taste; insoluble in water and ether, slightly in alcohol, soluble in fixed and essential oils.
Peucedanum officinale. The root.	*Peucedanin*, $C_{24}H_{12}O_6$, colorless rhombic prisms, without taste or odor; melts at 167° F.; insoluble in water, soluble in hot alcohol, ether, fixed and volatile oils. Probably angelicate of oreoselon, $C_{14}H_6O_3,C_{10}H_7O_3$.
Imperatoria ostruthium.	*Imperatorin*, identical with peucedanin.
Athamantum oreoselinum. The root.	*Athamantin*, $C_{24}H_{15}O_7$, colorless, rectangular prisms, peculiar rancid odor on heating, taste rancid, bitter, acrid; melts at 174° F. Probably valerianate of oreoselon, $C_{14}H_6O_3,C_{10}H_{10}O_4$.
Araliaceæ. Panax, *U. S.* The root of Panax quinquefolium.	*Panaquilon*, $C_{24}H_{25}O_{18}$, amorphous, yellow powder; easily soluble in water and alcohol, insoluble in ether; precip. by tannin, red solution with SO_3; by strong acids converted into *panacon*, $C_{22}H_{19}O_8$.
Compositæ. Absynthium, *U. S.* Artemisia absynthium; the herb.	*Absynthin*, $C_{16}H_{11}O_5$, crystalline; soluble in alcohol, less in water and ether; acid reaction; with KO, golden color.
Lactucarium, *U. S.* From Lactuca virosa.	*Lactucin*, white pearly scales, combined with lactucic acid. *Lactucone*, $C_{40}H_{34}O_3$, white granules deposited from hot alcohol on cooling; insoluble in water, soluble in ether.
Taraxacum, *U. S.* Root of Leontodon taraxacum.	*Taraxacin*, colorless crystals, bitter, acrid, fusible; soluble in boiling water, alcohol, and ether.
Inula, *U.S.* The root of Inula helenium.	*Helenin*, long white needles. Probably a stearopten.
Caprifoliaceæ. Lonicera xylosteum. The berries.	*Xylostein*, crystalline, bitter principle; by dilute acids converted into sugar and other substances. (The seeds contain a volatile poison.)
Ericaceæ. Uva Ursi, *U. S.* The leaves of Arctostaphylos uva ursi.	*Arbutin*, $C_{24}H_{16}O_{14}+2HO$, bitter, colorless crystals. See page 425. *Ursin*, colorless needles, soluble in alcohol, water, ether, and diluted acids. Dose, one grain. See page 426. *Urson*, $C_{20}H_{17}O_2$, colorless, silky, tasteless, acicular crystals; insoluble in water, acids, and alkalies; fusible, inflammable; orange yellow with SO_3.
Oleaceæ. Olea Europæa (olive-tree). The gum.	*Olivil*, $C_{28}H_{18}O_{10}$, needles in starlike groups, bitter and sweet taste; melt at 250°; soluble in water, ether, and boiling alcohol.

Plant	Principle
Fraxinus excelsior. Common European ash. The bark.	*Fraxin*, yellowish needles, slightly bitter and astringent; soluble in boiling water; fluorescent, but blue color disappearing on adding acids.
Phillyrea latifolia (a species of privet.)	*Phillyrin*, $C_{54}H_{34}O_{22}+3HO$. Crystalline, nearly tasteless, soluble in hot water and alcohol, insoluble in ether. By diluted HCl and heat forms *phillygenin*; polymeric with *jalicin* and *caligenin*. Reputed antiperiodic.
Apocynaceæ. Apocynum cannabinum, *U. S.*	*Apocynin*, peculiar active principle.
Asclepiadeæ. Asclepias Syriaca. The milky juice.	*Asclepion*, $C_{40}H_{34}O_6$, white crystalline mass, odorless, tasteless; insoluble in water and alcohol, soluble in ether.
Gentianeæ. Gentiana, *U. S.* The root of G. lutea.	*Gentianin*, yellow powder, hygroscopic, very bitter; nearly insoluble in alcohol, soluble in water.
Menyanthes trifoliata. Herb. (Buck-bean.)	*Menyanthin*, amorphous, bitter; soluble in alcohol, water, and not in ether.
Convolvulaceæ. Jalapa, *U. S.* The root of Ipomœa jalapa.[1]	*Convolvulin*, $C_{62}H_{50}O_{32}$, white or transparent; insoluble in ether and water, soluble in alcohol; resinous.
Convolvulus Orizabensis.	*Jalapin*, $C_{68}H_{56}O_{32}$, white amorphous, resinous. (See page 426.)
Solaneæ. Capsicum, *U. S.* Capsicum annuum, and other species. The fruit.	*Capsicin*, white tufts of crystals; soluble in alcohol and ether. (See page 426.)
Physalis alkekengi. The leaves of the winter cherry.	*Physalin*, $C_{28}H_{16}O_{10}$, bitter, amorphous, yellowish; soluble in alcohol, chloroform, and ammonia.
Scrophularineæ. Digitalis, *U. S.* The leaves of D. purpurea.	*Digitaline*, $C_{22}H_{19}O_9$, white granules, inodorous though sternutatory; very bitter and poisonous. (See page 427.)
Gratiola officinalis. Hedge hyssop.	*Gratiolin*, $C_{40}H_{34}O_{14}$, bitter, white, crystalline; soluble in boiling water and alcohol; insoluble in ether. *Gratiosolin*, $C_{46}H_{42}O_{25}$, amorphous, yellow; insoluble in ether, soluble in water and alcohol. Products of decomposition numerous.
Scrophularia nodosa. The herb.	*Scrophularin*, crystalline scales, bitter; soluble in water.
Primulaceæ, Cyclamen Europæum.	*Cyclamin*, white, amorphous, inodorous; hygroscopic, becoming gelatinous. Poisonous.
Thymeleæ. Mezereum, *U. S.* The bark of Daphne mezereum.	*Daphnin*, brilliant colorless prisms, soluble in boiling water, alcohol, and ether; bitter, inodorous.
Laurineæ. Laurus nobilis. The leaves.	*Laurin*, $C_{22}H_{15}O_3$, white prisms tasteless, odorless; insoluble in water; soluble in alcohol.
Aristolocheæ. Aristolochia clematitis.	*Clematitin*, $C_9H_5O_6$, is extracted by boiling water.
Euphorbiaceæ. Cascarilla, *U. S.* The bark of Croton eleuteria.	*Cascarillin*, white crystals, bitter, inodorous; slightly soluble in water; soluble in alcohol and ether.
Urticeæ. Humulus, *U. S.* Strobiles of H. lupulus.	*Humulin* (impure?), amorphous, bitter, yellow, inodorous; insoluble in ether, soluble in alcohol, nearly insoluble in water.

[1] Ipomœa jalapa, *Nuttall;* Ipomœa Schiedeana, *Fucearind;* Ipomœa purga, *Schlectendale;* Convolvulus jalapa, *Schiede;* Convolvulus purga, *Wenderoth;* Convolvulus officinalis, *Pelletan;* Exagonium purga, *Bentham;* are all synonyms for true jalap.

Datisca cannabina. Leaves and root.	*Datiscin*, $C_{42}H_{22}O_{24}$, colorless, silky needles or scales; easily soluble in alcohol, less in ether and cold water; very bitter, fusible; soluble in alkalies with yellow color, precipitated by acids; by SO_3 forms sugar and *datiscetin*, $C_{30}H_{10}O_{12}$.
Amentaceæ. Populus tremula. Bark and leaves of the aspen.	*Populin*, $C_{40}H_{22}O_{16}+4$ aq, colorless prisms, sweetish taste; soluble in alcohol, slightly in water, by boiling with alkali forms salicin and benzoic acid.
Salix and populus, several species. The bark.	*Salicin*, $C_{26}H_{18}O_{14}$, neutral, very bitter; soluble in water and alcohol, yielding many derivatives. (See page 427.)
Piperaceæ. Cubeba, *U. S.* The berries of Piper cubeba.	*Cubebin*, $C_{34}H_{34}O_{10}$, white, crystalline, inodorous, insipid, not volatilizable by heat, cryst. from alcohol; nearly insoluble in water, soluble in ether, acetic acid, fixed and volatile oils; with SO_3 carmine red; deposited in extract. cubebæ fluid.
Coniferæ. Pinus sylvestris and Thuja occidentalis.	*Pinipikrin*, $C_{44}H_{36}O_{22}$, bitter, amorphous, light yellowish brown; soluble in water and alcohol, insoluble in ether, liquid at 212°; with dilute SO_3 ? ericinal sugar and a resin.
Orchideæ. Vanilla aromatica. Prepared unripe capsule.	*Vanillin*, $C_{20}H_6O_4$, colorless four-sided needles, strong vanilla odor, hot biting task. (See page 426.)
Smilaceæ. Sarsaparilla, *U. S.* The root of Smilax officinalis.	*Smilacin* or *sarsaparillin*, $C_{18}H_{15}O_6$, colorless needles, disagreeable, bitter, acrid nauseous taste; soluble in boiling alcohol and ether, froths in solution, similar to *saponin*, slightly acid.
Liliaceæ. Aloe, *U. S.* Inspissated juice of Aloe socotrina and other species.	*Alöin*, $C_{34}H_{18}O_{14}$, sulphur-yellow crystals, insoluble in water, dissolved by alkalies. (See page 429.)
Scilla, *U. S.* The bulb of Scilla maritima.	*Scillitin*, bitter needles, insoluble in water, soluble in alcohol and ether; decomposed by alkalies, emetic, cathartic, and narcotic poison.
Lichenes. Variolaria amaralichen.	*Picrolichenin*, $C_6H_5O_2$, small, brilliant, rhombic, pyramidal crystals; very bitter, and said to be febrifuge.

2. *Quaternary or Nitrogenized Neutral Principles.*

Rosaceæ. The kernels, leaves, and flowers of many plants.	*Amygdalin*, $N,C_{40}H_{27}O_{22}$, white crystalline, inodorous, agreeably bitter, soluble in water and boiling alcohol, insoluble in ether. *Emulsin.* The peculiar vegetable albumen of this species of plants is a proteinic compound.
Leguminosæ. Also in malvaceæ and asparageæ. (Young beans, peas, asparagus, beets, liquorice root, &c.)	*Asparagin*, althæin, or malamid, $N,C_4H_4O_3+2HO$, octohedrons, colorless, inodorous, insipid; insoluble in ether, soluble in 58 parts water and less alcohol, by fermentation owing to impurities converted into succinate of ammonia, thus:— $2N,C_4H_4O_3+2HO_1+2H_1=2NH_4O,C_8H_4O_6$.

3. *Sulphuretted Neutral Principles.*

Cruciferæ. Sinapis alba, *U. S.*	*Sulpho-sinapisin*, $N_2C_{34}H_{25}S_2O_{10}$, crystallizable by the action of a ferment contained in the seed, converted into an acrid bitter principle, and probably hydro-sulpho-cyanic acid; by alkalies sinapic acid; by acids sinapin.

4. *Animal Neutral Principles.*

Cantharis, *U. S.* Cantharis vesicatoria. Cantharis vittata, *U. S.*, and other species.	*Cantharidin*, $C_{10}H_{6}O_{4}$, prepared by the evaporation of ether or chloroform tincture of the flies; crystallized from boiling alcohol, white scaly micaceous crystals, without odor or taste; when pure insoluble in water, slightly soluble in cold alcohol, soluble in ether, chloroform, benzole, fixed oils, &c., fusible and volatile; soluble in water in its natural state of combination. A powerful vesicant.
Castoreum, *U. S.*, from castor fiber.	*Castorin*, crystallizes from the boiling alcoholic tincture, purified by washing with cold alcohol, long fasciculated prisms, odor of castor, cuprous taste, insoluble in cold water and alcohol, soluble in volatile oils and 100 parts of boiling alcohol; Canadian castor contains 7 per cent.
Fresh meat. Chickens, game, etc.	Creatine, $C_{8}H_{9}N_{3}O_{4}+2$ aq. (See page 381.)

Remarks on some of the Neutral Principles.

Æsulin or polychrom, as shown in the syllabus, is the name given to a peculiar principle obtained from the bark of the horse chestnut tree.

The bark is exhausted by alcohol of eighty per cent., a little evaporated and set aside for several weeks, the powder washed with ice-cold water, and purified from a mixture of one part of ether and five of alcohol.

It is a colorless powder, microscopic needles, without smell, bitterish taste, little soluble in cold water, nearly insoluble in ether, soluble in alkalies. A very dilute solution, containing one-millionth part, opalesces with blue color in reflected light; acids destroy this property, alkalies restore it, chlorine destroys it, coloring the solution red.

By the action of dilute acids it is converted into sugar and æsculetin.

Rochleder's Formula.—$C_{42}H_{24}O_{26}+6HO=2C_{12}H_{12}O_{12}+C_{18}H_{6}O_{8}$; or, $C_{60}H_{33}O_{37}+3HO=2C_{12}H_{12}O_{12}+2C_{18}H_{6}O_{8}$, æsculetin.

Paviin may be obtained by the slow evaporation of the ethereal tincture in needles grown in star-like groups.

Its properties are similar to æsculin, but, while this fluoresces with sky-blue color, paviin shows a green color in solution; both usually occur together in the barks of this family; the genus *æsculus* containing *æsculin*, the genus *pavia*, *paviin*, in preponderance.

These principles, though little known except as scientific curiosities, are worthy a trial as antiperiodics. The bark has long been reputed to possess febrifuge properties.

Quassin, the active principle of the intensely bitter wood and barks of the quassias, is prepared by a very elaborate process, of which the following is the outline:—

The evaporated decoction is treated with lime, filtered, evaporated, exhausted by 85 per cent. alcohol, evaporated, dissolved in anhydrous alcoholic ether, by spontaneous evaporation from water it crystallizes in white, opaque granules, unalterable in air, intensely bitter, little soluble in water, more so in dilute acids, and alkalies, and salts (with several of which it is associated in the wood), melting like a resin; it is precipitated by tannin.

In Martinique and other neighboring islands, the wood of Bytteria febrifuga *Simarubeæ*, there called false simaruba, is employed for intermittents. Gerardias found its bitter principle to be quassin, of which it contains a much larger proportion than does quassia.

Colocynthin.—The fruit of colocynth, in fine powder, is to be mixed with and packed upon animal charcoal, is displaced with alcohol and evaporated spontaneously; a garnet colored, pulverizable mass, extremely bitter, soluble in water and alcohol, insoluble in ether.

Active cathartic in the dose of one and a half grain.

It is obtained pure by treating the aqueous solution of the alcoholic extract successively with acetate, and subacetate of lead, sulphuretted hydrogen and tannin; the latter precipitated, after dissolving in alcohol, again with lead and sulphuretted hydrogen; after being evaporated spontaneously, the residue is well washed with anhydrous ether. (Walz.)

By treating with dilute SO_3, it is converted into sugar and *colocynthein*, $C_{56}H_{42}O_{23}+2HO=C_{12}H_{12}O_{12}+C_{44}H_{32}O_{13}$.

Arbutin.—An aqueous decoction, is precipitated by acetate of lead, and the filtrate, after treating with HS, evaporated to a syrupy consistence; after some time, prisms of *arbutin* appear, colorless, bitter, at 212° losing water of crystallization, without becoming opaque. By emulsin it is converted into glucose and *arctusin*, colorless, sweetish-bitter needles.

According to Strecker, the products of the decomposition are sugar and *hydrokinone.* $C_{24}H_{16}O_{14}+2HO=C_{12}H_{12}O_{12}+C_{12}H_{6}O_{4}$.

Ursin.—The alcoholic solution of the aqueous extract of uva ursi is repeatedly treated with animal charcoal, and evaporated spontaneously.

Colorless needles, soluble in alcohol, water, ether, and dilute acids; neutral reaction. In the dose of one grain, this appears to be powerfully diuretic.

The resinoid principles of jalap have already been treated of in their practical relations among the concentrated or resinous extracts; in this connection it will be proper to refer to them as the neutral principles giving activity to that particular family of plants.

Convolvulin, formerly called Rhodeoretin.—To prepare this from the root of Convolvulus Schiedeanus (Ipomœa Jalapa), it is exhausted with boiling water, dried, exhausted with 90 per cent. alcohol, water added until precipitation commences, treated with animal charcoal, evaporated, exhausted with ether, the residue dissolved in alcohol, and precipitated by ether.

A white resinous substance, transparent in thin layers, without odor or taste, insoluble in ether, scarcely soluble in water, easily soluble in alcohol, also in alkalies, without being precipitated by acids, soluble in acetic acid.

The solution in alkalies contains convolvulic acid$=C_{62}H_{50}O_{32}+3HO$; soluble in water.

Convolvulin, dissolved in anhydrous alcohol, and treated with hydrochloric acid, is decomposed into an oily, crystallizing body, *convolvulinol* and sugar.

Convolvulic acid, in aqueous solution, treated with dilute SO_3, suffers the same decomposition. Convolvulinol, $C_{26}H_{24}O_{7}$, separated from its alkaline solution, has been converted into convolvulinolic acid.

The above three substances, by NO_5, are converted into ipomic acid.

Jalapin.—The root of Ipomœa Orizabensis, after exhaustion with boiling water, is treated with alcohol, water added until turbidity commences, boiled with fresh animal charcoal, filtered, precipitated with acetate of lead and a little ammonia, the filtrate treated with sulphuretted hydrogen, distilled, the resin treated with boiling water, and dissolved in ether.

White, without taste or smell, amorphous, melting point 300° F, little soluble in water, easily in alcohol and ether, soluble in wood spirit, benzol, turpentine, and acetic acid, slight acid reaction, soluble in alkalies and alkaline earths, changing into jalapic acid $=C_{68}H_{59}O_{35}$, which is tribasic.

Mineral acids decompose jalapin and jalapic acid into sugar and *jalapinol* (white crystalline) $=C_{32}H_{31}O_7$. Separated from its combinations with alkalies, it has been converted into *jalapinolic acid*, $=C_{32}H_{30}O_6$.

Jalapin, jalapic and jalapinolic acid, treated with NO_5, are converted into oxalic and ipomic acid, $=C_{20}H_{18}O_8$.

Capsicin.—In the winter of 1856 and '7, one of my pupils, H. B. Taylor, of Philadelphia, being about to prepare his thesis for the Philadelphia College of Pharmacy, pursued a course of experiments upon capsicum annuum, under my direction, which resulted in the discovery of a crystalline principle, which appears to be the true capsicin, though that name had before been applied to oily or soft resinoid products. The process was as follows: Powdered capsicum was treated with anhydrous ether and evaporated, the oleoresinous product was digested in alcohol of .809 sp. gr., the filtered alcoholic solution was treated with subacetate of lead, which threw down a copious precipitate; this was separated by filtration, and the clear tincture treated with sulphhydric acid; the precipitated sulphuret of lead was now removed, the solution boiled, again filtered, evaporated, and set aside, on an intensely cold day, to crystallize. On examination, the whole was found to have solidified into a mass of beautiful, nearly white, feathery crystals. Owing to the comparative insolubility of sulphhydric acid gas in alcohol, they were not completely free from lead salt, and were further purified and crystallized, though not with the same facility, from the change of temperature. These crystals seem analogous to a stearoptine; heated, they first melt, and then take fire, burning with a bright rose-colored flame, and giving off dense, suffocating fumes; heated with sulphuric acid, they blacken, and give off white fumes. The taste is excessively fiery, inflaming all parts with which it comes in contact; the odor is faint.

Digitaline.—This is associated in the leaves of the plant, with a variety of less important chemical products, one of which has been called *digitalin* by the French investigators, the termination in *ine* is therefore selected advisedly. It is prepared by treating the alcoholic extract with very dilute acetic acid heated to 110° F., treating this with charcoal, neutralizing by ammonia, and precipitating with concentrated infusion of galls; this precipitate is then treated with finely-powdered litharge, dissolved in alcohol, treated with charcoal, evaporated, and washed with pure ether. The yield is nearly one per cent. It precipitates from the alcoholic solution in granules, with no disposition to crystallize. It is white, inodorous, intensely bitter and irritating to the nostrils, little soluble in cold water, slightly in ether, more soluble in alcohol. It strikes an emerald green color with concentrated muriatic acid; it is freed from a resinous impurity which increases its solubility in alcohol, by washing on a filter with 70 per cent. alcohol, and recrystallizing from hot 85 per cent. alcohol. Digitaline is a powerful poison, given for the same sedative properties as the leaves. It has lately been much prescribed in the form of granules of sugar, which have been saturated with the tincture, so that each shall represent a given quantity of the medicine. The usual dose is one-thirtieth of a grain. Being among the most powerful of known poisons, it should be used with great care.

Salicin.—The bark of the following plants contain no salicin: S. alba, babylonica, bicolor, capræa, daphnoides, incana, fragilis, russiliana, triandra, viminalis and Populus angulosa, fastigiata, grandiculata, monilifera, nigra, virginica; all the other willows contain salicin, and it is probable that all the herbaceous kinds of spiræa, which yield salicylous acid (oil of spiræa), contain it originally.

Preparation.—The decoction of willow bark is evaporated to three times the weight of the bark employed, digested with oxide of lead, and the filtrate evaporated to syrupy consistence. After several days the crystals are purified by recrystallization. (Duflos.) There are several other processes.

It is obtained in white thin scaly crystals, very bitter, soluble in water, less in alcohol, insoluble in ether and oil of turpentine. Water at ordinary temperature dissolves 3½ per cent. No action on vegetable colors; deviates the plane of polarization to the left.

Concentrated SO_3 colors it blood red; water decolorizes it again, dissolving a peculiar acid (rufisulphuric acid). Cold diluted SO_3 or HCl converts it into sugar and saligenin. $C_{26}H_{18}O_{14}+2HO=C_{12}H_{12}O_{12}+C_{14}H_8O_4$—saligenin.

If treated hot, it is converted into sugar and *saliretin*, $2(C_{26}H_{18}O_{14})=2C_{12}H_{12}O_{12}+C_{28}H_{12}O_4$=saliretin.

Cold NO_5 of 1.16 specific gravity converts it into *helicin*. $C_{26}H_{18}O_{14}+O_2=2HO+C_{26}H_{16}O_{14}$=helicin.

If a more diluted NO_5, of 1.09 specific gravity, is used, the result is a compound between helicin and salicin, which has been called *helicoidin*. $2C_{26}H_{18}O_{14}+O_2=2HO+C_{52}H_{34}O_{28}$=(helicoidin)$=C_{26}H_{16}O_{15}+C_{26}H_{18}O_{14}$.

If salicin is heated with very dilute NO_5 just to the boiling point, and allowed to cool, or evaporated at a low temperature, salicylous acid is separated.

At the boiling point, nitrosalicylic acid is formed, and by continued influence picric and oxalic acids.

Melted with an excess of caustic potassa, it is converted into salicylate and oxalate of potassa.

Heated with binoxide of lead, formiate of lead is obtained; with black oxide of manganese and dilute SO_3, formic and carbonic acids; with bichromate of potassa and SO_3, carbonic, formic, and salicylous acids.

By dry distillation it yields, among pyro products, salicylous acid; and when taken internally it is found in the urine together with its products of decomposition—saligenin, salicylous, and salicylic acids.

Saligenin, $C_{14}H_8O_4$, pearly crystals, easily soluble in boiling water, alcohol, and ether, sublimes above 212°; colored red by concentrated SO_3; concentrated NO_5 oxidizes it to picric, dilute NO_5 to salicylous and nitrosalicylous acids, $C_{14}H_8O_4+2O=C_{14}H_6O_4+2HO$; heated with hydrate of potassa, it is converted into salicylic acid and hydrogen, $C_{14}H_8O_4+KO,HO=C_{14}H_5KO_6+4H$. Sesquisalts of iron impart an indigo-blue color. Dilute acids by boiling convert it into

Saliretin, $C_{28}H_{12}O_4=2C_{14}H_8O_4-4HO$, which is insoluble in water and ammonia, soluble in alcohol, ether, concentrated acetic acid, and fixed alkalies; concentrated SO_3 colors it blood red; concentrated NO_5 oxidizes it on boiling to picric, not to oxalic acid.

Helicin, $C_{26}H_{16}O_{14}$, white needles, without odor, bitterish taste, insoluble in ether, easily soluble in hot water and alcohol. By synaptase and boiling with alkalies is converted into sugar and salicylous acid—$C_{26}H_{16}O_{14}+2HO=C_{12}H_{12}O_{12}+C_{14}H_6O_4$.

Helicoidin is a derivative, having the composition $C_{52}H_{34}O_{28}=C_{26}H_{16}O_{14}$ (helicin)$+C_{26}H_{18}O_{14}$(salicin). By synaptase is decomposed into sugar, saligenin, and salicylous acid.

Salicin was formerly used to adulterate sulphate of quinia, which it resembles in appearance. It is tonic and febrifuge, though little used. Dose, three to thirty grains.

Vanillin.—Vanilla of commerce is exhausted with alcohol, evaporated to an extract, this exhausted by ether, which is to be evaporated, heated with boiling water, which, on evaporation, lets fall the principle; recrystallized and treated with animal charcoal, it is obtained in colorless four-sided needles, of strong vanilla odor, hot, burning taste; fuses at 195°, volatilizes at 302°; little soluble in cold water, very soluble in hot water, alcohol, ether, and the fixed and volatile oils.

Concentrated SO_3 dissolves it with yellow color; liq. potassæ dissolves it and deposits it again on being neutralized.

The crystals observed on the surface of the fresh bean of commerce are believed to consist of vanillin, not benzoic acid, as heretofore supposed.

Alöin.—This interesting proximate constituent of aloes has been prepared from several commercial varieties, especially from Barbadoes and Socotrine aloes. It was discovered by T. & H. Smith, of Edinburgh, who are still its principal manufacturers, and it has recently attained commercial as well as scientific interest from being pretty extensively prescribed as a mild and pleasant cathartic.

Preparation according to Groves.—Aloes is exhausted by boiling water, the decoction acidulated with muriatic acid, filtered, evaporated to a syrupy consistence, and set aside in a cool place to crystallize. The crystals, after a fortnight, are separated and purified by recrystallization from boiling water. Socotrine aloes yields 10 per cent. aloin. These crystals are to be dried by bibulous paper at a moderate heat; when thoroughly dry aloin is permanent in the air, but with moisture and heat conjoined, has a tendency to lose its crystalline form, assuming the amorphous character of aloes.

Alöin is in crystals of a sulphur-yellow color, bitter taste, and no odor, soluble in 60 parts of cold water, and in 5 parts of boiling water; extremely soluble in alcohol, muriatic and acetic acids, caustic potassa, and ammonia, giving a brown solution with alkalies. It is insoluble in ether, benzine, oil of turpentine, and chloroform, although softened by these into a mass. Heated in olive oil it fuses unchanged. It turns red by SO_3 and NO_5, and dissolves into a red solution. By heat it readily fuses, darkens in color, decomposes, and passes into a black voluminous charcoal.

Its purgative properties have been denied, but the experience of numerous practitioners here and in Europe, confirms its utility as a mild though pretty certain cathartic in doses of from two to three grains. (See *Extemporaneous Pharmacy.*)

Amygdalin.—This interesting principle is obtained from bitter almonds by the following process: Bitter almonds, powdered and expressed, to free them from fixed oil, are to be boiled in successive portions of alcohol till exhausted. The liquors thus obtained are placed in a still, and evaporated at a low heat, the alcohol being recovered. The syrupy residue is then to be diluted with water and mixed with yeast, and subjected to fermentation to separate sugar. Again evaporate, at a moderate temperature, to the consistence of syrup, cool, and add 95 per cent. of alcohol. The amygdalin will then precipitate, and may be collected on a strainer; it is then to be purified by repeated resolution in hot alcohol, and crystallization. Any oil it may contain may be separated by shaking the solution with ether before or after the fermentation. One pound of almonds yields at least two drachms of amygdalin. Heat decomposes it, giving off the odor of hawthorn; heated with alkaline solutions, it evolves ammonia and forms amygdalic acid.

Amygdalin seems destitute of active properties, except when mixed in solution with *emulsin*, a sort of vegetable albumen present in all almonds, producing grape sugar, oil of bitter almonds, and hydrocyanic acid, which is thus explained: $NC_{40}H_{27}O_{22}+4HO=2C_{12}H_{12}O_{12}+C_{14}H_6O_2+HNC_2$.

On the Decomposition of Organic Bodies.

On the foregoing pages the organic compounds have been treated of, and a number of pharmaceutical preparations derived from the organic kingdom. It is well known that such chemical and pharmaceutical compounds are subject to alterations by various influences, the study of which forms a most important part of chemistry. To many of these changes attention has been drawn in the appropriate places, and it remains now, without treating of the same in detail, to present them in a condensed form, conveniently arranged.

The decomposition of organic bodies may be treated of under four separate heads:—

I. *Oxidation by the Atmosphere.*—As a general rule, pure chemical compounds are not affected by dry or moist atmosphere, except perhaps to deliquesce or effloresce, or like the salts of some volatile organic acids, as acetic and valerianic, to evolve them in moist air. But oxidation is comparatively rare, and mostly met with in compounds destitute of oxygen and abounding in hydrogen; examples are the ternary alkaloids and the carbohydrogens of the volatile oils.

II. *Decomposition into simpler Compounds.*—1. *By air and water.* Complex organic bodies are subject to oxidation and ultimately break up into the inorganic compounds, carbonic acid, ammonia, and water; if this process of decomposition takes place slowly, it is called *decay;* if quicker in the presence of more water and with the evolution of an offensive smell, *putrefaction;* under similar circumstances, when the product is a useful compound, *fermentation;* of this last a distinction is made between *vinous* fermentation (see page 308) and *acid* fermentation, the latter being again subdivided in accordance with the acid obtained, and is then called acetic, lactic, butyric, succinic, &c. (see the acids named); the presence of a nitrogenated compound is necessary, to act as a ferment.

2. *By acids.* Of the concentrated acids, the action of sulphuric acid is the most violent; it abstracts water from all organic compounds, leaving a compound with a larger amount of carbon; or the carbon is oxidized, and the evolved gases contain carbonic oxide, and formic, carbonic, and sulphurous acids; compounds containing amide (NH_2) yield ammonia. Glacial phosphoric and arsenic acids have a similar action, but weaker.

Diluted acids act differently; they cause the combination with the elements of water (conversion of starch into sugar, p. 287), very seldom evolve carbonic acid (conversion of meconic into komenic acid), but very often decompose organic bodies into glucose and another compound of different behavior (see Tannic Acids, Salicin, &c.); the latter decomposition often takes place also by the influence of emulsin, synaptase, or similar ferments.

3. *By chloride of zinc.* Aided by heat, this is capable of abstracting water from organic compounds; it produces ether from alcohol, &c.

4. *By heat.* Organic compounds are called volatile if they may be distilled without suffering decomposition; others are decomposed, and the process is then termed *dry* or *destructive distillation*, and the products *pyro products.* These are, in the commencement of the distillation, highly oxygenated and of an acid nature (see p. 284), afterwards contain less oxygen, and at last are carbohydrogens (marsh gas, C_2H_4, olefiant gas, C_4H_4) or ternary alkaloids (see Artificial Alkaloids); water, tar, and charcoal generally accompany the products of the dry distillation of all complex bodies. Exposure to a continued red or white heat resolves them more or less completely into binary inorganic compounds and the elements.

III. *Artificial Oxidation.*—Many highly oxygenated inorganic compounds, when in contact with organic bodies, part with one or more equivalents of oxygen, which in its nascent state acts on the organic compound; such is the case with a number of acids, viz., nitric (see Oxalic Acid, p. 357, and Sugars, p. 289), chromic (see Valerianic Acid, p. 372), chloric, iodic acids, with peroxide of manganese (see Formic Acid, p. 361), binoxide of lead (see Tartaric Acid, p. 358), and the oxides of the noble metals. Many organic compounds, when in solution together with alkalies, are thereby rendered more prone to oxidation by the atmosphere.

IV. "*Integration*" *with Elements or Inorganic Compounds.*—A number of the nonmetallic elements may enter the combination of organic bodies as integral parts; the halogens by direct influence, sulphur by the influence of sulphuric acid or a sulphuric compound (see Artificial Volatile Oils, &c.). The integration of NO_4 has some importance in pharmacy; gun-cotton (p. 275) is such a compound.

Glycerin is decomposed by nitric acid into carbonic and oxalic acid, but if added very gradually to refrigerated strong nitric acid it is converted into a compound with NO_4, which has been called *Glonoin*, is insoluble in water, soluble in alcohol and ether, has a sweet aromatic taste, and is very poisonous; it is very explosive when heated, and its vapor causes violent headache. This substance has been proposed as a medicinal agent when a powerful action on the nervous system is required, but is as yet little known.

PART IV.

INORGANIC PHARMACEUTICAL PREPARATIONS.

CHAPTER I.

ON MINERAL ACIDS.

Preliminary Remarks.—In Part IV., the subject of pharmaceutical chemistry as pertaining to substances of inorganic origin is presented; those medicines which fall within the range of the dispensing office and shop, will be treated of in such detail as to render their preparation as easy and uniformly successful as possible, while the leading compounds used in the arts, and incidentally in medicine, and those prepared exclusively by the manufacturing chemist will be described with reference to their uses, and the modes of ascertaining their purity and genuineness.

The difference between that part of the *Pharmacopœia* called the List, in which the materia medica is presented, clothed in its appropriate nomenclature, and accompanied by well-ascertained standards whereby the genuineness and purity of many of the individual articles may be known; and that part occupied with formulæ or recipes designed to direct the apothecary and physician in the preparation of the crude articles of the list into eligible forms for use, has been fully presented on page 73 in an extract from the preface to the *Pharmacopœia* there inserted. This arrangement, however, includes among the preparations many articles which in this country are prepared exclusively in large manufacturing establishments; in fact, so generally has the manufacture of chemical preparations been concentrated in the hands of a few leading manufacturers, that even the largest dispensing establishments are in the habit of resorting to these for their supplies of all, except a few of the more readily prepared and extemporaneous articles. Owing to this fact, much of the space heretofore devoted in pharmaceutical works to descriptions and illustrations of apparatus and processes is now destitute of practical value to the largest class of students and readers.

In treating of these subjects, therefore, I have disregarded the divisions in the *Pharmacopœia*, and present such remarks on each preparation as have appeared to possess the most value to the classes to which this work is addressed.

It would not be inappropriate to preface this part of the work with an allusion to the value of practical chemical knowledge to the student or practitioner, whether of medicine or pharmacy. In no pursuit is a knowledge of chemistry unimportant; as the key which unlocks the physical sciences, and opens the most hidden secrets of nature, chemistry is invaluable to every industrial pursuit, and in every relation of life, and to no class is it more so than to the physician, the object of whose study is the highest and most intricate piece of nature's handiwork. The young man who would turn his attention in this direction may avail himself of numerous elementary works, adapted to impart accurate knowledge by means of experiments to be performed with cheap apparatus, and so arranged as to lead by gradual steps to the comprehension of facts which would otherwise be abstruse and difficult.

Of works of this description, it will be sufficient to name Bowman's Introduction to Practical Chemistry, Stockhart's Chemistry, and Francis's Chemical Experiments, while the more advanced student may consult with advantage the works of Fownes, Graham, Gmelin. and any of the numerous other leading modern chemists.

A knowledge of the principles of elective affinity, the peculiar force by which new compounds are formed from those previously existing, is not only of vast importance to the manufacturer and the analyst, but is even necessary to an understanding of the descriptions contained in a practical work like the present.

The great fact, which underlies the whole science of chemistry, that chemical substances combine with each other in certain definite proportions called equivalents, forming compounds, the equivalents of which are always equal to the sum of the equivalents of the elements they contain, is among the first to be thoroughly mastered by the student, and connected with this, he may find great advantage in the study or constant reference to a table of equivalent numbers, such as will be found in the appendix.

Nothing so facilitates the acquisition of scientific knowledge as an intelligible, concise, and familiar nomenclature, and though this has long been considered a stumbling block to students at the threshold of chemistry, it is confidently recommended as a necessary investment of time and energy which will yield ample returns in the subsequent prosecution of the science, whether in its theoretical or practical bearings.

Notwithstanding the elementary character of this work, I have not hesitated to employ in this and the last part the abbreviated method of notation now in universal use among chemists, and by which the composition of the most complex bodies is fully expressed by a few clear and intelligible symbols with numbers attached to designate the equivalent proportions of the elements they contain. The composition and relation of compound bodies can only be shown at a glance in this way, and it is earnestly desired of the pharmaceutical student that he will in no case neglect to address himself to a full comprehension of these chemical formulæ, as they are called.

The object of the present work is not to impart chemical principles, but to improve in its humble sphere the industrial application of the science to the healing art, and it would therefore be inappropriate to go further into these subjects in this place.

ACIDA.

All the inorganic acids employed in pharmacy are compounds, rich in oxygen, with the exceptions of muriatic, hydriodic, and some other hydracids, in which that element is wanting.

Acids are electro-negative compounds; they usually have a sour taste, change the blue color of litmus to red, and affect other vegetable colors similarly; with alkalies, whether vegetable or mineral, they form neutral salts in which the properties of both the ingredients are lost, while new properties are acquired. They also unite with the oxides of the metals proper, forming a great variety of valuable compounds which frequently exhibit slightly acid reactions; they usually retain the peculiarities of the metal from which they are prepared, modified by the nature of the acid ingredient.

The names of the mineral acids formed from the same element vary in their terminations according to the number of equivalents of oxygen they contain: thus, sulphur*ic* acid, SO_3, sulphur*ous* acid, SO_2, Nitr*ic*, NO_5, Nitr*ous*, NO_4, &c., the degree of acidification being marked by the terminations ic, and ous.

The strong acids act upon cork, and should be kept in ground stoppered bottles; those made of extra strength, of green glass, are called acid bottles. Unless the stopper and neck are very well ground and fitted to each other, they require to be cemented or luted together to prevent the escape of the acid; this may be done by warming the stopper in the flame of a spirit lamp, and inserting it in the neck of the bottle till the two surfaces are dried and warmed, then coating it with a thin stratum of melted wax, and inserting it securely in its place, and tying it over with kid or bladder. The more common mineral acids are found in commerce of three qualities; the commonest and cheapest used for manufacturing purposes, the medicinally pure, M. P., and the chemically pure, C. P. The use of the latter is chiefly in analysis. The specific gravity furnishes a ready means of testing the strength of the liquid acids, tables being given in chemical works showing the relation of the sp. gr. to the strength.

The mineral acids generally belong to the class of tonics with refrigerant and astringent properties. Externally, they are caustic, and require to be applied with care, as many know from experience who have used them, nitric acid especially, for warts. Nitric acid is also used as an alterative in syphilitic and other forms of disease.

They are apt to injure the teeth, upon which they also produce a very unpleasant and characteristic sensation. To obviate this in taking them, they should be largely diluted, and should be sucked through a small glass tube, which may be made by scratching a piece of the tube sold in the shops with a file; this enables the operator to break it at the point required, and then, by heating the sharp broken edges over an alcohol or gas flame till the glass melts, a rounded edge is left.

One of the most interesting and important facts in connection with the strong mineral acids, is their occasional use in poisonous doses. They are among the most powerful of poisons, owing to their corrosive properties producing the most painful and dangerous results. The best antidotes are large draughts of alkaline and oily liquids; the alkali to neutralize the acid, and the oil to obtund its action upon the delicate mucous surfaces. The most ready resort in such emergencies is frequently soap, which should be made into a very strong solution and given *ad libitum*.

Of the *mineral acids*, the following are used in medicine, and, except those in Italics, are officinal in the *U. S. Pharmacopœia*:—

	Sp. gr.	Dose.
Acidum Boracicum, HO,BO_3+2HO. Crystals.		gr. x to ʒj.?
" Carbonicum, CO_2. (See *Aquæ Medicatæ*.)		
" *Chromicum*, CrO_3. Crystals used as a caustic.		
" Muriaticum, gaseous, $HCl,+$water	1.16.	♏iij to v.
" Muriaticum dilutum, 1 part to 3 of water . . .	1.046.	♏xv to xl.
" Nitricum, liquid, HO,NO_5+4HO	1.42.	♏j to iv.
" *Nitroso-nitricum* " " $+NO_4$ . . .		♏j to iv.
" Nitricum dilutum, 1 part to 6 of water . . .	1.07.	♏xv to xl.
" Nitro-muriaticum, 1 part nitric to 2 muriatic acid .		♏iij to v.
" Sulphuricum, HO,SO_3	1.845.	♏j to ij.
" " dilutum, 1 part to 13 water . . .	1.09.	♏xv to xl.
" " aromaticum, alcoholic with aromatics .		♏xv to xxx.
" *Sulphurosum*, SO_2, used externally in skin diseases.		
" *Hydrosulphuricum*, HS, in solution, test liquid for metals.		
" *Phosphoricum, glacial*, HO,PO_5. (Variable). . .	solid.	
" " *dilutum*, 1 part to 10 of water . .	1.064.	♏xv to xl.
" *Hydriodicum*, HI. A colorless liquid		♏v to lx.
" *Chlorohydrocyanicum*, liquid, fumigation for the eye.		
" *Sulphohydrocyanicum*, do. do.		

Acidum Boracicum. (*Boracic or Boric Acid.*)

For medicinal purposes, this acid is prepared from borax. Mitscherlich recommends the following process: 1 part of borax is dissolved in four parts of boiling water, and decomposed by a quantity of muriatic acid sufficient to impart to the liquid a strong reaction on litmus paper; on cooling, boracic acid separates in shining scaly crystals, which are purified by recrystallization.

Muriatic acid is preferable to sulphuric acid, because the boracic acid can be easily purified from the former acid adhering to it, while sulphuric can only be entirely expelled by exposing the product to a strong heat, or by precipitating the hot solution with a sufficient quantity of nitrate of baryta.

The crystals are free of odor, have very little taste, dissolve in 20 parts of cold water, and 5 parts of alcohol. It reddens litmus paper and imparts to curcuma paper a peculiar brown color. On boiling the solution much acid evaporates with the aqueous vapor; its alcoholic solution burns with a green flame. Impurities which it may contain are detected by alcohol, which leaves most of them behind; sulphuretted hydrogen, if metallic salts are present; chloride of barium, if sulphuric acid, and by nitrate of silver, if muriatic acid, is present. Its salts are all soluble, and are decomposed when in solution by most acids.

Boracic acid is classified as a sedative; it is not much used in medicine, except in combination with soda, and with bitartrate of potassa.

For an interesting account on some borates see *Amer. Journ. of Pharm.*, xxxi. 241.

Acidum Chromicum.—To 100 parts, by measure, of cold saturated solution of bichromate of potassa, 150 parts of pure sulphuric acid are added and allowed to remain till cool; the sulphuric acid unites with the potassa, and the chromic acid crystallizes in deep red needles—very soluble and deliquescent. It is a powerful oxidizing and bleaching agent. In medicine its chief use is as a caustic application, which, it is said, "when rightly managed, does not spread beyond the prescribed limits, and so soon as its corrosive operation is finished passes into the state of inert pulverulent sesquioxide;" diluted with two parts of water, it has been used with great success as an injection in uterine hemorrhage.

Acidum Muriaticum, U.S. (*Hydrochloric or Chlorohydric Acid*, HCl.)

Prepared by the action of sulphuric acid and water on chloride of sodium (common salt), sulphate of soda and hydrochloric acid are formed. The latter gas is distilled over, the process being conducted in a retort or flask, connected with a receiver containing water, which absorbs it rapidly in proportion as it is refrigerated. A colorless or slightly yellow transparent liquid, giving off white acrid fumes on exposure to the air.

It should not dissolve goldleaf, as shown by the acid after digesting with it, giving no precipitate with protochloride of tin. The absence of saline impurities is shown by its being entirely volatile, and yielding no precipitate with chloride of barium or ammonia in excess.

Muriatic acid may be recognized, by the evolution of chlorine, on treating a muriate with SO_3 and black oxide of manganese; by the white precipitate occasioned by a soluble lead salt which is insoluble in ammonia and acids, but soluble in much hot water; by the white precipitate, produced in proto-salts of mercury which is rendered black by ammonia, dissolves very slowly in boiling muriatic or nitric acids, but readily in chlorine water and in aqua regia; by the white precipitate with nitrate of silver which acquires a dark, ultimately black color, in the sunlight, is insoluble in nitric acid, but readily soluble in ammonia.

Acidum Muriaticum Dilutum, U. S.

Is readily made by diluting the foregoing with water. The officinal recipe for making Oj is as follows:—

Take of Muriatic acid . . . . . f℥iv.
Distilled water . . . . . f℥xij.
Mix them in a glass vessel.

The specific gravity of this is 1.046. If the strong acid used is below the standard strength, it should be added in rather larger proportion, observing to reach exactly the specific gravity here named, as shown by a good hydrometer for liquids heavier than water, or by a 1000 gr. bottle.

Acidum Nitricum, U. S. (*Aquafortis, Nitric Acid*, HO,NO_5+3HO.)

Prepared by the action of sulphuric acid in excess upon nitrate of potassa (saltpetre) in a glass retort, when nitric acid and bisulphate of potassa are formed. The acid, being volatile, is distilled over by the application of heat. It is a colorless transparent liquid, with powerfully acrid odor, and is exceedingly corrosive, staining the skin yellow. The strongest acid, containing one equivalent of water, has the specific gravity 1.521; but, owing to the presence of water in the ingredients used in its preparation, and its mixing readily in all proportions with water, it is usually weaker, and has its specific gravity reduced in proportion to its dilution. In the *Pharmacopœia* of 1840, the officinal strength was 1.5, but it has been changed in the last edition to 1.42, as stated in the *Syllabus*, the object being to adapt it more nearly to the usual strength of the commercial article, and to establish a standard easily attained. The proportion added to water in making the diluted article has been changed to correspond. It fumes in the air like muriatic.

If nitric acid of a higher specific gravity than 1.42 be distilled, a stronger acid passes over first, and the boiling point of the residue in the retort gradually rises to 253°, when the officinal acid of 1.42 is distilled. An acid lighter than 1.42 likewise boils at a lower temperature, distilling an acid still weaker; the boiling point gradually rises to 253°, when it remains stationary; the officinal acid now distilling has the composition NO_5+4HO, and contains 60 per cent. NO_5 and 40 per cent. HO.

The principal impurities are, nitrous acid which is shown by a red color; sulphuric acid, which may be detected by adding to the diluted acid a solution of chloride of barium; and chlorine or muriatic acid, which would occasion a white precipitate with nitrate of silver. Nitric acid itself is remarkable for furnishing salts which are invariably soluble, except some basic salts of which the officinal subnitrate of bismuth is an example.

Cyanuret of potassium, mixed with a nitrate and heated on platina foil, causes detonation and ignition.

Copper filings, if mixed with a nitrate, will cause the evolution of red nitrous acid fumes after the addition of concentrated sulphuric acid.

The solution of a nitrate, to which concentrated sulphuric acid has been added, and afterwards a crystal of protosulphate of iron, acquires a deep brown color around the crystal, which disappears on agitation or on heating.

Nitrous acid (though, correctly speaking, the name is applied to a red-colored gas, having the composition NO_4, formed whenever binoxide of nitrogen, NO_2, escapes into the air) is commonly understood in trade to apply to fuming red-colored nitric acid, such as passes over chiefly at the commencement and close of the process of distilling nitrate of potassa with sulphuric acid as above. This kind of nitric acid contains nitrous acid fumes, which the manufacturers usually separate from the acid of commerce by boiling, thus rendering it colorless. The best and most distinctive name for the article under consideration is *nitroso-nitric acid.* Its chief use is in making Hope's camphor mixture, which is elsewhere spoken of as having peculiar value when made with this form of acid. As the preparation of nitric and nitroso-nitric acid may often be desirable to the physician or apothecary, I insert a view of the necessary apparatus. If the receiver

Fig. 194.

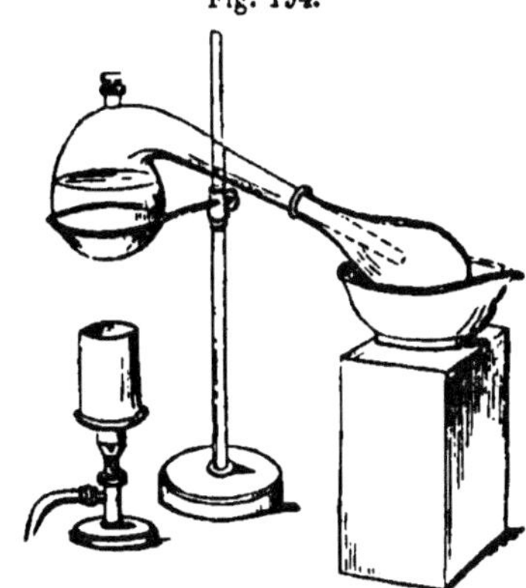

is well refrigerated, there will be no difficulty in collecting the acid. No luting of any kind is used. Nitrate of potassa, with half its weight of oil of vitriol, or one equivalent of each, is distilled at about 250°; the acid commences to pass over; afterwards the heat is increased, when the apparatus becomes filled with red fumes, which are absorbed by the nitric acid in the receiver, and with oxygen, which escapes; when acid ceases to come over, the process is completed.

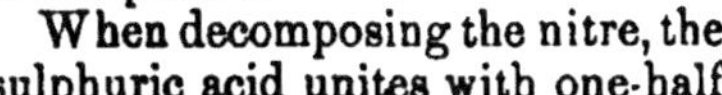

When decomposing the nitre, the sulphuric acid unites with one-half of the potassa, to form bisulphate of potassa, which, above 400°, acts on the other half of the nitre, setting nitric acid free, which is decomposed into nitrous acid and oxygen.

The red fuming acid should be put away for use in glass-stoppered bottles; if the colorless is preferred, it is heated or exposed to the air, to allow of the escape of the nitrous fumes.

An extemporaneous process for the production of nitrous fumes in nitric acid, is to drop, into a vial containing it, a few chips of some pure kind of wood; on this, part of the NO_5 will act, producing oxidation of the ligneous matter, and liberating NO_4. This process is only suggested where the last is impracticable.

Acidum Nitricum Dilutum, U. S.

Take of Nitric acid . . . . . f℥j.
Distilled water . . . . . f℥vj.
Mix them in a glass vessel.

The specific gravity of this is 1.07, and 100 grains saturate 20 grains of crystallized bicarbonate of potassa.

Acidum Nitromuriaticum, U. S. (*Aqua Regia*)

Take of Nitric acid . . . . . f℥iv.
Muriatic acid . . . . . f℥viij.

Mix them in a glass vessel, and, when effervescence has ceased, keep the product in a well-ground glass-stoppered bottle, in a cool and dark place. This forms a deep yellow, corrosive, fuming liquid, containing chlorine and nitric oxide in an unknown state of combination. The acid dissolves gold, from the free chlorine present. It should be made in small quantities, as required, care being taken, in dispensing it, to allow the effervescence to cease before securing the stopper in the bottle.

Acidum Sulphuricum, U. S. (*Oil of Vitriol, Sulphuric Acid*, HO,SO_3)

Made by burning sulphur and nitrate of potassa together in leaden chambers. Sulphur, when burned, forms sulphurous acid (SO_2), which, in contact, in the form of vapor, with nitrous acid from the burning nitre and water, becomes more highly oxidized into sulphuric acid, SO_3, which combines with one equivalent of water.

It is an oily-looking, very heavy liquid, without color when pure, having no odor, but an intensely acid caustic taste. It becomes darkened in color by contact with vegetable substances, which it chars by abstracting from them the elements of water. When mixed with water, it readily combines with it, disengaging heat; its strong affinity for water is one of its useful properties. When largely diluted with water, it is apt to deposit a white precipitate of sulphate of lead derived from the leaden vessels used in concentrating it.

It is easy to determine the nature of this acid, whether free or in combination; its characteristic reaction is a white precipitate with all soluble salts of baryta, which is insoluble in water, in acids and alkalies. Arsenic is an occasional impurity, which may be detected by sulphuretted hydrogen, giving a yellow precipitate when passed through it. Arsenic, if present in sulphuric acid may be removed by adding some muriatic acid, and heating, when, by double decomposition, water and chloride of arsenic are formed, the latter readily volatilizing; it is necessary to evaporate the excess of water from the acid afterwards (Buchner's method). To avoid this, Loewe proposed to add to the heated acid, gradually, chloride of sodium, as long as arsenical vapors are emitted; the sulphuric acid will be contaminated with a little sulphate of soda, which, however, does not render it unfit for any ordinary purposes. It is only prescribed internally in one of the officinal diluted forms which follow, though occasionally the strong acid is used in ointments.

Acidum Sulphuricum Dilutum, U. S.

Take of Sulphuric acid . . . . . f℥j.
Distilled water . . . . . f℥xiij.

Add the acid gradually to the water in a glass vessel, and mix them. The specific gravity of this is 1.09, and 100 grains of it saturate 25 grains of crystallized bicarbonate of potassa. Upon standing, the white precipitate at first formed (sulphate of lead) will be deposited, and the pure diluted acid may be decanted for use.

Acidum Sulphuricum Aromaticum, U. S. (*Elixir of Vitriol.*)

Take of Sulphuric acid . . . . . f℥iiiss.
Ginger, in coarse powder . . ℥j.
Cinnamon, do. . . ℥iss.
Alcohol . . . . . . q. s. (to make two pints).

Add the acid gradually to Oj alcohol, and allow the liquor to cool. Mix the ginger and cinnamon, and having put them into a percolator, pour alcohol gradually upon them until a pint of filtered liquor is obtained. Lastly, mix the diluted acid and the tincture. Formerly the tincture was made by treating the powdered aromatics directly with the mixed alcohol and acid. The present process is an improvement, giving a clearer and more elegant tincture. Elixir of vitriol is stronger than diluted sulphuric acid, though its dose in drops is usually about the same, the alcoholic liquid giving smaller drops than the aqueous.

This preparation is very extensively used as a refrigerant, tonic, and astringent. It is a popular remedy for night-sweats in phthisis, and for debility generally. In making solutions and pills of quinine, also in the compound infusion of cinchona, it has important pharmaceutical uses.

Acidum Sulphurosum, SO_2.—It is prepared by exposing to heat a mixture of one part concentrated sulphuric acid with one part of mercury, or one-third part of copper filings, washing the gas by passing it through a little water, and condensing it in water which is kept well cooled. Professor Procter directs the gas evolved from four ounces of copper turnings and eight fluidounces of sulphuric acid, to be condensed into four pints of water.

Sulphurous acid is a gas which dissolves largely in water, has the smell of burning sulphur, and has the composition SO_2.

It is free from sulphuric acid, if its solution causes a precipitate with acetate of baryta, which is entirely soluble in an excess of the boiling acid.

It has been used as a local application in certain skin diseases, usually diluted with three or more parts of water.

Acidum Hydrosulphuricum, Hydrothionicum, HS.—Sulphuretted hydrogen occurs naturally in the so-called sulphur springs, many of which have a high reputation as remedial agents. The White Sulphur Springs, in Virginia, and the far-famed Aix la Chapelle, Warmbrun, and Baden Springs, in Germany, and the springs at Harrowgate, in England, Moffat, in Scotland, Barèges, Cauterets, in France, and many others, owe their celebrity, in part, to sulphuretted hydrogen. These springs never contain it alone to the exclusion of other gases; nitrogen, oxygen, carburetted hydrogen, and carbonic acid, are often found in the same waters.

This acid is prepared artificially from black sulphuret of iron, by decomposing it with sulphuric acid in a flask, and conducting the gas through a glass tube into water. The iron, being oxidized by the oxygen of the water, liberates the hydrogen, which, in its nascent state, combines with the nascent sulphur, to form this gaseous acid, which, after being washed by passing it through a little water, is conducted into distilled water, kept well refrigerated.

Thus prepared, it is a colorless liquid, of a penetrating, disagreeable odor, like rotten eggs, and when inhaled acts as a poison. In contact with air, it is decomposed, hydrogen being oxidized to water, and sulphur precipitated. Hydrosulphuric or sulphohydric acid precipitates most metallic salts, and is, on that account, very much used as a test liquid in analytical researches.

It is free of sulphuric acid, if no precipitate occurs with chloride of barium, and of muriatic acid, if the filtrate from the precipitate with nitrate of copper occasions no precipitate with nitrate of silver.

The sulphur waters are much used in rheumatic and cutaneous diseases, externally, as baths, and also freely in large draughts.

Acidum Phosphoricum. (*Glacial or Monohydrated Phosphoric Acid.*)

This is prepared from calcined bones (bone phosphate of lime), by decomposing them with sulphuric acid, by which process a superphosphate of lime is produced (the article used as a basis for the manure known by that name). The superphosphate is neutralized by carbonate of ammonia, which generates phosphate of ammonia in solution with precipitation of phosphate of lime. By calcining phosphate of ammonia at a red heat, the volatile ingredient is expelled, and the solid HO,PO_5 remains combined with 1, 2, or 3 equivalents of water, or being a mixture of the tri, the bi, and the monobasic acid; the amount of water and the kind of acid being dependent on the temperature.

This acid hence exists in three allotropic modifications: 1, the ordinary or *c* phosphoric acid, as prepared by decomposition of bones is tribasic, cPO_5 being capable of uniting with three equivalents of a metallic oxide, and precipitating silver salts yellow; 2, pyro or *b* phosphoric acid, prepared by calcination of a c phosphate, bPO_5 unites with but 2 equivalents of a base, and precipitates silver salts white; 3, meta or *a* phosphoric acid, obtained by burning phosphorus in oxygen or atmospheric air; aPO_5 unites with only one equivalent of base, precipitates silver salts white, and has the property of coagulating albumen.

To obtain the glacial phosphoric acid pure, the fusion must take place at a considerable elevation of temperature in a platina vessel; vessels of clay, porcelain, and glass, which are generally employed by large manufacturers, are unsuitable for this purpose, as the resulting acid is invariably more or less contaminated with alumina, lime, silicic acid, &c., which render the crystals very slow of solution. Even silver vessels are corroded by the melted acid.

In aqueous solution the (*a*) meta and (*b*) pyro-phosphoric acids are soon converted into the tribasic acid, which is contained in the officinal diluted phosphoric acid and all the medicinal phosphates. It is in transparent glassy looking solid masses, of a very sour taste, and without odor, and freely soluble in water. (See *Compounds of Phosphorus.*)

Acidum Phosphoricum Dilutum.

This may be prepared by dissolving forty-five and a half grains of glacial phosphoric acid in one fluidounce of distilled water, about one part to ten by weight, or by the process of the *London Pharmacopœia*, by the action of nitric acid diluted with water upon phosphorus, by which the phosphorus is oxidized at the expense of the acid, and phosphoric acid results. It is a colorless liquid without odor, of an agreeable acid taste, sp. gr. 1.064. It is used in the dose prescribed in the syllabus as a tonic. It is employed in the preparation of the phosphatic lozenges and of the syrups of phosphate of lime and other preparations of the kind. (See chapter on *Phosphorous Compounds.*)

The vapors of boiling diluted phosphoric acid are without action on litmus paper; the acid is not rendered turbid by alcohol, and no precipitate is occasioned by the dilute solution of a baryta salt, which remains not entirely dissolved in an excess of phosphoric acid, nor is it soluble in nitric and muriatic acids, but freely in muriate of ammonia. Arsenic is sometimes present, either from the phosphorus or the sulphuric acid employed, and it is then in the state of arsenic acid; to detect it, the acid is first mixed with sulphurous acid and heated to expel the excess added, after which the addition of sulphuretted hydrogen causes a yellow precipitate. Solution of sulphate of lime produces a white precipitate soluble in acids. Magnesia salts in the presence of free ammonia cause a white precipitate insoluble in ammonia and ammonia-salts, but dissolving in acids.

A solution of a phosphate acidulated with muriatic acid, produces with a drop or two of sesquichloride of iron, and the subsequent addition of acetate of potassa, a gelatinous, white precipitate of phosphate of sesquioxide of iron.

Acidum Hydriodicum, HI.—Hydriodic acid is most conveniently made for medicinal purposes by the decomposition of iodide of potassium by tartaric acid. Dr. A. Buchanan, of Glasgow, uses 330 grains of the former and 264 grains of the latter, and dilutes the filtrate from the precipitate until it measures fifty fluidrachms, when each fluidrachm contains five grains of iodine combined with hydrogen, besides a small quantity of cream of tartar.

It is a colorless liquid, gradually eliminating free iodine when in contact with air; it has a peculiar acid taste and smell, which are not disagreeable in its diluted state.

It is considered to possess the medicinal properties of free iodine without its local irritating effects, if diluted with water; it has been given in doses commencing with a few drops, and gradually increasing it to half a fluidounce two or three times a day.

Acidum Chlorohydrocyanicum.—If fulminating silver is decomposed by muriatic acid, chloride of silver is precipitated, hydrocyanic acid evolved, and the liquid contains chlorohydrocyanic acid which has a sweetish acid taste—$2AgO,C_2NO+7HCl=2AgCl+HC_2N+4HO+C_2H_2NCl_5$. It was discovered by Liebig.

It has been employed by Drs. Turnbull and Turner in paralytic and torpid diseases of the eye and the ear, by exposing the diseased parts for half a minute to the vapors of one drachm of the acid contained in a sponge in a proper vial. It acts as a stimulant, producing a slight irritation and sensation of heat, and dilates the pupil less than hydrocyanic acid.

Acidum Sulphohydrocyanicum, Rhodanicum.—It has been found in the seed of mustard and other cruciferæ, and in the saliva of animals; but it is uncertain yet whether pre-existing or the result of a decomposition by reagents. To prepare it, powdered anhydrous ferrocyanuret of potassium is fused with flowers of sulphur at a moderate heat, dissolved in water, some oxide of iron precipitated by potassa, the filtrate evaporated, and the concentrated solution distilled with phosphoric acid.

It is a colorless liquid, of a sour taste, which, when concentrated, is readily decomposed on keeping, but keeps unaltered for a considerable time in a diluted state. Its characteristic property is to impart a blood-red color to all neutral persalts of iron and to assume the same color in contact with paper, cork, and other organic bodies containing oxide of iron.

It has been used by Dr. Turnbull in diseases of the eye, in a manner similar to chlorohydrocyanic acid.

CHAPTER II.

THE ALKALIES AND THEIR SALTS.

ALKALIES are electro-positive bodies; they may be divided into organic alkalies or alkaloids, which have already been considered, and inorganic alkalies which are oxides of peculiar, light, and very combustible metals. Ammonia forms a connecting link between these, and may be classed with either, though most conveniently with the latter. The three alkalies used in medicine, and to be presented in the present chapter, are, potassa, soda, and ammonia. They possess in common the property of turning vegetable reds to green or blue, and the yellow color of turmeric, and some other vegetable yellows, to brown. They neutralize acids, deprive them more or less of acidity, and form with them salts which are sometimes acid, sometimes alkaline, and sometimes neutral, according to the proportions and relative strengths of the acids employed.

The beautiful laws which govern the formation of salts have been very thoroughly studied, and are fully laid down in works on chemistry; a knowledge of these, in connection with the system of nomenclature found on them, is in the highest degree important, whether to the practical or theoretical chemist.

The plan of this work embraces only such reference to the laws of combination as the pharmaceutical history of some of the leading chemicals will necessarily bring into view. The officinal names are partly chemical and partly empirical, being, as more fully explained in the chapter on the Pharmacopœia and its Nomenclature, framed with a view to distinctness and adaptation to the purpose, rather than to chemical accuracy or elegance.

In chemical works, the classification of these is in accordance with their chemical relations and affinities. While in treatises on materia medica, they are arranged according to their therapeutical properties. In a pharmaceutical work like the present, it will be well, perhaps, to present yet a different arrangement, and bring them into view with reference to their commercial source and mode of preparation.

Potassa, soda, and ammonia, in their caustic condition (or combined with carbonic acid, which rather modifies than changes their medical properties), are used in medicine chiefly for neutralizing excess of acids existing in the secretions. In the case of ammonia, this use is combined with a powerful arterial stimulant property, adapting it to low forms of disease. The salts formed by these alkalies with the acids vary in their therapeutical properties. Some have a special tendency to the skin, some to the kidneys, some to the bowels, &c. Their physical properties are no less various; although they are mostly crystalline, some assume a pulverulent or amorphous form. The salts of potassa are generally disposed to deliquesce or become damp, while those of soda effloresce, or lose their water of crystallization, falling into powder. Those of ammonia, by decomposition, liberate their volatile and alkaline base, known by its pungency and by the production of a white cloud when brought in contact with vapor of muriatic acid.

The class of salts formed by muriatic acid, with the alkalies and earths, have been found to be compounds of chlorine with the metallic radicals of these, and might be considered with the so-called hydriodates among the halogen compounds, but are usually classed with the oxysalts.

The oxysalts of the alkalies are nearly all soluble. The bitartrates of potassa and ammonia, the antimoniate of soda, and the chloroplatinates, which occur as white crystalline precipitates, constitute tests for potassa and soda respectively. The great solubility of the alkalies and their compounds constitutes a prominent distinction between them and the earths, to be presented in another chapter. Most alkalies, both organic and inorganic, may be detected by all, forming with bichloride of platinum, especially in the presence of free muriatic acid, yellow crystalline double chlorides of platinum and the alkali, which, with the exception of soda and a few organic alkalies, are precipitated from a concentrated solution, by alcohol.

If a potassa salt is heated in the blow-pipe flame, the outer flame is colored violet; the same color is produced on igniting alcohol mixed with a salt; in both cases soda ought not to be present, as the color is obscured by it. Soda imparts an intensely yellow color to flame.

SALTS OF THE ALKALIES.[1]

GROUP 1.—*Starting with Wood-ashes.*[2]

Potash. Lixivium from ashes of forest trees evaporated to a dark hard mass.
Potassæ carbonas impurus. Ignited potash. Pearlash.
Salæratus. Dry pearlash subjected to gaseous CO_2. $2(KO),3(CO_2)$?
Potassæ carbonas, $2(KO,CO_2),3HO$. Solution of pearlash, filtered and granulated.
Liquor potassæ carbonatis. ℥xij to f℥xij water. Simple solution.
Potassæ bicarbonas, $KO,2CO_2,HO$. Passing CO_2 into solution of carbonate, &c.
Potassæ carbonas purus, KO,CO_2. Calcining bicarbonate and granulating.
Liquor potassæ. Boiling carbonate with hydrate of lime, sp. gr. 1.056.
Potassa, KO,HO. Evaporating liquor potassæ to dryness, and fusing.
Potassa, cum calce. Equal parts, potassa and lime, triturated, sometimes fused together.
Potassæ acetas, $KO,\overline{Ac}$. Neutralizing acetic acid with carbonate, and crystallizing.
Potassæ citras, $KO,\overline{Ci}$. Neutralizing citric acid with bicarbonate, and granulating.
Liquor potassæ citratis. A variety of extemporaneous processes.
Potassæ chloras, KO,ClO_5. Passing excess of chlorine through solution of potassa.
Sodæ chloras, NaO,ClO_5. Decomposing chlorate of potassa with bitartrate of soda.
Potassæ picras. Saturating picric acid with KO,HO.

Potash and pearlash, though important in their relations to the arts and to domestic economy, are seldom employed in medicine, except in the preparation of the other forms of caustic and carbonated alkali, and the other salts of potassa enumerated in the table.

[1] Those not officinal in Italics.
[2] See Non-metallic Elements, Phosphorous Compounds, &c.

Salæratus is a useful and tolerably pure sesquicarbonate of potassa, which occupies a position intermediate between the carbonate and bicarbonate, besides being distinguished from these by its anhydrous character; it is much used in baking to furnish the carbonic acid which raises the bread, rendering it light and porous. Light cakes made with it are generally considered less objectionable by dyspeptics than those made with yeast. Recently most of the salæratus of the shops is an imperfectly carbonated bicarbonate of *soda*.

Potassæ Carbonas, U. S.

Made by dissolving pearlash in a small quantity of water, filtering to separate insoluble matters, and evaporating to dryness, stirring actively so as to form a granular powder, which is very deliquescent, and contains water in the proportion of two equivalents to every three of salt. It is sometimes called *salt of tartar*, a name which is quite inappropriate. Dose, gr. x to ʒss.

Liquor Potassæ Carbonatis, U. S.

Made by dissolving in a mortar, or by agitation in a bottle, one pound of the carbonate in twelve fluidounces of water. Its uses are as an antilithic and antacid; it should be given in milk, or other bland and viscid vehicle. Dose, ♏x to fʒj.

When saturated with acetic acid, a precipitate with caustic alkalies shows the presence of earthy metallic oxides; with oxalate of ammonia the presence of lime; with sulphuretted hydrogen the presence of heavy metals.

Potassæ Bicarbonas, U. S.

Made by passing carbonic acid gas (generated by the action of muriatic acid on chalk or marble) into a solution of carbonate of potassa unto saturation, then crystallizing.

Fig. 195 shows the process of generating this gas in the bottle *a*, washing it by passing it through water in the bottle *b*, by means of the pipe *d*, which passes through a pipe *e*, of large bore to the bottom; and, finally, through *f*, conducting it into the solution of carbonate of potassa in *c*. The point of saturation may be judged proximately by the bubbles of gas leaving the pipe *f*, ceasing to diminish in size as they escape through *c*.

Fig. 195.

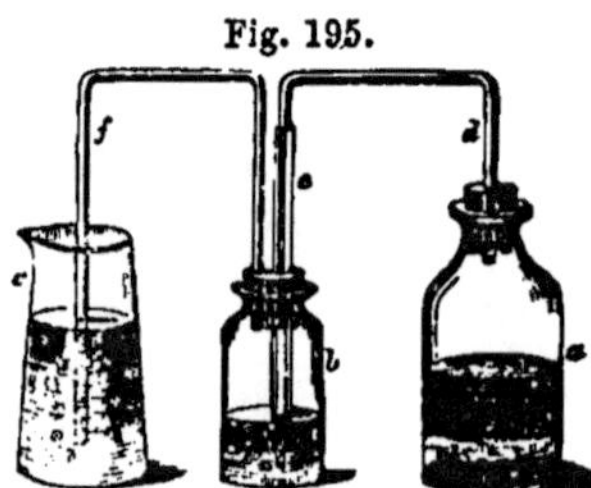

Bicarbonate of potassa is in large transparent crystals, with a mild alkaline taste, soluble in about four parts of water.

The bicarbonates do not precipitate sulphate of magnesia, by which they may be known if fully bicarbonated.

The presence of monocarbonate of potassa is proved by a reddish precipitate occasioned with corrosive sublimate.

A precipitate by an excess of caustic alkalies shows the presence of earthy or metallic oxides.

A residue after treating the salt with nitric acid, evaporating and redissolving in water, proves the presence of silicic acid; a precipitate in this solution, occasioned with silver or baryta salts, indicates muriatic or sulphuric acid.

By being calcined, this salt loses 30.7 grains of water and carbonic acid, forming the pure carbonate of the *Pharmacopœia.*

As a medicine, bicarbonate of potassa acts as a direct and efficient antacid; pleasanter and more efficient than bicarbonate of soda. It readily neutralizes free acid in the stomach, and the excess being absorbed renders the blood and urine decidedly alkaline, and is hence considered alterative in its action. It is used to liberate carbonic acid, and for making the saline preparations of potassa, is confined to carbonate, being pure. DOSE, ℈j to ʒj.

This salt is remarkable among the alkaline carbonates for its constancy of composition, being, in a crystalline form, invariably represented by the formula $KO,2CO_2+HO$, and is directed in the *Pharmacopœia* as the test to ascertain the strength of acids, which it neutralizes in the ratio of their strength. The following table exhibits the proportion of bicarbonate of potassa, which neutralizes 100 grains of each of the acids named:—

Acetic acid, 60	Diluted 7.5.
Citric acid, 150.	
Tartaric acid, 133.5.	
Nitric acid	Diluted, 20.
Sulphuric	Diluted, 25.

Potassæ Carbonas Purus, U. S.

The ignition of the potash forming pearlash deprives it of organic matter, and brings it more completely into the condition of a carbonate. The solution, filtration, and granulation of this deprives it of some inorganic impurities, but leaves it contaminated with silica. Charging it with a further dose of carbonic acid precipitates this impurity; and, finally, calcination at a red heat will drive off the additional dose of carbonic acid and the water of crystallization, and leave the pure carbonate. This is directed to be dissolved and granulated. The only use to which it is applied is as a test, and when absolute purity is required. An iron crucible is directed in the *Pharmacopœia* for this purpose, but a porcelain, or a platinum crucible (Figs. 196 and 197), will do in small operations.

Fig. 196. Fig. 197.

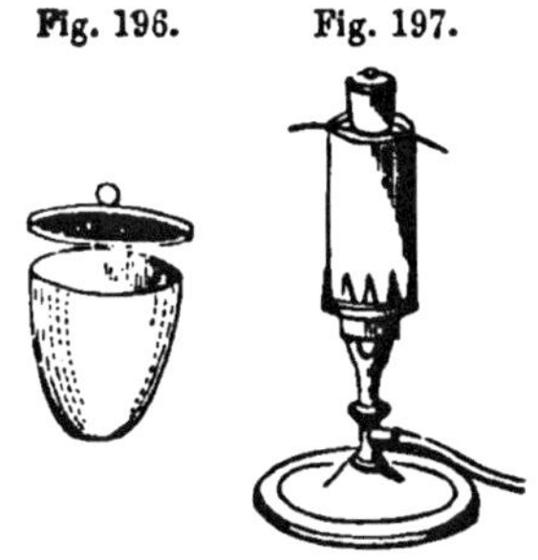

Fig. 197 shows the mode of suspending a crucible of small size over a gas lamp chimney by a bent wire; a similar arrangement may be adopted in using the Russian or other alcohol lamps. I have illustrated and described this more fully, because, on a small scale, it is readily practicable, and it is frequently difficult to obtain the chemically pure carbonate. Formerly this was directed to be prepared by igniting bitartrate of potassa, hence the name salt of tartar now frequently applied to both the carbonates.

Liquor Potassæ, U. S.

		(Reduced Quantity.)
Take of Carbonate of potassa	. .	℔j, or ℥iij, or ʒvj.
Lime	. . . . . .	℔ss, or ℥iss, or ʒiij.
Boiling distilled water	. .	Cong. j, or Oij, or f℥viij.

Dissolve the carbonate in one-half the distilled water. Pour a little of the water on the lime, and when it is slaked add the remainder. Mix the hot liquors and boil for ten minutes, stirring constantly; then set the liquor aside in a covered vessel till it becomes clear; lastly, pour off the supernatant liquor and keep it in well-stoppered bottles of green glass.

This process may be conveniently conducted with an ordinary evaporating dish over a spirit or gas lamp, care being taken that the carbonate of lime does not cake in the bottom of the dish while the heat is being applied; a glass rod should be used for stirring. When the boiling is finished, the whole may be conveniently poured into a precipitating glass, which should be covered by placing the dish over it, or into a salt mouth bottle into which the stopper should be introduced. On standing, the carbonate of lime will subside, and the *liquor potassæ* may be poured off clear. It will act upon filtering paper, so that filtration is not eligible. The use of the siphon, an instrument not before mentioned, will be convenient in drawing off the liquid from the carbonate, if any difficulty should occur in pouring it off clear. Figs. 199 and 200 repre-

Fig. 198.

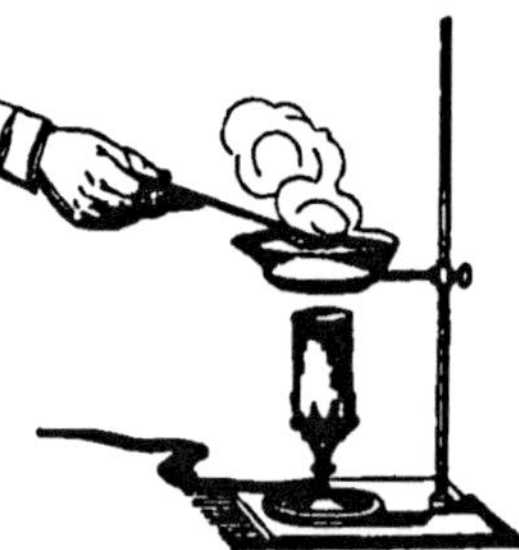

Fig. 199.

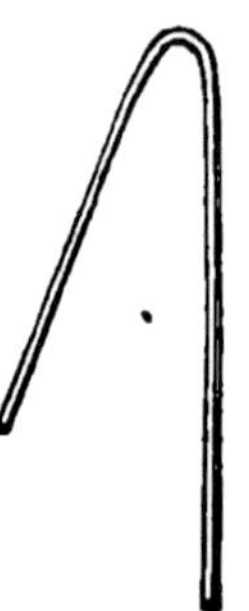

Plain siphon.

Fig. 200.

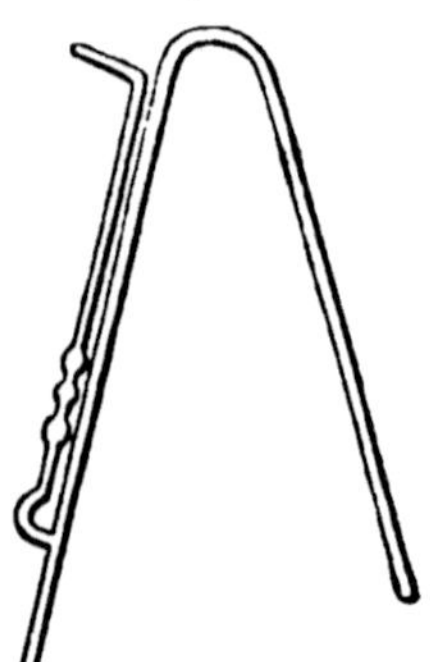

Siphon with suction tube.

sent siphons, the latter the most convenient kind; they are bent tubes, having one leg longer than the other. If the tube be filled and the short limb plunged into a vessel filled with some liquid which it is designed to draw off, the liquid will discharge itself from the end of the longer limb, and will continue to flow as long as this end of the tube is below the level of the liquid in which the end of the short limb is immersed. This current is caused by the unequal weight of the columns of liquid in the two limbs of the siphon. The plain siphon (Fig 199) is constructed by simply bending an ordinary piece of glass tube of the requisite size over a spirit or gas lamp. The inconvenience in its use arises from the difficulty of filling it with the liquid beforehand. It might be filled with water, but that would dilute the preparation. If a small quantity has been already drawn off, the siphon may be filled by inverting it, and pouring into its long end from a graduated measure, then applying the end of the finger to prevent its running out, and inserting the short limb in the liquid to be drawn off. In using the siphon, Fig. 200, the finger is placed at the end of the long limb, and the short limb being inserted in the liquid, the air is drawn out by applying the mouth at the end of the thin sucking tube attached for the purpose, till the apparatus is filled as far as the little bulbs. The current will then be fairly determined toward the receiving vessel, and the last drop of the clear liquid may be drawn off.

Liquor potassæ is a colorless liquid, with an intensely caustic taste, sp. gr. 1.056. It may be extemporaneously made by dissolving ℥ss of fused caustic potassa in f℥j of water, though this will not always make the solution precisely identical with the officinal.

It should not effervesce with acids or precipitate when mixed with two or three measures of strong alcohol. Metallic impurities are detected, as in the case of bicarbonate of potassa. It has a very strong affinity for carbonic acid and moisture, which it continually abstracts from the air. It attacks flint glass, hence the direction to keep it in green glass bottles. Its effect upon the skin is to produce an oily or soapy sensation, due to the destruction of the cuticle; it also destroys or greatly injures vegetable fibre.

Its use is chiefly confined to neutralizing free acid in the stomach and in the secretions. It is applied to the treatment of scrofulous and cutaneous affections, and to the arrest of the uric acid deposits in the urine. The dose is from ♏v to fʒss. When given internally, it should be largely diluted with milk. Dr. E. Wilson, of this city, has used it with success in a case of extreme obesity for reducing the accumulation of fat; by pushing the dose, diluted as above, to ♏xl three times a day, his patient, a female, lost 48 lbs. weight in a few months, so that from weighing 198 lbs. at the commencement of the treatment, she weighed only 150 lbs. at its close.

Potassa, U. S. (*Vegetable Caustic, Caustic Potassa, Hydrate of Potassa, Fused Potash.*)

This preparation is made from the foregoing by evaporating it to dryness, fusing it, and running it into moulds. It is usually found in the shops of two qualities—one in sticks somewhat thicker than a

And lastly

Citric acid,
Bicarbonate of soda, of each . . ʒj.

Cork and bottle immediately and securely. Dose, one bottle, as a cathartic.

Sodæ Chloras.

By mutual decomposition of solutions of chlorate of potassa and bitartrate of soda, bitartrate of potassa is precipitated while chlorate of soda is retained in solution, from which it crystallizes on evaporation; the mother liquor is best poured off from the first crystals formed, which are chiefly bitartrate of potassa; or the crystals are dissolved in the least possible quantity of cold water, so as to leave the crystals of cream of tartar behind.

It crystallizes in rhombohedrons, dissolves in alcohol, and in three parts of cold water, and is fusible, evolving some oxygen. It has been recommended as milder in its action than chlorate of potassa, and on account of its greater solubility.

The salt detonates when fused, if it contain tartaric acid.

Potassæ silicas, Silicate of potassa, is a transparent, vitreous mass, deliquescent and soluble in water; it is formed by fusing together silica and carbonate of potassa. It has been asserted to be a powerful solvent for arthritic calculi, composed of urate of soda; the dose is 10 to 15 grains twice daily, dissolved in much water.

Picrate of Potassa.

Picrate of Potassa, Potassæ Picras, vel Carbazotas.—This salt is obtained by neutralizing picric acid with potassa or its carbonate, and crystallizing from hot water. It appears in fine yellow needles of a persistent bitter taste, which are insoluble in alcohol, not very soluble in cold water; it requires 260 parts at 60° F., but dissolves with facility in boiling water; it contains no water of crystallization. It has been used by Braconnot as a substitute for quinia in intermittent fevers with good success; the dose is stated to be from two to five grains, in pills or powders on account of its sparing solubility.

Group 2.—*Alkaline Salts, starting with Common Salt.*

Sodii chloridum, $NaCl$. Obtained by evaporation of certain natural spring waters.

Sodæ sulphas, NaO,SO_3+10HO. By the action of sulphuric acid on common salt.

Sodæ carbonas, NaO,CO_2+10HO. By calcining sulphate of carbon, &c.

Sodæ carbonas exsiccatus, NaO,CO_2. By simple calcination of carbonate.

Soda, NaO. From carbonate of soda by lime.

Sodæ bicarbonas, $NaO,2CO_2+HO$. By passing gaseous CO_2 into a box containing effloresced crystals of the carbonate.

Sodæ phosphas, $2NaO,HO,PO_5+24HO$. By neutralizing superphosphate of lime with the carbonate, filtering and evaporating.

Liquor sodæ chlorinatæ. By treating carbonate, in solution, with chlorinated lime.

Sodæ hyposulphis, NaO,S_2O_2+5HO. From sulphur and carbonate of soda by combustion, &c.

Sodæ acetas, $NaO,\overline{Ac},+6HO$. An intermediate salt in the preparation of acetic acid.

Sodæ valerianas, $NaO,\overline{V}a$. An intermediate salt in the preparation of other valeriantes.

Sodæ choleinas. From ox-gall by purification.

Sodæ sulphovinas, $NO,C_4H_5S_2O_7+2HO$. From sulphovinate of baryta by NaO,SO_3+10HO.

Sodæ benzoas, $NaO,\overline{Bz}$. By neutralizing benzoic acid with NaO,CO_2.

Ammoniæ benzoas, $NH_4O,\overline{Bz}$. " " $NH_4O,+$ aq.

and when effervescence has ceased, strain and evaporate to dryness, stirring constantly after the pellicle has begun to form till the salt granulates, then rub it in a mortar (wedgewood), pass it through a coarse sieve, put it in a bottle, which should be kept closely stopped. This is a granular powder, slightly acid, soluble in twice its weight of water, from which alcohol precipitates a more concentrated solution, deliquescent, and in its effects refrigerant and diaphoretic. Its dose is from ℈j to ʒss.

Impure earthy and metallic oxides are detected by alkalies, sulphuretted hydrogen, and ferrocyanide of potassium; sulphuric and muriatic acids by the precipitates with baryta and silver salt; tartaric acid by the precipitate on addition of bisulphate of potassa, or of muriatic acid.

Among the diaphoretic solutions, under the head of *Extemporaneous Preparations*, this salt in various liquid forms will be again introduced.

Potassæ Chloras.

Chlorate of potassa is prepared by several modifications of the simple process of passing chlorine gas into a solution of potassa or its carbonate; at first, chloride of potassium and hypochlorite of potassa are formed; with these, a further proportion of chlorine produces changes resulting in the conversion of the hypochloric into chloric acid, which exists in combination with the potassa as chlorate of potassa (KO,ClO_5); this is separated by crystallization from the more soluble chloride of potassium. This salt has a cooling taste and diuretic refrigerant effect, being given in a variety of diseases in doses of gr. x to ʒss. In chemistry it is used to obtain pure oxygen, which it gives off, on the simple application of heat, leaving fused chloride of potassium in the flask or retort.

Soluble in two parts of boiling and sixteen parts of cold water; is very explosive when mixed with inflammable substances (sulphur, charcoal, &c.). If dropped in concentrated SO_3, the chloric acid of the salt is decomposed into hyperchloric and chlorous acids, which latter easily decomposes into chlorine and oxygen, thereby causing a violent explosion.

Its cold solution is not affected by any test except such as produce precipitates with potassa (tartaric acid, chloride of platinum). The presence of saltpetre is detected by the alkaline reaction of the salt after having been exposed to a strong heat.

Tartro-Citrate of Soda.

Tartro-Citrate of Soda.—This salt has been recently recommended, in solution, as furnishing a more permanent and cheaper purgative lemonade than the justly celebrated citrate of magnesia. I have had no experience with it as yet, but propose the following as a practicable formula for its preparation:—

Take of Tartaric acid . . . . . . ʒvj.
Bicarbonate of soda . . . . . ʒvss or q. s.
Water . . . . f℥xss.

Dissolve the acid in the water, and add the soda salt till it is nearly neutral, then filter and add

Simple syrup . . . . . . f℥iss
Tincture of fresh lemon peel . . fʒss.

Soda, Caustic Soda,

Is prepared precisely like caustic potassa; it is not used in medicine, but is employed in some chemical operations, where the presence of potassa is not admissible.

Sodæ Bicarbonas, U. S. (*Supercarbonate of Soda.*)

The best process for preparing this salt is a modification of that of Dr. Franklin R. Smith, of Bellefonte, Pa. The crystallized carbonate partly effloresced, or a mixture of the crystallized and dried, in proper proportion, is placed in a wooden perforated box, and carbonic acid gas (generated by the action of dilute sulphuric acid on marble) is passed into it. Owing to the strong affinity of the monocarbonate for a further dose of carbonic acid, the bicarbonate is generated in this simple way. As met with in the shops, it is a dry, white powder, slightly alkaline, permanent in the air, soluble in thirteen parts of cold water, decomposed by a boiling temperature. The commercial article I have generally found to contain some sesqui or monocarbonate. The taste betrays this, as also the fact of its readily precipitating carbonate of magnesia from a cold solution of Epsom salts, which well-made bicarbonate will not; also the formation of a reddish precipitate with corrosive sublimate. This impurity, the result of defective preparation, although not very important, renders this remedy less agreeable, and, in view of its employment in effervescing powders, &c., less effective. The proportion of carbonic acid given off from bicarbonate of soda by treating it with acids exceeds 50 per cent., so that it is one of the most productive articles for this purpose. It enters into soda, Seidlitz, yeast, and some other powders, in which tartaric acid is employed to decompose it; the proportion being thirty-five parts of the acid to forty of the bicarbonate.

Soda-salæratus is now employed in immense quantities as an adulteration of the proper salæratus, and as a substitute for bicarbonate of soda; it is, generally, an imperfect preparation, and a poor substitute for the officinal bicarbonate of soda.

Bicarbonate of soda is used in medicine as a mild antacid; it is very cheap, though, I think, inferior to bicarbonate of potassa for the purpose. DOSE, ℈j to ʒj in carbonic acid water, if at hand.

For effervescing powders, see *Extemporaneous Prescriptions*.

Sodæ Phosphas, U. S.

Phosphate of soda is formed by digesting bone-ash (phosphate of lime) in sulphuric acid, thus liberating phosphoric acid. The sulphate of lime being separated, carbonate of soda is added to the phosphoric acid till neutralized, and by crystallizing, the pure salt is produced in large, transparent, efflorescent, very soluble crystals.

It is a tribasic salt, consisting of one equivalent of phosphoric acid, two of soda, and one of water, and twenty-four of water of crystallization ($2NaO,HO,PO_5+24HO$). The enormous proportion of water, 62.3 per cent. of its weight, is a remarkable property of this salt.

It is a mild saline cathartic and diuretic. DOSE, from ʒij to ℥j, and is chiefly recommended by its taste, which resembles that of common salt. (See chapter on *Phosphorous Compounds.*)

Tests for Purity.—The precipitate with acetate of lead is soluble in nitric acid (absence of muriatic and sulphuric acids).

Lime is found by the white precipitate with oxalate of ammonia.

Sometimes it contains arsenate of soda, which is detected by saturating the solution with gaseous sulphuretted hydrogen, heating slightly, and afterwards carefully adding pure phosphoric acid, when sulphuret of arsenic will be precipitated.

Liquor Sodæ Chlorinatæ, U. S. (*Labarraque's Disinfecting Solution.*)

This may be conveniently prepared by the apothecary or physician by observing carefully the directions of the *Pharmacopœia*, as follows:—

			(Reduced.)
Take of	Chlorinated lime . . .	℔j.	℥j.
	Carbonate of soda . .	℔ij.	℥ij.
	Water	Cong. iss.	Oj.

Dissolve the carbonate of soda in three pints of the water by the aid of heat. To the remainder of the water, add, by small portions at a time, the chlorinated lime, previously well triturated, stirring the mixture after each addition; set the mixture by for several hours that the dregs may subside, then decant the clear liquid, and mix it with the solution of carbonate of soda. Lastly, decant the clear liquor from the precipitated carbonate of lime, pass it through a linen cloth, and keep it in bottles secluded from the light.

The necessity for the aid of heat in dissolving the carbonate of soda may be overcome by the use of the mortar and pestle, as directed in the chapter on Solutions. In the absence of a precipitating jar, wide-mouth packing bottles may be substituted, being well adapted to allow the undissolved portion of the first liquid, and the precipitated carbonate of lime of the last, to subside.

Labarraque's solution is a colorless alkaline solution, having a faint odor of chlorine, though somewhat modified, and an alkaline taste; it contains an excess of carbonate of soda. It owes its therapeutic and antiseptic value to containing hypochlorous acid, which is readily liberated on the addition of even a weak acid, and, on exposure to the air, by the absorption of carbonic acid. It is used in malignant fevers as an antiseptic and stimulant, and to correct fetid eructations and evacuations; it is a favorite addition to gargles in ulcerated sore-throat. One of its principal uses is to purify the air in sick-rooms, in which case it acts by decomposing sulphuretted hydrogen, against which gas when inhaled, it is also an antidote. The dose is f℥ss, diluted with water or mucilage. In gargles, f℥ss or f℥j may be used in Oss.

Hyposulphite of Soda.

Sodæ Hyposulphis, NaO,S_2O_2+5HO.—This salt, which is very extensively used by photographists for the solution of the unaltered iodide of silver, may be economically prepared by the following process: 16 oz. finely-powdered crystallized carbonate of soda are mixed with 5 oz. flowers of sulphur, and heated in a porcelain dish with constant agitation, until it takes fire and burns to sulphite of soda; this is dissolved in water and boiled with sulphur, by which another equivalent of this element is taken up, so as to form the hyposulphite acid; it is then evaporated to crystallization.

The crystals are large, colorless, rhombic prisms, of a cooling, afterwards bitterish, somewhat alkaline taste, and easily soluble in water; the solution gradually deposits sulphur, leaving sulphite of soda, or if in contact with the air, sulphate of soda in solution.

It has been recommended in various diseases as a resolvent, alterative, and sudorific, and also as a solvent for biliary concretions; ½ to 1 drachm of it are given in the course of day. Externally it has been employed as a bath in quantities of from 1 to 4 ounces dissolved in the necessary quantity of water, and with the subsequent addition of 3 fluidounces of diluted sulphuric acid for each ounce of the salt, so as to liberate the hyposulphurous acid which immediately decomposes into sulphur and sulphurous acid.

Sodæ Acetas, U. S.

This is officinal in the list with a view to the preparation of acetic acid by its decomposition, but it is also made as follows:—

Sugar of lead is decomposed by carbonate of soda, a precipitate of carbonate of lead is formed, and the acetate of soda remains in solution; or such a solution is obtained by neutralizing acetic acid with carbonate of soda; it is then evaporated to crystallization. The salt crystallizes in prisms of a salty, bitter taste, which effloresce in warm dry weather, and is fusible.

It has been used for the same purpose for which acetate of potassa is employed, and is said to act rather milder; the dose is about the same.

Metals are detected in the solution of this salt by sulphuretted hydrogen and ferrocyanuret of potassium; sulphuric acid (sulphate of soda) by the characteristic precipitate with acetate of baryta.

Sodæ Valerianas.

Valerianate of soda is made by saturating caustic soda with valerianic acid, as produced by the distillation of fusel oil from a mixture of sulphuric acid and bichromate of potassa, by which it is converted into valerianic acid, which combines with the soda. This salt is white, soluble, deliquescent, with the odor of valerian. Its only use is to prepare the other valerianates by double decomposition. It should be soluble in absolute alcohol. (See *Acidum Valerianicum.*)

Choleinate of Soda.

Sodæ Choleinas.—Under this name a preparation has been used which has no claim of being a pure chemical salt; the mode for preparing it from animal gall is as follows: The fresh ox-gall is evaporated to one-half, slimy and coloring matters are precipitated by an equal bulk of alcohol, the filtrate is treated with animal charcoal, the alcohol distilled off, and the residue washed with ether. The choleinate of soda then remains behind as a white, somewhat sticky mass, of a penetrating odor, and a peculiar, sweetish, afterwards bitter taste; it is easily soluble in water, and dissolves albumen and casein.

Being a natural constituent of bile, it has been employed with success in affections where a tonic with particular tendency to the biliary organs is desired. The dose is from 5 to 15 grains, two to four times a day.

Sulphovinate of Soda.

Sodæ Sulphovinas, $NaO,C_4H_5S_2O_7+2HO$.—Sulphovinate of soda is prepared by mixing about equal parts of concentrated sulphuric acid and strong alcohol and heating afterwards by means of a water-bath; water is then added, and carbonate of baryta to saturation; the solution of sulphovinate of baryta is then exactly decomposed by a solution of sulphate of soda, and the filtrate evaporated to crystallization. It crystallizes in hexagonal tables, is deliquescent and very soluble in water; it fuses at 187°, and is decomposed above 212°; its taste is pleasantly saline and sweet.

This salt has been recommended for delicate constitutions afflicted with weakness of the digestive organs and flatulency. The dose, as a laxative, is from ½ to 1 ounce.

The impurities might be baryta, detected by sulphuric acid, or sulphate of soda, detected by chloride of barium.

Sodæ Benzoas. (Benzoate of Soda.)

If benzoic acid is saturated with carbonate of soda, the solution yields, on evaporation and cooling, needles, which are little soluble in alcohol. It has been recommended in cases of gout on account of its being changed by the animal economy into hippuric acid.

Ammoniæ Benzoas. (Benzoate of Ammonia.)

The neutral salt has been employed in medicine; it is obtained by dissolving benzoic acid in strong ammonia by the aid of heat, not quite to saturation. It is very soluble in water, deliquescent in the air, loses ammonia and becomes solid again. Like benzoate of soda, it has been used in gout, also, as an antispasmodic, though in the latter case the activity may be due to the oil which it retains.

GROUP 3.—*Alkaline Salts, starting with Crude Tartar.*

Crude argols, or tartar. Deposited in the casks during the ripening of wines.

Potassæ bitartras, $KO,HO,2\overline{T}$. Purified by repeated recrystallizations, &c.

Sodæ et potassæ tartras, $KO,NaO,2\overline{T}+8HO$. Boiling carb. soda with bitartrate.

Potassæ tartras, $2KO,2\overline{T}=KO,\overline{T}$. Boiling carbonate of potassa with bitartrate.

Potassæ et boracis tartras, $KO,NaO,2\overline{T}+2(KO,BO_3,2\overline{T})+3HO$. Boiling borax with bitartrate; deliquescent.

Potassæ boracico-tartras, $KO,BO_3,2\overline{T}$. Boiling boracic acid with bitartrate; permanent.

Crude argols are imported from the wine-producing countries of two kinds, the red and the white tartar of commerce. Recently tartar has been produced, though not in large quantities, in the vicinity of Cincinnati, Ohio. It consists of potassa combined with an excess of tartaric acid, some tartrate of lime, coloring matters, &c., the lees and settlings of the wine which have separated during the conversion of the sugar of the grape juice into alcohol, and collected as a mass on the bottom and sides of the casks.

Potassæ Bitartras, U.S.

Cream of tartar is purified tartar made by treating argols with hot water, mixing with clay, which absorbs the coloring matters, purifying by crystallization, and reducing to powder. It is a white somewhat gritty powder, of an agreeable acid taste, sparingly soluble in the mouth, soluble in 184 parts of cold water, and in 18 parts of boiling water, which deposits it on cooling. It consists of one equivalent of potassa, one of water, and two of tartaric acid; the water contained in it is capable of being replaced by other bases, as in the two salts which follow it, and in the tartrate of iron and potassa, and the tartrate of antimony and potassa, described in subsequent chapters.

Cream of tartar in doses of ℥ss to ℥j, and in smaller quantities, is a very common and well-known hydragogue cathartic, refrigerent, and diuretic. It is usually given diffused in water, being sparingly soluble.

It is very liable to adulteration, which may be detected by its solubility as above, and by the following tests:—

Must be completely soluble in liquor potassæ and liquor ammoniæ.

Lime is discovered in the neutralized solution by a white precipitate with phosphate of soda, or neutral oxalate of ammonia.

Sulphuric acid, sulphate of lime, alum, and sulphate of potassa by an insoluble precipitate, in cold solution, with chloride of barium.

Metals (copper, iron, &c.,) by precipitates with sulphuretted hydrogen and ferrocyanuret of potassium.

Sodæ et Potassæ Tartras, U.S.

Rochelle salt is prepared by combining one equivalent of carbonate of soda with one of bitartrate of potassa. The soda of the carbonate uniting with the excess of tartaric acid of the bitartrate to form a neutral salt; carbonic acid is evolved. The crystals of this salt are usually large, transparent, slightly efflorescent, of a saline not very unpleasant taste, and very soluble in water. It is commonly sold in powder, and, combined with one-third its weight of bicarbonate of soda constitutes the so-called Seidlitz mixture. It is a mild and pleasant purgative. Dose, from ʒij to ℥j.

Tests.—Much tartrate of lime renders the solution, in 2½ to 3 parts of cold water, milky.

Lime, metals, and sulphuric acid, are detected as above, in the latter case, after acidulating with nitric acid.

Potassæ Tartras, U.S.

Soluble tartar is a salt in which the excess of tartaric acid in bitartrate of potassa is combined with potassa; by boiling one equivalent of the carbonate of that alkali with one equivalent of bitartrate, the carbonic acid escapes; the reaction closely resembles that last described, substituting potassa for soda. Tartrate of potassa is either in white crystals, or a granulated powder slightly deliquescent and freely soluble; it is less agreeable to the palate than the foregoing, which it resembles in medical properties and uses. The dose is from ʒj to ℥j.

Tests.—Milky solution in 2 parts cold water, shows the presence of tartrate of lime.

Lime is detected by phosphate of soda or neutral oxalate of ammonia.

Metals (iron, copper, tin), by ferrocyanuret of potassium and sulphuretted hydrogen, the latter after acidulating with muriatic acid.

Sulphuric and muriatic acids are found in the solution acidulated with nitric acid by the precipitate with nitrate of baryta and nitrate of silver.

Potassæ et Boracis Tartras.

The *tartarus boraxatus* of the German *Pharmacopœias* is prepared by dissolving 3 parts of crystallized pure cream of tartar in a solution of 1 part borax in 5 parts water, and evaporating with constant agitation to dryness. It is soluble in 2 parts of water, deliquescing in the air, and has a mild, agreeably sour taste. Its medicinal properties are similar to those of the other neutral tartrates.

In its solution metallic oxides, lime, and mineral acids are detected as above.

Potassæ Boracico-Tartras.

The *tartarus boraxatus* or *tartras borico-potassicus* of the French Codex, as originally prepared by Soubeiran, is prepared by dissolving 1 part of boracic acid and 4 of cream of tartar, in 24 parts of water, and evaporating to dryness at or near the boiling point, so as to prevent the premature separation of the excess of bitartrate of potassa. The salt resembles the foregoing in appearance and properties, except that it keeps in the air without attracting moisture.

Group 4.—*Alkaline Salts—Prepared from Natural Deposits.*

Potassæ nitras, KO,NO_5. From incrustations on the soil, in India and elsewhere.
Sal-prunelle, $KONO_5$, fused with a little sulphur, and containing a trace of sulphate.
Potassæ bisulphas, $KO,HO,2SO_3$. The residuum of the process for nitric acid.
Potassæ sulphas, $KOSO_3$. By adding KO to the residuum of the process for nitric acid.
Potassæ chromas, KO,CrO_3, from chrome iron ore and nitrate by fusion, &c.
" *bi-chromas*, $KO,2CrO_3$, from chromate by an acid.
Sodæ boras, $NaO,2BO_3+10HO$. Found native in Thibet and purified.
Sodæ nitras, NaO,NO_5. Found native in the desert in Peru.

Potassæ Nitras, U. S.

Nitre, or saltpetre, is imported from the East Indies, where it is extracted from the soils by mixing them with a little wood-ashes, lixiviating with water, and crystallizing. It is refined in this country by recrystallization, and then exists in large six-sided, nearly colorless prisms, freely soluble, and with a cooling rather sharp taste. Much of the saltpetre of commerce is adulterated with nitrate of soda and chloride of sodium (common salt). In the absence of these, 100 grains of the dry salt, treated with 60 grains of sulphuric acid, and the whole ignited in a crucible till it ceases to lose weight, yield 86 grains of sulphate of potassa. The presence of chlorides may be shown by treating a weak solution with a few drops of solution of nitrate of silver, which would throw down a white insoluble precipitate of chloride of silver. Among the uses of nitrate of potassa in pharmacy, are the preparation of nitric acid, of spirit of nitric ether, and of collodion. Owing to the immense consumption of it in a pure form by the manufacturers of gunpowder, they are resorted to for procuring the best qualities for medicinal use. Dupont, near Wilmington, Delaware, furnishes a fine article both in crystals and in the form of a granular powder. It is one of the most popular of the refrigerant, diuretic, and sedative medicines. DOSE, gr. v to ℈j. In over doses it acts as a corrosive poison.

Sal Prunelle.

This is fused saltpetre run into round moulds about the size of a filbert, of a white color, and possessing the properties of the nitrate. From the use of sulphur in its fusion, it often contains sulphate of potassa. It is used to dissolve in the mouth in affections of the throat.

Potassæ Chromas.

It is obtained in large manufactories as a preliminary step to the preparation of the bichromate, by melting powdered chrome iron ore with saltpetre, dissolving it out with water, evaporating and recrystallizing. For pharmaceutical use it may be conveniently made by adding carbonate of potassa to a solution of the bichromate until it has acquired a slight alkaline reaction. It occurs in lemon-yellow prisms of a bitter, almost styptic taste, requiring little more than two parts of water at 60° for its solution, which has an alkaline reaction; it is insoluble in alcohol.

It is an irritating resolvent, alterative and emetic; the dose is one-eighth grain every two or three hours; or from 2 to 4 grs. as an emetic. Externally it is mostly used in solution in water.

Potassæ Bichromas.

This salt is prepared from chromate of potassa, by adding to a solution of the latter some mineral acid, which abstracts part of the base, and leaves the bichromate in solution. As obtained in commerce it is sufficiently pure for medicinal purposes; it crystallizes in prisms, which are isomorphous with the anhydrous bisulphate of potassa, but the latter, owing to its greater solubility in water, can be easily removed by recrystallization if it should be present. Bichromate of potassa has a red color and a cooling bitter metallic taste; it is soluble in 10 parts of water at ordinary temperature, but is insoluble in alcohol.

It has been employed as a powerful alterative in the dose of $\frac{1}{20}$ to $\frac{1}{16}$ grain, repeated two or three times daily. In larger doses, ½ to 1 grain, it acts as an emetic, but its use is dangerous on account of its irritating poisonous properties. It has been externally employed as a caustic and irritant in the form of a nearly concentrated solution, and as powder.

Tests.—Muriatic acid or common salt is detected by nitrate of silver; sulphuric acid or sulphate of potassa by chloride of barium; soda of salts by antimoniate of potassa; lime and magnesia (as nitrates from imperfect purification), by carbonate of potassa; metallic oxides by sulphuretted hydrogen and ferrocyanide of potassium.

Potassæ Bisulphas. (*Bisulphate of Potassa.*)

Contained in the residuum of the preparation of nitric acid from nitrate of potassa, or obtained from the neutral sulphate by fusing it together with an excess of sulphuric acid, and recrystallizing it.

It is readily soluble in water, and has a bitter acid tastè; it contains 2HO. It is used occasionally in cases of constipation when the tonic effect of an acid is desired. The dose is one or two drachms.

Potassæ Sulphas, U. S. (*Vitriolated Tartar.*)

Sulphate of potassa is prepared from the residuum left after treating nitrate of potassa with sulphuric acid, for the distillation of nitric acid; it is also a residuary product in the manufacture of sulphuric and of tartaric acid. A supersulphate is the residuum in the first named case, which requires treatment to reduce it to the proper composition; the salt is then dissolved and crystallized. The crystals are hard, heavy, and usually regular in their shape, being six-sided prisms, terminated by corresponding pyramids. It is used in the preparation of Dover's powder, but in this country is rarely given alone or in any other combination. It is esteemed a cathartic in doses of ʒj to ʒij, and often prescribed as such in Europe, especially in cases of pregnancy.

Tests.—Lime or its sulphate is detected by oxalate of potassa; muriatic acid or chlorides by nitrate of silver; metallic oxides by sulphuretted hydrogen.

Sodæ Boras, U. S.

Borax is found native in Thibet, and imported in a crude condition from India, also manufactured in Tuscany. In its refined condition it is in large and handsome crystals, semi-transparent, with slight alkaline reaction, and slightly alkaline not disagreeable taste, soluble in water, especially when hot. The proportion of water of crystallization appears to vary with the process of crystallization. It is a diuretic and antacid, and by some is said to promote contraction of the uterus, to which end it is associated with ergot. It is a very favorite addition to gargles and mouth-washes—being much prescribed for the sore mouth of infants, triturated with sugar, 1 part to 7, and touched to the tongue, or blown in through a quill.

It is remarkable for its whitening effect upon ointments, upon which it seems to act by its sub-alkaline properties, partially saponifying them without materially diminishing their bland and emollient effects.

Tests.—Alum is detected by a white precipitate occasioned by carb. of potassa; metallic oxides by sulphuretted hydrogen; sulphuric acid by nitrate of baryta, if the precipitate is insoluble in water; muriatic acid by nitrate of silver, if the precipitate is insoluble in nitric acid.

Borax in solution precipitates the mucilage of gum Arabic, Iceland moss, salep, &c.; it colors curcuma paper brown, and dissolves in 2 parts boiling, and 12 cold water. Moistened with SO_3, it colors the flame of alcohol, &c., green.

Sodæ Nitras. (*Nitrate of Soda, Cubic Nitre.*)

The natural deposits of this salt in Peru contain chlorides and sulphates of soda, and other bases in variable proportions. The native salt, therefore, requires to be purified by recrystallization from twice its weight of boiling water, when it is generally sufficiently pure for medical purposes.

It crystallizes in rhombohedrons, detonates less violently than saltpetre upon burning charcoal, when it shows a yellow flame. Its solution in distilled water is not disturbed by any reagent, except those few precipitating the soda; impurities are detected as above.

Cubic nitre has medicinal properties similar to saltpetre, but is thought to be rather milder in its action, and is, therefore, much employed in Europe in infantile diseases. The dose is the same as saltpetre, but it may be given in much larger doses without inconvenience.

Group 5.—*Alkaline Salts—Preparations of Ammonia.*

Ammoniæ murias, $NH_3,H_2Cl=NH_4,Cl$. Neutral, odorless, much used in the arts.
Ammoniæ nitras, $NH_4O, NO_5=NH_3,HO,KO_5$. By heat furnished NO.
Liquor ammoniæ. Aqueous solution of caustic ammonia, sp. gr. .960.
" ammoniæ fortior. " " " sp. gr. .882.
Spiritus ammoniæ. Alcoholic solution of " " sp. gr. .831.
" ammoniæ aromaticus. Alc. solut. of carb. of ammonia with aromatics.
Ammoniæ carbonas. Hard, translucent, and pungent, $2NH_3,3CO_2+2HO$.
Ammoniæ bicarbonas. White, pulverulent, odorless, $NH_3,2CO_2+HO$.
Liquor ammoniæ acetatis. Neutral and mild solution of, $NH_3\overline{Ac}+HO$.
Ammoniæ citras, $NH_3,\overline{Ci},HO$. In solution a diuretic.
Ammoniæ valerianas, $NH_3,\overline{V}a$. Antispasmodic. Used in solution.
Ammonii sulphuretum, $NH_3+HS=NH_4S$. Test liquid forming sulphurets of metals.

Ammoniæ Murias, U. S.

Muriate of ammonia, sal ammoniac, or *chloride of ammonium*, is in the list of the *Pharmacopœia;* it is prepared on a very large scale in England from the residuary products of the destructive distillation of coal, and from other empyreumatic products containing ammonia. It is in white, translucent, fibrous masses, which are convex on one surface and concave on the other; it has a pungent saline taste, but no odor. It cannot be conveniently powdered by contusion or trituration, and is best reduced by dissolving, evaporating, and granulating. It is a very soluble salt; it is incompatible with strong acids, which liberate muriatic acid, and with alkalies, which disengage ammonia, as in some of the processes which follow. It is frequently prescribed, especially by German practitioners, as a stimulating alterative in catarrhs, combined with expectorants. Dose, from gr. v to xx.

The reactions of ammonia are similar to those of potassa; bichloride of platinum produces a yellow precipitate; tartaric acid a crystalline white precipitate, which is more soluble than cream of tartar.

The characteristic test to distinguish its salts from the potassa salts, is the evolution of ammonia on triturating them with hydrated lime, when the solution is heated with caustic potassa; ammonia is recognized by its peculiar odor and the white fumes occasioned with muriatic acid.

Muriate of ammonia must be perfectly white, and entirely dissipated by heat. Copper, lead, and tin are detected by sulphuretted hydrogen. Iron by ferrocyanuret of potassium. Sulphuric acid by chloride of barium.

Ammoniæ Nitras. (*Nitrate of Ammonia.*)

Nitric acid is saturated with carbonate of ammonia and evaporated. It occurs in prisms which are deliquescent and have a cooling salty taste.

It is given in similar complaints as saltpetre and nitrate of soda, in doses ranging from ½ to 2 scruples.

If thrown in a red-hot crucible it burns with a yellow flame, and had therefore received the name of nitrum flammans. When not too suddenly heated it is decomposed exactly into 4HO and 2NO, oxide of nitrogen or laughing gas.

Liquor Ammoniæ, U. S., *and Liquor Ammoniæ Fortior*, U. S.

Solution of ammonia (spirits of hartshorn), *and stronger solution of ammonia*, are obtained from muriate or any other common ammonia salt, by the action of quicklime, which combining with the acid, liberates the caustic alkali in the form of gas; this is passed by suitable contrivances into water, which absorbs it with intensity, especially if refrigerated.

The usual commercial strength is somewhat below that of the officinal *liquor ammoniæ*, which has the sp. gr. 960. The strongest marks 882, and requires diluting with two parts of water to bring it to the strength of the former; it is not, however, an economical mode of preparing the weaker to dilute the stronger.

Spiritus Ammoniæ, U. S.

The composition of spirit of ammonia is similar to the foregoing, except that alcohol is used as the solvent for the gas; it has nearly the strength of the officinal solution of ammonia, and has the sp. gr. .831.

The three officinal solutions of gaseous ammonia are used almost exclusively for external applications. They are too caustic to be given by the stomach unless largely diluted and modified by emollient or mucilaginous excipients. The dose of the officinal liquor ammoniæ (not fortior), or of spiritus ammoniæ, is ♏x to xxx. Several liniments introduced under the appropriate head contain one or other of these preparations; the only merit of *spiritus* over *liquor* ammoniæ, is, that it is miscible with certain tinctures, &c., which are decomposed by the aqueous ingredient in the former preparation. Liquor ammoniæ fortior is adapted to raise a blister suddenly.

Spiritus Ammoniæ Aromaticus, U. S. (*Aromatic Spirit of Ammonia.*)

Spt. sal volat. as this is also called is a very useful antacid stimulant. Unlike the foregoing caustic preparations, this contains carbonate of the alkali, and is well adapted to internal use. Some processes for preparing it require the solution of the solid carbonate in alcohol by the aid of a mortar and pestle, with the addition of aromatic essential oils, but our *Pharmacopœia* directs a different and somewhat more troublesome manipulation, as follows:—

Take of	Muriate of ammonia . .	Five ounces.
	Carbonate of potassa . .	Eight ounces.
	Cinnamon, bruised,	
	Cloves, bruised, each . .	Two drachms.
	Lemon-peel	Four ounces.
	Alcohol,	
	Water, each	Five pints.

Mix them, and distil seven pints and a half.

The two first ingredients decompose each other, forming chloride of potassium, which remains in solution in the retort or still used, and carbonate of ammonia, which in the form of vapor distils over with the alcohol and aromatics, and is collected in the receiver.

This preparation is given, alone or combined with other remedies, to treat a variety of indications in disease. DOSE, ♏xx to f℥j.

Ammoniæ Carbonas, U. S.

Carbonate of ammonia (sesquicarbonate) is prepared by treating a mixture of muriate or sulphate of ammonia and chalk (soft carbonate of lime). By double decomposition, chloride of calcium and carbonate of ammonia are formed; the latter, being volatile, sublimes, and is collected in a colorless almost transparent sublimate, with powerful pungent odor and acrid taste. Our markets are recently supplied with a fine article from New England, the ammonia salt being largely furnished from the refuse liquors of the gasworks. It is usually in irregular lumps from the breaking of a large dome-shaped mass at first obtained; it is very hard, and on that account liable to fracture a glass bottle in which it is placed.

The stimulant and antacid properties of this salt are very well known; it is given in various modes of combination, some of which will be noticed under the head of *Extemporaneous Preparations.* Its dose is gr. v.

Carbonate of ammonia in smelling bottles is much sought for to relieve headaches, and for this purpose may be most conveniently prepared as follows:—

Mix muriate of ammonia, granulated . . .	5 parts.
Carbonate of potassa " . . .	8 parts.

Moisten and flavor appropriately with *Liquor Ammoniæ.*

A pretty good Preston salt is made by combining with the above, 1 part of aromatic powder.

Ammoniæ Bicarbonas.

Bicarbonate of Ammonia.—By long exposure to the air, particularly in small fragments, the sesquicarbonate loses a portion of its pungency, falls into powder, and by the loss of gaseous ammonia becomes converted chiefly into bicarbonate. The use of this is as a milder and less stimulating diaphoretic and antacid. DOSE, gr. x to ℈j.

In using carbonate of ammonia for its direct simulating effect, care should be taken that it is free from the pulverulent, white bicarbonate; and where it has deteriorated by the formation of this on the surface of the lumps, they should be scraped away, and cracked, till the vitreous looking hard portion is reached. For saturating acids in the formation of neutral salts, the bicarbonate will answer a good purpose.

Liquor Ammoniæ Acetatis, U. S. (*Solution of Acetate of Ammonia. Spirit of Mindererus.*)

This excellent preparation is made very readily and conveniently by the officinal recipe, as follows:—

Take of Diluted acetic acid . . . Half a pint.
Carbonate of ammonia, in powder, A sufficient quantity.

Add the carbonate of ammonia gradually to the acid until it is saturated.

Diluted acetic acid, elsewhere stated, is made by adding one fluidounce of acetic acid to seven fluidounces of water, making eight. It will be found convenient and desirable to consume the bicarbonate or the partially bicarbonated sesquicarbonate, which falls readily into powder, and is almost useless for other purposes, in making this preparation. By making it in a tincture-bottle in which toward the last the stopper is kept, the solution will be made to absorb a large amount of gas, and to sparkle when decanted. The point of saturation may be determined proximately by the taste, and it is generally not desirable to continue adding the alkali till it is perfectly saturated, as it is far more agreeable to be a little acid than alkaline. This solution should always be made in small quantities, and is generally better to be prepared when required. It is very much prescribed as a mild stimulant and diaphoretic. Dose, f℥j to f℥ss. As an antidote to alcoholic liquids given while the patient is intoxicated, from f℥ss to f℥j.

Ammoniæ Citras. (*Citrate of Ammonia.*)

A solution of this salt has been used as a diaphoretic in similar cases as the acetate. It is best prepared extemporaneously by saturating lemon juice with carbonate of ammonia; the dose is ℥ss to ℥j.

Ammoniæ Valerianas. (*Valerianate of Ammonia.*)

To prepare the dry salt, valerianic acid is saturated with strong ammonia, evaporated below 150° to a syrupy consistence, and crystallized by spontaneous evaporation of its alcoholic solution. It is generally sold in the form of concentrated solution.

The crystals or hydrated liquid salt, have a sweetish taste, peculiar odor; soluble in alcohol and water. It is used in neuralgia, hysteria, and other nervous disorders in a dilute solution, proposed by Pierlot, which is made by dissolving one drachm of terhydrated valerianic acid in 32 drachms distilled water, saturating with carbonate of ammonia, and dissolving two scruples of alcoholic extract of valerian in the mixture.

It may be given in doses as high as one or two teaspoonfuls.

Ammonii Sulphuretum. (*Sulphuret of Ammonia.*)

Spirits of hartshorn is saturated with hydrosulphuric acid.

It is a yellowish liquid, of a disagreeable fetid smell, which is mostly used in analytical chemistry for the detection of some metals.

It has been recommended as a sedative and in diabetes in the dose of five or six drops largely diluted with water.

CHAPTER III.

ON THE EARTHS AND THEIR PREPARATIONS.

1st Group.—*Preparations of Lime.*

Marmor (Marble). Native hard carbonate of lime.
Creta (Chalk). Native soft carbonate of lime.
Creta præparata, CaO,CO_2. Levigated and elutriated nodules. Dose, gr. x to ʒj.
Testa (Oyster-Shells). The shell of ostrea edulis.
Testa præparata. Levigated and elutriated, small nodules.
Calx, CaO. Lime recently prepared by calcination.
Liquor calcis. Lime-water, contains 9.7 grs. to Oj.
Calcii chloridum, CaCl. Dissolving carbonate in HCl, and evaporating.
Liquor calcii chloridi. One part of CaCl in 2.5 of the solution. Dose, ♏xxx to f℥j.
Calcis carbonas præcipitatus. From CaCl by adding NaO,CO_2. Very white, fine powder.
Calx chlorinata, CaO,ClO+CaCl+CaO+Cl. Bleaching salt. Disinfectant.
Calcis phosphas, $3CaO,PO_5$. Calcined bones precipitated from solution in HCl.

Lime is the oxide of a light metal called calcium, its officinal name is *Calx*, symbol CaO. It exists to a very great extent in the mineral kingdom, being the most familiar type of the so-called alkaline earths. It is obtained from the soil by plants, and becomes incorporated into the structure of animals, entering specially into their bones, shells, and teeth.

Tests for the determination of Lime.—Soluble salts of lime impart to alcohol a yellowish-red color. The neutral salts are precipitated—

By carbonates and phosphates of the alkalies; the white precipitates are soluble in muriatic and nitric acids.

By oxalic acid; the precipitates soluble in muriatic and nitric acids; not in ammonia or excess of oxalic acid.

Sulphuric acid and soluble sulphates throw down a precipitate of sulphate of lime from concentrated solutions, soluble in much water and in diluted acids.

Only in very concentrated solutions does a precipitate take place by caustic potassa.

Marmor and *Creta* are the names given in the list to two native unorganized forms of carbonate of lime, while *Testa* is applied to the shell of the common oyster. Besides these, there is another form of hard carbonate of lime, called *limestone*, which, though not officinal, is employed for the preparation of lime.

Carbonate of lime for use in medicine requires to be prepared by the mechanical processes adapted to furnishing a pure and fine article. Chalk and oyster-shell are subjected to the process of elutriation; being powdered and diffused in water, to allow of the subsidence of crystalline particles, the turbid liquid is drawn off into other vessels, allowed to settle, and dried, by being dropped from a suitable orifice on to a drying slab, thus presenting the carbonate in nodules or small pyramidal amorphous masses, readily falling into a very fine, impalpable, white powder. In this way prepared chalk and prepared oyster-shell are produced. The precipitated carbonate of lime is very differently prepared, by means of a chemical process, described, along with the medical properties of the carbonate, on the next page.

Calx, U. S.

Lime itself is prepared from the carbonate, mostly from limestone, by calcinating along with carbonaceous matters. Sometimes with wood, furnishing wood-burnt lime; and at other times with coal, furnishing a more common article. The action of an intense heat drives off the carbonic acid which escapes, leaving the lime in its caustic state.

On the addition of water, lime becomes slaked, a high heat is produced, and it is found to have absorbed water. Lime is less soluble in hot than in cold water, is infusible before the blowpipe, and entirely soluble in muriatic acid. Silicic acid remains undissolved on the addition of this acid. Phosphate of lime, if the solution is acid, is thrown down on neutralization with ammonia. Alumina, magnesia, oxide of iron, are thrown down from this solution by a slight excess of ammonia.

Liquor Calcis, U. S.

Take of		
	Lime	Four ounces.
	Water	One gallon.

Upon the lime, first slaked with a little water, pour the remainder of the water, and stir them together, then immediately cover the vessel, and set it aside for three hours. The solution should be kept standing upon the undissolved lime in stopped glass bottles, and poured off clear when required for use.

Lime is soluble to a limited extent, and more so in cold than in hot water. The proportion contained in lime-water is from nine to ten grains to the pint; its dose is from f℥ss to f℥ij. It is particularly useful, in small doses, to allay irritation of stomach and nausea, and, as

30

an astringent antacid, is adapted to dyspepsia, accompanied with acidity of stomach and diarrhœa. Its taste and caustic properties are best disguised by admixture with milk; and a mixture of lime-water and milk is much used as food for infants.

Tests.—Lime-water of full strength is rendered turbid on application of heat. If prepared from lime obtained from common limestone, it is apt to contain caustic soda, from the decomposition, by lime, of some silicate of soda; it is recognized by passing carbonic acid (exhaled air) into it until the lime is precipitated, when the alkaline reaction will not have disappeared.

Calcii Chloridum, U. S. (*Chloride of Calcium*),

Is prepared by dissolving chalk or marble in muriatic acid, and evaporating to dryness, after which it may be fused. It is a white, amorphous mass or powder, with an acrid, bitter, saline taste, very soluble in water and alcohol, and so deliquescent as to be used for drying gases, and for depriving various liquid substances of water. It is also capable of crystallizing, when it absorbs six equivalents of water.

Metallic oxides, which may be present, are detected by precipitates in the solution with ammonia and sulphuretted hydrogen. A precipitate by solution of sulphate of lime would indicate baryta.

Liquor Calcii Chloridi, U. S.

Solution of chloride of calcium is directed, in the *Pharmacopœia*, to be made by obtaining the chloride as above, and dissolving it in water in about such proportion that 2.5 parts of the solution shall be equal to one part of the salt. It is rarely prepared or prescribed, although considered a deobstruent and alterative remedy, adapted to scrofulous diseases and goitre. DOSE, ♏xxx to f℥j.

Calcis Carbonas Præcipitatus, U. S.

Is prepared by adding to the solution of chloride of calcium as above, an equivalent proportion of carbonate of soda in solution. By double decomposition, carbonate of lime is formed and precipitated as a white powder, while chloride of sodium remains in solution and is separated by washing. The fineness of this precipitate is dependent upon the degree of concentration and the temperature of the solutions. If dilute and cold, the result would be the formation of a crystalline powder destitute of that softness and miscibility with liquids which adapts it to convenient use. The *Pharmacopœia*, therefore, directs strong solutions and a boiling temperature at the time of mixing them.

When properly made, this is a fine white powder, free from grittiness, insoluble in water, but soluble without residue in diluted muriatic acid, with abundant disengagement of carbonic acid. It is used as an antacid, with astringent properties, adapting it especially to diarrhœa. DOSE, from gr. x to ℨj.

As compared with prepared chalk, with which it is identical in composition, this is a far handsomer preparation, and, though less distinctly amorphous, is preferred for almost all prescription purposes. It is also well substituted for chalk in dentifrice.

Tests.—Sulphate of lime, which is an occasional adulteration, may be detected by washing the preparation with distilled water, in which chloride of barium and oxalic acid will produce precipitates.

Phosphate of lime is left behind on treatment with diluted acetic acid; it is dissolved by muriatic acid, in which solution the phosphoric acid is proved by perchloride of iron and acetate of potassa in excess.

Calx Chlorinata, U.S.

Under the name of chloride of lime, or bleaching powder, this substance is extensively manufactured and used as a bleaching agent. It is made from slaked lime by subjecting it to an atmosphere of chlorine gas till completely saturated. It is a whitish powder, having the odor of chlorine, which it gives off on exposure to the air. It is highly deliquescent, absorbing both moisture and carbonic acid from the air. A very moist consistence argues the presence of a considerable proportion of chloride of calcium, and is an indication of inferiority. Its composition varies, but it is, when of good quality, a mixture of hypochlorite of lime, CaO,ClO, chloride of calcium, CaCl, lime, CaO,HO, and free chlorine, Cl. It is only partially soluble in water.

For the full advantage of the liberation of chlorine the addition of an acid is necessary, though the spontaneous evolution of that gas is usually relied on for common disinfecting purposes. The chief popular use of chlorinated lime is as a disinfectant about cesspools, sewers, and places rendered offensive and unwholesome by the products of decomposition.

It is also used in the manufacture of chloroform and for the preparation of Liquor sodæ chlorinata, which is used as a substitute for it for internal and external use in medicine.

The *Pharmacopœia* gives the following test which shows an amount of chlorine available for disinfecting and medical purposes, of at least twenty-five per cent., and indicates a good commercial quality; though practically it is obtained only so strong as to contain one-third its weight of chlorine, theoretically it ought to have nearly one-half its own weight.

When forty grains, triturated with a fluidounce of distilled water, are well shaken with a solution of seventy-eight grains of crystallized sulphate of protoxide of iron, and ten drops of sulphuric acid in two fluidounces of distilled water, a liquid is formed which does not yield a blue precipitate with ferridcyanide of potassium.

This test is based on the oxidation of the iron under the influence of chlorine to sesquioxide; but aside from other objections, the difficulty of keeping the sulphate of iron entirely unaltered, renders this test inaccurate; a better result is obtained by treating thirty-six grains chloride of lime with fifty-three grains ferrocyanide of potassium, and after heating to the boiling point, testing with a salt of sesquioxide of iron, which must not furnish a blue precipitate.

By the influence of chlorine, the ferrocyanide is changed into the ferridcyanide of potassium; if less than 25 per cent. of chlorine is present, a part of the ferrocyanide remains unaltered, and reacts with the chloride of calcium, the resulting ferrocyanuret of potassium and calcium is taken up by boiling water, and throws down a precipitate of Prussian blue with sesqui-salts of iron.

Calcis Phosphas, U.S.

This salt, called bone phosphate of lime, is made by calcining bones and dissolving in muriatic acid, precipitating the phosphate by a solution of ammonia, washing, and drying.

It is a white insoluble powder, free from odor and taste; soluble in muriatic, acetic, and phosphoric acids.

This phosphate is used as a remedy for scrofulous diseases, defective nutrition, &c. DOSE, from gr. x to ʒss, repeated three times a day.

Tests.—Carbonate of lime, if present as an adulteration, is detected by its effervescing with acids.

Sulphate of lime is left behind on dissolving the salt in muriatic acid; the residue dissolves in much distilled water, and yields the characteristic precipitate with baryta and its salts.

(See chapter on *Phosphorous Compounds.*)

Calcis Bicarbonas

Cannot be obtained in the dry state. It is contained in all spring-water, to which it imparts the property of reacting acid on litmus and alkaline on logwood paper. A solution of this salt has been used in England, under the name of *Maugham's Carrara water*, which is made by dissolving Carrara marble, or any other pure carbonate of lime in water, saturated with carbonic acid.

It has been used as an antacid absorbent, alterative and a mild astringent in a number of diseases, particularly in various forms of dyspepsia. The dose of this water is one or two wineglassfuls and more, to the amount of about two quarts per day.

Calx Saccharatum, Syrupus Calcis.

Trousseau used the following proportion: 1 part of slaked lime, 10 parts water and 100 parts syrup are boiled together for a few minutes, strained and diluted with four times the weight of simple syrup.

This syrup has an alkaline taste and reaction, and is the solution of a chemical compound between sugar and lime. It is used for the same purposes as lime-water, but on account of its causticity it is necessary to dilute it considerably. It is given to children in the quantity of 20 to 30 grains during the day; adults take from 2 to 3 drachms during the same time.

Calçii Iodidum.

It may be prepared by dissolving lime or carbonate of lime in hydriodic acid, or by precipitating a solution of iodide of iron with lime, and evaporating the filtrate to crystallization.

It is a deliquescent salt, easily soluble in water, and has a bitterish taste. It has been used in scrofulous affections internally, in doses ranging from ½ to 2 grains three times daily, and externally in ointments, containing 2 drachms or less to the ounce.

Calcii Sulphuretum.

If lime diffused in water is decomposed by a current of sulphuretted hydrogen, a solution results, which on evaporation yields a white soft mass, of a sulphurous odor and taste.

It has been used as a depilatory by applying a paste formed with water to the parts, and washing it off after about a quarter of an hour.

The same compound in an impure state, prepared by dissolving flowers of sulphur in boiling milk of lime, and diluting the solution, has been employed for the cure of itch, by washing the body with such a solution, or by adding a sufficient quantity to a bath.

The sulphur springs generally contain more or less of this sulphuret, which, besides hydrosulphuric acid, forms the most active of their constituents.

2D GROUP.—*Of the Earths, &c. Preparations of Magnesia.*

Magnesiæ sulphas, MgO,SO_3+7HO, from native carbonate. Dose, ℥j.
" carbonas, $4(MgO,CO_2HO)$, $MgO,2HO$, from sulphate, by NaO,CO_2.
Magnesiæ carbonas ponderosum, $4(MgO,CO_2HO)$, $MgO,2HO$? do. do.
" *bicarbonas* (solution). Fluid magnesia.
Magnesia, MgO. By calcining the carbonate. Dose, ʒj.
Liquor magnesiæ citratis, ℥j of the salt in f℥xij bottle.
Magnesiæ citras, MgO, $\overline{Ci}$, 3HO ? By fusing citric acid and adding MgO.
Prepared citrate of magnesia. Effervescing powder, mixed citrate, bicarb. potassa, &c.
Moxon's effervescent magnesia, contains MgO,SO_3+7HO.
Magnesiæ acetas. In solution with orange syrup.
" *et potass, borotartras.* Soluble and mild salt.
" *sulphuretum.* Gelatinous alterative. Dose, 5 to 30 grains.

The salts of magnesia, like those of lime, have for their base the oxide of a metal. This has a brilliant gray color; and a sp. gr. of 2.2. It is rarely met with, except in the cabinet of the chemist.

Tests for the Detection of Magnesia.—Magnesia is precipitated by the fixed alkalies and their carbonates. The precipitate is soluble in ammonia; so is likewise the precipitate occasioned by oxalate of ammonia; phosphate of soda in conjunction with ammonia causes a crystalline white precipitate of $2MgO,NH_4O,PO_5$, which is insoluble in ammonia and ammoniacal salts, but dissolves easily in acids.

Magnesiæ Sulphas, U. S.

Epsom salt is made from a magnesian limestone, called by mineralogists, dolomite. By the action of sulphuric acid, the magnesia is converted into the soluble sulphate, which, on filtration and evaporation, yields that salt in crystals. By stirring, as it passes into a solid consistence, it is obtained in acicular crystals, which effloresce by exposure to the air, becoming white and pulverulent. Its sensible properties are familiar to most. In doses of from ℥ss to ℥j, Epsom salts is a brisk saline cathartic; in small doses, a diuretic. It is much combined with senna, senna and manna, &c., in well-known and very disagreeable infusions.

Tests.—Its solution is not colored nor precipitated by ferrocyanuret of potassium, and gives off no hydrochloric acid on the addition of sulphuric acid. The *Pharmacopœia* also directs the following test of this salt: 100

grains dissolved in water and mixed with sufficient boiling solution of carbonate of soda completely to decompose it, yield a precipitate of carbonate of magnesia, weighing, when washed and dried, 34 grains.

Magnesiæ Carbonas, U. S.

The carbonate, called also magnesia alba, is usually made from sulphate by adding carbonate of soda, and boiling the mixed solutions. Sulphate of soda and carbonate of magnesia result from the play of affinities; the former is soluble and is washed out, while the latter is collected, pressed into oblong squares, called bricks, dried at a moderate heat, and wrapped in paper for sale. It is very light, pulverulent, insoluble, tasteless, soft, though somewhat granular. It is a compound of about 1 part of hydrated magnesia and 4 of hydrated carbonate of magnesia, as shown in the syllabus.

By boiling it with pure water, this does not acquire an alkaline reaction, nor yield a precipitate with chloride of barium or nitrate of silver. It is wholly dissolved with effervescence by diluted sulphuric acid, and the solution is not precipitated by oxalate of ammonia.

Heavy Carbonate of Magnesia.

This is the result of a similar process to the foregoing, except that the solutions are much more concentrated, or are boiled together until effervescence ceases. It is heavier than the common carbonate, and is found in a white rather dense powder, preferred from its small bulk.

Carbonate of magnesia is used chiefly as an antacid, in doses of ℈j to ʒj, though liable to the objection of liberating carbonic acid gas in the stomach, producing eructations and distension.

Bicarbonate of Magnesia

Is a salt quite soluble in water, but which is not permanent, and exists only in solution. The so-called fluid magnesias, of which Murray's, Dinneford's, and Husband's, are the best known, are solutions of this salt. They are conveniently prepared by passing a stream of carbonic acid gas into freshly precipitated hydrated carbonate of magnesia, or preferably by forcing the gas into a strong fountain such as is used for mineral water, containing the freshly precipitated carbonate. The quantity contained in these solutions is necessarily small, and they have a tendency to deposit the salt as they lose the free carbonic acid; their usefulness is limited to the case of children, and to the treatment of acidity of stomach in adults. The taste is more alkaline and disagreeable than that of the insoluble carbonate, or of magnesia itself.

According to Graham, the crystals deposited from such solutions are compounds of mono-carbonate of magnesia with one, two or four equivalents of water.

Magnesia, U. S.

Usually prepared by calcining the carbonate at a high heat, until it presents a peculiar luminous appearance, called brightening. This preparation is very various in its physical properties, owing to the various modifications of the process for its preparation; it will not be necessary in this work to describe these. The reader is referred, for an account of some interesting experiments made in my laboratory by Thos. H. Barr, of Terre Haute, Ia., and by Thos. Weaver, of Philadelphia, in the *American Journal of Pharmacy*, vol. xxvi. p. 193, and vol. xxviii. p. 214.

Common calcined magnesia is a very light white powder, almost insoluble and tasteless, but imparting a sensation of grittiness to the tongue, which renders it a disagreeable medicine to most persons. It should be entirely soluble in diluted muriatic acid, without effervescence. The presence of lime would be shown by a white precipitate with sulphuric or oxalic acid, by which acids magnesia is not precipitated. When moistened it changes turmeric paper brown, but water which has been boiled on it should not be alkaline, nor give a precipitate with chloride of barium or nitrate of silver.

The four best varieties in commerce are the English ponderous magnesia, sold in bulk, and Henry's, Husband's, and Ellis's, sold in bottles.

The *ponderous* is not much used in this country; it has the advantage of smallness of bulk, but lacks the extreme softness of the bottled article. *Henry's* leaves nothing to desire; it is very heavy, soft and smooth, and is highly esteemed among the more wealthy classes; its price, which is enhanced by the payment of duty, almost puts it out of the reach of the middle and poorer classes. *Husband's* is somewhat cheaper and equally good, though, as would be inferred from the ascertained composition, it requires a little larger dose. *Ellis's* is the most recent make; it maintains the same price in bottles as the last named, and approaches it in quality. This is also obtainable by the pound at a somewhat reduced price.

The following is Weaver's process for a dense and soft magnesia; it is practicable on a small or large scale.

Take of	Sulphate of magnesia . . .	℥iv and ʒij.
	Bicarbonate of soda . . .	℥iij.
	Nitric acid,	
	Carbonate of soda,	
	Water, of each . . .	Sufficient.

Dissolve the sulphate of magnesia in six ounces of water, add a few drops of nitric acid, and boil for fifteen or twenty minutes; then add sufficient carbonate of soda, dissolved in a little water, to produce a slight precipitate, and continue boiling for some time, filter, and set aside to cool. Triturate the bicarbonate of soda with about eight ounces of cold water and add it to the cold solution of sulphate of magnesia; after frequent agitation filter, transfer to a porcelain capsule and boil quickly till reduced to a small bulk, collect the precipitate, wash thoroughly, and when nearly dry transfer to a crucible free from iron and calcine, at a low heat just approaching to redness. The first part of this process is designed to separate traces of iron as sesquioxide, which it accomplishes most effectually and economically, and the last, to decompose the sulphate at such a temperature as to insure a soft and heavy product. The elevation of the heat above redness seems to produce the grittiness characteristic of common qualities of magnesia.

In presenting a formula for this very popular cathartic beverage, I shall depart from the usual custom of following the *Pharmacopœia.* It is to be regretted that, from taking the officinal directions, some pharmaceutists have been so unsuccessful as to give up the preparation of the solution, and purchase it of other apothecaries or druggists, so that its manufacture is thrown very much into a few hands. One druggist in Philadelphia has frequently sold a gross of bottles of the citrate per day, on an average, for thirty days in succession. The recipe below is that I have used for some years; it is original with myself, and I believe seldom fails to furnish a satisfactory article.

	To make one doz.	To make one bottle.
Take of Citric acid . . .	℥ix (offic.)	ʒvj.
Magnesia . . .	℥ij+ʒv, or sufficient	ʒj+gr. xlv.
Syrup of citric acid .	12 fluidounces	f℥j.
Water	1 gallon, or sufficient	f℥xss.

The following abridgment of Barr's table of the composition of these three kinds will show the relative purity of the specimens examined:—

	Henry's. Sp. gr. 3.404.	Husband's. Sp. gr. 3.326.	Ellis's. Sp. gr. 3.386.
Magnesia	94.40	84.306	94.04
Water	.50	11.400	.80
Sulphate of magnesia and soda, iron, &c.	5.81	3.608	4.41

The dose of magnesia as a cathartic is about ʒj, or, of the common kind, near a tablespoonful, of the heavy kinds, about a teaspoonful; as an antacid, smaller doses are used.

Liquor Magnesiæ Citratis, U. S.

Make an acid solution of citrate of magnesia with the citric acid, magnesia, and 3 pints of the water (f℥iv in making a single bottle); to this add the lemon syrup, and divide the whole among 12 f℥xij bottles (or put into one bottle if the smaller quantity), fill these with the remainder of the water, adjust the corks, and add to each bottle about ℈ij of crystallized bicarbonate of potassa.

The quantity of magnesia here indicated is adjusted to an article of average purity; sometimes this weight is found too much and must be diminished to 95 or 100 grains; if, on the other hand, the magnesia is rather poorly calcined, and contains some carbonate, it may be best to increase the proportion from 105 to 110, or even 120 grains to the bottle, though this must be done with great caution, as the slightest excess may occasion the precipitation of a large amount of the hydrated citrate. If the preparation is not decidedly acid, it will be disagreeable to take, and will possess no advantage over the common saline cathartics, but if too strongly acid, it will be almost equally objectionable. The bicarbonate of potassa has the great advantage of neutralizing a portion of the acid, while it forms a very soluble and agreeable salt. If carbonate of magnesia were used, in the proportion of the *Pharmacopœia* formula, the tendency to deposit would be increased, which is the greatest practical difficulty with this solution.

The size of the bottle is another point to be observed; it must not fall short of f℥xij. The so-called pint-inks are very suitable; porter bottles will do to substitute for them. Bottles are made for the purpose both with and without the label blown in the glass, which are very convenient.

Although the above recipe is perfectly satisfactory for one or two dozen bottles when they are to be sold in a few weeks, it does not answer the purpose of the wholesale manufacturer, or the pharmaceutist who prepares it for use on shipboard. We are indebted to F. Stearns, of Detroit, for the following practical recipe adapted to these purposes.

Precipitate sulphate of magnesia by adding to it a hot solution of carbonate of soda (12 lbs. of the carbonate suffices for 10¼ lbs. of the sulphate), wash the precipitated carbonate of magnesia upon a linen filter, drain, and having ascertained the amount of water contained in a sample of known weight by drying and calcining it, introduce the moist hydrate into a suitable apparatus; and to every 1.280 grains of anhydrous magnesia the moist hydrate contains, add one gallon of clean soft water (allowing of course for the water already mechanically combined with the hydrate), then subject the whole to the action of carbonic acid gas under a pressure of ten atmospheres for 24 hours or until the magnesia is dissolved.

Having drawn it off, filter and prepare the solution of the citrate as follows: introduce into f℥xij strong bottles, ten and a half fluidounces of the solution, and one and a half ounce of lemon syrup, not acidulated, and having the corks ready and softened, introduce into each 366 grains of citric acid in crystals, cork and wire immediately—a bottling machine greatly facilitates this operation.

Each bottle of the solution as made by either of these recipes holds about ℥j of the salt, and is a full cathartic dose; divided portions may be taken for its refrigerant and aperient effects, the cork being always carefully secured, and the bottle inverted in the intervals of taking the doses.

Soluble Citrate of Magnesia.

Citrate of magnesia is insoluble in water as precipitated from a solution, but is more soluble if made by the direct union of its constituents in a dry condition. The proportion employed must be varied according to the purity of the magnesia and the condition of the acid. Citric acid is what is called a tribasic acid, having three equivalents of water of combination (see page 298); as found in commerce, it is liable to contain, in addition, either one or two equivalents of water of crystallization, so that its saturating power is not uniform. The basic citrate ($3MgO, \overline{Ci}$) is the neutral and soluble salt aimed at, and the proportion contained in the following recipe will furnish it in a tolerably eligible form with the use of the commercial acid and magnesia.

Take of	Citric acid (crystallized)	100 grains.
	Calcined magnesia	35 grains.
	Water	15 drops.

Dissolve the acid in the water, and its water of crystallization by the aid of heat, then stir in the magnesia; a pasty mass will result, which soon hardens, and may be powdered for use. The chief practical difficulty in the process results from the great comparative bulk of the magnesia, and the very small quantity of the fused mass with which it is to be incorporated. A portion of the magnesia is almost unavoidably left uncombined, and the salt is, con ntly, not neutral. This uncombined magnesia should be dusted mass before powdering it. Care must be taken to avoid a high ten which renders the salt less soluble.

M. E. r et suggests the following formula and manipulation.

Take of Citric acid	35¼	parts.
Carbonate of magnesia	21¼	parts.
Boiling water	10⅜	parts.

Powder the citric acid and dissolve it in the boiling water. When the solution is cold and before it crystallizes pour it into a wide earthen vessel, and by means of a sieve distribu rbonate of magnesia evenly and rapidly over its surface without stir the reaction takes place slowly; when it ceases beat the mixture rapi o long as it retains its pasty consistence.

According to this authority the el of temperature occurring during this process is due to a change in the mo ular condition by which the salt becomes insoluble; for this reason he re mmends that the dish should be placed in a vessel of cold water, and that he salt should be dried at a temperature not exceeding 70° Fahr.

The citrate thus prepar ible when at first made, though not rapidly so; it also dily soluble by keeping, and is liable to run into mass rd and unmanageable. Some mix powdered citric acid and, perhaps, a little carbonate, and sell it as solid citrate; but olves very slowly, and seems a very poor substitute for the efferves g solution.

The *prepared citrate of magnesia*, of Charles Ellis & Co., is made from the salt as prepared by fusion, so combined as to furnish an effervescing draught, which though not clear contains the undissolved portion so nicely suspended as to be taken without inconvenience. The recipe is as follows:—

Take of Powdered citrate of magnesia	℥iv.
Powdered sugar	℥viij.
Powdered citric acid	℥iiss.
Powdered bicarbonate of soda	℥iij.
Oil of lemons	♏x.

Combine the acid and sugar and rub into a fine powder; dry all the water of crystallization from the acid over a water bath. Add the citrate of magnesia and oil of lemons, and mix intimately; then add the bicarbonate of soda and triturate the whole into a fine powder, which must be preserved in bottle properly excluded from the air. The dose for an adult is from one to three tablespoonfuls mixed in a tumbler of water and drank in a state of effervescence.

Moxon's Effervescent Magnesia.

The following recipe for a good effervescing aperient is from Gray's Supplement; though less agreeable than the above, it answers a good purpose, and is popular with some:—

Take of Carbonate of magnesia . . . . . . ℥j.
Sulphate of magnesia . . . . . . ℥ij.
Tartrate of potassa and soda . . . . . ℥ij.
Bicarbonate of soda . . . . . . ℥ij.
Tartaric acid . . . . ℥ij.

To be perfectly freed from water of crystallization, and mixed and kept in a well-corked bottle.

Dose, from a teaspoonful to a tablespoonful dissolved in water and drank immediately.

Acetate of Magnesia.—This is very deliquescent and difficult to crystallize; in the dry state it is generally known as a gummy mass. It has been proposed as a substitute for citrate of magnesia. Renault recommends to dissolve 120 parts of carbonate of magnesia in acetic acid and evaporate to 300 parts, which solution, when wanted for use, is to be mixed with 3 times its weight of orange or some other agreeable syrup. It is more agreeable if, like citrate of magnesia, it contains a quantity of free carbonic acid.

Garrot recommended a *syrup of acetate of magnesia*, prepared by dissolving 10 parts calcined magnesia in 50 parts acetic acid, and adding 150 parts of some agreeable fruit syrup. Of similar composition is the *elixir of acetate of magnesia*, prepared by dissolving 10 parts calc. magnesia in 40 parts acetic acid, and adding 40 parts alcohol and 70 of an aromatic syrup.

Magnesii Sulphuretum.—If a boiling solution of sulphate of magnesia is mixed with a concentrated solution of sulphuret of potassium, a white gelatinous mass of sulphuret of magnesium is precipitated, which, on account of its weaker taste and smell, and milder action, has been recommended for internal use in cases of itch, instead of the other sulphurets, in doses of 5 to 10 grains for children. It likewise operates slightly as a laxative.

Magnesiæ et Potassæ Borotartras.—100 parts of boro-tartrate of potassa, 24 parts carbonate of magnesia, and 600 parts of water are to be gradually mixed and evaporated. Dissolved with citric acid it has been recommended as a purgative, for which purpose Garrot has proposed the following formula: Take of borotartrate of magnesia and potassa ʒj, citric acid ʒss, lemon syrup ℥ij, water ℥x.

3D GROUP.—*Preparations of Baryta.*

Barytæ carbonas, BaO,CO_2. Native witherite. Soluble in strong acids.
Barii chloridum, $BaCl,2HO$. Poisonous; used only in solution.
Liquor barii chloridi, ℥j to ℥iij water. Dose, five drops.
Barii iodidum. Poisonous. Dose, ¼ to 1 grain.

Test for Baryta.—The best and most reliable test for baryta is the precipitate which its solutions throw down with free sulphuric acid and all soluble sulphates, even with sulphate of lime. Sulphate of baryta is insoluble.

Barytæ Carbonas, U.S.

Carbonate of baryta, which, like the other earths, has a metallic base, is a rather rare mineral, being chiefly imported from Sweden, Scotland, and the North of England. It is usually in masses of a light grayish color and fibrous texture. It is soluble in the strong acids with effervescence, forming salts, which, if soluble, furnish in solution the best tests for sulphuric acid, throwing down a white precipitate insoluble in boiling nitric acid.

Barii Chloridum, U.S. (*Muriate of Baryta.*)

When muriatic acid is added to carbonate of baryta, by simple elective affinity, the muriatic acid displaces the carbonic with effervescence, and with the baryta forms chloride of barium and water. By evaporation, the chloride may be obtained in flat, four-sided crystals.

It is a white, freely soluble, permanent salt, with a bitter acrid taste, and imparts a yellow color to flame. If the crystals deliquesce the presence of another earthy chloride may be inferred. It is poisonous, as are all the other baryta salts; it is chiefly used in medicine in the form of

Liquor Barii Chloridi, U.S.

Take of Chloride of barium	. . . . .	℥j.
Distilled water	. . . .	f℥iij.

Dissolve the chloride in the water, and filter if necessary.

This solution is almost too strong for convenient use; it is stated to be deobstruent and anthelmintic. The dose is about five drops, but it is very rarely prescribed. It is, however, much employed as a test for sulphuric acid or soluble sulphate, forming the very insoluble sulphate of baryta.

Barii Iodidum

Is obtained by dissolving carbonate of baryta in hydriodic acid, or by adding to an alcoholic solution of iodide finely-powdered sulphuret of barium, and evaporating the filtrate by a moderate heat.

It occurs in colorless, deliquescent needles, which are decomposed by the carbonic acid of the atmosphere. It is very poisonous, and has been recommended as a discutient and alterative in scrofulous diseases, internally, in the dose of one-eighth to a grain twice daily, and externally in ointments containing 20 to 30 grains to the ounce.

4TH GROUP.—*Preparations containing Alumina.*

Alumen (Potassa-alum), $KO,SO_3+Al_2O_3,3SO_3+24HO$. Manufactured from alum earths.
Alumen (Ammonia-alum), $NH_4O,SO_3+Al_2O_3,3SO+24HO$. From sulphate of ammonia, &c.
Alumen exsiccatum. Deprived of its water of crystallization by heat.
Alumina, $Al_2O_3,3HO$. Precipitated by KO from alum.
Aluminæ sulphas, $Al_2O_3,3SO_3+18HO$, by dissolving alumina and SO, and crystallizing.
Aluminæ acetas, $Al_2O_3,Ac+HO$?

Aluminum is the name of the metallic radical of the earth *alumina*, a white, faintly bluish metal, which has recently attracted much attention from the discovery of an economical process for its extraction. Its extraordinary lightness, beauty of color, and indifference to oxidizing influences, fitting it to displace silver, and even platinum, for many purposes in the arts.

Tests for Alumina.—Alumina is recognized by being precipitated white by alkalies, redissolved by an excess of the same, and re-precipitated by chloride of ammonium. Compounds of alumina, ignited upon charcoal before the blowpipe, and then moistened with a little protonitrate of cobalt and ignited again, yields an unfused mass of a deep sky blue color.

Alumen, U.S. (*Alum.*)

This complex salt is found in commerce in large crystalline masses, very cheap and abundant, being largely produced for use in the arts. Formerly it was produced from a peculiar ore or schist occurring largely in many parts of the world, and had the composition given in the syllabus as that of potash alum. The alum now most common, as far as my observation extends, is a double sulphate of alumina and ammonia; this is made by the use of sulphate of ammonia, as prepared from the residuary liquor of the gas-works, instead of a salt of potassa, as in the old processes, and its composition varies accordingly. The properties of the two are so similar that they are seldom distinguished from each other.

Alum is slightly efflorescent in dry air from the loss of a portion of its large amount, nearly one-half its weight, of water of crystallization; it is very soluble; it is incompatible with alkalies and their carbonates. It is, also, incompatible with vegetable astringents.

Alumen Exsiccatum, U.S. (*Dried Alum.*)

Take of alum, in coarse powder, a convenient quantity. Melt it in a shallow iron or earthen vessel, and maintain it at a moderate heat until ebullition ceases and it becomes dry, then rub it into powder.

Dried or burnt alum differs from the crystallized salt in containing no water; 474.5 grains of the crystals should yield 258 grains of the anhydrous salt, which is consequently nearly double its strength. Care should be taken not to push the heat so far as to drive off a portion of the sulphuric acid. Dried alum is less soluble in water than alum, but no portion of it should be wholly insoluble.

Alum is an astringent, and in the dried condition a mild escharotic. In large doses it is a cathartic. It is much used as a gargle for sore throat, as an injection for leucorrhœa, &c. Internally, it is used in hemorrhages, in hooping-cough, &c. Burnt alum is used exclusively as an external application.

Iron alum, iron and ammonia alum, chrome alum, and manganese alum are compounds in which the alumina is substituted by other bases composed of 3O to 2 equivalents of the metal, and combined with either potassa or ammonia.

Alumina.

Dissolve alum in six times its weight of boiling water, add solution of carbonate of soda in slight excess, agitate for a few minutes, filter and wash the precipitate with distilled water, the product is hydrate of alumina. It may be further purified by dissolving in diluted muriatic acid, precipitating with ammonia, and again washing with water; dried on bibulous paper, it retains its combined water, but by a high heat it becomes anhydrous.

Pure ammonia alum, by calcining to a white heat, becomes converted into anhydrous alumina. The hydrated precipitate is freely soluble in diluted acids and in caustic potassa solution.

Alumina is much used as a base for coloring matters, as in the lake pigments. In medicine it is used as an antacid and astringent, with which it combines the properties of an absorbent; it has been used in purulent and catarrhal affections of the eye. The dose is five to twenty grains three or four times daily.

Sulphate of Alumina.

Saturate diluted sulphuric acid with hydrated alumina, evaporate and crystallize. It is in thin flexible plates of a pearly lustre, sweet and astringent taste. Soluble in twice its weight of cold water, but not in alcohol.

Its chief use is as an antiseptic, in foul ulcers, &c. A solution of one pound in two pints of water is used to preserve dead bodies; as a lotion it may be used in a somewhat less concentrated form.

Under the name of *benzinated solution of alumina*, Mentel proposed the following preparation as a styptic and, largely diluted with water, as an injection in leucorrhœa and various ulcerated affections: eight ounces of sulphate of alumina are dissolved in sixteen ounces of water, and saturated with hydrated alumina; six drachms of selected benzoin balsam is digested with it for six hours, then cooled and filtered. It has a very agreeable odor, and a balsamic astringent taste.

Aluminæ Acetas.

A solution of this salt is obtained by saturating acetic acid with hydrated alumina, and cannot be evaporated without the loss of acetic acid. It has a faint smell of acetic acid and a sweetish taste, and possesses antiseptic properties.

It has been used medicinally on account of its astringent properties, in diarrhœa and gleet in doses of a half to one drachm within twenty-four hours, and as an injection in various affections requiring astringent applications.

CHAPTER IV.

ON THE NON-METALLIC ELEMENTS AND THEIR MEDICINAL PREPARATIONS.

Of the non-metallic elements, chlorine has been referred to under the head of medicated waters. Carbon has been considered as a derivative of lignin, and of the remainder it will only be necessary to consider in this chapter iodine, bromine, and sulphur, reserving the new and interesting compounds of phosphorus for a distinct chapter. The distinction as here made between the closely allied groups and non-metallic elements, and of metals, is one of convenience merely. Arsenic, which is one of the so-called intermediate elements, will be more conveniently considered among the metals.

1st Group.—*Preparations of Iodine.*[1]

Iodinium, I. Solid crystalline scales, sp. gr. 4.95.
Potassii iodidum, KI. In cubical crystals. Dose, gr. ij to gr. v.
Sodii iodidum, NaI. Cubical crystals. Dose, gr. ij to v.
Ammonii iodidum, NH_4+ I Very deliquescent. Dose, gr. v to x.
Tinctura iodinii. ℥ss to f℥j alcohol, externally used.
" iodinii composita, I, gr. xv, KI, ℥ss to f℥j. ♏ xv to xxx.
Liquor iodinii compositus, I, gr. xxijss, KI, gr. xlv to f℥j. ♏ x to xx.

Iodinium, U.S. (*Iodine.*)

This non-metallic element is procured for use in medicine from the fused and vitrified ashes of sea-weed called kelp, which is prepared in the Western Islands, North of Scotland, and Ireland. The kelp being broken and lixiviated, yields about half its weight of soluble soda, potassa, and magnesia salts. The common salt, and carbonate and sulphate of soda, are crystallized out on evaporation. The mother liquor contains iodides of sodium, potassium, and magnesium, to which sulphuric acid is added, liberating carbonic acid, sulphuretted hydrogen, and sulphurous acid, by effervescence, and sulphur, which is deposited. The acid lye is next distilled from peroxide of manganese, which liberates the iodine, and it is condensed in cooled glass receivers. (See Essay on the Manufacture of Iodine, *Proceedings Amer. Pharm. Ass.*, 1857, page 110.)

Iodine is in bluish black crystalline scales, with a metallic lustre, sp. gr. 4.948, fusing at 225°, boiling at 347°, and evaporating at ordinary temperature, especially when damp. Its vapor is of a splendid violet color. Odor like chlorine, melts when heated, then sublimes in very heavy violet vapors, soluble in ether and alcohol, but very sparingly in water, although by the addition of iodide of potassium or chloride of sodium, it is rendered very soluble. Free iodine precipitates starch in the cold, of a dark blue color, which reaction is its most familiar and delicate test. It dissolves in alkaline solutions, forming iodides and iodates. With the metals and most of the non-metallic elements, it combines with avidity, and several of its combinations are officinal; of these, the iodides of mercury, of lead, zinc, cadmium, iron, arsenic, and sulphur, are considered under the head of their metallic elements, while several preparations which seem to owe their value exclusively to iodine, are introduced here. Locally applied, iodine is an irritant and vesicant, staining the skin brown or orange color, causing itching, redness, and desquamation. Applied by inunction, it is absorbed, producing its characteristic stimulating effect; inhaled as vapor, it exercises its alterative effect on the mucous membrane of the respiratory passages. Its influence is chiefly exerted on the glandular and absorbent systems. It is used both internally and topically for an immense number of diseases requiring alterative treatment. The salts of iodine are much used for their several alterative effects; when given internally, it is always in solution or combination.

[1] Most of the iodine salts are described under the several heads of their metallic bases.

Potassii Iodidum, U. S. (*Iodide of Potassium.*)

This salt was formerly directed to be made by combining iodine with iron, and decomposing the iodide of iron with carbonate of potassa, precipitating the carbonate of iron, filtering and crystallizing; this process, which is, in some respects, the most convenient to the pharmaceutist, has been superseded in the *Pharmacopœia* by the plan of adding iodine directly to a solution of potash, thus forming the mixed iodide of potassium, and iodate of potash ($6KO + I_6 = 5KI + KO,IO_5$). This being heated to redness in contact with charcoal, the iodic acid, IO_5, parts with its oxygen, and the iodate is reduced to iodide of potassium.

This salt is in white, shining, semi-opaque cubes, with a characteristic marine odor, an acrid saline taste, resembling common salt. Soluble in two-thirds its weight of cold water, and freely in alcohol. Nitric acid decomposes its solution, yielding iodine; and if starch be subsequently added, it yields the characteristic blue iodide of amylum.

Tartaric and other acids do not liberate iodine immediately, but the peculiar acid compound, hydriodic acid (HI) before described; hence the old name of the salt hydriodate of potassa.

Iodide of potassium is liable to adulteration with bicarbonate or carbonate of potassa; the latter renders it very damp, and they both occasion effervescence with acids, and throw down a precipitate with sulphate of iron. Chloride of platinum should color its solution reddish-brown, without causing a precipitate. The presence of a chloride may be determined with nitrate of silver, which throws down nothing from the pure salt but iodide of silver, which is almost insoluble in ammonia, while chloride of silver is readily soluble in it. The iodide of silver, precipitated from 10 grains of iodide of potassium, weighs, when washed and dried, 14.1 grains. When acetate or nitrate of lead is added to iodide of potassium, it throws down a yellow iodide of lead, soluble in boiling water. Bromide may be detected by adding nitric acid, and observing the vapors that arise; those of bromine are red; those of iodine purple. Sometimes iodate of potassa is present, which may be detected by tartaric acid liberating iodine, perceptible by the starch test.

This salt contains no water of crystallization. Every four grains contain about three grains of iodine. The aqueous solution is capable of taking up a large quantity of iodine, forming a liquid of a deep brown color.

Iodide of potassium is considered to possess the same medicinal virtues as iodine, though preferred by some physicians to obtain the constitutional effects of the alterative. It is used very extensively, both alone and combined with iodine, and with other alterative remedies; it is incompatible with the preparations of mercury generally, greatly increasing their activity. DOSE, gr. ij to gr. v.

Iodide of Sodium.

Sodii Iodidum.—The best process for preparing this salt is from a freshly-prepared solution of iodide of iron or zinc, by precipitating it with pure carbonate of soda, evaporating, and allowing it to crystallize at a temperature exceeding 120° F. Below this temperature, it crystallizes with four equivalents of water in deliquescent, flat, hexagonal prisms; crystallized as above, it forms cubes which contain no water, and are very soluble in water, and also in alcohol.

It has been used as a substitute for iodide of potassium, but is objectionable on account of its proneness to deliquescence; its greatest advantage over the potassium salt consists in its having 85 per cent., while the other has only 76 per cent. of iodine in combination.

Ammonii Iodidum. (*Iodide of Ammonium.*)

Hydriodic acid is supersaturated with ammonia and evaporated with the precaution of keeping the ammonia slightly in excess.

It crystallizes in cubes, and is very deliquescent. It has been used as a substitute for iodide of potassium, being more irritating than this salt on account of the looseness with which the iodine is confined.

Internally it has been used in doses as high as 10 grains; externally held in combination in ointments of from ℈j to ʒj to an ounce of lard.

Tinctura Iodinii, U. S. (*Simple Tincture of Iodine.*)

		To make Oj.	To make f℥j.
Take of	Iodine	℥j.	ʒss.
	Alcohol	Oj.	f℥j.

Dissolve the iodine in the alcohol. This is best done by triturating it with successive portions of alcohol in a glass or porcelain mortar. This tincture contains one grain in 16 minims, or about 35 drops; it is not adapted to internal use, as, on the addition of water, the iodine is precipitated, and exercises its peculiar irritating topical effect on the coats of the stomach. It is applied to the skin as a powerful irritant in cutaneous and subcutaneous inflammation. In treating erysipelas, and when the surface to be treated is circumscribed, it is applied with a camel-hair brush.

Tinctura Iodinii Composita, U. S. (*Compound Tincture of Iodine.*)

		To make Oj.	To make f℥j.
Take of	Iodine	℥ss.	gr. xv.
	Iodide of potassium	℥j.	ʒss.
	Alcohol	Oj.	f℥j.

Dissolve the iodine and iodide of potassium in the alcohol.

This is adapted to the same use as the foregoing; by the presence of the iodide of potassium, the precipitation of iodine on contact with aqueous liquids is prevented. It may also be used internally in doses of ♏xv to xxx.

These tinctures are included under the general head, *Tincturæ*, U.S., while the following is placed under the head *Iodinium*:—

Liquor Iodinii Compositus, U. S. (*Lugol's Solution.*)

		To make Oj.	To make f℥j.
Take of	Iodine	ʒvj.	gr. xxijss.
	Iodide of potassium	℥iss.	gr. xlv.
	Water	Oj.	f℥j.

Lugol's solution, as originally proposed, contained twenty grains of iodine, and forty of iodide of potassium, to f℥j of water; the present officinal preparation is adjusted to the proportions convenient for a pint, and, as is seen above, is somewhat stronger.

In iodine and compound iodine ointments we have nearly the same proportions as in the tinctures, substituting lard for alcohol and water. (See *Extemporaneous Preparations.*)

2D GROUP.—*Bromine Preparations.*

Bittern. The mother liquor after the crystallization of common salt.
Brominum. Heavy, very volatile liquid, sp. gr. 2.96.
Brominii chloridum. Br,CL$_4$. Very powerful caustic, &c.; fluid.
Potassii bromidum, KBr. White cubical crystals. Dose, gr. v to x.
Liquor ferri bromidi. Solution of bromide with excess of bromine. Dose, ♏v to x.

Brominum, U. S. (*Bromine.*)

Bromine is a heavy liquid, non-metallic element, of a red color, stifling odor, and acrid taste; very volatile and fuming, soluble in ether and alcohol, and to a small extent in water; it precipitates starch of an orange color. Associated with iodine in sea-water and numerous mineral springs, it is largely extracted from bittern, the liquor left after the crystallization of common salt, whether from sea-water or from certain salt springs. At the salt works, in Western Pennsylvania, this bittern is preserved for the extraction of the bromine, and the American bromine prepared there is fully equal to the imported article. The principal consumption of bromine is in the daguerreotype process, in which large quantities are consumed annually. The mode of its extraction, which is rather complex, is detailed in chemical works. The vast quantities of bittern thrown away at a single salt manufactory, render it a cause of regret that there is not some use to which it can be profitably applied.

Care should be taken in handling bromine, especially in warm weather, or near a fire; it boils at about 117° F., liberating stifling red fumes, which have the sp. gr. 5.39. Few vapors are so corrosive or so dangerous to those exposed to their inhalation. An aqueous solution of bromine, containing one part to forty, has been administered in doses of six drops three times a day, being adapted to cases in which Iodine has lost its effect from habitual use.

Chloride of Bromine.

This compound is prepared by passing a stream of chlorine gas through bromine in a freezing mixture, or at a low temperature. It is a reddish liquid, very fluid and volatile, soluble in water, and having a penetrating odor and disagreeable taste.

It has been used externally as a caustic, in combination with chlorides of zinc, antimony, &c., and internally in doses of a fraction of a drop, as a powerful stimulant to the lymphatic system.

Iodine forms two compounds with bromine, but they are little known, and not used in medicine. (See *Salts of Iron*, &c.)

Bittern, as obtained from the salt works, is a heavy liquid, without color, and having a caustic taste and highly stimulating properties. Its chief medical use is to produce redness, and, by continued rubbing of the part, a pustular eruption. It is a good application in rheumatism, and in glandular swellings, being absorbed, and producing the alterative effects of the iodine and bromine salts.

Potassii Bromidum, U. S.

Bromide of potassium is obtained by similar processes to iodide, substituting an equivalent quantity of bromine for the iodine. It closely resembles the iodide in most of its properties, and, like it, is an anhydrous salt. It is believed to possess very similar medicinal properties to iodide, acting as a powerful alterative, adapted to scrofulous and syphilitic complaints, chronic skin diseases, &c. It is directed in rather large doses—gr. v to gr. x.

Tests.—It is very soluble in cold water, more so in hot, slightly soluble in alcohol. By heat it decrepitates, and at a red heat fuses without decomposition or loss of weight. Its aqueous solution does not affect the color of litmus or turmeric, and is not precipitated by chloride of barium. When mixed with starch and heated with SO_3 it becomes yellow; 10 grains of it require 14.28 grains of nitrate of silver for complete precipitation, and the precipitate formed has a yellow color. If iodine is present it will be shown by adding a few drops of chlorine water to the solution, and then introducing starch paper, which will show the characteristic blue color caused by iodine.

Liquor Ferri Bromidi.

This preparation was introduced to notice by Dr. Gillespie, of Freeport, Armstrong Co., Pa., who, besides being a practitioner of medicine, is engaged in the bromine manufacture, in connection with the salt springs near that place. Dr. G. recommends this solution very highly as a tonic alterative, and it has been successfully used by numerous other practitioners. It is made by macerating iron filings with bromine under water, till they have combined; an excess of bromine being used. The solution, as made by Dr. Gillespie, is given in the dose of ♏v to x, three times a day, increased to ♏xxv.

3D GROUP.—*Sulphur Preparations.*

Sulphur. Sublimed sulphur, S. Yellow crystalline powder. DOSE, gr. x to ʒij;
" lotum. Thoroughly washed with water, " " "
" præcipitatum. A light and very fine powder, " "
Sulphuris iodidum, IS_6. Blackish crystalline masses, used in ointment.

Sulphur, U. S. (*Flowers of Sulphur.*)

Sulphur is a very abundant substance in the mineral kingdom, existing in direct combinations with the metals, as sulphurets; and with their oxides, as sulphates. Virgin sulphur is a native, tolerably pure form, abundant in Naples, Sicily, and the Roman States, from whence it is imported. By fusion, and running into moulds, roll sulphur or rolled brimstone is prepared, while flowers of sulphur is the result of subliming and condensing it in suitable chambers.

Sulphur has a characteristic yellow color, sp. gr. 1.98, is entirely volatilized by heat, and combustible, burning with a characteristic blue color, yielding sulphurous acid gas, which is a powerful disinfectant and bleaching agent.

Flówers of sulphur, or sublimed sulphur, is a crystalline powder, of a harsh and gritty character; wholly insoluble in water, alcohol, and ether; tasteless, and nearly odorless; it is the form of sulphur much administered as an alterative and laxative remedy in small doses; being absorbed, it enters the circulation and is given off from the skin as sulphuretted hydrogen. Externally, it is used as a slight stimulant to the skin, and has the power of destroying the acarus scabiei, or itch insect, for which it is popularly known as the remedy.

DOSE, as an alterative, gr. x to ʒss; as a laxative, ʒss to ʒij, alone or combined with bitartrate of potassa.

Sulphur Præcipitatum, U. S. (*Milk of Sulphur.*)

Made by boiling sulphur and lime together till they combine, forming bisulphuret of calcium, and hyposulphite of lime, then adding muriatic acid, which abstracts the calcium, forming chloride, while the sulphur is precipitated as a bulky, light powder; the result of the reaction between S_2O_2 and 2HS, being water and sulphur. This has a soft and very fine consistence, and is adapted to suspending in liquids, though little used internally. Dose, the same as the foregoing. It should be completely volatilized by heat. Very considerable quantities have been consumed recently, in the preparation of the following excellent application to the hair, which is also a remedy for skin diseases, blemishes of the complexion, &c.

Twiggs's Hair Dye.

Take of Precipitated sulphur,
Acetate of lead, of each . . . . ʒj.
Rose water . . . . f℥iv.

Triturate together in a mortar. This is not an instantaneous dye, but should be applied twice a day till it gradually restores the color to its natural shade.

Sulphuris Iodidum, U. S.

Take of Iodine . . . . ℥iv.
Sulphur . . . . ℥j.

Rub the iodine and sulphur together in a glass, porcelain, or marble mortar till they are thoroughly mixed. Put the mixture into a matrass, close the orifice loosely, and apply a gentle heat so as to darken the mass without melting it. When the color has become uniformly dark throughout, increase the heat so as to melt the iodide, then incline the matrass in different directions, in order to return into the mass the portions of iodine which may have condensed on the inner surface; lastly, allow the vessel to cool, break it, and put the iodide into bottles, which are to be well stopped.

Fig. 201. Fig. 202.

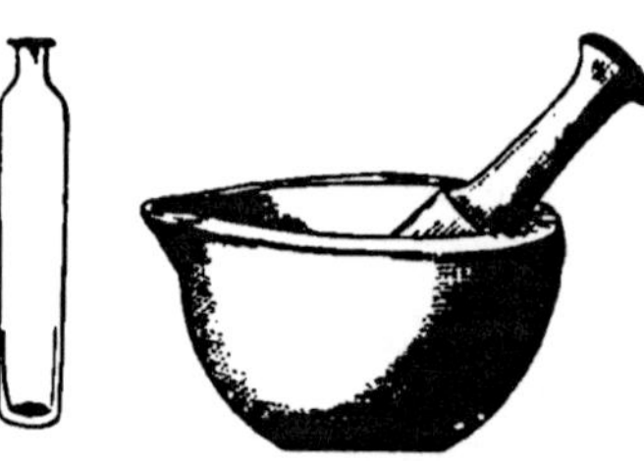

Apparatus for making iodide of sulphur.

A suitable vessel for a small operation is a test tube or a common, very cheap bottle, such as are shown in Fig. 201, should be selected with thin glass at the bottom. The iodide is in bluish-black crystalline masses, in odor reminding of iodine, staining the skin yellow. Two equivalents of sulphur are combined with one of iodine, so that it is a bisulphuret (IS_2).

Internally, this is rarely or never prescribed, but it is much used in the form of ointment applied to chronic and obstinate skin diseases.

CHAPTER V.

ON THE COMPOUNDS OF PHOSPHORUS USED IN MEDICINE.

PHOSPHORUS was discovered by an alchemist in 1669; it has ever since been regarded as a substance of considerable interest, though until our time little used in the arts, and to meet only limited and unusual indications in medicine; its manufacture has, of latter years, received a great impulse from its use in the odorless matches now so extensively introduced. Phosphorus exists in the mineral, vegetable and animal kingdoms variously combined, the phosphates of lime, lead, iron, copper, and manganese, being its principal native mineral compounds. Phosphate of lime, potassa and iron, and free phosphoric acid, are extensively diffused in plants, and from these sources it is furnished as a constituent of animal tissues. The bones of animals contain a large proportion of tribasic phosphate of lime, and are used for the preparation of phosphoric acid and phosphorus. The albuminous and fibrinous tissues, "proteine compounds," and the brain, contain the element phosphorus, though in minute quantity and in an uncertain state of combination. This element, as is well known, is a constituent in animal excrements, and especially in urine; it is diffused in the air, combined with hydrogen, and is a very important ingredient in a certain class of manures.

The application of physiological science to the theory and practice of medicine has recently given rise to numerous experiments upon the usefulness of phosphorous compounds, as nutritive tonics designed to remedy abnormal conditions of the secretions, and to supply the elements wasted in disease.

Prof. Samuel Jackson, of the Chair of Institutes in the University of Pennsylvania, whose progressive ideas have had considerable influence upon the methods of practice pursued in this country, has for the last eight or ten years been in the habit of prescribing certain preparations containing the phosphates of lime, iron, soda, and potassa, in the treatment of anemic and other low forms of disease. The popularity reached by these preparations has led to the extensive introduction of other remedies, prepared on the same principles; and, more recently, the announcement by Dr. J. Francis Churchill, of Paris, of a specific agency on the part of certain phosphorous compounds, in checking the progress of pulmonary consumption, has swelled the tide of popularity of the metallic and earthy phosphates, pyrophosphates, and hypophosphites, till they have become, for the time being, leading articles of pharmaceutical manufacture, and I have thought it necessary to devote an entire chapter in the second edition, to the full and complete illustration of the subject.

Phosphorus.

This element is obtainable from bones, by calcining, treating with oil of vitriol, and then subliming the mass with charcoal. The phosphorus is thus collected, and being cast into moulds, is found in commerce nearly colorless, in translucent, or white pipes, having a peculiar, almost waxy consistence, and by light assuming a red tint. It is luminous in the dark, from forming phosphorous acid (PO_3), and is kept under water to prevent gradual oxidation, and to guard against accident from its ready inflammability. It should be handled with care, and not intrusted to children, who frequently procure it for experiment, without due precaution. Its sp. gr. is 1.77. Melting point, 108° F.; at 217° it begins to emit a slight vapor, and boils at 550°, being converted into a colorless vapor. It is soluble in ether, oils, naphtha, and bisulphuret of carbon, but not in water or alcohol. By combustion it yields phosphoric acid, the acid which is combined with lime in bones, &c. It is readily powdered by fusion in a vial or flask of moderately warm water, and shaking up as it cools.

Phosphorus, when taken internally, enters the circulation and, according to Magendie, Orfila, Tiedemann, and others, imparts to the breath, urine, and sweat, a garlic smell, and makes these secretions luminous in the dark; it is absorbed by the skin, and after its solution in a fixed oil has been rubbed upon the stomach, all the exhalations are luminous.

On account of its very energetic action, phosphorus is now seldom employed internally. In small doses it acts as a stimulant, diuretic, and diaphoretic; in larger doses, one grain and more, as a corrosive poison; ether and fixed oils in which phosphorus is soluble increase and hasten its action. Externally in the form of liniment, it has been employed with marked success in severe rheumatisms, gouts, and similar affections. Great caution is necessary in its use.

Red phosphorus is an allotropic variety which is not poisonous, but may be administered in considerable doses. If the ordinary kind is kept for several days at a temperature between 465° to 480°, red phosphorus is found at the bottom of the vessel, while the supernatant mass is a mixture of both varieties, from which the ordinary kind may be extracted by bisulphide of carbon.

Red phosphorus is much less inflammable, fusible, and luminous than the ordinary kind; in the presence of moisture and oxygen it is gradually oxidized to an acid liquid, but without phosphorescence; after having been so oxidized, it appears not to be convertible into the translucent or ordinary kind.

Tests.—To detect impurities in phosphorus, it is best to oxidize it by nitric acid; antimony then remains undissolved, while arsenic, lead, bismuth, copper, and iron may be detected by their various tests; arsenic will produce a yellow precipitate with sulphuretted hydrogen; sulphur has been converted into sulphuric acid, and nitrate of baryta causes an insoluble precipitate. The metals are left behind if phosphorus is purified by dissolving it in bisulphide of carbon; sulphur is not detected in this way, but if pieces of phosphorus are just covered with water, sulphuretted hydrogen will be emitted, which produces a black color with acetate of lead.

Phosphorus combines in four proportions with oxygen:—

1. Phosphoric acid, PO_5 (three modifications). See page 439 and page 488.
2. Phosphorous " PO_3. By gradual oxidation of phosphorous in the atmosphere.
3. Hypophosphorous acid, PO. By the decomposition of the phosphuret of an alkaline earth by water.
4. Phosphoric oxide, P_2O. By the oxidation of phosphorus under water.

The existence of this last compound is denied by many chemists who assert it to be merely amorphous (red) phosphorus.

The following are the salts of phosphoric and hypophosphorous acids which have been used in medicine:—

The phosphates of potassa, soda, ammonia, lime, manganese, iron, zinc.
The hypophosphites of potassa, soda, quinia, lime, iron, manganese.

Phosphoric Acid.

The compounds of phosphoric acid, from their having been longest in use, may first claim attention. Under the head of the mineral acids, allusion has already been made to the tribasic character of this acid, and the fact of its forming three hydrates, the tribasic, bibasic, and monobasic acids, expressed by the formulæ $3HO,PO_5$, $2HO,PO_5$ and HO,PO_5. In the study of the salts of phosphoric acid, the importance of this fact becomes apparent, for these are of three kinds throughout, according as they contain one or other of these modifications of the acid.

The officinal phosphate of soda is made, as already stated, by digesting calcined bones in sulphuric acid to liberate the tribasic phosphoric acid $3HO,PO_5$, and adding carbonate of soda, which separates the lime as carbonate, leaving the acid in combination with soda, in solution. It is a very soluble crystalline salt, having the composition $2NaO,HO,PO_5+24HO$, by decomposition with acetate of lead forming an insoluble phosphate of lead, and decomposing this with sulphuretted hydrogen, the tribasic phosphoric acid may be obtained in a state of purity; it gives a yellow precipitate with nitrate of silver, and it invariably forms salts having three equivalents of base to one of the acid. This class of salts are the old phosphates, and they are perhaps not improperly termed the common phosphates.

Of the three equivalents of base, one or two may be substitued by water, thus forming three distinct classes of the common phosphates. Those salts which like the above soda salt, contain one equivalent of basic water, are termed *neutral* phosphates; if they contain two equivalents of basic water, for instance $NaO,2HO,PO_5$ they are called *acid;* and *basic,* if they contain no basic water like the basic phosphate of soda $3NaO,PO_5$. Of the common phosphates only the so-called neutral salts are employed in medicines.

If the phosphate of soda, as above, is heated to redness it is completely changed, and after being dissolved in water affords crystals of a new salt, which have been called pyrophosphate of soda. If this salt be now treated with acetate of lead, and the lead salt washed and heated as in the other case, an acid liquid is obtained which contains bibasic phosphoric acid, 2HO, gives a white precipitate with nitrate of silver, and invariably forms salts which contain two equivalents of base; these have been termed *pyrophosphates*, though bibasic phosphates would be a more correct term.

If the biphosphate of soda be heated to redness, a salt is formed which, treated in a similar manner with the last, gives an acid liquid containing the monobasic phosphoric acid, HO,PO_5. The glacial phosphoric acid, according to Graham, is in general composed almost entirely of this monobasic acid (protohydrate); this is characterized by producing a white precipitate in solution of albumen, which is not disturbed by the other hydrates, and in solutions of the salts of earths and metallic oxides, precipitates which are remarkable semi-fluid bodies, or uncrystallizable soft solids—all these salts, of course, contain only one equivalent of base to one of acid, corresponding in composition with the acid, considered as a protohydrate of phosphoric acid. The term *meta-phosphates* has been applied to these salts.

The mode of designating the three varieties by the letters, *a*, *b*, and *c*, though indicated in the article on phosphoric acid, page 439, is not convenient or definite for the purposes of this chapter, and will be substituted by the more familiar terms phosphoric acid, $3HO,PO_5$, pyrophosphoric acid, $2HO,PO_5$, and metaphosphoric acid, HO,PO_5, and the same mode of designating the salts will be adopted. The quantity of fixed base, such as soda, with which phosphoric acid combines in the humid way is entirely regulated by the proportion of water previously in union with the acid, which is simply replaced by the base. The influence of temperature or the circumstances of exposure, however, produce a remarkable effect in modifying the nature of these compounds, some of which, by simple solution, pass from the meta into pyro, and from the pyro into the common phosphates, while the common phosphates, as phosphate of soda, as we have seen above, by heat alone are converted into pyrophosphates. These changes, however, do not exclusively pertain to temperature, as, in combination by fusion with phosphoric acid, the use of one, two, or three equivalents of the base determines the character of the salt.

There are many curious properties of phosphoric acid compounds which show them to occupy an intermediate place among chemical agents, between mineral and organic bodies, to possess most unusual polymeric properties, and a pliancy of constitution, which, to use the language of Graham, "peculiarly adapts the phosphoric above all other mineral acids to the wants of the animal economy."

Phosphate of Potassa.

Of the three phosphates of potassa, that corresponding in composition to the medicinal phosphates of soda and ammonia, $2KO,HO,PO_5$, is the one used in medicine. It may be prepared by boiling glacial phosphoric acid, to change it into $3HO,PO_5$, and then adding two equivalents of carbonate or bicarbonate of potassa, or by decomposing bone phosphate of lime with sulphuric acid as in the officinal process for phosphate of soda, page 452, and adding carbonate of potassa; the proper proportions are given below:—

Take of Bone, burnt to whiteness and powdered	.	Ten parts.
Sulphuric acid	. . . . . .	Six parts.
Bicarbonate of potassa	. . . . .	Sufficient.

Mix the powdered bone with the sulphuric acid, in an earthen vessel; then add ten parts of water, and stir them well together, digest for three days, occasionally adding a little water, and frequently stirring; then pour on ten parts of boiling water, and strain through linen; set by the strained liquid that the dregs may subside, from which pour off the clear solution, and boil it down to eight parts; to this add bicarbonate of potassa previously dissolved in hot water until effervescence ceases; filter, and evaporate to dryness.

This salt is slightly acid to test paper, though called the neutral phosphate, it is white, amorphous, deliquescent, and freely soluble. It has been given as an alterative in scrofula and phthisis in the dose, 10 to 20 grains, and as an ingredient in some of the compounds used as tonics.

Phosphate of Ammonia.

This has a similar composition to the foregoing; its formula is $2NH_4O,HO,PO_5$. It may be made by saturating a strong solution of phosphoric acid with ammonia, applying heat, and setting the solution aside that crystals may form; or it may be made by saturating the excess of acid in the superphosphate of lime as produced in the last process, with carbonate of ammonia, and procuring the salt by evaporation and crystallization, previously adding ammonia to a slight alkaline reaction. It is a white salt in efflorescent, rhombic prisms, losing water and ammonia, very soluble in water, but insoluble in alcohol. It was formerly much in vogue as a remedy for gout and rheumatism. DOSE, 10 to 40 grains.

Precipitated Phosphate of Lime.

Although bone phosphate of lime, as already mentioned, is the source of most of the phosphoric acid preparations, it is not the form of phosphate most in use; this is obtained in a fine powder by precipitation, and is officinal in the Dublin *Pharmacopœia*, see page 468. This forms the basis of several of the preparations now so popular; it is said to be essential in animals, as well as plants, to the formation of cells, and seems to be useful in certain pathological states of the system, characterized by defective nutrition. It is insoluble in water, soluble in nitric, sulphuric, hydrochloric, and carbonic acids; its solution in nitric acid is precipitated by oxalate of ammonia; the neutralized nitric solution should give a yellow precipitate of phosphate of silver. It should not effervesce with acids.

Phosphate of Manganese.

This salt is prepared by mixing solutions of sulphate of manganese four parts, and phosphate of soda five parts, washing the precipitated phosphate till the sulphate of soda is completely removed, and drying at a moderate heat. It is a white, nearly insoluble powder, and may be made into pills, lozenges, or syrup.

A phosphatic salt of manganese is deemed peculiarly eligible, therapeutically.

Ferri Phosphas, U. S.

The officinal phosphate of iron is formed by double decomposition between solutions of 2 equivalents of sulphate of protoxide of iron, and 1 equivalent of phosphate of soda. Its composition as thus prepared is variable, being a mixture of phosphate of protoxide of iron, and phosphate of sesquioxide in different proportions. Wittstein gives a very accurate account of it, with specific directions for its preparation. As first precipitated it is white, and is then nearly pure phosphate of protoxide, $2FeO,HO,PO_5$, resembling in composition the officinal phosphate of soda; the reaction is thus represented $2(FeO,SO_3)+2NaO,HO,PO_5=2FeO,HO,PO_5+2(NaO,SO_3)$; the soluble sulphate of soda being washed away and the salt dried, it is found to have acquired a slate color, more or less green, the protoxide of iron having become partially changed, as before stated, into sesquioxide, and combined with phosphoric acid in the salt $2Fe_2O_3,3HO,3PO_5$. It is soluble in acids like phosphate of lime, but not in water.

Phosphate of iron has long been in use in medicine for the general purposes to which the ferruginous salts are applicable, though until the recent introduction of several preparations containing it in solution, it has been little known to practitioners. DOSE, gr. v to x.

Phosphate of sesquioxide of iron, Fe_2O_3,PO_5+4HO, is the white precipitate occasioned by phosphate of soda in sesquisalts of iron; it has been used in medicine in cases like the foregoing, and in similar doses.

Pyrophosphate of Iron.

The fact has been already adverted to that when the officinal phosphate of soda is heated to redness it undergoes a change, the phosphoric acid it contains being converted into bibasic or *pyro*-phosphoric acid, so that by recomposition it would furnish a different class of salts, it now remains to advert to the salt formed by decomposing this with a sesquisalt of iron. By precipitating a solution of sesquisulphate of iron with one of pyrophosphate of soda, taking care to operate at a temperature below 59° F., we obtain a gelatinous precipitate, which has the property of dissolving with facility in excess of pyrophosphate of soda. If obtained at the boiling temperature, the solution in excess of the soda salt would be unstable, acquiring a black color, and a disagreeable taste; the proportion of pyrophosphate of soda required to dissolve it under the most favorable circumstances is 4 parts to 16 of the gelatinous ferruginous precipitate representing three parts of the salt dried at 212° F. When prepared in the cold, this solution keeps tolerably well in close vessels though not entirely eligible, blackening after frequent or long exposure to the air, and acquiring a disagreeable saline and metallic taste. The citrate of ammonia has, therefore, been proposed as a solvent, and is highly recommended by M. Robiquet, who first called attention to this compound as a remedial agent, with the asserted advantage of its ready assimilation in the system and the entire absence of any tendency to disorder the stomach or bowels.

In the absence of any evidence from practitioners who have tried the two preparations, I am inclined to the opinion that the ordinary phosphate of sesquioxide is equally advantageous; it furnishes just as nice and tasteless a solution with citrate of ammonia, as the pyrophosphate; citrate of sesquioxide of iron is not precipitated by the ordinary phosphate of ammonia, and it would seem that there can be little difference in a medicinal point of view, whether pyro or common phosphate is used. In case of need, a very similar solution may be obtained extemporaneously by dissolving together 4 parts phosphate of ammonia, and 10 parts citrate of sesquioxide of iron, which would furnish in perfect solution very nearly 6 parts of phosphate of iron and 8 parts of citrate of ammonia, without calculating the water of crystallization.

A beautiful salt in scales like those of citrate of iron, but of lighter color, is manufactured by the General Apothecaries Company, London, labelled soluble pyrophosphate of iron; it is probably made by precipitating the pyrophosphate, dissolving in citrate of ammonia, boiling the solution and evaporating to syrupy consistence, spreading on plates of glass with a brush and drying in a stove. DOSE, gr. v to gr. x.

Phosphate of Zinc.

This salt which has the composition $ZnO2HO,PO_5+2HO$, is obtained in minute silvery plates, which are nearly insoluble on mixing dilute solutions of phosphate of soda and sulphate of zinc. It is a remedy of considerable reputation in the treatment of epilepsy. It is given in doses of 2 to 3 grains in powder or pill.

SYRUPS AND OTHER FLUID PREPARATIONS OF THE PHOSPHATES.

In 1853, the following recipe was published in the *American Journal of Pharmacy*, vol. xxv. p. 411, by A. B. Durand, of Philadelphia.

Durand's Syrup of Phosphate of Lime.

Take of	Precipitated phosphate of lime	128	grains.
	Glacial phosphoric acid . .	240	"
	Sugar, in coarse powder . .	7½	oz. (offic.)
	Distilled water . . .	4	fluidounces.
	Essence of lemon . . .	12	drops.

Mix the phosphate of lime with the water in a porcelain capsule, over a spirit or gas lamp, or in a sand bath; add gradually the phosphoric acid until the whole of the phosphate of lime is dissolved. To this solution add sufficient water to compensate for the evaporation, then dissolve the sugar by a very gentle heat, and, when perfectly cold, add the essence of lemon. The syrup of phosphate of lime, thus prepared, is colorless, transparent, of an acid taste, and contains two grains of the phosphate of lime and nearly four grains of phosphoric acid to each teaspoonful. When diluted by the patient previously to its being taken, it forms a phosphoric lemonade not unpleasant to the taste. DOSE, a teaspoonful.

In a paper in the *American Journal of Pharmacy*, vol. xxvi. p. 112, noticing the above, T. S. Weigand remarks upon the acidity of the preparation as an objection to its use in some cases, and proposed the following modified recipe:—

Wiegand's Syrup of Phosphate of Lime.

℞.—Calcis phosphatis præcip.	℥j.
Acidi chlorohydrici	f℥iv.
Aquæ, q. s. ft.	f℥vij.
Sacchari, q. s. ft.	f℥xij.

Dissolve the phosphate of lime, previously mixed with an ounce of water by means of the acid filter, then add the remaining water to this; add the sugar until the bulk is increased to twelve fluidounces, and strain.

Wiegand's Compound Syrup of Phosphates.

Take of Protosulphate of iron	Four drachms and two scruples.
Phosphate of soda (crystallized	Seven drachms and a half.
Phosphate of lime (recently precipitated)	Four drachms.
Phosphate of potassa	
Glacial phosphoric acid	One ounce.
Sugar, in coarse powder	Eight ounces (offic.).
Water	A sufficient quantity.

Dissolve the sulphate of iron, and five and a half drachms of the phosphate of soda, severally, in three fluidounces of the water, and mix the solutions; wash the precipitated phosphate of iron with (cold) boiled water, mix it with the phosphate of lime and half a pint of water in a porcelain capsule, apply heat, gradually add the phosphoric acid, continuing the heat until a clear solution is obtained, and dissolve in it seven ounces of the sugar; then dissolve the phosphate of potash, two drachms of the phosphate of soda, and an ounce of sugar in a fluidounce of water, acidulate the solution with phosphoric acid, and add it to the syrupy solution first obtained. A slight cloudiness is occasioned by mixing the solutions, which may be entirely removed, and the syrup rendered permanently transparent, by adding forty drops of hydrochloric acid.

Each teaspoonful of this syrup contains about one and two-fifths grain of protophosphate of iron, two and a half grains of phosphate of lime, one and one-fifth grain each of the alkaline phosphates, and four and a half grains of free phosphoric acid, which may be considered the dose.

As some of the preparations in use were colored with cochineal and flavored with orange-peel, which rendered them less disagreeable, this syrup was recommended to be so treated by rubbing up six grains of cochineal with a little sugar, and adding ten drops of the oil of orange-peel, adding the mixture to the syrup, and filtering.

To the information already collected and furnished upon this subject, Prof. Procter added the following contributions which appeared in the *American Journal of Pharmacy.*

Syrup of Phosphates of Lime and Iron.

Take of	Protochloride of iron (in crystals) .	ʒj.
	Chloride of calcium (fused) . .	ʒiss.
	Phosphate of soda (crystallized) . .	ʒvij.
	Phosphate of potassa . . .	ʒj.
	Glacial phosphoric acid . . .	ʒiij.
	Syrup of lemons,	
	Distilled water, of each . . .	f℥iv.

Triturate the chlorides of iron and calcium, six drachms of the phosphate of soda, and the phosphoric acid, together with a little water, until a homogeneous liquid is obtained, and then add the rest of the water gradually; dissolve the phosphate of potassa and the remainder of the phosphate of soda in the syrup, and add it to the first solution, and mix. The result is a syrupy, acid, saline liquid, holding a portion of gelatinous phosphate of lime in suspension. This may be entirely dissolved by using more phosphoric acid, or by adding a little hydrochloric acid.

The reactions that occur in the above formula are, first, the production of phosphate of lime, phosphate of iron, and chloride of sodium: next, the immediate solution of the first two through the agency of the free phosphoric acid. When the syrup containing the phosphates of soda and potassa is added, a portion of the free acid is attracted by them, and a small part of the phosphate of lime is precipitated in a hydrated form. Sulphate of iron may be substituted for the chloride in the above formula by using two drachms instead of one, and first triturating the soda, salt, and chloride of calcium alone with a little water till double decomposition ensues, then adding the *sulphate* of iron, and again triturating, and lastly the phosphoric acid. By observing this order, no sulphate of lime is formed, and the mixed hydrated phosphates of lime and iron at first formed are readily dissolved by the free acid. When sulphate of iron is used, of course both sulphate of soda and chloride of sodium exist in the preparation.

Syrup of Undissolved Phosphates.

The phosphates of iron and lime of commerce are often so granular and dense that their solution and absorption in passing along the alimentary canal must be much interfered with. This difficulty may be avoided, when the free phosphoric acid is objectionable, by presenting the insoluble phosphates in a hydrated form, thus:—

Take of	Protosulphate of iron (cryst.) . . .	℥ij.
	Chloride of calcium (fused) . . .	℥iss.
	Phosphate of soda (cryst.) . . .	℥vij.
	Syrup of ginger,	
	Distilled water, of each	f℥iv.

Triturate the chloride of calcium with the phosphate of soda and three fluidounces of the water, till the decomposition is complete and a smooth mixture is obtained, then add the syrup, and finally the sulphate of iron, previously dissolved in a fluidounce of the water. The resulting mixture consists of the hydrated phosphates of iron and lime, with about two drachms of sulphate of soda, and a little common salt, the whole suspended and rendered palatable by the syrup.

The enterprising firm of Blair & Wyeth, Pharmaceutists, of this city, were the first to give to this combination any considerable commercial importance; they issued the preparation, as they produced it, under the ingenious and popular name of *chemical food*, and a demand was soon created for it, which led to efforts on the part of several pharmaceutists to improve upon the published recipes; it was in this stage of the affair that my name became connected with it by an application from Prof. Procter, editor of the *American Journal of Pharmacy*, to furnish him with my recipe for the preparation, as I had attained considerable practical acquaintance with it. In responding to this request from one to whom our profession is indebted for so many contributions to its available resources, I was influenced by no desire to prejudice the interests of the house who at that time were the principal manufacturers of this preparation, but acted on the principle, fully recognized in the Ethics of the Philadelphia College of Pharmacy and American Pharmaceutical Association, that "any discovery which is useful in alleviating human suffering, or in restoring the diseased to health, should be made public for the good of humanity, and the general advancement of the healing art;" a principle of reciprocity which, while in some instances it may occasion inconvenience, is in so many ways useful to the profession and to every member of it, that it is worthy of universal adoption.

The recipe then furnished was published, with my name attached, on the responsibility of the editor of the journal, and has since been adopted by numerous pharmaceutists in this country and also in Great Britain, where it has attained considerable popularity; experience has shown that the quantity of sugar then prescribed is too large, and in copying it for insertion here, I have modified it so as to avoid that cause of precipitation. I have also substituted a flavoring ingredient which I find an improvement on the oil of orange at first employed.

Parrish's Compound Syrup of Phosphates.

Take of	Protosulphate of iron	ʒx.
	Phosphate of soda	ʒxij.
	Phosphate of lime	ʒxij.
	Phosphoric acid, glacial	ʒxx.
	Carbonate of soda	℈ij.
	Carbonate of potassa	ʒj.
	Muriatic acid,	
	Water of ammonia, of each . .	Sufficient.
	Powdered cochineal	ʒij.
	Water	Sufficient.
	Sugar	℔ij ℥viij, offic.
	Orange-flower water	f℥j.

Dissolve the sulphate of iron in f℥ij of boiling water, and the phosphate of soda in f℥iv of boiling water. Mix the solutions, and wash the precipitated phosphate of iron till the washings are tasteless. Dissolve the phosphate of lime in four fluidounces of boiling water with sufficient muriatic acid to make a clear solution; when cool precipitate it with water of ammonia, and wash the precipitate.

To the freshly-precipitated phosphates as thus prepared, add the phosphoric acid previously dissolved in water; when clear add the carbonates of soda and potassa, previously dissolved in water, and muriatic acid to dissolve any precipitate. Now dilute with water till it reaches the measure of twenty-two fluidounces, add the sugar, and towards the last, the cochineal; dissolve by the aid of heat, strain, and when cool add the orange-flower water.

As thus made, each teaspoonful contains about 2½ grains of phosphate of lime, 1 grain of phosphate of iron, with fractions of a grain of phosphates of soda and potassa, besides free phosphoric and hydrochloric acids. The solution is perfect, the taste agreeably acid, and the flavor pleasant. The disposition to precipitate a bulky sediment of the insoluble phosphates is one of the greatest annoyances in this preparation, when made on a large scale, and can be obviated best by substituting hydrochloric acid for a suitable portion of the phosphoric acid used, taking care to separate the liquid into two portions, and adding the carbonate of soda and potassa to that consisting exclusively of the phosphoric acid solution, lest portions of chloride of sodium and chloride of potassium should be formed and contaminate the resulting solution.

Scheffer's Process.

Owing to the uncertain strength of phosphoric acid of commerce, sometimes being strictly monobasic, and at others a mixture as before described, there is some uncertainty about the proportions to be employed, and besides, the expensiveness and occasional scarcity of the glacial acid operates against its use. These considerations have induced the trial of a method by double decomposition, which should always furnish a uniform strength of acid from a cheap and accessible source.

E. Scheffer, of Louisville, Ky., has proposed to take 49.25 drachms of phosphate of lime, 34.125 sulphuric acid,[1] diluted with three times its weight of water, put them in a thin dish and heat on a water-bath for half a day. By this process only 37.25 drachms of phosphate of lime will be decomposed by the sulphuric acid which combines with the lime with these 37.25 drachms to form sulphate of lime, while the phosphoric acid is set free and holds the other twelve drachms of phosphate of lime in solution. After it has cooled, the magma is pressed, macerated with fresh water, and again pressed, and the liquid evaporated if necessary to twenty fluidounces, cooled and filtered. The phosphate of iron and carbonate of potassa and soda are now added as in the recipe, and the whole made into a syrup *secundem artem.*

The washing of the precipitated sulphate of lime is best performed in a funnel, the water being thrown upon the middle in a kind of a reservoir formed by raising the precipitate on the sides of the funnel; the last portions are collected separately and evaporated until, with the stronger portion, they have the desired measure.

Richardson's Method of Preparation.

Joseph G. Richardson, of Philadelphia, has proposed to use citric acid as the solvent for the phosphates in the compound syrup, this substitution, though probably modifying the therapeutic properties of the preparation, furnishes it in a very agreeable form, and is worthy a more extended trial. The following is the recipe from the *American Journal of Pharmacy*, vol. xxx. p. 19:—

℞.—Solutions of persulphate of iron, U. S. P. (containing ℥iv in Oj)	f℥x.
Pyrophosphate of soda	℥ss.
Phosphate of lime,	
Phosphate of soda (rhombic),	
Phosphate of potassa, of each	℈iv.
Hydrochloric acid	f℥ij.
White sugar	℥xij.
Citric acid,	
Solution of ammonia, of each	Sufficient.

Precipitate the solution of persulphate of iron by the pyrophosphate of soda, dissolved in about f℥viij of water, wash the precipitate, triturate it with ʒij citric acid, and gradually add ammonia, until the liquid becomes clear and slightly alkaline, then dissolve the phosphate of lime in the hydrochloric acid, precipitate with liquor ammoniæ, filter, wash the precipitate, and while still moist triturate with ℈viij citric acid, and let it stand till it becomes clear; mix with this the foregoing solution of pyrophosphate of iron, neutralize with liquor ammoniæ and slightly acidify with eight grains of citric acid, pulverize the phosphates of soda and potassa and dissolve them in this liquid, filter if necessary, add the sugar, the solution of which is to be effected by

[1] Monohydrated sulphuric acid is made by heating the pure acid of commerce in a porcelain capsule in a sand bath until acid vapors begin to rise.

agitation without the aid of heat, and lastly, dilute with sufficient water to make the whole measure 16 fluidounces.

If preferred, the solution may be colored with cochineal, and flavored to taste.

Syrup of Phosphate of Iron and Ammonia, by Joseph Roberts, Baltimore.

Take of	Sulphate of iron	278 grains.
	Phosphate of soda	359 grains.
	Glacial phosphoric acid . . .	396 grains.
	Liquor ammoniæ	Sufficient.
	Sugar	5½ ounces.
	Water	Sufficient.

Dissolve the phosphate of soda and the sulphate of iron separately. Mix the solutions and wash the resulting precipitate of phosphate of iron. Then to one-half the phosphoric acid dissolved in one ounce of water, add liquor ammoniæ until it is saturated. To the other half of the phosphoric acid dissolve, in a like quantity of water, add the moist phosphate of iron and dissolve by a gentle heat, then add the solution of phosphate of ammonia and the sugar, and evaporate to seven fluidounces. This preparation contains 4½ grains of phosphate of iron, 4¾ grains of phosphate of ammonia, and 3½ grains of phosphoric acid, to a fluidrachm or teaspoonful.

The peculiarity of this preparation is the large amount of the ferruginous phosphate held in perfect solution, a result accomplished by the use of the citrate of ammonia.

Syrup of Phosphate of Manganese.

℞.—Sulphate of manganese (in crystals) . .	℥iss, gr. xvij.
Phosphate of soda	℥iiss or q. s.
Muriatic acid	fʒiv.
Water, q. s., to make	f℥vij.
Sugar, q. s., to make, with the foregoing .	f℥xiiss.

Dissolve the salts separately, each in half a pint of water, and add the solution of phosphate of soda to the solution of sulphate of manganese, as long as it produces a precipitate, which wash with cold water, and dissolve by means of the muriatic acid; dilute till it measures seven fluidounces, then add sugar sufficient to make up the bulk of twelve and a half ounces. Each fʒ contains 5 grains of the salt.

Syrup of Pyrophosphate of Iron.

After what has already been said of the pyrophosphate of iron, it will only be necessary to append a working formula for its preparation in this form. Prof. Procter's is as follows:—

Take of	Pyrophosphate of soda . . .	120 grains (3 equivalents.)
	Solution of persulphate of iron .	(to contain 2 equivalents.)
	Water	Sufficient.
	Citric acid	40 grains.
	Liquor ammoniæ	Sufficient (about fʒiss).
	Syrup of orange flowers . .	2 fluidounces.
	Syrup	Sufficient.

Dissolve the pyrophosphate in 4 fluidounces of water, add solution of persulphate of iron till it ceases to precipitate, then wash the white gelatinous iron salt on a filter till the washings pass tasteless. Triturate the iron salt in a mortar with the citric acid previously powdered, and the ammonia gradually added with constant stirring, until a transparent reddish brown liquid is obtained, then add the syrup till 14 fluidounces are attained. This has no ferruginous taste. DOSE, a teaspoonful.

Syrup of Superphosphate of Iron.

This syrup is prepared by adding freshly-precipitated phosphate of iron to saturation in a boiling solution of metaphosphoric acid (glacial). On cooling it congeals into a soft mass which is freely soluble in water in all proportions, and free from inky taste.

The syrup is made from this by dissolving five grains in each fluidrachm of simple syrup. DOSE, a fluidrachm or less.

SALTS OF HYPOPHOSPHOROUS ACID.

Hypophosphorous acid, as already shown, is a compound of phosphorus and oxygen, one equivalent of each, PO. It requires, however, no less than three equivalents of water to form the liquid acid, and of these, two equivalents enter into its salts, one only being replaced by bases. When heated, these salts emit phosphuretted hydrogen, a peculiar self-inflammable gas (fire-damp) of an odor reminding, some, of garlic. They are permanent in the air, but in solution, by heat, are liable to absorb oxygen; they are all soluble in water, and a few are crystalline. Several processes have been used to produce these salts. Rose recommends boiling phosphorus in a solution of caustic baryta till all the phosphorus disappears, and the vapors have no longer the garlic odor. Lime is found to answer the same purpose, and is commonly used. Hypophosphite of lime is perhaps the most important of these salts; by oxidation in the animal economy, it is probably converted into readily assimilable nascent phosphate of lime, and by decomposition it furnishes the other salts of this acid. It is, moreover, one of the salts most highly recommended by Dr. Churchill, to whose suggestion, in the first instance, the employment of these remedies may be traced.

Prof. Procter has brought to this subject his admirable talent for research, and has simplified it in an article in the *American Journal of Pharmacy*, vol. xxx. p. 118, from which portions of what follows are quoted.

Hypophosphite of Lime.

When phosphorus is boiled with milk of lime it gradually disappears, with evolution of spontaneously inflammable phosphuretted hydrogen, which explodes as it reaches the atmosphere with the formation of water and phosphoric acid. When the strong odor of phosphuretted hydrogen ceases to be given off, the liquid contains, besides the excess of lime, nearly half of the phosphorus as phosphate of lime, and the remainder, deducting the considerable portion which has escaped into the air as phosphuretted hydrogen, is hypophosphite of lime. According to Wurtz, more than one equivalent of water is decomposed, and the phosphuretted hydrogen is accompanied by free hydrogen. If this be true, the source of the super-oxidation of so much of the phosphorus is traceable to the resulting oxygen; but Rose is of the opinion that this oxygen is derived from the atmospheric air in contact with the boiling liquid. When the process is conducted in a flask, it requires a constant ebullition of the liquid to prevent the explosion consequent upon the entrance of the atmospheric air. To avoid this result, it has been found safer to employ a deep, open vessel. The constant evolution of gas and vapor, which keeps a froth on the surface, excludes the atmosphere in a great degree, so that the yield is not much diminished, whilst the safety and easiness of the process are greatly increased. The process should be conducted under a hood with a strong draught, or in the open air, to avoid the disagreeable fumes which are evolved.

Take of		
	Lime, recently burned	4 lbs. av.
	Phosphorus	1 lb. "
	Water	5 gals.

Slake the lime with a gallon of the water, put the remainder in a deep boiler, and as soon as it boils add the slaked lime, and mix to a uniform milk. The phosphorus is now added, and the boiling is kept up constantly, adding hot water from time to time, so as to preserve the measure as nearly as may be, until it is all oxidized and combined, and the strong odor of the gas has disappeared. The mixture froths much, and but little of the phosphorus reaches the surface. Then filter the solution through close muslin, wash out that portion retained by the calcareous residue with water, and evaporate the filtrate till reduced to six pints. The concentrated liquid should now be re-filtered to remove a portion of carbonate of lime which has resulted from the action of the air on the lime in solution, and again evaporated till a pellicle forms, when it may be crystallized by standing in the drying-room, or the heat may be continued with stirring till the salt granulates, when it should be introduced into bottles.

Hypophosphite of lime is a white salt with a pearly margarin-like lustre, and crystallizes in flattened prisms. Its composition, according to Wurtz, is $CaO,+2HO,PO$, the water being essential to the salt. It is soluble in six parts of cold water, and in not much less of boiling water; it is soluble slightly in diluted alcohol, but insoluble in alcohol sp. gr. .835.

E. Scheffer prepares this by a modification of this process, which, he says, saves the great waste occurring in the above process, and has the advantage of liberating very little of the offensive gas produced by the other. He first oxidizes the phosphorus by fusing it under water, and pumping atmospheric air into it; the phosphorus burns somewhat, and swells up, having become partially converted into oxide of phosphorus, P_2O, and now combines with milk of lime without boiling, most readily at 130° F., the gas given off being chiefly hydrogen, and not, as in the other case, the offensive compound of phosphorus and hydrogen, the production of which is so great an annoyance in the neighborhood of chemical manufactories.

Hypophosphite of Soda.

This is prepared by double decomposition between hypophosphite of lime and crystallized carbonate of soda.

Take of	Hypophosphite of lime . .	6 oz.
	Crystallized carbonate of soda .	10 oz.
	Water	A sufficient quantity.

Dissolve the hypophosphite in four pints of water, and the carbonate in a pint and a half, mix the solutions, pour the mixture on a filter, and lixiviate the precipitate of carbonate of lime, after draining, with water, till the filtrate measures six pints. Evaporate this liquid carefully till a pellicle forms, and then stir constantly, continuing the heat till it granulates. In this state the salt is pure enough for medical use; but if desired in crystals, treat the granulated salt with alcohol sp. gr. .835, evaporate the solution till syrupy, and set it by in a warm place to crystallize.

Hypophosphite of soda crystallizes in rectangular tables with a pearly lustre, is quite soluble in water and in ordinary alcohol, and deliquesces when exposed to the air. Its composition is NaO+2HO,POa.

Hypophosphite of Potassa.

This is prepared by the same process as that given above for the soda salt, substituting five and three-quarters ounces of granulated *carbonate of potassa*, in place of ten ounces of crystallized carbonate of soda, and using half a pint instead of a pint and a half of water to dissolve it.

Hypophosphite of potassa is a white, opaque, deliquescent salt, very soluble in water and alcohol. Its greater tendency to absorb moisture renders it less eligible for prescription than the soda salt. Its composition is KO+2HO,PO.

Hypophosphite of Ammonia.

This is prepared from hypophosphite of lime and sulphate or carbonate of ammonia.

Take of	Hypophosphate of lime	6 oz.
	Sesquicarbonate of ammonia (translucent)	7.23 oz.
	Water	A sufficient quantity.

Dissolve the lime salt in four pints of water, and the ammonia salt in two pints of water, mix the solutions, drain the resulting carbonate of lime, and wash out the retained solution with water. The filtrate should then be evaporated carefully to dryness, then dissolved in alcohol, filtered, evaporated, and crystallized.

This salt is deliquescent in the air, very soluble in alcohol and water, and when carefully heated evolves ammonia, and leaves hydrated hypophosphorous acid. The composition of this salt is NH_3+2HO,PO.

Hypophosphites of Iron.

There are two hypophosphites of iron in use in the preparations which follow, hypophosphite of sesquioxide, Fe_2O_3,3PO, as suggested by Prof. Procter, and hypophosphite of protoxide, FeO,2HO,PO, proposed by W. S. Thompson, of Baltimore. The first of these is directed to be prepared by precipitating a solution of hypophosphite of soda or ammonia with solution of sesquisulphate of iron. It is necessary to avoid the presence of an alkaline carbonate or the precipitate will be contaminated with free sesquioxide of iron. After washing the gelatinous precipitate thrown down by the mixed liquids, which must be done with care, as in this state it is soluble, it may be dried into an amorphous, tasteless white powder, freely soluble in hydrochloric and hypophosphorous acids.

The hypophosphite of protoxide of iron is present in one of the syrups for which recipes are given below, and is recommended in this form of preparation by being more permanent than the sesquisalt, which, as observed by W. S. Thompson, continually tends to pass into proto-salt in saccharine solution; the proto-salt is also more soluble.

Hypophosphorous Acid.

So far as I am aware, this acid has not been prescribed in a free state, but it is highly probable that it may come into use. Any claims which phosphoric acid may possess as an agent to supply the waste of phosphorus and phosphates in the human economy, will be more than equalled by this acid. Hypophosphite of baryta is the salt which is most eligible for the preparation of this acid, but it is convenient to prepare it from the lime salt, viz:—

Take of	Hypophosphite of lime . . .	480 grains.
	Crystallized oxalic acid . . .	350 grains.
	Distilled water	9 fluidoz.

Dissolve the hypophosphite of lime in six ounces of the water and the acid in the remainder, with the aid of heat; mix the solutions, pour the mixture on a white paper filter, and when the liquid has passed, add distilled water carefully, till it measures ten fluidounces, and evaporate this to eight and a half fluidounces.

The solution thus prepared contains about ten per cent. of terhydrated hypophosphorous acid (HO+2HO,PO), a teaspoonful representing six grains of the acid, which contains two and a quarter grains of phosphorus. The dose of this acid solution will probably vary from ten minims to a teaspoonful.

Hypophosphite of Manganese.—A preparation containing this salt having been prescribed, it is appropriate to mention it in this place, though, as it is not sold in a separate state, it need not be separately treated of in this place. (See *Syrup of Hypophosphite of Manganese.*)

Hypophosphite of Quinia.

This elegant salt introduced to notice by Prof. J. Lawrence Smith, of Louisville, Ky., is made with facility by dissolving one ounce sulphate of quinia in water, by the aid of diluted sulphuric acid, then precipitating the alkaloid with ammonia, washing, digesting in hypophosphorous acid with heat; the quinia in excess, after filtering, it evaporates spontaneously till it crystallizes. It may also be made by double decomposition between hypophosphite of baryta and sulphate of quinia. It is in elegant tufts of feathery crystals, soft to the touch, soluble in 60 parts of water, and more so in hot water. It loses water at 300°, melts and turns brown. DOSE, one to five grains.

Eligible Combinations of the Hypophosphites.

The following preparations have all been suggested within a recent period as eligible combinations for administering these remedies. I also insert my own recipes, which have not before appeared in print.

Procter's Syrup of Hypophosphite of Lime.

Take of	Hypophosphite of lime	1 ounce.
	Water	9½ fluidounces.
	White sugar	12 ounces.
	Fluid extract of vanilla . .	½ fluidounce.

Dissolve the salt in the water, filter, add the sugar, dissolve by aid of heat, and add the vanilla. The dose is from a teaspoonful (three and a half grains) to a tablespoonful (fourteen grains), according to the circumstances of the case, three times a day.

Procter's Compound Syrup of Hypophosphites.

Take of	Hypophosphite of lime	256 grains.
	Hypophosphite of soda	192 "
	Hypophosphite of potassa	128 "
	Hypophosphite of iron[1] (recently precipitated) .	96 "
	Hypophosphorous acid solution . q. s. or	240 "
	White sugar	9 ounces.
	Extract of vanilla	½ ounce.
	Water	A sufficient quantity.

Dissolve the salts of lime, soda, and potassa in six ounces of water; put the iron salt in a mortar, and gradually add solution of hypophosphorous acid till it is dissolved; to this add the solution of the other salts, after it has been rendered slightly acidulous with the same acid, and then, water, till the whole measures twelve fluidounces. Dissolve in this the sugar, with heat, and flavor with the vanilla.

Without flavoring, this syrup is not unpleasant.

[1] This quantity, 96 grains, of hypophosphite of iron is obtained when 128 grains of hypophosphite of soda, dissolved in two ounces of water, is decomposed with a slight excess of solution of persulphate of iron, and the white precipitate well washed on a filter with water.

Wm. S. Thompson's Syrup of Hypophosphites. (Containing the Protosalt of Iron.)

Take of	Hypophosphite of lime	256 grains.
	Hypophosphite of soda	192 "
	Hypophosphite of potassa	128 "
	Protosulphate of iron, crystallized	185 "
	Carbonate of soda	240 "
	Hypophosphorous acid, sp. gr. 1.036	3½ fl. ounces.
	Sugar	12 ounces.

Dissolve the protosulphate of iron and carbonate of soda, each separately, in four fluidounces of water, and mix the solutions. Wash the precipitated carbonate of iron thoroughly with sweetened water, and drain it on a muslin filter. Having placed the salts of lime, soda, and potassa in a suitable porcelain dish, add about two fluidounces of water, and one fluidounce of hypophosphorous acid; heat the mixture gently, and add the moist carbonate of iron, in small portions, from time to time, alternately with the hypophosphorous acid, until the solution is complete. Add water enough to make the whole measure ten fluidounces; pour it into a bottle containing the sugar and agitate as before.—*Journ. and Trans. of Maryland College of Pharm.*, June, 1858.

Parrish's Syrup of the Hypophosphites.

The presence of preparations of iron in these compounds was not called for by the original discoverer of their therapeutic value, who considers the alkaline and earthy hypophosphites as superior to any of the ordinary "*hæmatogens*," and in practice I believe the following very simple preparations have been found fully equal to those in which *iron* is introduced with an excess of hypophosphorous acid.

Take of	Hypophosphite of lime	℥iss.
	" soda	℥ss.
	" potassa	℥ss.
	Sugar (com.)	℔j, 12 oz.
	Hot water	Oj f℥iv.
	Orange-flower water	f℥j.

Make a solution of the mixed salts in the hot water, filter through paper, dissolve the sugar in the solution by the aid of heat; strain and add the orange-flower water. DOSE, a teaspoonful, containing nearly five grains of the mixed salts.

The *glycerole of hypophosphites* has the same composition as the foregoing, except that the solution is formed with a less proportion of water, to which a smaller portion of sugar is added, and the quantity made up with glycerin. We modify the flavor, also, by the use of a little oil of bitter almonds, to distinguish it from the corresponding syrup.

Some pharmaceutists omit the sugar altogether, and propose this course in making all glyceroles, using glycerin as the solvent, as well as for its nutritive and remedial properties. I do not find this to furnish a

[illegible] ingredients have, perhaps, [illegible] solution, and in view of [illegible] I think a teaspoonful a [illegible] is usual with such pre- [illegible]. The proportion of gly- [illegible] be charged for the prepa- [illegible] must be placed at some [illegible].

[illegible] in this preparation, [illegible] they are apt to acquire

[illegible] preparations, which have been [illegible] published formulæ as yet exist.

[illegible] of Iron.

[illegible]	185 grains.
[illegible]	240 "
[illegible] sp. gr. 1.036	f℥iijss or q. s.
[illegible]	12 ounces.

[illegible] and carbonate of soda, each separately, [illegible] the solution. Wash the preci- [illegible] with sweetened water, and drain [illegible] a small portion of [illegible] acid till it forms a clear [illegible] eight fluidounces, and add the [illegible]. This contains very nearly one grain of [illegible] the ounce.

[illegible] supplied for physicians'

[illegible] of Manganese.

[illegible] manganese	[illegible] grains.
[illegible]	[illegible] grains.
[illegible]	[illegible]
[illegible]	[illegible]
[illegible]	[illegible]
[illegible]	℥ss.

[illegible] in separate portions of [illegible] evaporate to one pint, dis- [illegible] and add the orange-flower [illegible] grains of hypophosphite

[illegible] dwelt upon in this chapter, [illegible] than the pharmaceutist. They [illegible] general remark and discus- [illegible] of learning the estimate [illegible] their patients.

[illegible] have long been known and occasionally used. The former, according to Dr. Pareira, "increases incontestably the presence of calcareous salts in the bones, the blood, and the urine," and is hence useful in rickets; and the latter, in addition to the well-known general effects of the ferruginous salts, has enjoyed a high reputation in Europe as an alterative, both internally and externally used.

The chief practical difficulty about the use of these preparations has been their insolubility, and their present popularity is undoubtedly due to their being scientifically combined with the alkaline phosphates, in such proportion as the study of the healthy secretions, and the normal composition of the tissues indicates, and, above all, their being in perfect solution in an eligible form, commending itself to the taste of the patient. The capability of assimilation of medicinal substances has long been known to depend greatly upon their state of division, and no degree of comminution of a solid substance seems so favorable to this object as perfect solution. That the so-called chemical food is a useful and elegant tonic, meeting a want constantly experienced by practitioners in treating chronic cases, is attested by thousands who have used it.

The value of the salts of hypophosphorous acid has been much more zealously called in question, but can no more admit of a doubt; the extraordinary claim set up by Dr. Churchill, of a specific property possessed by these salts of curing consumption, even after it has progressed beyond its incipient stage, is certainly not established by general experience, but there is a cloud of witnesses to the utility and singular efficiency of these remedies in the treatment of many cases of nervous and general debility and ill health.

This is not the place to dwell upon this subject, but the remarks here made may serve as answers to the numerous inquiries addressed to me by physicians, though they must be taken as the opinion of a pharmaceutist, whose position and pursuits do not qualify him to pronounce upon a purely therapeutical question.

CHAPTER VI.

IRON AND MANGANESE.

FERRUM. (IRON.)

Ferri Ramenta (*Iron Filings*). *Ferri Filum* (*Iron Wire*).

THIS indispensable metal is too well known to require description. Its purest common form is that of wire, or preferably card teeth. The filings (Ramenta), when obtained as a residuum from the manufactories, are apt to be contaminated with other metals. They are also liable to rust, which is objectionable in some cases.

The salts of iron used in medicine are numerous, including salts of the protoxide, of the sesquioxide, and of the black or magnetic oxide, and also halogen salts. The salts of protoxide are now generally termed by chemists ferrous salts, and are accordingly named ferrous sulphate, ferrous carbonate, &c. While the salts of the peroxide (sesquioxide) are named ferric salts, as ferric sulphate, ferric oxalate, &c. While the salts of the black oxide, which may be regarded as a compound of the proto and sesquioxide, are named ferroso-ferric salts, and the chlorides, iodides, &c., follow the same rule. This rule, which gives simplicity and accuracy to the nomenclature of this and of the other metals, is not yet adopted in the *Pharmacopœia*, and the terms are only employed in this work as synonyms. The officinal names of the halogen and analogous compounds are likewise different in some instances from those adopted by modern chemists, for while the compounds of chlorine are called chlorides, those of sulphur and cyanogen have the termination, *uret*.

Iron is conveniently recognized in its *protosalts*, by the following tests. They have a green color in solution, potassa and soda throw down a white hydrate, which becomes black on boiling from loss of water; this oxide undergoes changes by exposure to the air to gray, green, bluish-black, and then to the red sesquioxide. Alkaline carbonates affect it similarly. These salts are not precipitated by sulphuretted hydrogen, as many metallic salts are, but give a black precipitate with alkaline sulphurets. They give a white precipitate when free from sesquisalts, with ferrocyanide of potassium; by exposure this becomes blue; by ferricyanide an intense blue is immediately produced. Tannic acid only blackens these salts when they contain sesquisalts.

The *sesquisalts* of iron have generally a yellow tint, but by dissolving in excess of ferric-oxide become red. (*Graham.*) Alkalies and alkaline carbonates throw down a red-brown precipitate of hydrated sesquioxide; sulphuretted hydrogen converts them into protosalts with precipitation of sulphur; ferrocyanide of potassium throws down Prussian blue, but the ferricyanide has no effect, except upon protosalts. Tannic acid produces a bluish-black precipitate, the basis of common black ink.

The well-known tonic "*hæmatogenic*" properties of the iron salts, of which the officinal and unofficinal preparations are presented in the order in which they are treated in this chapter (the unofficinal in *Italics*), are much modified by the combinations in which it exists, and its salts have a wide range of therapeutic action.

PREPARATIONS OF IRON.

Name.	Comp.	Dose.	Remarks.
Ferri pulvis	Fe	gr. j—gr. iij.	Steel gray powder.
Ferri sulphas	FeO,SO_3+7HO	gr. v.	Green crystals.
Ferri et quiniæ sulphas		gr. j to iv.	Octohedrons.
Ferri et ammoniæ sulphas		gr. iij to vj	
Ferri sulphas exsiccat.	FeO,SO_3+HO	gr. iij.	Whitish powder.
Syrupus ferri protocarbonatis	10 per ct., FeO,CO_2	Dose, fʒj.	Colorless.
Ferri subcarbonas	$Fe_2O_3,2HO+FeO,CO_2$?	gr. v—℈j.	D'k brown powder.
Ferri sesqui chloridi	Fe_2Cl_3		Styptic.
Tinct. ferri chloridi	gr. xxxij (Fe_2Cl_3) to f℥j	♏x—xxx.	Clear yel'w liquid.
Spiritus ferri chlorati æthereus		♏xxx.	Used in Europe.
Ferrum ammoniatum	15 per ct., Fe_2Cl_3	gr. iv—x.	Orange col. grains.
Liq. ferri per sulphatis	$Fe_2O_3,3SO_3+Aq.$		Light b'wn liquid.
Ferri oxidum hydratum	$Fe_2O_3,3HO$	fʒj—f℥ss	Moist b'wn magma.
Liq. ferri citratis		♏iij—v.	fʒj contains ʒj.
Ferri citras	$Fe_2O_3,C_{12}H_5O_{14}$	gr. iij—v.	Garnet col. scales.
Ferri et quiniæ citras	Variable	gr. ij—v.	" "
Ferri et strychniæ citras	"	gr. iij.	" "
Ferri et zinci citras	"	gr. ij to v.	Greenish scales.
Syr. ferri citratis	ʒj in each f℥j	♏xx—fʒj.	f℥j contains ʒj.
Syr. ferri protocitratis	"	♏xxx—fʒj.	" "
Ferri et ammon. citras		gr. v.	Garnet scales.
Ferri et magnesiæ citras		gr. v.	Greenish scales.
Ferri acetas	In solution and tinct.		See page 516.
Ferri tannas		gr. x.	Black, insoluble.
Ferri lactas	$FeO,\overline{L},3HO$	gr. j—gr. v.	White plates or powder.
Ferri proto-tartras	$2FeO,C_8H_4O_{10}$	gr. v to x.	Crystalline powd.
Ferri et ammoniæ tartras	$NH_3,Fe_2O_3,C_8H_4O_{10}+4aq$	gr. v to x.	Garnet col. scales.
Ferri et potassæ tartras	$Fe_2O_3,KO,2C_8H_4O_{10}$	gr. x—℈j.	" "
Ferri ferrocyanuretum	3Cfy,4Fe	gr. v—xv.	Prus'n blue, cakes.
Liq. ferri nitratis	$Fe_2O_3,3NO_5+Aq.$	♏x—xx.	{ Astring't in bowel complaints.
Syr. ferri protonitratis	$FeO,NO_5+Syr.$	♏xv—xx.	
Liq. ferri hypochloratis	$Fe_2O_3,3ClO_7$	♏x.	1-12th of its weight
Ferri iodidum	FeI	gr. ij—v.	Decomposes spontaneously.
Liq. ferri iodidi	gr. vij (FeI) to fʒj	♏xx—xl.	Light green syrup.
Ferri bromidum	Fe,Br	gr. ij—v.	Brick red powder.
Syr. ferri bromidi		♏xx—xl.	Greenish syrup.
Liq. ferri bromidi	(Gillespie's)	♏v—x.	See *Bromine*.
Ferri sulphuretum	FeS	gr. v—x.	{ Externally in baths.
Ferri et potassii sulphuretum	$FeS,2KS_3+KS_2O_3$	gr. v.	
Ferri valerianas	$Fe_2O_3,3\overline{Va}.$	gr. j.	Red, amorphous.

Ferri Pulvis, U. S. (*Iron by Hydrogen. Quevenne's Iron.*)

Prepared by passing a stream of hydrogen over the calcined subcarbonate (dry sesquioxide), contained in a gun-barrel heated to low redness, by which the oxygen of the oxide combines with hydrogen, forming water, and leaves the metal in a very fine condition.

[1] See Phosphorus Compounds, &c.

It is an impalpable powder, of a steel gray color, soluble in dilute hydrochloric and sulphuric acids, with rapid evolution of hydrogen. It oxidizes when exposed to damp air, and should be kept in bottles. It is usually contaminated with a little carbon, black oxide, and occasionally sulphuret of iron. The latter impurities give it a dull black color. When well prepared, it will burn on the application of a lighted taper; and a small portion of it, struck on an anvil with a hammer, forms a scale having a brilliant metallic lustre.

Metallic iron possesses in a high degree the property of restoring to the blood this essential ingredient, when, from disease, it is deficient. From its extreme 'fineness, it is readily soluble in the stomach, and the only objection to its use is that occasionally it produces eructations of hydrogen, or if it contains sulphuret of iron, sulphuretted hydrogen is evolved.

This, like other iron preparations, is apt to produce astringent effects, though less so than the persalts; hence the occasional use of mild purgatives during its administration. It also blackens the stools.

Iron, in powder, is usually given in the dose of two grains. It is conveniently given in lozenges, made with chocolate, though it has more taste than the subcarbonate. In pills it is much combined with the tonic extracts. (See *Extemporaneous Pharmacy.*)

Ferri Sulphas, U.S. (*Sulphate of Iron. Green Vitriol.*)

Prepared by dissolving iron wire in diluted sulphuric acid. One eq. of iron decomposing one of water, combines with its oxygen, and forms a protoxide, which last unites with one eq. of sulphuric acid to form sulphate of protoxide of iron. The hydrogen is liberated in a gaseous form, and may be collected for experiment. Green vitriol of commerce, which is used in the arts, is an impure sulphate, containing peroxide. It is prepared from the native sulphuret, and may be purified by crystallization.

When pure, sulphate of iron is in light bluish green rhomboidal prisms, having an astringent, styptic taste. Composition, FeO,SO_3+7HO. It dissolves in about one and a half times its weight of cold water; is insoluble in alcohol; when exposed to air and moisture, it oxidizes, and becomes covered with a brownish yellow peroxide. It also effloresces, becoming white on the surface.

Owing to the large amount of water in its crystals, it is inconvenient to dispense, in combination with vegetable substances in the form of powder or pill; and hence, in the Edinburgh and Dublin Pharmacopœias, is directed to be exposed to a moderate heat till it is converted into a dry whitish mass, which is to be reduced to powder, and is called *Ferri Sulphas Exsiccatum.* By this it loses six equivalents of water, and is consequently much stronger than the crystallized salt. In addition to the "hæmatic" virtues common to the iron salts, this preparation is decidedly astringent. It is much prescribed internally in cases attended with immoderate discharges, and is also used externally, in injections, &c., though less frequently than sulphates of zinc and copper. DOSE, in crystals, 5 grains; dried, 3 grains.

The presence of copper in this salt may be detected by placing a clean polished spatula in the solution. If copper is present, it will be precipitated with its characteristic color on the surface of the iron.

Ferri et Quiniæ Sulphas. (Sulphate of Iron and Quinine.)

As a first step to the preparation of this salt, it is necessary to prepare the sesquisulphate of iron; 125 grains crystallized protosulphate of iron, is in the usual way made into a solution of the sesquisulphate, which is then mixed with a solution of 480 grains crystallized sulphate of quinia and the mixture set aside. In several months colorless octohedrons crystallize out, of a strongly bitter taste, and nearly insoluble in water.*

The salt combines the medicinal virtues of iron and quinia, and is used in doses of from one to four grains. It is more astringent than the citrate of these bases.

Ferri Subcarbonas, U. S. (*Precipitated Carbonate of Iron.*)

Made by decomposing the sulphate of iron by means of an alkaline carbonate, as the carbonate of soda. When first formed, it is a bulky greenish, almost white, precipitate, which may be converted, by admixture with sugar, into Vallette's mass, which see; but when dried in air, it becomes much darker, and finally brown, from more or less conversion into the sesquioxide and loss of carbonic acid. If the drying is carried on at a low temperature, this change is only partial, and the preparation effervesces rapidly when thrown into acids, and has a dark brown color. This is a much more soluble form, and to be preferred to the bright red colored powder produced by heating.

The subcarbonate of iron is one of the most popular of the chalybeate salts. It has the properties attributed to the powder of iron, with a more agreeable effect from swallowing it. The carbonate is not astringent, and produces little or no action upon the mucous membranes of the alimentary canal. DOSE, gr. v to ℈j.

Syrup of Protocarbonate of Iron.

The facility with which protocarbonate of iron dissolves in simple syrup makes this liquid form of administration particularly eligible, especially as the solution is nearly colorless, and the presence of sugar completely protects the salt from further oxidation and change. It may be made as follows:—

Take of Sulphate of iron . . . . . ℥ij.
Crystallized carb. soda . . . . ℥iiss.
Water . . . . Oij.
White sugar . . . . . . ℥iv.

First, dissolve the sulphate of iron and two ounces of the sugar in 16 oz. of the water, with ebullition, and filter; then the carbonate of soda with the remaining sugar in the remainder of the water, with ebullition, and filter; when the solutions have cooled, mix them in a glass vessel and shake for a moment; allow the precipitate to collect during twenty-four hours, and decant. Afterwards,

Take of White sugar . . . . . . ℥iiss.
Water . . . . f℥x.

Dissolve with ebullition, and filter. To this, when cold, add the precipitate, allow it to subside, and decant. Repeat the process, to remove sulphate of soda, resulting from the double decomposition. This should be done quickly to avoid unnecessary solution of the precipitate. Subsequently agitate the precipitate from time to time in a fresh portion of a like saccharine solution; it will dissolve in a few days. Lastly,

Take of White sugar	. . . . .	℥xxxviiiss.
Water	. . . .	f℥xix.

Add the saccharine-ferruginous solution, and boil to sp. gr. 1.262 (at boiling point), and flavor with tincture of fresh lemon or orange-peel. The product will be sixty-four fluidounces of an almost colorless, clear syrup of protocarbonate of iron, containing 9.90 per cent. of oxide of iron.—*Am. Journ. Pharm.*, vol. xxx. p. 459. (See *Pil. Ferri Carbonatis.*)

Tinctura Ferri Chloridi, U. S. (*Tincture of Muriate of Iron*)

This is one of the preparations usually made by the apothecary. It is placed among the preparations of iron in the *Pharmacopœia*, though also adapted to be inserted among the tinctures:—

Take of Subcarbonate of iron	. .	Three ounces.
Muriatic acid	. . . .	Half a pint.
Alcohol	. . . . .	A pint and a half.

Pour the acid on the subcarbonate of iron in a glass or porcelain vessel. Mix them, and when effervescence has ceased, apply a gentle heat, and continue it, stirring occasionally until the powder is dissolved; then filter the solution, and mix it with the alcohol. It is an equally good plan to mix the dissolved chloride before filtering; the quantity of liquid to be filtered is thus larger, but the filter is less likely to break. As a small portion of the powder will be apt to remain undissolved, the wash-bottle may be used, as shown in Fig. 204, to spirt a strong jet of alcohol into the dish and thus carry all the contents on to the filter.

Fig. 203.

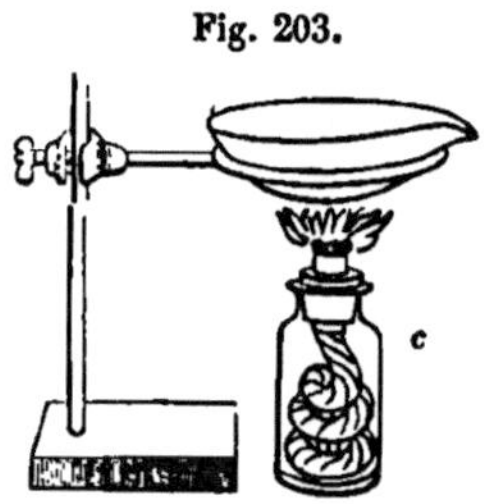

Fig. 204.

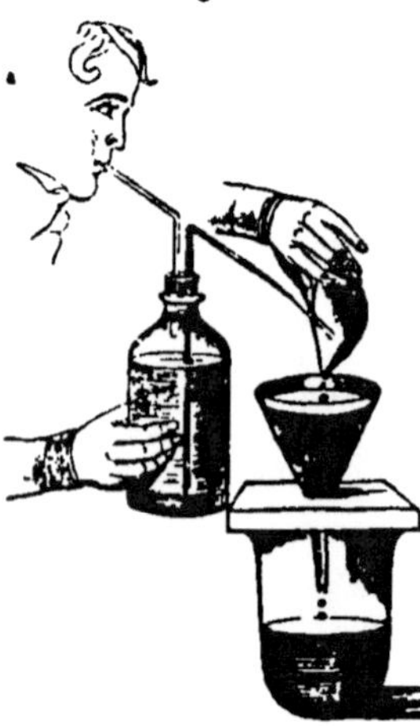

The tincture of chloride of iron is a solution of the sesquichloride (Fe_2Cl_3) in alcohol; it should contain about thirty-two grains of that salt to f℥j. If a considerable proportion of subcarbonate remains undissolved, from its peculiar insoluble molecular condition, or from deficiency of strength in the muriatic acid, a little more acid should be added before withdrawing the heat, or preferably, adopting the suggestion of A. P. Sharpe, of Baltimore, muriatic acid gas, generated by heating commercial muriatic acid in a flask, should be passed through a glass tube into the liquid, until a perfect solution is effected. Dr. Squibb, finding so much difficulty in dissolving the subcarbonate, which, unless recently prepared, and dried without a high heat, is exceedingly unsuitable for the purpose, proposes an entirely new formula, which preserves the officinal proportions, and insures the perfect solution of the salt. It is as follows:—

Take of Iron filings	℥xviij.
Muriatic acid (sp. gr. 1.16)	f℥x.
Nitric acid (sp. gr. 1.42) .	f℥ivss, or sufficient.
Alcohol	f℥xxx.
Distilled water . . .	f℥vj.

To the iron filings, in a suitable flask, add f℥viss of the muriatic acid, and ℥j of distilled water. When the reaction has subsided, boil gently for four hours, add f℥ij of distilled water, heat again to boiling, and strain off the hot solution. Wash the flask and residue with f℥j of distilled water, and add the washings to the original solution. To the strained solution now add the remainder of the muriatic acid and heat the mixture. Add the nitric acid by degrees until it falls into the hot mixture without effervescence. Now make up the measure to f℥x by adding water, and mix with the alcohol.

The protochloride is at first produced by the action of muriatic acid on the iron, is completely converted into sesquichloride by the nitric acid, the color changing, at the same time, from green to brown. One fluidounce contains 32.04 grains (7 per cent.) of sesquioxide, or 64.8 grains (14.2 per cent.) of sesquichloride of iron.

In prescribing this preparation, it should be remembered that the drops are very small, so that, although its dose is from ten to thirty minims, twice that number of drops may be given. It should not be prescribed with strong mucilage, which it has the property of gelatinizing. It is most frequently presented alone, dropped into water.

It is one of the most popular of the iron preparations. Besides the properties which are common to these, it is astringent, used in passive hemorrhages, and a diuretic which adapts it to a variety of cases. It is also one of the best solvents and vehicles for sulphate of quinia.

Solution of Sesquichloride of Iron and Pravaze's Solution.—This salt has lately become very popular with surgeons as a local remedy for aneurisms, and as a general styptic. The process prescribed by M. Burin du Buisson is to saturate as quickly as possible pure colorless muriatic acid with gelatinous hydrated peroxide of iron; evaporate the solution to somewhat less than one-half over a gentle fire, and then continue the evaporation by means of a salt-water bath, taking care to remove the aqueous vapors which would cause the formation of muriatic acid, and a deposition of insoluble oxychloride. When the solution has attained the consistence of a thick syrup, cease evaporating, and add an excess of the gelatinous hydrate diluted with a little water, agitate for a quarter of an hour, and afterwards allow the liquid to rest for several hours. Next add distilled water, sufficient to bring the solution to the density of 30° Beaumé, sp. gr. 1.261, and allow it to stand for eight days in contact with an excess of the hydrate, after which filter and allow it to stand again for two weeks. This strength is used for the cure of varices, but it is to be diluted for injection into aneurismal tumors, to sp. gr. 1.160 to 1.115.

This solution may be made from the dry sesquichloride of iron, by dissolving from 12 to 30 per cent. of it in water, as may be required.

The *Prussian Pharmacopœia* directs an aqueous solution of sesquichloride of iron, which contains ten per cent. of its weight of iron; this is probably never used internally, but kept as a convenient solution for readily obtaining the peroxide of iron, and for the preparation of the following:—

Spiritus Ferri Chlorati Æthereus; Bestucheff's Nervine Tincture; Lamotte's Golden Drops.—It is prepared by mixing one part (by weight) of solution of perchloride of iron with one and a half parts strong alcohol, and one-half part of ether, exposing the mixture in well-corked white bottles to the sun until it becomes colorless, and subsequently allowing it to oxidize again in contact with the air until it has obtained a yellowish color.

It probably contains some chloric ether and acetic acid, and nearly the whole of the iron as a protosalt. This remedy acquired much celebrity during the last century, and is still much used in Europe as a mild ferruginous preparation, agreeably modified by the presence of ether. Its medium dose is ♏xxx.

Ferrum Ammoniatum, U. S. (*Ammoniated Iron. Flores Martiales.*)

Subcarbonate of iron is mixed with muriatic acid in a glass vessel; water and sesquichloride of iron are formed; a solution of the latter is then evaporated along with a solution of muriate of ammonia; a mixture of the two salts is the result, in about the proportions of fifteen per cent. of the former to eighty-five of the latter.

It is met with in the shops in the form of small orange-colored pulverulent grains, sometimes quite crystalline, having a feeble odor and a styptic saline taste. It is deliquescent and soluble in diluted alcohol and water. It also sublimes almost without residue.

In consequence of the small proportion of iron present, it is a compound of little value. The large amount of muriate of ammonia contained in it renders it alterative, and in large doses aperient. It has been used with advantage in amenorrhœa, scrofula, &c. Also as a deobstruent in glandular swellings. Dose, gr. iv to x.

Liquor Ferri Persulphatis.

Under this head I prefer to introduce to notice the first step in the preparation of the officinal *hydrated oxide of iron*, because it is in the condition of a solution of the undecomposed sulphate of sesquioxide that the sesquioxide is best kept for extemporaneous precipitation, and because this solution is also useful for other purposes in pharmacy. The following formula for its preparation is compiled from that of the *Pharmacopœia*:—

Take of	Sulphate of iron .	One ounce.
	Sulphuric acid .	Fifty-three minims.
	Nitric acid . .	A fluidrachm and a half, or sufficient.
	Water . .	Half a pint.

Dissolve the sulphate of iron in the water, adding also the sulphuric acid (this may be done in a flask or evaporating dish); boil the solution; then add the nitric acid, a few drops at a time, continuing the boiling after each addition till it ceases to produce a dark color; then filter the liquid, if necessary, or pour it off into an appropriate bottle for preservation and future use.

The following process yields the same results with greater facility, and in a very short time:—

Take of Sulphate of iron . . One ounce.
Sulphuric acid . . Fifty-three minims.
Nitric acid . . . A fluidrachm and a half.

Triturate the sulphate of iron with the sulphuric acid into a pasty mass. Add the nitric acid, little by little, and continue the trituration till red fumes cease to be given off. Then dissolve in water half a pint, and filter if necessary.

In this process the nitric acid, by its facility of yielding oxygen to metallic oxides, converts the protoxide of the protosulphate into sesquioxide, but the sesquioxide requires a larger dose of acid to form the salt, hence the addition of sulphuric acid. The solution has a reddish-brown color, and rather styptic ferruginous taste; its composition is shown in the syllabus.

Monsel's Persulphate of Iron.

A concentrated solution of persulphate of iron, free from excess of acid, is much employed under this name as a styptic both internally and externally.

The following is the formula for Monsel's solution, rendered in officinal weights and measures:—

Take of Distilled water, three fluidounces.
Sulphuric acid, two drachms and a half (offic.).
Protosulphate of iron, twenty-five drachms (offic.).
Nitric acid (35° B.), four drachms (offic.).

Add the sulphuric acid to the water in a porcelain capsule, and heat it to boiling; powder the sulphate of iron, and add one-half of it to the acidulated water; when dissolved, pour in the nitric acid, little by little. When the red fumes cease to be developed, add the remainder of the sulphate of iron, and stir with a glass rod till dissolved, and the effervescence ceases. Continue the heat until the solution, which at first is dark-colored, has become reddish-brown, and measures three fluidounces and three fluidrachms. The nitric acid must not exceed 35° B.

The specific gravity of this solution is 1.522. When it is carefully evaporated in a capsule, removing the pellicle which forms on the surface from time to time, it gets exceedingly tough like an extract, and when dried on glass in transparent laminæ, it is very difficult to remove it, owing to strong adhesion; it is so deliquescent that the drying cannot be well performed in the open air, but requires a stove heat. (See *Am. Journ. Pharm.*, vol. xxxi. p. 403.)

Ferri et Ammoniæ Sulphas. (*Ammonio-Ferric Alum.*)

This elegant styptic remedy has recently been much prescribed, especially in leucorrhœa; it is made as follows:—

Take of Crystallized protosulphate of iron . . ℥viij.
Sulphuric acid . . . . . . fℨvij.
Nitric acid . . . . f℥iss.
Sulphate of ammonia . . . . ℥ij, ℨij.

Boil the sulphate of iron in two pints of water and add to it the sulphuric acid; when dissolved add the nitric acid gradually, boiling for a minute or two after each addition, until the nitric acid ceases to produce a black color; boil violently to separate deutoxide of nitrogen and reduce the liquid to about one half, then add the sulphate of ammonia and a little sulphuric acid and set it aside to crystallize. Wash the crystals thoroughly in a little cold water to which a small portion of sulphuric acid has been added.

This salt is in elegant violet-tinted crystals of a more or less octohedral form. Its peculiar merit consists in its marked astringency without the stimulating properties of some of this class of salts. It is easily assimilated when taken internally. DOSE, 3 to 6 grains, and while it controls excessive discharges, is often useful in correcting their cause. Though called an alum, this salt contains no alumina; it is similar to the double sulphate of potassa and iron, which is called iron alum, though this is more soluble.

Ferri Oxidum Hydratum, U. S. (*Hydrated Oxide of Iron. Ferri Sesquioxidum Hydratum. Hydrated Ferric Oxide.*)

This is made by adding ammonia in excess to the solution of the persulphate as above. The alkali neutralizes the sulphuric acid and throws down the oxide of iron as a reddish-brown precipitate. This, if designed for use as an antidote for arsenic, is to be collected on a strainer, water being passed through it to dissolve out the sulphate of ammonia, and then squeezed out, and the moist brown magma transferred to a wide-mouth bottle and kept under a super-stratum of water. It has been ascertained, however, that by long standing, under these circumstances, the hydrated oxide loses wholly or in part its power of neutralizing arsenious acid, hence the necessity of keeping the solution of persulphate and reserving the addition of ammonia till the emergency requiring its use shall occur. As will appear in several of the recipes which follow, the hydrated sesquioxide comes in play in making some of the persalts of iron; it is also an eligible medicine for producing the usual tonic effects of the iron preparations, and may be dried at a temperature not exceeding 180° F., without losing its constitutional water; at a red heat it becomes anhydrous.

Its dose in the form of magma is f℥j; as an antidote f℥ss every five or ten minutes till a large excess has been given.

Ferri Citras, U. S. (*Citrate of Sesquioxide of Iron. Ferric Citrate.*)

Of the several citrates of iron, the citrate of the sesquioxide is most commonly used. It is made by saturating a solution of citric acid in an equal weight of water with freshly-precipitated moist hydrated sesquioxide of iron; this is evaporated at 150°, to the consistence of a syrup, spread on glass or porcelain plates, where it speedily dries in thin layers, which are separated and broken into fragments. If evaporated at too high a temperature, it is apt to become adhesive, and cannot be separated in scales.

It is in beautiful garnet red-colored plates, slightly soluble in cold water, readily in boiling, and has an acid ferruginous taste. DOSE, gr. iij to v.

Liquor ferri citratis is a name appropriate to the solution of the above salt, which it is convenient to keep on hand for dispensing. This salt is more soluble when freshly prepared than when old, and although it is slowly and imperfectly soluble in cold water, under ordinary circumstances, it is readily obtained and kept in a very concentrated solution, which, being of known strength, may be readily diluted to the point desired.

In the process of making the citrate, as above, the evaporation of the liquid obtained by adding the sesquioxide to solution of citric acid, may be dispensed with, and the liquid further diluted, if necessary, so that each fluidrachm shall contain a drachm of the citrate, and each minim a grain; this requires that for a drachm of citric acid, used, there should be about a fluidrachm and a half of the resulting solution.

Ferri et Quiniæ Citras. (*Citrate of Quinine and Iron.*)

This very popular salt, as met with in commerce, is of uncertain strength, partly in consequence of there being no authoritative formula for its preparation; the usual composition, founded on the relative doses of its two principal ingredients, is five grains of citrate of iron to one of citrate of quinia. The salts are to be mixed while the former is in solution, and afterwards concentrated and dried in scales, like the simple citrate of iron, which it resembles, except in taste; it has the bitter taste of the quinia.

The dose of citrate of quinia and iron is gr. ij to gr. v.

Ferri et Strychniæ Citras. (*Citrate of Iron and Strychnia.*)

Take of Acid citrate of iron	℥j.
Strychnia	gr. x.
Water	f℥iv.

Triturate the citrate of iron with a portion of the strychnia and add it with the remainder to the water previously heated, stirring till it is dissolved, filter if necessary, evaporate to a syrupy consistence, and pour it out upon glass to dry into scales. Dose, 3 grains.

These proportions were suggested by Prof. Procter, as giving a suitable dose of the strychnia with the dose of iron salt usually prescribed; the proportion is 1 grain in 49 of the salt. C. A. Heinitsh, of Lancaster, Pa., and Jos. Abel, of Pittsburg, Pa., have since recommended a preparation of about half the proportion of strychnia. 1 part to 100 of citrate of iron. Used in atonic dyspepsia, chorea, and suppressed menstruation. Dose, 3 to 6 grains.

Ferri et Zinci Citras.

If carbonate of zinc is added to a solution of citric acid, it begins to precipitate an insoluble salt before the point of saturation is attained, this precipitate being collected before it contains an excess of carbonate, and ammonia and citrate of iron added, a dark green solution is formed, which, concentrated and dried on glass, gives brownish-green scales, very soluble in water. The quantity of citrate of iron may be varied from the equivalent proportions, to four parts of citrate of iron and one of citrate of zinc, with a similar product. The latter proportion exists in the "modified wine of iron," of which a formula is given on page 143.

Syrupus Ferri Citratis. (*Syrup of Citrate of Magnetic Oxide of Iron.*)

Take of	Citric acid	ʒv.
	Sulphate of iron	℥j.
	Water,	
	Solution of ammonia, of each . . .	Sufficient.
	Sugar	℥viij.

By either of the processes given for liquor ferri persulphatis, convert ℥ss of the sulphate of iron into sulphate of the sesquioxide; mix this in solution with the remaining ℥ss of the sulphate, and add the solution of ammonia until it ceases to throw down a precipitate of the black or magnetic oxide. Having collected and washed this, add it to the citric acid, dissolved in f℥j of water, heat to about 150° F. and filter; dilute the filtered liquid with water to make f℥v; in this dissolve the sugar and a clear dark-colored syrup will be the result.

This contains ʒj of the salt to f℥j, and is a very eligible preparation in the dose of ♏xx to fʒj. It is apt to deposit the citrate if kept very long.

Syrupus Ferri Protocitratis. (*Syrup of Proto-Citrate of Iron.*)

Take of	Sulphate of iron	ʒiiiss.
	Carbonate of soda	ʒiv.
	Sugar,	
	Water, of each	Sufficient.
	Citric acid	℥ss.
	Simple syrup	f℥iv.

Dissolve the sulphate of iron and carbonate of soda in equal portions of water, and add the one to the other in a beaker or precipitating glass. Wash the precipitated protocarbonate of iron with water, in which a small portion of sugar has been dissolved, and add it to a concentrated solution of the citric acid; evaporate to a greenish, deliquescent mass, and dissolve in the syrup. This is a greenish-brown liquid, containing nearly ʒj of the salt to f℥j. Dose, ♏xxx to fʒj. It is liable to deposit the salt by long keeping.

The syrup of citrate of iron of *Beral* is a saccharine solution of the citrate of ammonia and sesquioxide of iron.

Ferri et Ammoniæ Citras. (*Ammonio-Citrate of Iron.*)

This salt is prepared like the following, substituting carbonate of ammonia for that of magnesia; it dries into garnet-red scales, of a pleasant ferruginous taste. It is used in doses of about five grains, like the other mild preparations of iron.

Ferri et Magnesiæ Citras.

It appears in greenish-yellow scales, which are obtained by dissolving freshly-precipitated oxide of iron in citric acid, saturating with carbonate of magnesia, and evaporating.

It has a sweetish, slightly ferruginous taste, and is soluble in water. It is much used in some places as a mild chalybeate, which is easily assimilated; it is given in doses of from three to twelve grains.

Ferri Acetas. (*Acetate of Iron.*)

The *Dublin Pharmacopœia* has a tincture of this salt, prepared by double decomposition between sesquisulphate of iron and acetate of potassa, in alcoholic solution, and removing the crystalline precipitate of sulphate of potassa; it has a deep-red color, and a strong ferruginous taste. A much pleasanter preparation is the *tinctura ferri acetatis ætherea*, of the *Prussian Pharmacopœia*, which, as a first step, orders an aqueous solution of this salt, prepared by dissolving fresh sesquioxide of iron in acetic acid, so that the solution contains 8 per cent. of iron, or 11.43 of oxide of iron, and has a sp. gr. of 1.143. To make the ethereal tincture, nine ounces of this liquor, two ounces strong alcohol, and one ounce (all by weight) of acetic ether, are mixed. It is a very agreeable preparation, and largely employed in Europe in doses of about ℥ss.

Duflos has proposed a basic acetate as an antidote to arsenious and arsenic acid, especially when combined with alkalies. It is prepared by completely saturating acetic acid with sesquioxide of iron. The solution contains $Fe_2O_3,\overline{Ac}$, and in cases of poisoning by arseniates or arsenites, is freely used, largely diluted with warm water.

Rademacher's tinctura ferri acetici is prepared by boiling an intimate mixture of 2 oz. 7 dr. protosulphate of iron, 3 oz. acetate of lead, 6 oz. of distilled water, and 12 oz. wine-vinegar, in an iron vessel, and, after cooling, adding 10 oz. alcohol. This mixture is set aside for several months, and when it has assumed a deep red color, is filtered and preserved. Age improves this tincture in taste and smell. It is used in the same cases as other mild ferruginous preparations, in doses of from thirty to sixty drops.

Ferri Lactas. (*Lactate of Iron, Ferrous Lactate.*)

Obtained by digesting metallic iron with dilute lactic acid, or preferably, by decomposing the lactate of lime with sulphate of protoxide of iron.

It is, when pure, in the form of very white crystalline plates, sparingly soluble in water, with acid reaction, and ferruginous taste, though, as generally met with in this country, it is a greenish white, or gray powder; it has the advantage of less solubility than some of the other salts, and hence a less powerful taste.

This is regarded as a superior preparation, on the supposition that all the combinations of iron are converted into lactates upon their entrance into the stomach. It has been incorporated with flour in the preparation of bread, and is well adapted to the form of lozenge, of chocolate drops, &c.

The lactate has been found beneficial in chlorosis, and the kindred forms of disease, in which iron is indicated, and is said to possess a marked influence upon the appetite; it is, however, rarely prescribed in this country. Dose, gr. j to gr. v, repeated at suitable intervals.

Ferri Tannas. (*Tannate of Iron.*)

All sesquisalts of iron, if not too acid, are precipitated by tincture of galls or tannic acid; the precipitate is of a bluish-black color, insoluble in water, and tasteless. It has been highly recommended as a chalybeate, which is well adapted to weak stomachs. Dose, in chlorosis, ten grains or more.

A syrup has been proposed, containing 2½ drachms citrate of iron, 1 drachm extract of galls, to 4 ounces raspberry syrup, and twelve ounces simple syrup. The dose is a tablespoonful several times a day.

Ferri et Potassæ Tartras, U. S. (*Tartrate of Iron and Potassa.*)

This double salt is directed to be prepared by heating together, to 140° F., hydrated sesquioxide of iron with bitartrate of potassa. The excess of tartaric acid in the latter salt is saturated by the ferric oxide, forming a neutral, uncrystallizable salt. This is obtained by evaporation in a thick, syrupy liquid, which is poured on plates of glass, to dry. As thus prepared, it forms garnet scales, having the physical characters of the citrate; soluble in seven times its weight of water, and becoming damp on exposure. Its astringency is much less than the ferruginous preparations generally, and its stimulating influence less obvious. From its slight taste, and ready solubility, it is one of the best preparations for children. DOSE, gr. x to xx.

Ferri Prototartras. (*Prototartrate of Iron.*)

Is obtained as a crystalline powder, by digesting iron filings with tartaric acid in solution; or in larger crystals, by mixing hot concentrated solutions of protosulphate of iron and tartaric acid. It is little soluble in water, has a mild ferruginous taste, and contains 13 per cent. water of crystallization.

It may be used like the other milder forms of iron.

Ferri et Ammoniæ Tartras. (*Ammonio-Tartrate of Iron.*)

It is best prepared by saturating a solution of bitartrate of ammonia with freshly precipitated oxide of iron, and evaporating, and drying it upon slabs. It appears in brownish-red scales, of a sweet ferruginous taste, soluble in water, and is given in doses of five grains and more.

Ferri Ferrocyanuretum, U. S. (*Ferrocyanuret or Ferrocyanide of Iron. Prussian Blue.*)

Obtained by a double reaction ensuing upon mixture of solutions of ferrocyanuret of potassium and sulphate of iron, the latter being first converted into a tersulphate by addition of NO_5 and SO_3.

It is an insipid, inodorous substance, in porous, oblong, rectangular cakes, of a rich velvety blue color. Insoluble in water, alcohol, and mineral acids, excepting sulphuric, which forms with it a white, pasty mass, decomposed by water; alkalies decompose it, dissolving sesquioxide of iron, and precipitating an alkaline ferrocyanide. Red oxide of mercury, boiled with Prussian blue, affords the soluble cyanide of mercury, with an insoluble mixture of oxide and cyanide of iron.

Tonic and sedative. Has been recommended in intermittent and remittent fever; also in epilepsy and facial neuralgia. DOSE, gr. v–xv.

Hydrocyanate of iron is the name given to a preparation manufactured and sold by Tilden & Co., of New Lebanon, New York. It appears to be a mixed compound, of ferrocyanide of potassium, and ferrocyanide of iron, probably made by adding an excess of cyanide of potassium, to protosulphate of iron in solution, and either omitting the washing, or washing imperfectly. The dose is smaller than the foregoing; ½ gr. to 1 gr.

Liquor Ferri Nitratis, U. S. (*Solution of Pernitrate of Iron, or Ferric Nitrate.*)

Take of Iron wire, cut in pieces	℥j.
Nitric acid	f℥iij.
Distilled water	Sufficient.

Mix the acid with a pint of distilled water, add the iron, and agitate occasionally, until gas ceases to be disengaged, then filter the solution, and add to it sufficient distilled water to make it measure thirty fluidounces.

This solution, which is at first of a clear red color, and powerful styptic taste, is apt to throw down, upon standing, a bulky precipitate of subnitrate of sesquioxide. This may be prevented by the addition of a little muriatic acid, or by observing the following directions of Prof. Procter:—

Mix the acid with ten fluidounces of the distilled water in a thin, wide-mouth bottle, which should be surrounded by water. Add the iron gradually, about a drachm at a time, waiting until active effervescence has ceased, after each addition, before making the next. When all the iron has thus been thrown in, filter the solution through paper, heat it gently in a capsule or flask, and carefully drop in nitric acid, followed by stirring or agitation, until a drop of the solution, tested with ammonia, yields a red precipitate, without any tinge of black. Then add distilled water until the liquid measures thirty fluidounces. The solution should have a bright, Madeira wine color. It is used as an astringent in diarrhœa, and in hemorrhages from the bowels, uterus, &c., in individuals of pale and feeble constitutions. As a remedy in dysentery, it has no superior. A gentleman of considerable experience writes: "I regard it as much a specific as quinine is for ague." Dose, ♏v to xv.

Syrupus Ferri Protonitratis. (*Syrup of Ferrous Nitrate.*)

It requires a particular course of manipulation to dissolve iron in nitric acid, without, as in the above preparation, a large portion passing to the higher stage of oxidation. If, however, instead of adding the iron in divided portions to the nitric acid, we add the nitric acid more diluted to the iron in great excess, the acid gradually becomes saturated, the solution has a light-greenish color when filtered, and is precipitated of a greenish color by ammonia. It is necessary for the solution to stand on the iron for several hours after the last addition of acid.

Take of		
	Iron wire (card teeth), in pieces .	Two ounces.
	Nitric acid (sp. gr. 1.42) . .	Three fluidounces.
	Water	Thirteen fluidounces.
	Sugar, in powder	Two pounds.

Put the iron in a wide-mouthed bottle, kept cool by standing in cold water, and pour upon it three fluidounces of water. Then mix the acid with ten fluidounces of water, and add the mixture in portions of half a fluidounce to the iron, agitating frequently until the acid is saturated, using litmus paper. When all the acid has been combined, filter the solution into a bottle containing the sugar and marked to contain thirty fluidounces. If the whole does not measure that bulk, pour water on the filter until it does. When all the sugar is dissolved, strain, if necessary, and introduce the syrup into suitable vials, and seal them.

This preparation is, I believe, used for nearly the same purposes as the foregoing. Dose, ♏v to xv.

Liquor Ferri Hyperchloratis

Has been recommended in certain forms of disease, on account of the large quantity of oxygen it contains. It is prepared by dissolving sesquioxide of iron in hyperchloric acid. The solution contains $Fe_2O_3,3ClO_7$, and one-twelfth of its weight of iron. It is given in mucilaginous liquids, in doses of about ten drops.

Ferri Iodidum, U.S. (*Iodide of Iron. Ferrous Iodide.*)

Take of Iodine	℥ij.
Iron filings	℥j.
Distilled water	Oiss.

Mix the iodine with Oj water, in a glass or porcelain vessel, and gradually add the iron filings, stirring constantly. Heat the mixture gently, until of a light-green color. Filter, and pour upon it the remaining Oss of water, boiling hot. Evaporate the filtered liquor at a temperature not exceeding 212°, in an iron vessel, to dryness. Keep in a closely-stopped bottle. One eq. of iron is here made to unite directly with one eq. of iodine, forming a protiodide, FeI. It is in the form of green, or grayish-black, tabular crystals, sometimes amorphous masses, exceedingly deliquescent, and possessed of a styptic, chalybeate taste. It should be perfectly soluble in water when freshly prepared, imparting to a solution the odor and taste of iodine. By exposure to the atmosphere, it decomposes into free iodine and sesquioxide of iron.

Iodide of iron produces the valuable effects of the ferruginous salts, in addition to those of iodine: it is peculiarly applicable to the treatment of scrofulous diseases in anæmic patients, and is very much prescribed. It should be remembered that the proportion of iron, in the iodide, is small, and that it is a comparatively powerful preparation. DOSE, gr. j to ij. Owing to its liability to decompose and its extraordinary deliquescence, it is rarely prescribed, except in the form of the syrup next described, or in that of pilulæ ferri iodidi, introduced among extemporaneous preparations.

Liquor Ferri Iodidi, U.S. *Syrupus Ferri Iodidi.* (*Syrup or Solution of Iodide of Iron.*)

		Reduced quantity.
Take of Iodine	℥ij.	℥ss.
Iron filings	℥j.	ʒij.
Sugar, in powder	℥xij.	℥iij.
Distilled water	Sufficient.	Sufficient.

Mix the iodine with f℥v of distilled water (f℥iss, reduced quantity), in a porcelain or glass vessel, and gradually add the iron filings, stirring constantly. Heat the mixture gently, till all the iodine is dissolved, or until the liquid acquires a light greenish color. Then having adjusted a bottle to the measure of twenty fluidounces, or made ready the bottle shown in Fig. 205 (mark f℥v on a vial for the reduced quantity); then introduce the sugar into the bottle, filter the solution on to it, adding fresh water upon the filter above, occasionally shaking the bottle, until the resulting syrup measures f℥xx (f℥v for the reduced quantity).

It is well to transfer this to small vials, f℥ss and f℥j, as by frequent opening and restopping a large bottle, it will undergo a change—becoming brown. This may be partially obviated by leaving a few strips of iron in the bottom of the bottle. The use of heat in this preparation is unnecessary, the reaction, which is the same as that in the process for making the solid iodide, will take place satisfactorily in the cold.

Fig. 205.

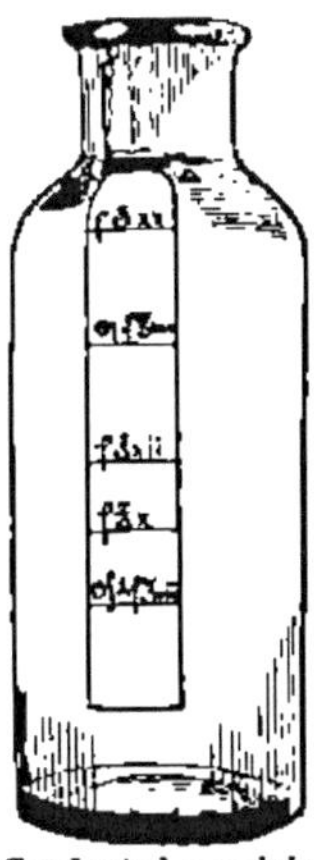

Graduated receiving bottle.

The use of sugar as a preservative of this delicate salt, is an important improvement, introduced about the year 1840, and has brought the iodide of iron within the reach of the practitioner in a very permanent and eligible form. This solution contains about 7½ grains of salt to f℥j. Dose, ♏xx to xl.

It dissolves small proportions of the iodides of mercury, copper, &c., and is incompatible with most chemical agents, but may be mixed with the syrups and fluid extracts of the vegetable alteratives, or, what is perhaps better, prescribed in a separate vial, to be dropped into the syrup at the time of taking it.

The inconvenience of a change of composition in this syrup by time, with the liberation of iodine, has been the subject of numerous pharmaceutical notes. A good practical method of obviating this is suggested by Dr. Battey, of Georgia, who secures a coil of fine iron wire to the cork of the bottle in which it is kept, so that it reaches down below the middle of the mass of liquid. The action of the sun's rays upon this syrup bleaches it so that from a light green color, it comes to be quite colorless.

A preparation is sometimes prescribed in this city under the name of *Dr. Hays's Syrup of Iodide of Iron;* the formula is published in the *Amer. Journ. of Med. Sciences*, for 1840, p. 449. It is made from 400 grains of iodine, and 160 of iron, and 2 ounces of sugar to f℥iv. Dose, ♏v.

Bromide of Iron.

This salt is obtained by adding bromine to iron filings in excess under water, and submitting them to a moderate heat. When the liquid assumes a greenish-yellow appearance, it is filtered and evaporated rapidly to dryness in an iron vessel. Bromide of iron is a brick red, very deliquescent salt, of an acrid styptic taste, and requires to be kept closely stopped in glass vials. This bromide has been used quite extensively in Pittsburg, Pa., as a tonic and alterative, and is considered by some physicians a highly efficacious preparation. An eligible form for administration of bromide of iron is the following:—

Syrup of Bromide of Iron.

Take of Bromine	200 grains.
Iron filings	85 grains.
Water	f℥ivss.
Sugar	℥iij.

Make a solution in the manner directed for preparing the officinal solution of iodide of iron. Dose, ♏xx, three times a day, gradually increased. (See *Medical Examiner*, vol. vii. p. 162.)

For the preparation of a solution of bromide of iron with excess of bromine, see Bromine.

Sulphurets of Iron.

Several sulphurets have been proposed, as stimulating alteratives, and as antidotes against the poisonous action of arsenic, lead, mercury and other metals, which are precipitated by hydrosulphuric acid. As this latter acid may be set free by the intestinal acids, and in larger quantities has itself a poisonous action, the free use of these sulphurets seems to require care.

Ferri sulphuretum, called black sulphuret of iron, is prepared by fusing together iron and sulphur. If well prepared, it has a yellowish-gray or blackish color, without odor or taste, and is wholly soluble in diluted acids, with evolution of sulphuretted hydrogen. It is chiefly used for the preparation of this gas, but has been given in scrophulous and chronic skin diseases, in doses of 5 or 10 grains, twice a day.

Ferri et potassii sulphuretum, prepared by fusing together equal parts of iron filings and carbonate of potassa, with ½ part of flowers of sulphur, is a brown mass of the odor of sulphuretted hydrogen. It has been recommended as an antidote against arsenic, and also as a powerful alterative in doses of 5 grains, and in larger doses, diluted, in cases of poisoning; externally it has been employed as an addition to baths in the quantity of 1 to 3 ounces.

Valerianate of Iron.

This preparation is made by the decomposition of valerianate of soda by tersulphate of sesquioxide of iron; it is a dark red amorphous powder, having a faint odor and taste of valerianic acid. Its composition is thus shown, $Fe_2O_3,3\overline{Va}$. It is insoluble in cold water, decomposed by hot water, and is soluble in alcohol. In hysterical affections complicated with chlorosis, it is prescribed in doses of about a grain repeated several times a day.

MANGANESE.

This is a metal resembling iron in its therapeutical as well as in some of its chemical properties. It forms several oxides, of which the protoxide, MnO, is present in its most important oxysalts, which have a rose color, or are colorless. The salts of manganese are not incompatible with vegetable astringents, which is their chief pharmaceutical merit. None of them are officinal.

Tests for Protoxide of Manganese.—The salts in which oxide of manganese forms the base are recognized as follows:—

Sulphuretted hydrogen produces in alkalies and sulphuret of ammonium, in neutral solutions, a flesh-colored precipitate of MnS, turning to brown in contact with air, soluble in acids.

Alkalies cause a whitish precipitate of MnO,HO; carbonates of the alkalies a similar precipitate of MnO,CO_2. By exposure to the air, they are partly oxidized, and turn brown.

Carbonate of soda, fused with compounds of manganese in the outer flame before the blowpipe, assumes from NeO,MnO_3, a green color, turning to a turbid blue green after cooling.

PREPARATIONS OF MANGANESE.[1]

Manganesii oxidum nigrum, MnO_2. Native impure mineral.
Manganesiæ sulphas, $MnO,SO_3,+4HO$. Pale rose-colored crystals, soluble.
Manganesiæ carbonas, $2MnO,CO_2+HO$. Whitish insoluble powder.
Manganesii chloridum, $MnCl+4HO$. Milder than sulphate. Dose, gr. v.
Manganesiæ acetas, $MnO,\overline{A}c$. By dissolving carbonate in $\overline{A}c$.
Manganesiæ lactas, $MnO,\overline{L}+4HO$. Dose, gr. j. Rose-colored cryst.
Syrupus manganesii iodidi. Contains ʒj MnI, to each f℥j.
Syrupus ferri et manganesii iodidi. Same strength as Liq. Fer. Iod., *U. S.*
Potassæ permanganas, KO,Mn_2O_7. Purple cyst, or green powder.

The native impure form of manganese in commerce, that of black oxide, is used to prepare all the rest; it is imported in lumps and in powder, and should have a dark, shining, crystalline appearance.

Sulphate of Manganese. (Manganous Sulphate.)

This salt may be prepared as follows:—

Mix in a sand crucible the black oxide of manganese with sulphuric acid until of a thick pasty consistence. Cover with a smaller crucible and expose the mixture to a red heat for half an hour. At the end of this interval, remove the crucible from the fire, and when cool reduce the dark brown mass to a coarse powder. Introduce this into a crucible, and saturate as before with sulphuric acid. Again apply heat and continue it till white vapors cease to be expelled. The mass remaining contains the sulphate, which may be obtained impure by solution and evaporation. To purify this from iron, the following directions are given: The filtered solution is to be heated in a porcelain capsule, and when nearly boiling, drop into it carbonate of manganese in small portions at a time until all the iron shall have been precipitated and the liquid changes from a dark red to a pale rose tint. Now evaporate and crystallize. Some processes recommend the heating of black oxide with carbon previous to adding the sulphuric acid, others direct the addition of the moist carbonate to diluted sulphuric acid. These crystals are of a pale rose color, containing when formed below 42° F. 7HO, above that temperature 4HO; they have a styptic taste, are freely soluble in water, and may be given as a tonic in a dose of gr. v; as a cholagogue cathartic, ʒj to ʒij is required.

Carbonate of Manganese.

This is made by precipitating sulphate with a carbonated alkali, or directly from the native black oxide, as follows:—

Take of black oxide of manganese ℔j, in powder, put it in a porcelain dish on a sand bath or other source of heat; pour on it muriatic acid Oij, and stir well. Chlorine is evolved, which makes it necessary to operate in the open air or under a chimney. Muriatic acid should

[1] See Phosphorous Compounds, chap. v.

be added until it is nearly dissolved. To get rid of free muriatic acid and sesquichloride of iron, and carbonate of soda, boiling, after each addition, as long as the carbonate precipitated is contaminated with iron, or until a portion of the solution tested with yellow prussiate of potassa does not produce a blue color. The solution of chloride of manganese, being now separated from the oxide of iron by filtration, will furnish, on the addition of an excess of carbonate of soda, a bulky white precipitate, which, being washed in cold boiled water and dried, constitutes carbonate of manganese. It is a white or pale rose-colored powder, insoluble in water, and liable to pass into a higher state of oxidation; it may be given in powder, dose, gr. v, or in the form of saccharine powder, or made into a mass with honey.

Manganesiii Chloridum.

Its medicinal properties are similar to those of the sulphate, but it is considered a milder preparation. It is soluble in water and alcohol, and is given in doses of about five grains.

Manganesiæ Acetas.

By dissolving the carbonate in acetic acid and evaporating, colorless or rose-colored prisms are obtained, which are permanent in the air, have an astringent metallic taste, and are soluble in alcohol, and in three and a half parts of water. It is considered one of the mildest medicinal salts of manganese, and is given like the other.

Manganesiæ Lactas.

Prepared by dissolving carbonate of manganese in lactic acid, and evaporating; crystallizes in four-sided prisms of a pale rose color, is efflorescent, and contains 4HO. It has been used together with lactate of iron in doses of one grain, in chlorosis.

Syrup of Iodide of Manganese.

Take of Sulphate of manganese	℥ij.
Iodide of potassium	℥ij, ʒiij.
Sugar	℥xij.
Water,	
Syrup, of each	Sufficient.

Dissolve the sulphate and iodide each in f℥iij of cold water, to which f℥ij of syrup have been added, mix them in a glass-stoppered bottle, and, after the crystals of sulphate of potassa cease to precipitate, throw the solution on a filter of fine muslin, and allow it to pass into a pint bottle containing the sugar; add sufficient water to the filter to bring up the measure of the resulting syrup to exactly a pint. This contains about ʒj of the iodide to each f℥j. Dose, ♏x.

Syrup of Iodide of Iron and Manganese. (Procter.)

This preparation nearly represents the officinal solution of iodide of iron, and is used for the same purposes, and in the same doses.

Take of Iodide of potassium	1000 grains.
Protosulphate of iron	630 "
Protosulphate of manganese	210 "
Iron filings (free from rust)	100 "
White sugar (in coarse powder)	4800 "
Distilled and boiled water	q. s.

Triturate the sulphates and the iodide separately to powder, mix them with the iron filings, add half a fluidounce of distilled water, and triturate to a uniform paste. After standing a few minutes, again add half a fluidounce of distilled water, triturate, and allow it to rest fifteen minutes. A third addition of water should now be made and mixed. The sugar should then be introduced into a bottle capable of holding a little more than twelve fluidounces, and a small funnel, prepared with a moistened filter, inserted into its mouth. The magma of salts should then be carefully removed from the mortar to the filter, and when the dense solution has drained through, distilled or boiled water should be carefully poured on in small portions, until the solution of the iodides is displaced and washed from the magma of crystals of sulphate of potash. Finally, finish the measure of twelve ounces, by adding boiled water, and agitate the bottle until the sugar is dissolved. The solution of the sugar may be facilitated, when desirable, by standing the bottle in warm water for a time, and then agitating.

Each fluidounce of this syrup contains fifty grains of the mixed anhydrous iodides in the proportion of three parts of iodide of iron to one part of iodide of manganese, and the dose is from ten drops to half a fluidrachm.

For paper on the preparations of manganese and iron, including effervescing powders, lozenges, pills, chocolate, and syrup, see *Am. Journ. Pharm.*, vol. xxv. p. 174, also vol. xxii. p. 297.

Permanganate of Potassa.

This salt, which is sometimes called *hypermanganate of potassa*, may be made by mixing equal parts of very finely-powdered deutoxide of manganese and chlorate of potassa with rather more than an equal part of caustic potassa, dissolving in a little water, evaporating to dryness, and exposing to a temperature just short of redness. The mass, on treatment with hot water, yields a deep purple solution of this salt, which on evaporation crystallizes, or, if evaporated to dryness, the salt is obtained as a dark green powder. The crystals are purple, and dissolve in 16 parts of water.

The uses of this preparation are, internally as a remedy in diabetes, dose 3 grains 3 times a day, gradually increased, and externally as a caustic and "deodorizer" in treating foul ulcers. It is applied in powder, dusted on to the part, or in solution, from 1 to 10 grains to the ounce.

CHAPTER VII.

PREPARATIONS OF COPPER, ZINC, NICKEL, AND CADMIUM.

CUPRUM. (COPPER.)

THE properties of metallic copper are generally familiar; it furnishes, by oxidation and combination with acids, some important medicines, which are also, in excessive doses, corrosive poisons. The best antidote is white of egg, or milk and other bland liquids; magnesia will aid in the case of sulphate, by decomposing that salt. Copper is apt to contaminate stewed fruit, from the use of copper vessels in their preparation: it may be detected by immersing a clean spatula in the suspected liquid, which deposits a film of metallic copper.

The presence of copper is also detected by the following reactions of the solutions of its oxide.

Potassa and its carbonate cause a blue precipitate soluble in an excess of the precipitant in the presence of some organic bodies. If grape sugar is present the clear solution on boiling precipitates red suboxide of copper.

Ammonia precipitates them greenish, an excess redissolves the precipitate with a beautiful blue color.

Sulphuretted hydrogen and sulphuret of ammonium produce a black or deep brown precipitate, soluble in NO_5.

Iodide of potassium causes a white precipitate, free iodine is liberated at the same time.

Ferrocyanuret of potassium causes a brown red precipitate soluble in alkalies.

Copper Preparations.

Cupri carbonas, CuO,CO_2+CuO,HO. Pale green powder. Dose, gr. x?
" *oxidum*, CuO. Black color. Dose, $\frac{1}{4}$ to 1 gr.
" *nitras*, CuO,NO_5+3HO. Blue deliquescent crystals. Dose, $\frac{1}{8}$ to $\frac{1}{4}$ gr.
" *chloridum*, $CuCl,+2HO$. Green soluble needles. Dose, $\frac{1}{16}$ to $\frac{1}{8}$ gr.
" sulphas, CuO,SO_3+5HO. Blue vitriol. Dose, tonic, $\frac{1}{4}$ gr., emet. gr. v.
Cuprum ammoniatum, $CuO,SO_3,HO+2NH_3$. Blue amorphous moist powder, or prismatic crystals. Dose, $\frac{1}{2}$ gr.
Cupri subacetas, $2CuOAc+6HO$. (?) Verdigris; amorphous green masses. Externally.
Cupri acetas, $CuO,Ac+HO$. "Distilled verdigris," crystals.
Cuprum aluminatum. Lapis divinus.

Cupri Sulphas, U. S. (*Blue Vitriol. Blue Stone.*)

Four methods are in use for obtaining this salt. 1st. By evaporating the waters which flow through copper mines, and which hold it in solution. 2d. Roasting copper pyrites, lixiviating the residuum to dissolve the sulphate, and evaporating so as to obtain crystals. Both the S and the Cu of the pyrites abstract O from the air, and become, the one SO_3, and the other CuO; and these uniting form sulphate of copper. 3d. Another mode is to sprinkle plates of copper with sulphur, which are next heated to redness and plunged into water; the sheets are entirely corroded; a sulphuret is formed, which, by the action of heat and air, gradually passes into a sulphate; this is dissolved in water, and crystals obtained by evaporation. 4th. By dissolving the scales, obtained in the process of annealing sheet copper, in diluted sulphuric acid, evaporating and crystallizing. The salt is in large, rhombic, blue crystals, with a styptic metallic taste; it contains five equivalents of water, and is represented by CuO,SO_35HO. It effloresces slightly in dry air; soluble in water, precipitated by ammonia, but redissolved in an excess, forming a rich blue solution. The impurities contained in it, when in crystals, seldom affect its value as a medicine.

Sulphate of copper is much used as a tonic and astringent (dose gr. $\frac{1}{4}$ to gr. $\frac{1}{2}$), and as a prompt and powerful emetic in five grain doses; as an injection in gonorrhœa, &c., it is dissolved in water in the proportion of 2 to 8 grains to f℥j. A crystal polished by trituration on a damp cloth, is applied as an astringent to inflamed or granulated eyelids, &c.

If it contains iron, its precipitate with ammonia leaves a brown residue on being dissolved in an excess of the precipitate.

Zinc is detected by the white precipitate produced by sulphuretted hydrogen in a solution previously precipitated by potassa.

Cupri Carbonas.

Sulphate of copper is precipitated by carbonate of soda; the precipitate is a pale green tasteless powder, which is to be washed and dried at a moderate temperature.

It has been used in neuralgia in doses amounting to about one drachm (?) in twenty-four hours.

It is wholly soluble in muriatic acid; the solution yields no precipitate with chloride of barium.

Cupri Oxidum.

If the carbonate or the nitrate of copper is heated to redness, until it ceases to lose weight, the salt has been converted into the oxide, which is of a fine black color.

This oxide, which is also much employed in elementary organic analysis, has been recommended in preference to the carbonate in doses of ¼ to 1 grain three or four times a day, and for indurated glands, in ointments containing 1 drachm to the ounce.

It is wholly soluble in dilute muriatic acid, and the solution, after precipitating the copper by sulphuretted hydrogen, and filtering, leaves no residue on evaporation.

Cupri Nitras.

It is obtained by dissolving copper, its oxide or carbonate, in nitric acid, and evaporating to crystallization, when it crystallizes in deep blue prisms, which are deliquescent and soluble in alcohol. It acts as a caustic, dissolved in mucilaginous liquids it has been given in doses of ⅛ grain; externally as injections in gonorrhœa and similar complaints. In substance or in concentrated solution it has been employed as a caustic in ulcerated throat, in syphilis, &c. From the deliquescent nature of the salt, care is necessary to prevent its spreading.

The solution yields no precipitate with nitrate of baryta (SO_3), nitrate of silver (HCl), sulphuric or muriatic acids (lead, &c.).

Cupri Chloridum.

Muriatic acid dissolves oxide and carbonate of copper; the solution by evaporation yields green needles, which are easily soluble in alcohol and water.

It has been occasionally used as a powerful alterative in doses commencing with $\frac{1}{16}$ grain.

Cuprum Ammoniatum, U. S. (*Ammoniated Copper. Ammonio-Sulphate of Copper.*)

Sulphate of copper, ℥ss, and carbonate of ammonia, ʒvj, are rubbed together in a glass mortar until effervescence ceases; the ammoniated copper is wrapped in bibulous paper, and dried with a gentle heat.

When thus rubbed together, these salts give out part of their water of crystallization, by which the mixture becomes moist, and, at the same time, a portion of the carbonic acid of the sesquicarbonate escapes, producing effervescence, and the compound assumes a deep azure blue color.

Its composition, as thus prepared, is $NCuH_3O,SO_3+NH_3,HO$, with a variable excess of carbonate of ammonia. A salt of the above composition is obtained in beautiful blue crystals from a solution of sulphate of copper, precipitated and dissolved by ammonia, if alcohol is poured over the surface and set aside; gradually the water is abstracted by the alcohol and the salt crystallizes.

It may be considered pure if it has the proper color, and dissolves in twice its weight of water without residue.

Ammoniated copper is regarded as a tonic and antispasmodic. It is occasionally prescribed in combination with assafœtida in pill. Dose, gr. ½ repeated.

Cupri Subacetas, U. S. (*Ærugo. Impure Subacetate of Copper. Verdigris.*)

Made by exposing copper plates to the action of the fermenting refuse of the wine-press, or to pyroligneous acid, when this salt forms on the surface.

It is obtained in powder, or amorphous masses, or consisting of very minute crystals, of variable color, with a peculiar metallic odor, and styptic metallic taste; resolved by water into a soluble neutral acetate, and insoluble tris-acetate; when treated with sulphuric acid, gives off acetic acid fumes; from the solution, ammonia precipitates the oxide, but redissolves it when in excess.

Verdigris, as it occurs in commerce, is of variable composition and shade of color. The light green appears to be a mixture of various basic salts, while that of a greenish-blue color has the composition $2CuO,\overline{A}c+6HO$ (Berzelius). It is used exclusively in the shape of ointment.

Verdigris ought to be nearly soluble in dilute acetic acid, and the solution, if precipitated by ammonia, must be wholly taken up by an excess of it.

Cupri Acetas.

The neutral acetate is prepared by dissolving the above in dilute acetic acid and evaporating to crystallization. It is met with in commerce under the name of *distilled verdigris*, and occurs in dark green crystals, soluble in 5 parts of boiling water. Rademacher uses a tincture of this salt prepared by double decomposition from 3 ounces sulphate of copper, and 3¾ ounces acetate of lead, to 30 ounces (weight) diluted alcohol. But it is scarcely ever used.

Cuprum Aluminatum.

The European Pharmacopœias have a preparation under this name and the synonyma *Lapis divinus*, *Lapis ophthalmicus St. Yves*, for which the Prussian Pharmacopœia gives the following directions:

sulphate of copper, nitrate of potassa, and alum, of each two ounces, are fused by a moderate heat in a copper or earthen vessel, and after mixing in one drachm powdered camphor, the mass is poured out upon a cold slab and kept in well-stoppered bottles. It is used externally.

ZINCUM, *U.S.* (ZINC.)

This metal occurs in nature in two principal forms: as a sulphuret, *blende*, and as a carbonate or silicate, *calamine*, from which the metal is extracted, by distilling them with carbonaceous matters.

It is a bluish-white crystalline metal, soluble in dilute hydrochloric and sulphuric acids, with evolution of hydrogen, also in nitric acid; melted and dropped into water, it constitutes granulated zinc. It is used in pharmacy for the preparation of the sulphate, acetate, and chloride, which are officinal, and numerous other salts.

From its salts, oxide of zinc is precipitated by alkalies and their carbonates, white; soluble in an excess of alkali. Sulphuretted hydrogen, from neutral or alkaline solutions, white. Sulphuret of ammonium, white; the last two are insoluble in alkalies, soluble in acids. Ferrocyanuret of potassium, white; insoluble in dilute HCl.

PREPARATIONS OF ZINC.[1]

Calamina. Native, impure carbonate of zinc. A gray coarse powder.
" Præparata. Calcined, powdered, and levigated.
Tutia. A product of smelting lead ores containing zinc. Slate colored.
Zinci sulphas, ZnO,SO_3+7HO. Small, white, efflorescent crystals. Emetic gr. x.
" carbonas præcipitatus, $8ZnO,3CO_2+6HO$. (?) A pure white, very light powder.
" oxidum, ZnO. A pure, white powder, not effervescing with acids.
" acetas, $ZnO,\overline{Ac}+7HO$. Micaceous, freely soluble crystals.
" chloridum, ZnCl. White, translucent plates or masses. Very deliquescent.
" *cyanuretum*, ZnCy. White powder, insoluble, poisonous. Gr. ¼ to j.
" *ferrocyanuretum*, $(2KCy+FeCy)+3(2ZnCy+FeCy)+12HO$.
" *iodidum*, ZnI. White, deliquescent, caustic.
" *lactas*, $2ZnO,\overline{L}+6HO$. White, styptic, crystals or plates.
" *valerianas*, $ZnO,\overline{Va}$. White, pearly scales, soluble in alcohol. Dose, gr. j to ij.

Calamina, U.S. (*Calamine. Native Impure Carbonate of Zinc.*)

This mineral is found abundantly in Germany, England, and the United States. It is, however, as recently procured, very impure, and seldom contains a considerable proportion of carbonate of zinc. For use, it must be brought to the condition of an impalpable powder, when it constitutes—

Calamina Præparata, U.S. (*Prepared Calamine.*)

Obtained by heating the impure carbonate to redness and pulverizing the product, which is then levigated and elutriated.

It is in the form of a pinkish or gray powder, of an earthy appear-

[1] The unofficinal preparations, as in the other tables, in Italic.

ance. It should be almost entirely soluble in sulphuric acid, and the precipitate thrown down by ammonia and potassa should be redissolved by these reagents. The calcination of calamine drives off a quantity of CO_2 and water, so that little remains except oxide of zinc, and earthy impurities. The precipitated carbonate or oxide of zinc may be substituted with advantage.

It is only used externally as a dusting powder and exsiccant, or in the form of cerate as a mild astringent.

Tutia. (*Impure Oxide of Zinc. Tutty.*)

This oxide is formed during the smelting of lead ores containing zinc; it is, as I have seen it, usually in little nodules, like those of prepared chalk, of a bluish or slate-color. It is said to be much adulterated, some specimens factitious, and is very properly substituted by the officinal oxide of zinc.

Zinci Sulphas, U.S. (*Sulphate of Zinc. White Vitriol.*)

Prepared by dissolving zinc in dilute sulphuric acid, evaporating and crystallizing.

Water is decomposed in the presence of the acid and metal, hydrogen is liberated, the zinc oxidized, and the oxide formed combines with the sulphuric acid.

Usually in small, four-sided colorless prisms, of the same form as sulphate of magnesia, possessing a disagreeable, metallic, styptic taste, very soluble in water, insoluble in alcohol, slightly efflorescent, precipitated, and again redissolved by ammonia. When heated, it dissolves in its water of crystallization, and by prolonged ignition, the acid is all expelled, and oxide of zinc is left. Its composition is thus represented, ZnO,SO_3+7HO.

Iron is detected by a bluish precipitate with ferrocyanuret of potassium; copper by the dark precipitate with sulphuretted hydrogen; magnesia by the residue left on dissolving it in caustic potassa.

In small doses it acts as an astringent and tonic; in large doses as a quick, direct emetic; externally, as a powerful astringent. It is used as a tonic, chiefly in diseases affecting the nervous system, and when gradually increased, tolerance soon becomes established; sometimes it is given as an astringent in chronic passive discharges. As an emetic, it is used when the rapid emptying of the stomach is desired without the production of much depression, as in narcotic poisoning. Externally, in solutions of different strengths, it is employed as a lotion or injection, in ophthalmia, gleet, &c.

DOSE, gr. ss to ij in pill. As an emetic, gr. x. The strength of a solution for external employment, may be from gr. j to x to f℥j water.

Zinci Carbonas Præcipitatus, U.S. (*Precipitated Carbonate of Zinc.*)

Solutions of carbonate of soda and sulphate of zinc in equal parts are mixed together; a double decomposition takes place; sulphate of soda is formed in solution, and carbonate of zinc is precipitated. A white flocculent powder resembling magnesia subsides, which is frequently washed till the washings are tasteless; the powder is dried by a gentle heat. It must be wholly soluble in diluted acids; impurities are then detected as with oxide.

Uses same as those of calamine. In the form of the officinal cerate, it is much used as a dressing for burns.

Zinci Oxidum, U.S. (*Oxide of Zinc. Flowers of Zinc.*)

This is made by exposing the precipitated carbonate to a strong heat, by which CO_2 is driven off, and the residue is the oxide of zinc.

In the solution in nitric acid, the following impurities may be detected:—

Lead or copper, by a black precipitate with sulphuretted hydrogen; cadmium, tin, antimony, or arsenic, by a yellowish precipitate by the same reagent; earthy oxides, by the white precipitate with carbonate of ammonia, insoluble in an excess of the precipitates; sulphuric and muriatic acids, by baryta and silver salts; iron, by a bluish precipitate with ferrocyanide of potassium.

It is a white or yellowish-white powder, without odor or taste; insoluble in water, but soluble in diluted hydrochloric and other acids without effervescence, and in ammonia and potassa.

Oxide of zinc is a tonic, especially to the nervous system; also somewhat astringent; used in chorea, epilepsy, and neuralgia. Locally, it is slightly astringent and desiccant, and constitutes an excellent application to excoriated surfaces, and to chapped or cracked nipples. An ointment of oxide of zinc is officinal.

Zinci Acetas, U. S. (*Acetate of Zinc.*)

It may be procured in either of the following ways: 1. By dissolving oxide of zinc in acetic acid, and crystallizing the saturated solution. 2. By double decomposition between a solution of sulphate of zinc and a solution of acetate of lead. 3d. The officinal process, granulated zinc ℥ix, is added to a solution of ℔j of acetate of lead in water Oiij, and agitated occasionally till no precipitate is formed on the addition of iodide of potassium. The familiar experiment of forming the zinc, or lead-tree, leaves this salt in solution. In concentrating the solution to one-fifth its bulk, previously to crystallizing, a little of the acetic acid is apt to be dissipated, and should be replaced by dropping in a small excess of the acid.

When carefully crystallized, it is in the form of very handsome pearly or silky hexagonal crystals, which effloresce in a dry air. As found in the shops, it is sometimes in white micaceous scales; very soluble in water, moderately soluble in alcohol, and has an astringent, metallic taste.

When heated, it fuses and gives out an inflammable vapor, having the odor of acetic acid; the mineral acids decompose it.

It is used as a topical remedy, in the form of collyrium, in ophthalmia, and as an injection in gonorrhœa, gleet, leucorrhœa, &c.

Zinci Chloridum, U. S. (*Chloride of Zinc. Butter of Zinc.*)

Take of Zinc, in small pieces . . . ℥iiss.
Nitric acid (sp. gr. 1.42),
Prepared chalk, each . . . ʒj.
Muriatic acid . . . . A sufficient quantity.

To the zinc, in a glass or porcelain vessel, add gradually sufficient muriatic acid to dissolve it; then strain, add the nitric acid, and evaporate to dryness. Dissolve the dry mass in water, add the chalk, and, having allowed the mixture to stand for twenty-four hours, filter and again evaporate to dryness.

This beautiful preparation is well prepared by the above process of the *Pharmacopœia*. The chloride of zinc being first formed by the action of the muriatic acid on the metal, the next step is to separate the iron derived from the muriatic acid, and from the zinc; this is done by the use of nitric acid, which peroxidizes the iron, and, on evaporation to dryness, dissolving, and filtering, it is left behind. The pure chloride is now digested with chalk, to free it more completely from iron, by neutralizing any free acid. Another method, which is effectual in removing iron, is to add to the solution, as at first formed, a little freshly-precipitated hydrated carbonate of zinc; filter and evaporate.

The final concentration of the liquid requires care, as, by pushing the heat too far, the chloride is decomposed, and contains a portion of insoluble subchloride or oxide; on the other hand, care must be taken to free it entirely of water, otherwise it will not harden into solid and dry masses. The proper point is ascertained by dipping into it a glass rod, on which it should thicken into a hard, dry condition. There are two ways of finishing this operation. In one case, the mass, in its fused condition, is poured on to a dry marble slab, and, when nearly cool, is broken into fragments, and put immediately into dry salt-mouth bottles, usually of ℥j capacity. Another plan is to warm the bottles thoroughly in a sand bath, and drop the fused mass, a little at a time, into them; if in the proper condition, the separate concretions will not run together, but remain in a convenient shape for removal from the bottle when required.

Chloride of zinc, as thus prepared, is white, crystalline, and semi-transparent, rapidly absorbing water, if exposed to the air; soluble in alcohol and water. If a large amount of sediment is present in the aqueous solution, it may be inferred that, by the intense heat employed in its concentration and fusion, a portion has been reduced to the condition of oxide as above. The addition of a little dilute HCl will dissolve this sediment.

It is used as a powerful escharotic, and as a remedy for toothache. In solution, it is an antiseptic, especially adapted to dissecting-room purposes; it is convenient to employ a solution of zinc in the muriatic acid, without either purifying or concentrating it. A mixture of chloride and oxide hardens by time, and is used as a filling for the cavities of teeth.

The following solution is the best antiseptic for this purpose with which I am acquainted:—

Take of	Granulated zinc	℔ iv.
	Hydrochloric acid . . .	℔ iv or q. s.
	Water	9 quarts.

Dissolve, avoiding excess of acid. The solution contains one part of chloride of zinc in twelve.

Zinci Cyanuretum. (*Cyanide of Zinc.*)

It may be prepared by double decomposition between solution of cyanuret of potassium and sulphate of zinc, or by conducting gaseous hydrocyanic acid in a solution of acetate of zinc. The latter is the best process.

It is a brilliant white powder, insoluble in water, soluble in dilute mineral acids; it is tasteless and inodorous, but, when well triturated, the odor of prussic acid is given off.

It combines the properties of hydrocyanic acid with those of zinc, and has been used in epilepsy, chorea, and similar diseases, in doses of one-half to one grain.

It is wholly soluble in muriatic acid, precipitated white by carbonate of ammonia, dissolved again in an excess; and in this solution, no precipitate is caused by phosphate of soda, a white precipitate by sulphuret of hydrogen.

Zinci Ferrocyanidum. (*Ferrocyanuret of Zinc.*)

This salt has sometimes been mistaken for the former one, and care is necessary to distinguish them, as the cyanide is poisonous in the medicinal doses of the ferrocyanide. This is prepared by precipitating sulphate of zinc by ferrocyanide of potassium.

It is a white powder, similar in appearance to the former, but little soluble in boiling muriatic acid. It has been used in similar complaints as the former, in doses of two grains and more.

It may be considered pure, if it is of a purely white color, and yields nothing to cold muriatic acid.

Zinci Iodidum.

Two parts iodine, one part zinc, and four parts water, are digested until the color of iodine has disappeared; after filtration, it is evaporated until, when poured upon a cold slab, it hardens; a little iodine has then been expelled.

It is in white, very deliquescent pieces, forming a turbid solution with water and alcohol. It must be wholly soluble in carbonate of ammonia.

It is caustic and poisonous, and used only externally in aqueous solution, or in ointments, containing gr. xv to xxx to the ounce.

Zinci Lactas. (*Lactate of Zinc.*)

It is prepared by dissolving carbonate of zinc in lactic acid, or by double decomposition between hot concentrated solutions of lactate of potassa or lime and chloride of zinc.

It crystallizes in four-sided prisms, of an acid reaction, and a sour styptic taste; they require 58 parts of cold water for solution, and are nearly insoluble in alcohol.

It is used in epilepsy in doses of two grs. three times a day, gradually increasing the dose.

Valerianate of Zinc.

Prepared by decomposing sulphate of zinc with valerianate of soda in solution at 200° F. On evaporation, crystals of the valerianate collect on the surface, and are skimmed off, washed with cold water to separate adhering sulphate of soda, and dried. The salt is in pearly scales with a faint valerian odor, astringent metallic taste; sparingly soluble in water, more so in alcohol. It is a good deal prescribed, perhaps more than any other salt of valerianic acid, being adapted to a variety of nervous affections. DOSE, gr. j to ij in pill, repeated at intervals.

CADMIUM.

Cadmium is a scarce metal which usually accompanies the zinc ores; it was discovered in 1817 as an impurity in medicinal preparations of zinc. It has a white tin color, a high metallic lustre, is very malleable, and oxidizes slowly in the air; its specific gravity is 8.6. Its salts are isomorphous with the corresponding salts of zinc. Its compound with oxygen is oxide of cadmium, CdO.

Tests for Oxide of Cadmium.—Sulphuretted hydrogen and sulphuret of ammonium cause a bright yellow precipitate, insoluble in an excess; ammonia a white precipitate, easily soluble in excess; potassa and the alkaline carbonates a white insoluble precipitate; zinc precipitates the metal. The compounds of cadmium when mixed with oxalate of potassa and exposed to the inner flame of the blowpipe, produce a brownish yellow incrustation without any metallic globules.

PREPARATIONS OF CADMIUM.

Cadmii sulphas, CdO,SO_3+4HO, colorless crystals, soluble in water.
Cadmii iodidum, CdI, soluble in alcohol and water.

Sulphate of Cadmium.

Granulated cadmium is dissolved in dilute sulphuric acid; the solution may be much accelerated by adding small portions of nitric acid; it is then evaporated to dryness to expel the excess of nitric acid; redissolved in water and crystallized.

The crystals are six-sided prisms, easily soluble in water, insoluble in alcohol, and containing 25 per cent. of water.

It is used almost exclusively in nervous inflammatory diseases of the eye and ear, in solutions containing a grain to an ounce or two of rose-water, or about five grains to a drachm of ointment; for injections to the ear, somewhat stronger.

It may be considered pure when sulphuretted hydrogen causes a purely yellow precipitate, the filtrate from which leaves no residue on evaporation.

Iodide of Cadmium.

This salt has been proposed as a substitute for iodide of lead, the intense yellow color of which is sometimes objectionable. It is prepared by dissolving iodine with granulated cadmium under water, and evaporating the solution.

It crystallizes in colorless six-sided tabular crystals, soluble in alcohol and water, and fusible on the application of heat.

NICKEL.

This is a rare metal obtained from an ore of arsenic found in Westphalia. It is fixed in the fire, and is hence left behind after the distillation of arsenic, and when purified is found in commerce as a white, hard, malleable magnetic metal, capable of receiving a lustre rivalling silver, sp. gr. 8.82; it is not oxidized by the air, or is little attacked by acids, except in the presence of nitric acid which dissolves it freely; most of its salts possess a pale green color.

Nickel is recognized by the following tests: Caustic alkalies give a pale apple-green precipitate, insoluble in excess, but soluble in solution of carbonate of ammonia, yielding a greenish-blue liquid. Ammonia gives a similar precipitate, soluble in excess, and yielding a deep purplish-blue solution. Ferrocyanide of potassium gives a greenish-white precipitate. Sulphuretted hydrogen occasions no change in solutions of nickel containing the mineral acids, but in alkaline solutions gives a black precipitate.

Sulphate of Nickel. (*Niccoli Sulphas.*)

This salt is formed by dissolving carbonate or oxide of nickel in dilute sulphuric acid, and gently concentrating by evaporation so that crystals may form.

It is in emerald-green prismatic crystals, efflorescent, soluble in 3 parts of cold water, insoluble in alcohol and ether. It has a sweet, astringent taste, composition NiO,SO_3+7HO.

This salt is used as a tonic. Prof. Simpson employed it successfully in a case of obstinate periodic headache. The dose is from ½ grain to 1 grain, three times a day, given in the form of pill or simple solution.

COBALT.

This metal is found like the foregoing in ores of arsenic, and the crude mineral, sold as fly-stone by druggists, appears to be one of these cobalt and arsenic ores. The metal itself is white, brittle, strongly magnetic, unchanged in the air, feebly acted on by dilute hydrochloric and sulphuric acids.

Solutions of the salts of cobalt are known as follows: Solution of ammonia gives a blue precipitate, slightly soluble in excess, giving a brownish-red color. Solution of potassa a blue precipitate, turning to violet and red when the liquor is heated. Sulphuretted hydrogen produces no change in acid solutions, but with ammonia gives a black precipitate. Melted with borax before the blowpipe it gives a bead of magnificent blue color.

Protoxide of Cobalt.

This is the only compound used in medicine; it has been employed as a remedy in rheumatism. It is formed by precipitation from the nitrate or chloride with carbonate of soda, washing and igniting. Its chief use is in forming beautiful blue colors in glass, enamels, &c.

CHAPTER VIII.

ON LEAD, SILVER, BISMUTH.

PLUMBUM. (LEAD.)

METALLIC lead is not used in medicine, nor is it officinal for use in preparing any of its salts. It is abundantly diffused in the form of galena, a native sulphuret, which is extensively worked in this country for the production of the metal. Exposed for a long time to its influence, individuals exhibit symptoms of slow poisoning, called lead colic. In over-doses its salts are poisons.

Lead is a soft bluish-colored metal, very malleable and fusible; its properties are familiar to most. It forms five oxides, of which the one most important in a pharmaceutical point of view is the protoxide.

The lead salts show the following reactions:—

A brown or black precipitate by sulphuretted hydrogen and sulphuret of ammonium; a white precipitate by muriatic acid and soluble chlorides, soluble in much water; a yellow precipitate by iodide of potassium, soluble in boiling solutions of alkaline chlorides and iodides; a yellow precipitate by chromate of potassa, scarcely soluble in dilute nitric acid; a gray metallic precipitate by tin and zinc; a white precipitate by ferrocyanuret of potassium.

PREPARATIONS OF LEAD.

Plumbi oxidum semivitreum, O, litharge. Yellow or reddish flakes or powder.
Emplastrum plumbi. See fixed oils, also plasters.
Plumbi oxidum rubrum, 2(or 3)$PbO+PbO_2$. Red lead. Bright red powder.
Plumbi acetas, $PbO,\overline{Ac},3HO$. Matted acicular crystals, whitish by efflorescence.
Liquor plumbi subacetatis. A clear heavy liquid, depositing white carbonate.
Liquor plumbi subacet. dilutus. f℥ij liq. plumb. subacet. to Oj.
Plumbi carbonas, PbO,CO_2. A heavy, white, opaque powder.
Plumbi nitras, PbO,NO_5. White crystals, soluble in water, disinfectant.
Plumbi iodidum, PbI. A bright yellow amorphous powder, used in ointment.
Plumbi chloridum, PbCl. Flat needle-shaped crystals, used externally.
Plumbi tannas, cataplasm de cubitum.

Plumbi Oxidum Semivitreum, U. S. (*Semivitrified Oxide of Lead, Litharge.*)

Generally obtained as a secondary product in the cupellation of argentiferous galenas, when the oxide becomes fused or semivitrified, and is driven off in hard particles of a scaly texture. English litharge is the best. It is in the form of small red or orange red scales, devoid of smell or taste; soluble, or almost entirely so, in dilute nitric acid. It is much contaminated with iron and copper, and usually contains a little carbonic acid. If carbonate of lead is present, effervescence takes place with dilute nitric acid; this solution has a green color if copper, and a yellow or brownish color if iron is present. It is chiefly used for its effect on fixed oils, with which it combines, and hence occasions paint, to which it is added, to dry and harden rapidly. (See *Emplastrum Plumbi.*)

Plumbi Oxidum Rubrum. (*Red Lead.*)

The yellow protoxide of lead, which is commercially known by the name of massicot, is introduced into a reverberating furnace, there to be calcined for 48 hours, heated to redness and allowed to cool slowly. Or the hot massicot is cooled by being sprinkled with water, and after levigation heated in closed tin boxes to redness; the slower the product is allowed to cool, the finer will be the color.

It is a heavy scaly powder of a bright red color, which appears yellow when rubbed upon paper. Before the blowpipe upon charcoal it is wholly reduced to the metallic state; exposed to the light it is blackened somewhat, by being partially reduced.

Its chief use is as a red paint; it enters into the composition of a few ancient plasters. (See *Emplastrum.*)

Plumbi Acetas, U. S. (*Saccharum Saturni. Sugar of Lead.*)

Made by dissolving litharge in dilute acetic acid, evaporating the solution, and crystallizing; also by the direct action of vinegar upon sheets of lead partially exposed to the air, so as to become oxidized, when the oxide being dissolved in the acid, the salt may be obtained in spongy masses composed of interlaced acicular crystals, possessing an acetic odor, and sweet metallic taste; exposed to the air it effloresces slightly, is soluble in four times its weight of cold water, and much less of boiling water, communicating a turbidness to the solution from taking up CO_2, which ordinary water generally holds; this turbidness may be removed by the addition of a little acetic acid or vinegar.

It is precipitated as a white carbonate by carbonate of soda, a yellow iodide by iodide of potassium, and a black sulphuret by sulphuretted hydrogen. It is also incompatible with all acids, and with numerous soluble salts. If sugar of lead contains iron, ferrocyanuret of potassium will cause a bluish precipitate; if copper is present, the precipitate will have a reddish color.

Sugar of lead is very extensively employed, both internally and externally. It ranks as a sedative astringent, checking morbid discharges, diminishing the natural secretions, and is capable by various combinations of filling a variety of indications in disease. DOSE, gr. ss to iij in pill, care being taken not to induce its poisonous effects. Externally, it is used in solution from gr. j to gr. viij to f℥j as a sedative, astringent, and desiccant to inflammed parts.

Liquor Plumbi Subacetatis, U. S. (*Solution of Diacetate of Lead. Goulard's Extract. Strong Lead Water.*)

			Reduced.
Take of	Acetate of lead	℥xvj	℥ij.
	Semivitrified oxide of lead, in fine powder	℥ixss	ʒixss.
	Distilled water	Oiv	Oss.

Boil them together in a glass or porcelain vessel for half an hour, occasionally adding distilled water so as to preserve the measure, and filter through paper; keep the solution in closely-stopped bottles. By the action of litharge on acetate of lead, the diacetate is formed by an additional equivalent of the oxide entering into the composition of the salt.

This is one of the simple preparations readily prepared, even by the country practitioner. The litharge should be in very fine powder before commencing the process, and care should be taken to prevent its caking, and the consequent fracture of the vessel, by constant stirring; an evaporating dish will be found convenient, and in filtering, a covered funnel will be useful. It may be well to mention as necessary,

Fig. 206.

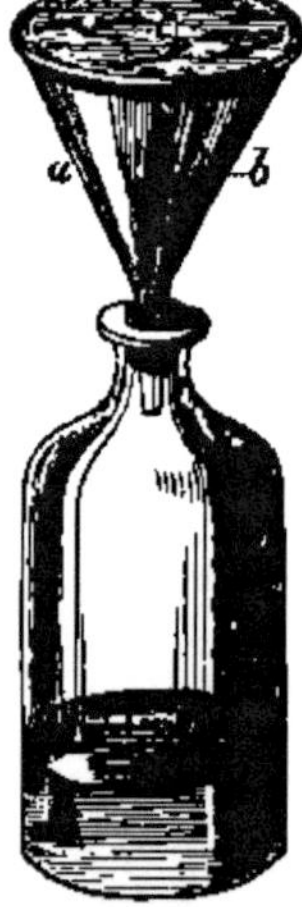

Closed filter.

Fig. 207.

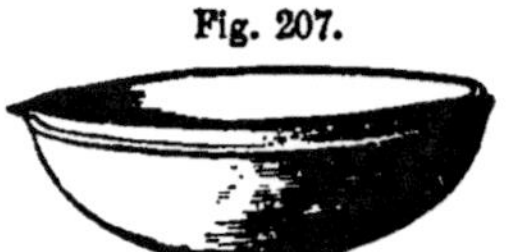

Evaporating dish.

in this case, that the filter should be strengthened by a little plain filter set into the funnel at its narrowest part, in which the plaited filter may rest.

Solution of subacetate of lead is a clear colorless liquid, sp. gr. 1.267, with an alkaline reaction, and sweet, metallic astringent taste; agrees with the acetate in most of its properties, except that it precipitates arabin from solution. It is remarkable for its great affinity for carbonic acid, which occasions a precipitate of carbonate of lead, merely on exposure to the air. If this solution should be contaminated with copper, this metal will be removed by immersing a strip of bright metallic lead in it. Diluted with water, it is applied as a sedative lotion to sprains, bruises, &c. (See *Ceratum, and Linimentum Plumbi Subacetatis.*)

Liquor Plumbi Subacetatis Dilutus, U. S. (*Lead-Water.*)

Take of	Solution of subacetate of lead . . .	fʒij.
	Distilled water	Oj.

Mix them.

The water containing carbonic acid will produce a precipitate of carbonate of lead, which exposure to the air will increase so that the preparation is liable to become inert, and should be mixed when required. Lead-water is generally regarded as a very weak preparation, and but for its popular employment as a cooling wash, might be made much stronger, as may be readily done by extemporaneous prescription.

Plumbi Carbonas, U.S. (*White Lead.*)

This important substance, which, as ground in oil, is extensively used as a pigment, is obtained by two methods: 1. By passing a stream of CO_2 through a solution of subacetate of lead. The CO_2 combines with the excess of PbO, and precipitates as PbO,CO_2, while a neutral acetate of lead remains in solution; this is boiled with a fresh addition of PbO, and again brought to the condition of subacetate, and treated as before with CO_2. This plan is pursued by the French and Swiss manufacturers. 2. Our own manufacturers cast the lead into thin sheets, which are then rolled into cylinders, five or six inches in diameter, and seven or eight high; each cylinder is placed in an earthen pot, containing Oss vinegar, the lead being supported by projecting pieces from contact with the vinegar. Strata of these pots are arranged in sheds, with refuse stable materials, which are giving off CO_2, and have a certain elevation of temperature due to fermentation. At the end of six weeks, the stacks are unpacked, and the sheet lead is found almost entirely converted into a flaky, white, friable substance, which is the white lead. This is separated, and reduced to fine powder. Carbonate of lead is a heavy, opaque substance, in powder or friable lumps, insoluble in water, of a fine white color, inodorous, and nearly insipid.

Carbonate of lead, to furnish a cheaper paint, is often mixed with sulphate of baryta, lime, or lead, or with carbonate of lime (chalk); the last impurity will remain behind when the article is dissolved in caustic potassa; the former are all insoluble in diluted nitric acid, which readily dissolves the carbonate of lead.

This is regarded as the most poisonous of the lead salts; it is employed externally as a dusting powder in excoriations of children, and as an astringent and sedative dressing to ulcers and inflamed surfaces.

Plumbi Nitras, U.S. (*Nitrate of Lead.*)

Litharge is dissolved in nitric acid, by the aid of heat; the liquid filtered, and set aside to crystallize; the PbO unites directly with the NO_5 to form the nitrate, which is an anhydrous salt, in beautiful white, nearly opaque, octahedral crystals, permanent in the air, of a sweet astringent taste, soluble in water and alcohol.

It is an effectual disinfectant, decomposing sulphuretted hydrogen, and the hydrosulphurets contained in putrescent animal fluids.

Ledoyen's Disinfecting Fluid, which is greatly esteemed abroad, is a solution of this salt in water ʒj to f℥j. It may be made directly by dissolving carbonate of lead, or litharge, in diluted nitric acid, to saturation, and will be found extremely useful in sick chambers, where the urine discharges are fetid, and infectious.

Plumbi Nitras Fusus.—If nitrate of lead is fused at a temperature not high enough to decompose much of it, it may be moulded like lunar caustic, and applied in a similar manner.

Plumbi Iodidum, U. S. (*Iodide of Lead.*)

Take of Nitrate of lead,
Iodide of potassium, each . ℥iv.
Distilled water . . . A sufficient quantity.

With the aid of heat, dissolve the nitrate of lead in Oiss, and the iodide of potassium in Oss of the distilled water, and mix the solutions. Having allowed the insoluble matter to subside, pour off the supernatant liquid, wash the precipitate with distilled water, and dry it with a gentle heat.

This process may be readily accomplished with the apparatus usually pertaining to a country practitioner's outfit; in fact, it is one of the easiest processes of the *Pharmacopœia*. The two salts dissolved separately, may be mixed in a wide mouth bottle, the precipitate collected in a plain filter (Fig. 208).

Fig. 208.

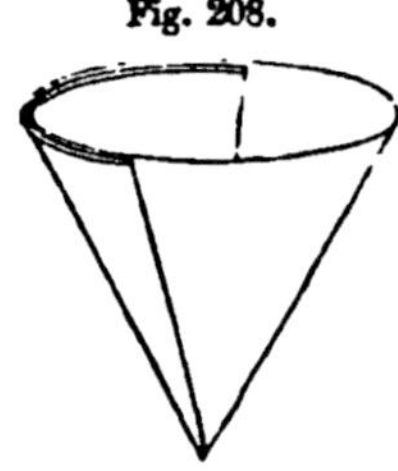

Plain filter for collecting precipitates.

Iodide of lead is a bright yellow, heavy, tasteless, inodorous powder, very sparingly soluble in cold, but readily soluble in boiling water, acetic acid, and alcohol. Fuses and sublimes yellow, but soon gives off violet vapors from decomposition.

It may be considered pure for medicinal use if two grains of it dissolve in one fluidounce of boiling water, and separate on cooling in brilliant crystalline powder.

This preparation is supposed to have the resolvent properties of iodine, combined with those peculiar to lead, and hence it is used in ointment to reduce indolent tumors, scrofulous and syphilitic.

Plumbi Chloridum.

Chloride of lead is obtained by precipitating a soluble lead salt, and may be crystallized from its hot solution in anhydrous flat needles, soluble in 135 parts of cold water.

It has been recommended as preferable to chloride of zinc in some diseases, especially cancer; externally as fomentations by dissolving from one-half to one drachm in a quart of water, and in ointments containing about ℈j or ʒss to the ounce.

Plumbi Tannas.

Under the name of *cataplasma ad decubitum*, the Prussian Pharmacopœia prepares tannate of lead in the following manner: 2 oz. oak bark boiled with a sufficient quantity of water down to eight ounces, is mixed with two ounces of solution of subacetate of lead, the precipitate separated by filtration, and used while still moist, mixed with two drachms of alcohol.

The tannate of lead is also prepared by precipitating tannic acid or an infusion of galls by acetate of lead. The precipitate is much darkened during washing and drying; it is made into an ointment by using one drachm of it to an ounce.

Argentum, *U. S.* (Silver.)

This well-known metal is placed in the list of the *Pharmacopœia* on account of its use in preparing the several salts. It is found most abundantly as sulphuret combined with copper, lead, and antimony; the argentiferous galena, already referred to as furnishing litharge, is the most abundant source of silver.

Its physical properties are sufficiently familiar. It is very malleable and ductile; its hardness is between that of copper and gold; sp. gr. 10.475 to 10.500.

Silver is freely soluble in nitric acid, and dissolves in sulphuric acid by the aid of heat. Its surface is rapidly tarnished by sulphuretted hydrogen. Its nitric acid solution should be nearly colorless, and when heated with an excess of chloride of sodium, should give a white precipitate with ammonia entirely soluble in an excess, and the filtered liquor should not be discolored by sulphuretted hydrogen. The alkaline carbonates, oxalates and ferrocyanides precipitate solutions of silver white, the alkaline arsenites and phosphates yellow. The arseniates red—the fixed alkalies brown—on the surface of metallic copper or zinc it is thrown down pure silver. All silver salts are more or less blackened by the influence of light, hence their use in photography.

Preparations of Silver.

Argenti nitras, AgO,NO_5 (crystals). Colorless; soluble in water; staining the skin.
Argenti nitras fusus. In sticks; thickness of a quill wrapped in paper.
Argenti oxidum, AgO. A blackish insoluble powder; soluble in ammonia.
Argenti cyanuretum, $AgCy$. A white, odorless, tasteless, insoluble powder.
Argenti chloridum, $AgCl$. White curdy precipitate changing color.
Argenti iodidum, AgI. Pale yellow, less soluble in ammonia.

Argenti Nitras, U. S. (*Crystallized Nitrate of Silver.*)

This salt is made by dissolving silver in nitric acid, evaporating the solution, and crystallizing. It is a new officinal, as in former editions of the *Pharmacopœia* the name was applied to the fused article in sticks. It is in crystals, which are anhydrous and colorless. Its purity is proven by precipitating its solution in distilled water with muriatic acid; the filtrate or evaporation must leave no residue. It is soluble in its weight of water, stains the skin black, and, when moistened and applied, acts as a caustic, which is its chief use. The crystallized article is preferred for solution, being less liable to be adulterated, and to decompose by the action of light, than the fused and wrapped article. Internally, it is given in pill with a tonic extract, preferably extract of quassia, as an astringent and alterative affecting the nervous system. When administered a long time it is capable of staining the whole surface of the body blue or lead color. Dose, gr. ¼ to gr. j.

Argenti Nitras Fusus, U. S. (*Lunar Caustic.*)

This is made as the preceding, except that instead of crystallizing it, the evaporation is carried further, and after becoming dry it is fused, and when it runs like oil is poured into moulds. It is thus obtained in sticks of suitable sizes for application as a caustic; it is, however, crystalline in structure, and very brittle. When the sticks have cooled, they are wrapped tightly in paper, in which they are sold. The crystals are more economical to the purchaser from having less paper weighed with them. The high heat applied in the fusion of nitrate of silver is apt to reduce a portion to the metallic condition, so that it has a gray color, and is not entirely soluble. The fusible nature of this salt enables us to introduce it readily into silver catheters and other surgical instruments, and also, by a very ready expedient, to point the sticks and alter them in size thus: Heat a half dollar held in a pair of pincers over a lamp, and apply to it the end of the stick of caustic, rotating it at such an angle as to give the requisite sharpness; if the coin is hot enough, it will fuse at the point and take the shape desired.

The extensive use of the nitrate and its high price lead to the admixture of nitrate of potassa, especially with the fused article; this adulteration may be detected as described in the case of the crystallized article, or by passing a stream of sulphuretted hydrogen into its solution till it ceases to throw down sulphuret of silver, then filtering and evaporating; there should be no residue. If 17 grains of the nitrate are dissolved in water, it should precipitate entirely the chlorine of 6 grains of common salt.

Chloride of silver is much introduced of latter years for the purpose of rendering the fused nitrate less brittle. This admixture should always be distinctly announced on the label. It renders the salt only partially soluble in water.

The stain of nitrate of silver on the fingers and on articles of clothing is sometimes very inconvenient; it may generally be removed by a little cyanide of potassium, or by moistening the part with tincture of iodine and immediately applying iodide of potassium, or ammonia, and then washing it off.

So numerous are the incompatibles of nitrate of silver that it should generally be prescribed in pill, and singly except with some vegetable excipient as white turpentine. It generally forms a white cloud, with the purest undistilled water, from the presence of chlorides, and in water containing organic matter throws down a brown precipitate.

Argenti Chloridum.

When a silver salt is brought in contact with muriatic acid, or a solution of a chloride, the result is always a white curdy precipitate of chloride of silver, which is insoluble in nitric acid, but dissolves freely, without residue, in ammonia.

It has been used in syphilis, epilepsy, dysentery, and other diseases, in doses from one to three grains several times a day.

Argenti Iodidum.

It is a pale yellow precipitate, caused in solution of silver by hydriodic acid or iodides; insoluble in nitric acid, and nearly insoluble in ammonia.

It has been used in similar complaints as the chloride, when the effect of iodine is desired. The dose is one or two grains.

Argenti Oxidum, U. S.

			Reduced.
Take of	Nitrate of silver . . .	℥iv.	℥ss.
	Distilled water . . .	Oss.	f℥j.
	Solution of potassa . .	Oiss, or q. s.	f℥iij.

Dissolve the nitrate of silver in the water, and add the solution of potassa as long as it produces a precipitate; wash the precipitate repeatedly with water, until the washings are nearly tasteless. Lastly, dry the powder, and keep it in a well-stopped bottle, protected from the light. This is a dark brown or black powder, insoluble in water, but soluble in ammonia and in acids. It may be considered pure if it is wholly soluble in ammonia and in nitric acid, and if the latter solution, when treated like the nitrate, leaves no residue. It is used instead of nitrate of silver for the tonic effects of the silver salts. Dose, gr. ss to gr. ij.

Argenti Cyanuretum, U. S. (*Cyanide of Silver.*)

The salt has been described in connection with its use in preparing hydrocyanic acid. It is a tasteless, white powder, insoluble in water, soluble in ammonia and in cyanide of potassium; and when decomposed by muriatic acid, the solution must not contain any fixed matter. When heated, it yields cyanogen and metallic silver.

Bismuthum, *U. S.* (Bismuth.)

This is a rare metal, of a pinkish-white color, found native; very brittle; fuses readily, and crystallizes; soluble in diluted nitric acid, and the nitrate is precipitated by water. It is chiefly prepared in Germany, whence it is exported; it generally contains both arsenic and copper, to free it from which, the following process is recommended: Heat to redness, in a covered crucible, a mixture of oxide or subnitrate of bismuth, with half its weight of charcoal, or mix sixteen ounces of the metal, powdered, with two ounces carbonate of soda, and two drachms of sulphur; mix, fuse for an hour, and separate the metal from the scoriæ.

It is little affected by the air; burns when strongly heated; sp. gr. 9.8 to 9.9. Sulphuretted hydrogen gives a black precipitate with its salts; the nitric solution is not precipitated by sulphuric acid. Chromate of potassa gives a yellow precipitate, differing from that of lead by being soluble in NO_5, and insoluble in KO. By alkalies a white precipitate is thrown down, insoluble in an excess; by carbonate of potassa, white; by ferrocyanuret of potassium, white; by iodide of potassium, brown; by iron, zinc, copper, cadmium, tin, and lead, in the metallic state. The soluble salts of bismuth are remarkable for dazzling white precipitate, produced on throwing their solution into a large amount of water.

Bismuth is used in the composition of type metal, solder, pewter, and fusible metal. Its medicinal salts are not numerous, but remarkable for rather unusual therapeutic properties.

Preparations of Bismuth.

Bismuthi subnitras, BiO_3,NO_5. Insoluble powder. Dose, gr. j to gr. vj.
Bismuthi subcarbonas, BiO_3,CO_2. Insoluble powder. Dose, gr. j to gr. vj.
Bismuthi valerianas. Remedy in neuralgia. Dose, gr. ss to gr. ij.

Bismuthi Subnitras, U. S.

By adding diluted nitric acid to bismuth, red fumes are given off; the metal is oxidized, and the oxide dissolved by the undecomposed acid, forming a solution of ternitrate of teroxide ($BiO_3,3NO_5$); this is thrown into water and decomposed. Four equivalents are resolved into three of neutral, generally called subnitrate (BiO_3,NO_5), and one of the nine nitrate ($BiO_3,9NO_5$); the latter remains in solution, while the officinal salt goes down as heavy white powder, almost insoluble, tasteless, odorless. It is darkened by sulphuretted hydrogen.

Impurities are detected in the nitric acid solution as follows:—

Sulphuric and muriatic acid by nitrate of baryta and of silver; baryta by sulphuric acid; magnesia in the filtrate from the precipitate by carbonate of ammonia in excess by phosphate of soda; lead or zinc by the black or white precipitate occasioned by sulphuretted hydrogen in the alkaline liquid from digesting the powder with caustic potassa; arsenic from the same solution, after supersaturating with muriatic acid, by a yellow precipitate caused by sulphuretted hydrogen.

It is a tonic and antispasmodic. Dose, gr. j to vj, and is employed as a cosmetic, and with asserted advantage in skin diseases.

Prof. Rogers, of the University of Pennsylvania, has ascertained that nearly all the subnitrate of bismuth of commerce contains arsenic, a fact which has induced a favorable disposition towards the substitution of subcarbonate for it in medicine. In toxicological investigations, the liability to the presence of arsenic from this source should not be forgotten.

Bismuthi Subcarbonas.

It is formed when a soluble salt of bismuth is gradually added to an alkaline carbonate. It is a white, tasteless powder, which, after being dissolved in nitric acid, is tested for its purity like the nitrate.

It is employed instead of the nitrate, being much more soluble in the gastric juice, besides being, from its mode of preparation, less liable to be contaminated with arsenic.

Bismuthi Valerianas.

By adding gradually the aqueous solution of nitrate of bismuth to valerianate of soda; the white precipitate is washed with water containing a small quantity of valerianic acid.

It has been brought to the notice of the medical profession as a remedy for neuralgic affections, in doses of from one-half to two grains three or four times a day.

CHAPTER IX.

ANTIMONY AND ARSENIC PREPARATIONS.

ANTIMONY.

THIS metal is imported from France under the name of *Regulus of Antimony;* it is a brittle metal, usually of a lamellated texture, of a bluish white color; its Latin name, *Stibium*, as abbreviated Sb, furnishes its symbol. It forms four combinations with oxygen, suboxide, Sb_2O_6 teroxide, SbO_3, antimonious acid, SbO_4, and antimonic acid, SbO_5. Teroxide and the tersulphuret enter into the officinal compounds.

Tests for Antimony.—In its soluble salts, *antimony* is recognized by the following tests:—

Sulphuretted hydrogen and sulphuret of ammonium cause in acid solutions an orange colored precipitate; alkalies and their carbonates, a white, bulky one; zinc, a black powder of the metallic antimony; zinc and sulphuric acid evolve antimoniuretted hydrogen, SbH_3, which burns with a bluish-green color; on a porcelain cup, held in the flame, a black spot of very little lustre is deposited; if the antimoniuretted hydrogen is passed through a tube, the middle of which is heated to redness, a bright metallic mirror is formed in the cooler part of the tube; this mirror will disappear if a stream of dry sulphuretted hydrogen is passed through the tube, while the metallic mirror is heated, and sulphuret of antimony of a reddish or blackish color will make its appearance; this disappears entirely if through the tube be passed a stream of dry muriatic acid gas, by which chloride of antimony is carried over and may be condensed in water, there to be recognized by the precipitates with the above tests. Before the blowpipe, oxide of antimony, when mixed with carbonate of soda and cyanide of potassium, yield globules, and a white pulverulent and crystalline incrustation of the oxide.

Antimonic Acid.—Its salts are insoluble with the exception of antimoniate of potassa, which is a test for soda salts. This antimoniate may be recognized by yielding precipitates with the soluble salts of all other bases; these precipitates when mixed with chloride of ammonium and heated, are decomposed into water, chloride of antimony, chloride of the metallic base and ammonia; the chloride of antimony is volatile. For the quantitative determination of antimonic acid, H. Rose uses the antimoniate of soda, and calculates from the remaining chloride of sodium the equivalent quantity of antimonic acid. If insoluble antimoniates are boiled with muriatic acid, with the addition of some tartaric acid, terchloride of antimony enters into solution, there to be recognized like the salts of oxide of antimony.

Preparations of Antimony.

Antimonii sulphuretum, SbS_3. Native black sulphuret or crude antimony.
Antimonii sulphuretum præcipitatum, SbO_3+5SbS_3+16HO. (?) Reddish-brown powder.
Kermes mineral, SbO_3+2SbS_3. Dark-brown powder.
Sodii et antimonii sulphuretum, $3NaS+SbS_5+15HO$. Colorless crystals.
Antimonii quinque sulphuretum, SbS_5. Orange-colored powder. Golden sulphur.
Calcii et antimonii sulphuretum. Mixture of SbO_3,SbS_3,CaS. Light-brown powder.
Antimonii et potassæ tartras, $SbO_3,KO,C_8H_4O_{10}+3HO$. Translucent crystals.
Vinum antimonii. Gr. ij to f℥j white wine =¼ gr. to f℥j.
Pulvis antimonialis. Variable mixture of SbO_3,SbO_5 with CaO,PO_5, &c.
Antimonii chloridum, $SbCl_3$. Colorless or yellowish liquid (butter of antimony).
Antimonii oxidum, SbO_3. White inodorous powder.
Potassæ antimonias, KO,SbO_5+HO. White insoluble powder.

Antimonii Sulphuretum, U. S. (*Black Sulphuret of Antimony.*)

This drug should be procured in powder somewhat purified by fusion and levigated, in which condition it is kept by the druggists; it may then be considered as tolerably pure SbS_3; it should be soluble in boiling muriatic acid, giving off sulphuretted hydrogen, terchloride remaining in solution.

It often contains arsenic, which may be found out by fusing it in small quantities with pure saltpetre, and testing the solution with nitrate of silver; antimoniate of silver is white, the arseniate has a reddish-brown color.

Antimonii Sulphuretum Præcipitatum, U. S. (*Precipitated Sulphuret of Antimony.*)

This officinal salt is made by boiling black sulphuret of antimony with a solution of potassa, straining it, and while yet hot, dropping into it diluted sulphuric acid as long as it produces a precipitate, which, being washed and dried, and rubbed into a fine powder, constitutes the officinal precipitated sulphuret.

In this process, the alkali decomposes a portion of the black sulphuret, forming sulphuret of potassium, and holds in solution both the undecomposed tersulphuret and the teroxide liberated by the alkali. On the addition to this of an acid, the sulphuret of potassium being decomposed and the excess of potassa neutralized, the mixed tersulphuret and teroxide are thrown down, so that this powder has the complex composition represented in the syllabus. According to Liebig it is amorphous, hydrated, tersulphuret of antimony, which loses part of its water by drying, the other part is only given off by exposure to a temperature of 480°.

This powder is of a color varying from yellowish-red to reddish-brown, insoluble in water, but nearly soluble in solution of potassa. It is used as an alterative and diaphoretic, especially in combination with calomel and guaiacum, as in Plummer's pill, or with extract of conium or hyoscyamus in the treatment of chronic rheumatism.

As its action depends very much upon the amount of acid in the stomach, it is of varying activity. Its dose is from gr. j to iij, twice a day.

Kermes Mineral. (*Oxysulphuret of Antimony.*)

If the solution obtained by boiling the black sulphuret in potassa, instead of being treated with sulphuric acid as in the foregoing process, be allowed to cool after filtration, a dark brown powder will fall, which will consist, according to Berzelius and H. Rose, of tersulphuret of antimony, with some antimonio-sulphuret of potassium or sodium; if soda had been used instead of potassa, and if the boiling has been long continued, also oxide of antimony usually in microscopic six-sided prisms. If precipitated sulphuret of antimony had been used, and the boiling continued for about an hour, the precipitate on cooling, besides a small quantity of alkaline sulphuret, is principally, according to Liebig, $2SbS_3+SbO_3$. There are modifications of the process of manufacture adapted to yielding this preparation, and the result is by no means uniform. A process yielding a large proportion of kermes is by fusing crude antimony with carbonate of soda or potassa, boiling the fused mass repeatedly with water, and filtering while yet hot. It likewise contains variable proportions of crystallized oxide of antimony. To obtain a uniform result, Dulk has proposed to make this preparation by fusing together precipitated sulphuret, and teroxide of antimony and rubbing the mass into a fine powder. The dose, in view of this various composition, may be stated at from gr. ½ to gr. iij.

Sodii et Antimonii Sulphuretum. (*Antimonio-Sulphuret of Sodium.*)

This double salt, which is officinal in the *Pharmacopœias* of Slesvie-Holstein, Saxony and others, has been discovered by Schlippe, and is remarkable for its readiness to crystallize with an unvariable composition, and for its use in the preparation of golden sulphur.

It is prepared by slaking 2 parts of burned lime in an iron vessel, and dissolving in it 2 parts of sulphur by boiling with 40 parts of water; the clear liquid is decomposed by 6 parts of crystallized carbonate of soda; the filtrate boiled with 2 parts of finely-powdered black sulphuret of antimony, evaporated, a little caustic soda added and crystallized.

Another method is to fuse for half an hour a mixture of equal parts of anhydrous sulphate of soda, sulphuret of antimony, and a quarter part of charcoal, and after separating the metal and powdering the mass, boiling it in water and crystallizing as above.

It occurs in colorless or yellowish tetrahedrons, easily soluble in water, insoluble in alcohol, and decomposed by acids, alkalies and metallic salts. It contains 45.29 per cent. of SbS_5.

Golden Sulphuret of Antimony. (*Golden Sulphur.*)

Antimonii sulphuretum aureum, as formerly prepared, was deposited on the addition to the solution from which kermes has been precipitated, of an acid; it varies in composition and in color according to the degree of change which has taken place spontaneously, and the consequent proportion of sulphur thrown down with the antimonial sulphuret and oxide.

As now prepared, it is of a uniform composition, being the *quinque sulphuret of antimony*, which contains 61.8 per cent. metallic antimony. Schlippe's sulphuret of antimony and sodium is dissolved in 6 parts of distilled water, and the solution gradually added to a mixture of $\frac{1}{10}$ strong sulphuric acid and 10 of water; the precipitate is well washed and rapidly dried.

It is a dark orange-colored powder, nearly tasteless and inodorous, insoluble in water and alcohol; by alkalies it is decomposed, an antimonio-sulphuret being dissolved and antimoniate of alkali left behind; it is soluble without residue in sulphuret of ammonium. The quinque sulphuret of antimony is given in doses of $\frac{1}{4}$ to 1 grain.

Calcii et Antimonii Sulphuretum.

This soluble sulphuret, as used by Hufeland, was an uncertain preparation, containing sulphuret of antimony and calcium, sulphate and antimoniate of lime. It was prepared by exposing to a red heat a mixture of carbonate of lime, sulphur and sulphuret of, or metallic, antimony.

No double sulphuret with calcium has yet been obtained resembling the foregoing antimonio-sulphuret of sodium. Duflos proposes to mix intimately 1 part of Liebig's kermes with 4 parts of sulphuret of calcium, by which process a brownish powder is obtained, almost entirely soluble in water, and decomposed by acids into sulphuretted hydrogen, and a bright red sulphuret of antimony.

It is a mixture of the two sulphurets with oxide of antimony, and has no claims to the rank of a chemical compound. It has been used in various skin diseases, &c., in larger doses than the other antimonials.

Antimonii et Potassæ Tartras, U. S. *Antimonii Potassio Tartras.* (*Tartar Emetic.*)

This preparation, as its name implies, is a double salt, consisting of the oxide of antimony, and potassa, united, each with an equivalent of tartaric acid. The first step in its preparation is the precipitation of teroxide of antimony, SbO_3; this is accomplished by boiling the black sulphuret with muriatic acid, forming chloride of antimony, and liberating sulphuretted hydrogen; the chloride is then thrown into water, which, as already stated, decomposes it, precipitating oxychloride (oxide of antimony contaminated with chloride, $9SbO_3 + 2SbCl_3$). The second step is to boil this oxychloride with bitartrate of potassa. The oxide unites with the excess of tartaric acid of the bitartrate, forming a double tartrate of oxide of antimony and potassa, in the same way that oxide of iron is combined, so as to form, with the bitartrate, the double tartrate of iron and potassa, &c. (See, also, *Sodæ et Potassæ Tartras*, and *Potassæ Tartras.*) The chloride of antimony present in the oxychloride is decomposed by water, during the boiling, into oxide and free muriatic acid, the former aiding in the production of the tartar emetic, and the latter by its presence preventing the precipitation of iron and other metallic impurities, which would otherwise contaminate the product.

Arsenic if present in the sulphuret of antimony employed, is easily prevented from contaminating the product, by allowing the hot solution to drop into half its measure of strong alcohol, by which tartar emetic is at once precipitated in a crystalline powder.

Tartar emetic crystallizes in beautiful colorless, rhombic, octahedral crystals, which effloresce and become opaque by exposure to the air. It is wholly soluble in 15 parts of water. Its solution does not yield a precipitate with chloride of barium, or, if very dilute, with nitrate of silver. The watery solution is remarkable for decomposing rapidly, forming algæ.

It is incompatible with acids, alkalies, and alkaline carbonates. Astringent solutions precipitate it in an insoluble form.

Internally administered, tartar emetic, in doses of gr. ij to iv, is a powerful emetic; in doses of gr. 1/16 to 1/4, it is a diaphoretic and expectorant; gr. 1/8 to gr. j, is a decided sedative. It is very much prescribed, and in a great variety of diseases, both alone and combined with other remedies. Externally, it is applied in ointment to raise a peculiar pustular eruption.

If arsenic should be present, it may be discovered by fusing a sample of the tartar emetic with pure nitrate of potassa, and testing the neutralized solution with nitrate of silver, which by producing a reddish-brown precipitate, shows a contamination with arsenic.

Vinum Antimonii, U. S.

Take of Tartrate of antimony and potassa	℈j.
White wine	f℥x.

Dissolve the tartrate of antimony and potassa in the wine. This is best done by trituration in a mortar, as explained under the head of Solution. It is regarded an improvement by some to dissolve the antimonial with an ounce of water, and then bring up the quantity to the required measure by the addition of wine.

DOSE, as an expectorant diaphoretic, ♏x to xxx, at intervals; its chief use is to furnish a convenient method of giving very divided doses of the salt; f℥j contains 1/4 grain.

Pulvis Antimonialis. Pulvis Jacobi. (*James' Powder.*)

This is directed to be made by mixing tersulphuret of antimony with horn shavings, throwing into a red-hot crucible, and stirring till vapor no longer rises, then rubbing the residue to powder and heating it to redness for two hours. Reduced to a fine powder, the resulting compound is constituted chiefly of a mixture in variable quantities of teroxide of antimony (SbO_3), antimonic acid (SbO_5), with phosphate of lime. It is a white, inodorous, tasteless, insoluble powder, which was formerly much in use as an alterative and diaphoretic, and was officinal previous to 1830. Its dose is gr. iij to gr. x, every three or four hours, in fevers.

Antimonii Chloridum. (*Butter of Antimony.*)

In accordance with the *Prussian Pharmacopœia*, this preparation is made by dissolving 1 lb. of black sulphuret of antimony in 4 lbs. of crude muriatic acid. Sulphuretted hydrogen is evolved, which makes it necessary to operate in the open air, or conduct the gas into water or a chimney. After filtration, it is evaporated to 1½ lb., and a mixture added of ¾ lb. muriatic acid, and 1½ lb. water.

It is a colorless or yellowish liquid, sp. gr. 1.4, free from arsenic and lead, and is decomposed by water, oxide of antimony with some chloride being precipitated; this precipitate was formerly employed in medicine under the name of *Pulvis Algaroth.*

Powder of chloride of antimony has been used as a caustic, producing a white scab with little pain; it may be made into ointments containing one drachm to the ounce, or if intended for diseases of the eye, from 10 to 15 grains to an ounce.

Antimonii Oxidum. (*Teroxide of Antimony.*)

If the precipitate occasioned by throwing the chloride into water, is digested with a weak solution of carbonate of soda and subsequently well washed, oxide of antimony remains behind as a white, insoluble, inodorous powder.

It is used for preparing tartar emetic, but has been also employed in medicine; the following preparations are enjoying an increased reputation in Philadelphia:—

Tyson's Antimonial Powder, No. 1.

Take of Teroxide of antimony . . . 2 grains.
Phosphate of lime . . . 18 grains.

Mix well.

Tyson's Antimonial Powder, No. 2.

Take of Teroxide of antimony . . . 2 grains.
Phosphate of lime,
Sulphate of potassa, of each . 9 grains.

Mix well.

These powders are used in doses of from 5 to 10 grains.

Potassæ Antimonias.

Formerly preparations were employed in medicine under the name of *antimonium diaphoreticum non-ablutum* and *ablutum*, which were of variable composition. A preparation similar to the last named is officinal in the *Prussian Pharmacopœia*, which is nearly pure antimoniate of potassa. It is prepared by throwing into a red-hot crucible, small quantities of an intimate mixture of 1 part metallic antimony and 2 parts nitrate of potassa, continuing the heat for half an hour, and washing with water.

It is a white inodorous and tasteless powder, which is a good diaphoretic in doses of ½ to 1 grain.

Arsenicum, U. S.

This metal, which is made officinal on account of its use in preparing its iodide, exists in nature in combination with nickel and cobalt. Owing to its volatile and oxidizable character, it is conveniently collected as arsenious acid, during the smelting of these ores. When pure, metallic arsenic is brittle and granular, steel-colored, but usually dull and blackish on the surface. When heated, it sublimes, giving off a garlicky odor, and if exposed to the air, absorbing oxygen and passing into arsenious acid, AsO_3. It forms, by higher oxidation, arsenic acid, AsO_5; and also combines readily with sulphur.

Pure metallic arsenic may be readily obtained by mixing, in a suitable reduction tube, arsenious acid and charcoal, and applying heat, when the metal will be sublimed.

Arsenic may be detected in minute quantities; though its detection requires many nice and difficult manipulations.

It is well for the inexperienced to avoid the responsibility of such examinations in important cases, as there are many precautions necessary to an accurate and definite result.

The following are the most important reactions:—

Tests for Arsenious Acid.—Nitrate of silver produces a yellow precipitate, soluble in nitric acid and ammonia; sulphate of copper causes a yellowish green precipitate; alkaline arsenites with an excess of alkali, throw down, when boiled with a few drops of sulphate of copper, a red precipitate of suboxide of copper, oxidizing at the same time the arsenious to arsenic acid; sulphuretted hydrogen and sulphuret of ammonium cause in acid solutions a yellow precipitate of AsS_3, soluble in alkalies, their carbonates, bicarbonates, and sulphurets, nearly insoluble in muriatic acid, decomposed and dissolved by nitric acid, and depositing a metallic mirror, if mixed with carbonate of soda and suddenly subjected to an intense heat in a glass tube through which a current of perfectly dry hydrogen passes.

Compounds of arsenious acid, if subjected to the influence of water, zinc and sulphuric acid, yield arseniuretted hydrogen, AsH_3, which burns with a bluish color, the flame at the same time giving off white vapors of garlic odor, which condense upon cold objects. Upon a porcelain dish held in the flame, metallic arsenic will be deposited in blackish-brown spots, of a bright metallic lustre. Arseniuretted hydrogen passed through a tube heated to redness, yields a bright metallic mirror; this in a feeble stream of sulphuretted hydrogen is converted into yellow sulphuret of arsenic, which is not affected by a current of muriatic acid gas.

Compounds of arsenious acid, if mixed with carbonate of soda and cyanide of potassium, and heated to redness in a glass tube, through which a slow stream of dry carbonic acid passes, yields in the colder parts a beautiful metallic mirror; this is a most delicate test for arsenious acid.

Before the blowpipe upon charcoal, arsenious acid, whether free or in compounds, is reduced and reoxidized, thus producing a characteristic garlic odor.

Tests for Arsenic Acid.—Sulphuretted hydrogen and sulphuret of ammonium cause in acid solutions a yellow precipitate of AsS_5; nitrate of silver produces a reddish-brown precipitate, sulphate of copper a greenish-blue; sulphurous acid reduces it to arsenious acid; before the blowpipe, with cyanide of potassium and with zinc and sulphuric acid the reactions are as above.

PREPARATIONS OF ARSENIC.

Acidum arseniosum, AsO_3. White opaque, sometimes translucent masses.
Liquor potassæ arsenitis, AsO_3 and KO,CO_2, 64 grains each to Oj; gr. iv. AsO_3=f℥j.
Liquor sodæ arsenitis, AsO_3 and NaO,CO_2, 60 grains each to Oj; gr. $3\frac{3}{4}$ AsO_3=f℥j.
Acidum arsenicum, AsO_5; not used in medicine.
Ammoniæ arsenias, $2NH_4O,HO,AsO_5$; colorless rhombic prisms.
Liquor ammoniæ arseniatis, gr. j to f℥j; contains one-eight-hundredth As.
Sodæ arsenias, $2NaO,HOAsO_5+24HO$; isomorphous with phosphate of soda.
Liquor sodæ arseniatis, gr. j to f℥j; contains one-seven-hundredth As.
Ferri arsenias, $2FeO,AsO_5+2Fe_2O_3,AsO_5+12HO$; dark green powder.
Arsenici iodidum, AsI_3. A soluble orange-red salt.
Liquor hydrargyri et arsenici iodidi. AsI_3 and HgI_2, of each 70 grains to Oj.

Acidum Arseniosum, U. S. (*White Arsenic.*)

As before stated, this compound is a collateral product in the smelting of cobalt ores. These ores, which are worked extensively in Bohemia and Saxony, furnish the supplies of arsenic to commerce. It comes in broken masses; sometimes translucent and sometimes opaque, white or buff-colored. Soluble in about 100 parts of cold water; more soluble in boiling water, which, on cooling, deposits octahedral crystals. It should be preferred for chemical uses in mass, though the powder, which is liable to adulteration, answers well for common purposes.

In medicine, it is used as an alterative and febrifuge. DOSE, $\frac{1}{16}$ to $\frac{1}{8}$ grain.

Externally it is occasionally applied in cancerous affections. Arsenious acid is well known to be a violent corrosive poison, and being cheap and abundantly sold as a poison for rats and for other purposes, is apt to be taken accidentally or with criminal design. The best antidote is *hydrated peroxide of iron*, which is described in its appropriate place. It should be given in tablespoonful doses, repeated every ten minutes, till a large excess has been given.

Liquor Potassæ Arsenitis, U. S. (*Fowler's Solution.*)

Take of Arsenious acid, in small fragments,

Pure carbonate of potassa, each	. Sixty-four grains.
Distilled water	. A sufficient quantity.
Compound spirit of lavender .	. Half a fluidounce.

Boil the arsenious acid and carbonate of potassa in a glass vessel or porcelain capsule, with twelve fluidounces of distilled water, till the acid is entirely dissolved; to the solution, when cold, add the spirit of lavender, and afterwards sufficient distilled water to make it fill exactly the measure of a pint.

This very popular medicine is so simple in its mode of preparation as to be conveniently made by the country practitioner. It will be found to facilitate its completion, to triturate the arsenic into a fine powder before introducing it into the flask or capsule. The officinal recipe directs pure carbonate of potassa, KO,CO_2; but it is more common to use the ordinary granulated article $2(KO,CO_2)\,3(HO)$, which, although usually contaminated with a little silica, and differing in its combining proportion by reason of the water it contains, is quite satisfactory. Fowler's Mineral Solution has a characteristic reddish, almost opalescent appearance, a faint odor of lavender, and very little taste; by some it is stated to be a solution of arsenious acid in the alkaline solution; by others, a solution of arsenite of potassa. Four grains of arsenious acid are used to each fluidounce. DOSE, ♏iij to xv.

Liquor Sodæ Arsenitis. (*Harle's Solution.*)

This preparation is very similar to Fowler's solution; the principal difference being the substitution of soda for potassa. 30 grains of arsenious acid and dry carbonate of soda are digested with 6 ounces of distilled water, and after solution, sufficient cinnamon water is added to make the whole measure eight fluidounces.

It is used for the same purposes and in the same doses as Fowler's solution.

Arsenic Acid.

If arsenious acid diffused in water is heated, and nitric acid in small quantities added until nitrous acid fumes cease to be given off, the solution contains arsenic acid. An addition of muriatic acid to the water accelerates the reaction, but is not indispensably necessary.

When evaporated to dryness and fusion without carrying the heat too high, arsenic acid appears as a colorless or white vitreous mass, free of water of crystallization, deliquescent, and sometimes forming crystals containing water. It is exceedingly poisonous, has not been used in medicine in its free state, but the following compositions have of late been employed.

Ammoniæ Arsenias. (*Arseniate of Ammonia.*)

To prepare the dry salt, a concentrated solution of arsenic acid is mixed with concentrated ammonia until a precipitate commences to appear; on setting aside, colorless oblique rhombic prisms are deposited; they are efflorescent in the air, and lose ammonia.

It is a very poisonous salt, exhibiting in a high degree the alterative effects of arsenic; the dose is $\frac{1}{24}$ to $\frac{1}{18}$ grain.

Liquor Ammoniæ Arseniatis. (*Biette's Arsenical Solution.*)

One grain of arseniate of ammonia is dissolved in one ounce of water; the dose is 20 minims to half a drachm.

Sodæ Arsenias. (*Arseniate of Soda.*)

A diluted solution of arsenic acid is saturated with a solution of carbonate of soda, and evaporated to crystallization. It is isomorphous with the corresponding phosphate of soda, and, like it, crystallizes with 24 and 14 equiv. of water. It is efflorescent, and not used in medicine.

Liquor Sodæ Arseniatis. (*Pearson's Arsenical Solution.*)

Arseniate of soda is allowed to effloresce by exposure to the air; after it ceases to lose weight, it is dissolved in distilled water in the proportion of one grain to the ounce.

This solution contains rather more arsenic than Biette's liquor; it is considered milder than it, and given in the same doses; in minute doses, it is asserted to be a reliable remedy against salivation.

Ferri Arsenias.

Arseniate of soda or ammonia produces in the solution of protochloride of iron a white precipitate, which, during washing and drying, assumes a dirty green color by being converted into a ferrosoferric salt. In cancer, psoriasis, &c., it has been given in doses of $\frac{1}{16}$ to $\frac{1}{12}$ grain, usually combined with phosphate of iron; externally it is used in ointments containing about half a drachm to an ounce.

Arsenici Iodidum, U. S. (*Iodide of Arsenic.*)

Take of Arsenic (the metal) . . . A drachm.
Iodine . . . . . . Five drachms.

Rub the arsenic in a mortar until reduced to a very fine powder free from metallic lustre, then add the iodine, and rub them together till they are thoroughly mixed, then put the mixture into a small flask or test-tube, loosely stopped, and heat it very gently until liquefaction occurs, then incline the vessel in different directions in order that any portion of the iodine which may have condensed on its inner surface may be returned into the fused mass. Lastly, pour the melted iodide on a porcelain slab, and when it is cold break it into pieces and put it into a bottle, which is to be well stopped. This is an orange-red crystalline solid, readily reduced to powder, entirely soluble in water, and wholly volatilized by heat. It is seldom prescribed extemporaneously, being little known to practitioners, although doubtless capable of valuable therapeutic applications.

It is made officinal for the purpose of furnishing a ready means of forming the solution which follows:—

Liquor Arsenici et Hydrargyri Iodidi, U. S. (*Donovan's Solution.*)

Take of Iodide of arsenic,
Red iodide of mercury, each . . Thirty-five grains.
Distilled water . . . . . Half a pint.

Rub the iodides with half a fluidounce of the water used, and when they have dissolved, add the remainder of the water; heat to the boiling point, and filter. According to my experience, there is no utility in the application of heat to this solution, at least in a majority of cases. Of course, the mixed powder should be entirely dissolved.

Donovan's solution is a clear, very pale straw-colored, or colorless liquid, with a slightly styptic taste. It should not be prescribed with other chemical preparations, as a general rule. It is a powerful alterative, said to be particularly adapted to the treatment of venereal diseases. Dose, ♏v to xx. Each f℥j contains about ⅛ grain of arsenic estimated as arsenious acid.

CHAPTER X.

MERCURY.

HYDRARGYRUM, *U. S.* (MERCURY.)

MERCURY is obtained chiefly from its bisulphuret, native cinnabar, by distillation with lime; sometimes it is met with in its metallic state, and rarely, combined with chlorine. Very rich cinnabar is found in California, from which a considerable proportion of our mercury is obtained.

When pure, mercury is a brilliant white, metallic liquid, becoming solid at —39° F., boiling at 662° F.; sp. gr. 13.5; entirely vaporized by heat; when small globules of it are rolled slowly on a sheet of paper, not a particle should adhere. It dissolves many metals, as tin, bismuth, zinc, silver, and gold, forming amalgams with them. It may be separated from these when they contaminate it, by distillation. It is not attacked by muriatic nor by cold sulphuric acid, though the latter acid, at a boiling temperature, forms with it a bisulphate of the deutoxide, sometimes called bipersulphate. Nitric acid also dissolves it, forming a nitrate of the protoxide, and a binitrate of the deutoxide. Mercury forms numerous salts, a number of which are officinal preparations.

In the two classes of salts formed by the protoxide and deutoxide or binoxide of mercury, these oxides are recognized in the following way:—

Tests for the Protoxide.—Sulphuretted hydrogen and sulphuret of ammonium cause a black precipitate, insoluble in diluted acids; alkalies cause a black precipitate; muriatic acid throws down a white precipitate of calomel; protochloride of tin precipitates the metallic mercury.

Tests for the Binoxide.—Sulphuretted hydrogen and sulphuret of ammonium at first produce a white precipitate, which on the further addition of the precipitant turns yellow, orange, brown and black; fixed alkalies in the absence of ammonia, cause a reddish-brown precipitate, which is yellow with an excess of the precipitant; the precipitate caused by ammonia is white; protochloride of tin at first throws down calomel; when in excess, the metal is reduced.

The following convenient test for the mercurials is very delicate, and well adapted to pill masses, &c. :—

On to a copper coin brightened with a little NO_5, a small portion of the suspected substance is placed and moistened with a drop or two of water into a pasty consistence; a small fragment of KI is added to it, and on washing it a mercurial stain will remain. Numerous so-called "vegetable," and other "quack" pills will be found to show the presence of calomel in this way. The reaction in the case of blue mass is less rapid, though equally certain.

MERCURIAL COMPOUNDS.

Off. Name.	Comp.	Uses.	Dose.
Hydrargyri chloridum corrosivum	$HgCl_2$	Alterative, antiseptic, &c.	1/16 to 1/4 gr.
Hydrargyri chloridum mite	$HgCl$	Cathartic and alterative.	1/12 to 20 grs.
" sulphas flavus	$3HgO_2,2SO_3$	Emetic and errhine.	Emetic, 3 grs.
" iodidum rubrum	HgI_2	Alterative in syphilis, &c.	1/16 to 1/4 gr.
" iodidum	HgI	"	1/4 to 1 gr.
" *sesquiiodidum*	Hg_2I_3	"	1/8 to 1/4 gr.
Iodide of calomel	$2HgCl+HgCl_2+HgI_2$	"	1/16 to 1/4 gr.
Biniodide of calomel	$HgCl_2+HgI_2$	"	1/16 to 1/4 gr.
Potassii et hydrargyri iodidum	$KI,2HgI_2$	"	1/12 to 1/4 gr.
Syrup of iodohydrargyrate of potassium and iron	HgI_2 1/16 gr. and FeI_2 3/4 gr. to fʒj	Alterative.	fʒj.
Hydrargyri bibromidum	$HgBr_2$	"	1/16 to 1/4 gr.
" *bromidum*	$HgBr$	Cathartic and alterative.	1/12 to 6 grs.
" cyanuretum	$HgCy_2$	Alterative.	1/16 to 1/8 gr.
" sulphuretum rubrum	HgS_2	Alterative fumigations.	
" sulphuretum nigrum		Mild alterative.	gr. v to ʒj.
" oxidum rubrum	HgO_2	Externally, stimulant.	
" " nigrum	HgO	Alterative, sialagogue, &c.	1/4 to 3 grs.
" *acetas*	$HgO,\overline{A}o$	Alterative.	1/8 to 1 gr.
" *protonitratis liquor*	HgO,NO_5	"	gtt. iij.
" *binitratis liquor*	$HgO_2,2NO_5$	"	
" *phosphas*	$2HgO,HO,PO_5$	"	1/2 to 2 gr.
Hydrargyrum ammoniatum	$HgCl,NH_2$	Externally in ointment.	
" cum creta	3 parts Hg+5 p. CaO,CO_2	Antacid and alterative.	1/2 to 3 grs.

The composition stated in the syllabus is that generally adopted by pharmacologists in this country; it is founded on the view that the combining equivalent of mercury is 202. Supposing the equivalent to be 101, as European chemists generally do, we should call corrosive chloride, protochloride ($HgCl$); calomel, subchloride (Hg_2Cl), and so on.

Hydrargyri Chloridum Corrosivum, U. S. (*Corrosive Sublimate.*)

By the action of boiling sulphuric acid on mercury, the bipersulphate ($HgO_2,2SO_3$), is first formed. When this is heated with common salt, mutual exchange takes place, and bichloride of mercury and sulphate of soda, the former of which sublimes, are produced. The changes are represented in the formula $HgO_2,2SO_3+2NaCl=HgCl_2+2(NaO,SO_3)$. Corrosive sublimate is in heavy white crystalline masses, of a styptic and metallic taste; soluble in about twenty parts of cold water; much more so in alcohol; soluble also in ether; it melts and entirely sublimes when heated. Its watery solution, precipitated by alkalies or lime-water, throws down the red or yellowish binoxide. (See *Extemporaneous Prescriptions.*) When this precipitate is heated, it gives off oxygen, and runs into globules of metallic mercury; a solution of corrosive sublimate precipitates albumen, and forms with it a definite insoluble compound, to which property its use as an antiseptic is due.

It is a very powerful irritant; when taken in large doses, it causes burning at the epigastrium, vomiting and purging; applied to the skin, it is corrosive. It is less apt to produce salivation than the other preparations of mercury, and in very small doses it is useful as an alterative in chronic affections, syphilitic or not; externally it may be used as a lotion, gargle, injection, or ointment, in chronic skin diseases, ulcerated sore throats, and chronic discharge, from mucous membranes.

DOSE, $\frac{1}{16}$ gr. to $\frac{1}{4}$ gr. in solution, or pill with crumb of bread. The solution for external use is usually made in the proportion of $\frac{1}{4}$ or $\frac{1}{2}$ gr. to f℥j of water. It is much used in solution with muriate of ammonia, which increases its solubility, as a poison for bedbugs; the proportions to be used are one ounce of corrosive sublimate, half an ounce of muriate of ammonia to two pints water. When taken in poisonous doses, recourse should be had immediately to albuminous liquids; eggs, if at hand, should be administered freely, or a thin paste of wheat flour or milk, care being taken to evacuate the bowels and to carry off completely the precipitated material, which, though comparatively insoluble, is by no means inert.

Hydrargyri Chloridum Mite, U. S. (*Calomel.*)

To prepare this, the bipersulphate of mercury first formed, as explained under the bichloride, is afterwards, by being rubbed with a second equivalent of the metal, reduced to a condition capable of forming, when heated, the neutral protosulphate (HgO,SO_3); and this, by the action of the common salt, is converted into the protochloride of mercury, sulphate of soda being produced at the same time.

Calomel, when sublimed, occurs in cakes, with a crystalline structure; but as a drug, it is met with in the form of a white, or yellowish white, heavy powder, without odor or taste; sublimes with heat; treated with potassa, it is blackened, from the precipitation of the protoxide, which, when heated, runs into metallic globules.

Under the name of English or hydro-sublimed calomel, a preparation has appeared in commerce, which is preferred by some physicians to the kind made in the manner described above; it is prepared in accordance with Wœhler's suggestion, by conducting the calomel vapors during the process of sublimation into a chamber, through which steam is passed; or, as proposed by Dann, by condensing the calomel in a current of cold atmospheric air. Any corrosive sublimate present in the vapors, is washed out by the condensed water of Wœhler's process.

Calomel must be entirely free of corrosive sublimate; if treated with alcohol or boiling water, the filtrate must yield no precipitate with sulphuretted hydrogen and nitrate of silver. Calomel is entirely volatile; most foreign admixtures are left behind on heating upon platina foil.

By the action of nitric and muriatic acids, calomel is slowly converted into corrosive sublimate; soluble chlorides, and even continued boiling with water or alcohol, alone have a similar action. Chlorine, hypochlorites, iodine, iodides, hydrocyanic acid, and cyanurets, decompose calomel with the production of corrosive sublimate; it should therefore not be prescribed at the same time with muriate of ammonia or nitro-muriatic acid, which last is specially indicated in torpor of the liver; symptoms of violent gastric irritation have been unexpectedly produced from neglecting this precaution.

The peculiarities of calomel as a mercurial agent, are, that it produces little local irritation; it acts as a purgative by increasing the secretion of bile and other intestinal fluids, and hence is much relied on in affections of the liver, and obstructions to the portal circulation. It is much combined with other remedies, being greatly modified in its effects by judicious combination with sedatives, cathartics, astringents, &c.

DOSE, as a purgative, 5 grs. to ℈j; to produce ptyalism, $\frac{1}{2}$ grain to 1 grain, frequently repeated. It has become customary to administer exceedingly minute quantities of this preparation, so low as the $\frac{1}{24}$ of a grain repeated every hour or two, the constitutional effects being perceptible after a grain has been given in this way. I am informed that its power to salivate is greatly increased by long trituration with sugar of milk, perhaps on account of the extremely fine division to which it is thus brought, and of some chemical change not yet investigated.

Hydrargyri Sulphas Flavus, U.S. (*Turpeth Mineral.*)

The bipersulphate of mercury, formed by the action of boiling sulphuric acid on the metal, and mentioned in the two preceding formulæ, is readily decomposed by reducing it to powder and submitting it to the action of warm water, which changes its composition and properties, producing a yellow-colored insoluble subsalt, $3HgO_2+2SO_3$. This is used almost exclusively as an errhine, variously diluted with snuff, powdered liquorice root, lycopodium, &c.

Hydrargyri Iodidum Rubrum, U.S. (*Biniodide or Red Iodide of Mercury.*)

The two iodides of mercury resemble the two chlorides in their relative medicinal activity. This is, like corrosive sublimate, a powerful poison; it is one of the preparations easily made from ingredients always at hand. The following is the officinal process in detail:—

Take of Corrosive chloride of mercury . .	Half an ounce.
Iodide of potassium	Five drachms.
Hot distilled water	A pint.

Dissolve the chloride of mercury in twelve fluidounces of hot water by trituration in a mortar, adding small quantities of this solvent at a time, and pouring it into a precipitating jar, Fig. 209, till the salt is completely taken up; then dissolve the iodide of potassium in four fluidounces of hot water by shaking them together in a vial. Now pour the solution of iodide into the solution of chloride contained in the precipitating jar, both liquids being hot at the time of mixing them; this will produce immediately a brilliant scarlet-colored precipitate of biniodide of mercury, leaving in solution the very soluble chloride of potassium. Now fold a plain filter, Fig. 211; having poured off the supernatant liquid from the precipitated biniodide,

Fig. 209. Fig. 210. Fig. 211.

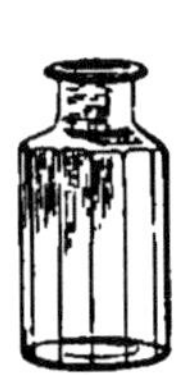

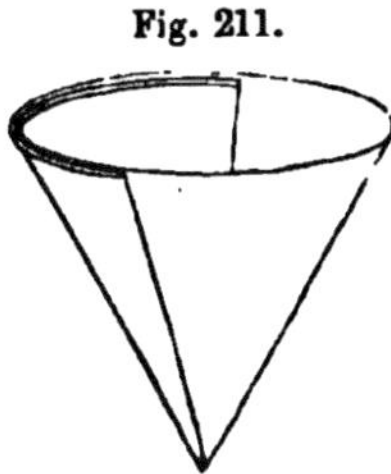

Precipitating jar. 4 oz. fluted vial. Plain filter.

throw the latter on the filter in a funnel and wash it by adding repeatedly fresh portions of pure water. Wrap the filter up in soft paper, and lay it away with a weight on it in a warm place to dry.

Biniodide of mercury is a beautiful scarlet-colored powder, or in fine crystals, if the boiling hot solution has been allowed to cool slowly. Insoluble in water, but soluble in alcohol, and in solutions of iodide of potassium and chloride of sodium. It is wholly sublimed by heat, condensing in scales which are at first yellow, but afterwards red. It is conveniently given in pill, but perhaps more frequently in solution of iodide of potassium with or without the addition of vegetable alterative preparations. DOSE, $\frac{1}{16}$ to $\frac{1}{4}$ gr. (See *Extemporaneous Prescriptions.*)

Hydrargyri Iodidum, U.S. (*Protiodide, or Green Iodide of Mercury.*)

Conveniently made by the apothecary or physician as follows:—

Take of Mercury	. . . . .	An ounce.
Iodine	. . . . .	Five drachms.
Alcohol	. . . . .	Sufficient.

Rub the mercury and iodine together, adding sufficient alcohol to form a soft paste, and continue the trituration till the globules disappear. Then dry the iodide in the dark with a gentle heat, and keep it in a well-stopped bottle, covered with dark paper to protect it from the light. By this process, though a slight excess of mercury may be used, a small quantity of the red iodide is formed, which remains mixed with the protiodide. It may be removed by dissolving it out with alcohol, moderately heated.

The mercury is conveniently weighed by balancing a small paper pill-box on the scales, and giving to one side of it a little crimp, as shown in Fig. 212; so that a small stream of the metal may be poured out conveniently. The accurate adjustment of the quantity is troublesome. The iodine also requires care in weighing, owing to its corrosive action on the metals. The most convenient method is to balance a pair of watch-glasses by filing away the heavier of the two, or by pasting on to the lighter a small piece of tin foil, and then to lay them away for weighing corrosive substances. In the absence of this, a piece of thick

Fig. 212.

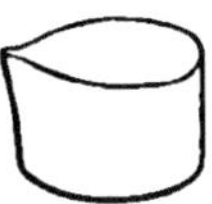

and well glazed writing-paper may be put on to each plate and balanced. If the scales are kept in a case, as shown in the first chapter, they should be taken out whenever iodine is to be weighed on them, as the vapor becoming diffused through the air inside the case will corrode the metal.

Iodide of mercury is a greenish-yellow powder, insoluble in water, alcohol, or solution of chloride of sodium, but soluble in ether. Heated quickly, it sublimes in red crystals, which afterwards become yellow by age; it is converted into sesquiodide, which has a yellow color, and is believed to be more active. It is used as an alterative, usually in pill. DOSE, ¼ gr. to 1 gr.; it is incompatible with iodide of potassium, which converts it into biniodide with separation of mercury.

Hydrargyri Sesqui-iodidum. (*Yellow Iodide of Mercury.*)

Owing to the instability of the protiodide of mercury, it is not very reliable as a medicine for internal use; as a substitute for it, the sesqui-iodide has been proposed, which is unalterable by exposure and age. It is made by precipitating protonitrate, or some other protosalt of mercury, by iodide of potassium, to which one-sixth of its weight of iodine has been previously added.

It is a bright lemon-yellow powder, insoluble in water and alcohol; it sublimes when heated in red crystals, which turn yellow on cooling. It is decomposed by hydriodic acid and by iodides which are incompatible with it. It is given in doses of one-eighth to one-quarter grain.

Iodides of Calomel.

Boutigny has proposed for medicinal use two preparations, which have been called respectively iodide and biniodide of calomel. The former is prepared by heating four equivalents of calomel in a retort until it commences to sublime, when gradually two equivalents of iodine are added. According to the mode of preparation, the obtained salt appears to be a mixture of two equivalents of calomel, one of biniodide, and one of bichloride of mercury, thus $4HgCl+2I=2HgCl+HgCl_2+HgI_2$.

The biniodide of calomel is prepared in a similar manner from equal equivalents of calomel and iodine, and must therefore contain one equivalent each of bichloride and biniodide of mercury, $2HgCl+2I=HgCl_2+HgI_2$.

Gobley (see *Am. Journ. Pharm.*, xxx. 168) prepares these iodides by triturating the material together, introducing it into a retort, and heating it in a sand bath to fusion.

It is evident that the two preparations must be of different intensity in their medicinal properties. They have been given in doses of one sixteenth to one-eighth grain, and employed externally in the proportion of a scruple to half a drachm to one ounce of ointment.

Potassii et Hydrargyri Iodidum. (*Iodohydrargyrate of Potassium.*)

A hot solution of iodide of potassium dissolves three equivalents of biniodide of mercury, one of which crystallizes out on cooling, afterwards yellow prisms are separated having the composition stated in the syllabus. They are soluble in alcohol and ether, but decomposed by water, which takes up a salt of the composition KI,HgI_2.

It is said to be less apt to produce salivation than other mercurial preparations. It is given in doses of one-twelfth to one-eighth grain, and in ointment of the same strength as the other mercurial iodides. When intended for use in solution, it has been recommended to make it extemporaneously with an excess of iodide of potassium, or dissolve it in a solution of this iodide.

Syrup of Iodohydrargyrate of Potassium and Iron.

J. E. Young, of Williamsburg, N. Y., offers this preparation, made by combining sixty-four grains of iodine in three drachms of water with iron, and filtering the solution into three and a half fluidounces of syrup; two grains of red iodide of mercury and one and a half grains iodide of potassium are dissolved in one drachm of water and added to the syrup, the whole to measure four fluidounces. Some orange-flower-water may be added to improve the taste. The dose is a teaspoonful.

Hydrargyri Bibromidum. (Bibromide of Mercury.)

This corrosive poison is prepared by combining two parts of bromine with five parts of mercury under water.

It crystallizes from water in white shining scales, from alcohol in needles; is soluble in water, more in alcohol and ether, and sublimes when heated.

In its action it is stated to be analogous to corrosive sublimate, and is employed in the same doses.

Hydrargyri Bromidum. (Bromide of Mercury.)

Nine parts of bibromide of mercury are mixed with five parts of mercury and sublimed, or a protosalt of mercury is precipitated by bromide of potassium.

It appears as a soft white powder or in thin prismatic crystals, insoluble in water and alcohol, but decomposed by the continued action of bromides or iodides.

It is said to resemble calomel in its action, and is given in medium doses of four to five grains.

Hydrargyri Cyanuretum, U. S. *(Bicyanide of Mercury.)*

By boiling ferrocyanuret of iron with red oxide of mercury, till the mixture becomes of a yellowish color, filtering and crystallizing, this may be made with great facility by following, literally, the officinal directions. It is in freely soluble, permanent, transparent crystals, which evolve hydrocyanic acid, on the addition of hydrochloric acid. By heat it is decomposed, giving off cyanogen, and leaving a black residuum containing metallic mercury.

Bicyanide of mercury is, like the bichloride, a powerful poison, differing from that remedy in producing no epigastric pain in its operation. Some practitioners prefer it to bichloride in the same doses, and for the same purposes.

The solution must not be precipitated by muriatic acid or caustic potassa.

Hydrargyri Sulphuretum Rubrum, U.S. *(Red Sulphuret of Mercury. Artificial Cinnabar.)*

When melted sulphur is brought in contact with mercury, direct union ensues; and if the compound is afterwards sublimed, it consists of dark scarlet, shining, crystalline masses, forming, when powdered, a beautiful scarlet color known by the name of vermilion; insoluble in water or alcohol. Volatilizes entirely when heated alone, but with potassa it is reduced to metallic globules.

When the fumes are brought into contact with the surface of the body, the drug acts as a topical alterative, and becomes absorbed, affecting the system the same as other mercurials. It is used as a fumigation in some syphilitic skin diseases; ℨss, thrown on a hot iron and placed beneath the patient, wrapped in a blanket, will effect the object. The vapor should not be allowed to enter the lungs.

Hydrargyri Sulphuretum Nigrum, U.S. (*Ethiops Mineral.*)

Made by rubbing mercury and sulphur together till the globules disappear and a powder is formed.

Ethiops is an insoluble black powder which is rarely used for any purpose. It may be safely given in doses of from gr. v to ℨj, though marked by no very active properties.

Hydrargyri Oxidum Rubrum, U.S. (*Peroxide of Mercury. Red Precipitate.*)

Prepared by dissolving, with heat, mercury, ℔iij, in a mixture of nitric acid, f℥xviij, and water, Oij; evaporating the liquor, and triturating what remains to a powder. This is put into a very shallow vessel, and heated till red fumes cease to rise.

Red oxide is in orange-red, shining, crystalline scales; when strongly heated, it yields oxygen and metallic mercury, without the production of red fumes. It is insoluble in water, but soluble in nitric and hydrochloric acids. It is used only externally, as a stimulant and escharotic; it is much applied as an ointment to the eye; as an escharotic, in powder, alone, or mixed with sugar, to specks in the cornea, over chancres, and fungous ulcers.

The directions of our *Pharmacopœia* enjoin great care in reducing the red oxide of mercury to a very fine powder; as it is very apt to be gritty from containing crystalline portions.

The preparation is rendered uniform, smooth and satisfactory by employing the product of the following formula of T. S. Weigand:—

Take of Bichloride of mercury . . . 550 grains.
Caustic potassa, in solution . . 116 "

Dissolve the chloride in one pint of boiling water, and pour the solution into the solution of caustic potassa, diluted with two pints of water; wash with water till there is no taste, and dry on a porous tile; the powder is smooth, dense, and well suited for the purpose of admixture with fatty matters.

Hydrargyri Oxidum Nigrum, U.S. (*Black Oxide of Mercury.*)

Made by triturating calomel with a solution of caustic potassa. The protoxide of mercury precipitates, while chloride of potassium remains in solution, and is separated by washing.

Black oxide of mercury is in powder, which becomes olive-colored by the action of light. It is wholly dissipated by heat, metallic globules being sublimed. It is insoluble in water, but is wholly dissolved by acetic acid.

As a medicine, it is like calomel in its action, and is sometimes substituted for it, but is said to be liable, from occasionally containing deutoxide, to operate harshly. ʒij, placed on a hot iron, answers the purposes of a mercurial vapor bath. Triturated with lard, it substitutes mercurial ointment. Its dose, as an alterative, is a quarter to a half grain daily; as a sialagogue, gr. j to iij, three times a day, in pill.

Hydrargyri Acetas. (*Protacetate of Mercury.*)

This salt crystallizes from a hot solution of protoxide of mercury in acetic acid, or from a mixture of the hot solutions of the protonitrate of mercury and acetate of potassa.

It separates in soft scales, is slightly oxidized by the air, and blackened by the light while moist.

It is used in similar complaints as the other mercurial salts in the dose of one-sixth to one grain.

Liquor Hydrargyri Protonitratis.

The Prussian *Pharmacopœia* contains a solution of the protonitrate of mercury, prepared by digesting mercury in excess with nitric acid and water, equal parts, and diluting the solution until it has the specific gravity of 1.1, and contains in twelve parts one part of mercury. It is used in venereal diseases in the medium dose of two drops.

If the solution should contain binoxide, this may be detected by precipitating it with chloride of sodium, and testing the filtrate with sulphuretted hydrogen, which will produce a yellowish precipitate changing to black.

Liquor Hydrargyri Binitratis.

This is officinal in the Dublin *Pharmacopœia*, and may be prepared, according to Professor Procter, by dissolving two ounces of mercury in three and three-quarters ounces (offic.) of nitric acid, specific gravity 1.34, by the aid of heat, and evaporating to two and a half fluidounces.

The Prussian *Pharmacopœia* has a similar but weaker preparation.

Hydrargyri Phosphas. (*Protophosphate of Mercury.*)

The solution of a protosalt of mercury is precipitated by phosphate of soda, and the precipitate well washed.

It is a white crystalline powder, insoluble in water, and has been employed in doses of about one grain, once or twice a day.

Hydrargyrum Ammoniatum, U.S. (*White Precipitate of Mercury.*)

When ammonia is added to a solution of corrosive sublimate, a peculiar compound, and not the oxide of mercury, is precipitated. This is a white, amorphous powder, in irregular masses, frequently bearing the impression of the fabric on which it is drained and dried. It sublimes when heated; is insoluble in water; dissolves in hydrochloric acid without effervescence; and, when heated with potassa, gives off ammonia, and becomes yellow from the formation of the binoxide of mercury. Generally considered as a compound of amidogen or amide (NH_2) with chloride of mercury. This salt is never used internally; it is applied externlly, to chronic skin affections in the form of ointment.

Hydrargyrum cum Creta, U.S. (*Mercury with Chalk.*)

Made by triturating three parts of mercury with five parts of prepared chalk, till it loses its fluidity and metallic lustre, and assumes the form of a dark-gray powder.

This process is one of great labor; and other modes of preparation have been employed. Those which proceed upon the principle of oxidizing the mercury are objectionable, as rendering this very mild powder drastic and violent in its action. It is much less used than blue mass, which it resembles in its action. The proportion of mercury is, partly from its defective preparation, larger than in blue mass, but it is said to be equally mild when well made. A good substitute is formed by mixing powdered blue mass with prepared chalk, extemporaneously.

Its chief use is in treating the complaints of children, the chalk neutralizing acid in the stomach, while the mercury increases the biliary secretion. Dose for a child, from a half to gr. iij.

For other mercurial preparations, see *Pills and Ointments.*

CHAPTER XI.

PREPARATIONS OF GOLD AND PLATINUM.

Aurum. (Gold.)

Gold is a soft metal, of a peculiar yellow color, and a lustre which is not affected by exposure to the air or heat; it is extremely malleable, being readily drawn into very fine wire, or beaten into leaves of $\frac{1}{200000}$th of an inch in thickness, or, if plated on to silver, not exceeding the one twelve-millionth part of an inch. Its specific gravity is 19.5; its fusing point 1300° F. It is not attacked by acids, except by nitromuriatic acid, which solution is the starting-point for all preparations of gold. Our gold coins, though not chemically pure gold, are sufficiently so for preparing its compounds for medicinal use; during the operation, the foreign metals are mostly separated.

Gold leaf, like silver leaf, is used for coating pills containing nauseous or strong-smelling substances.

It combines with oxygen in two proportions, forming a suboxide, AuO, and a peroxide, AuO_3.

Tests for Peroxide of Gold.—Sulphuretted hydrogen and sulphuret of ammonium cause a black precipitate, soluble in sulphuretted alkaline sulphurets; potassa produces a reddish-yellow precipitate; ammonia a precipitate of a similar color, which is fulminating gold; protochloride with a little perchloride of tin, throws down a purple red precipitate, insoluble in muriatic acid.

Preparations of Gold.

Auri pulvis, Au. Obtained by precipitation or by mechanical division.
Auri oxidum, AuO_3. Anhydrous blackish brown powder, easily decomposed by heat.
Auri chloridum, $AuCl_3$. Yellow or reddish; crystalline, combining with metallic chlorides.
Sodii et auri chloridum, $NaCl,AuCl_3+4HO$. Yellow crystals, not deliquescent.
Auri iodidum, AuI_3. Dark green; readily decomposed, combining with iodides.
Auri cyanidum, AuCy. Yellow, crystalline, insoluble; combining with alkaline cyanurets.

Auri Pulvis. (*Pulverized Gold.*)

If the solution of gold in nitromuriatic acid is mixed with a solution of protosulphate of iron, a pulverulent precipitate of a cinnamon-brown color is produced, which is metallic gold, *aurum præcipitatum.* By filing of pure gold, it may likewise be obtained in a pretty fine powder, *auri limatura*; or by rubbing gold leaf with sulphate of potassa to a fine powder, and dissolving out the potassa salt, *aurum præparatum.*

Gold, in its metallic form, is supposed to act as a tonic and alterative, and to be considerably milder than any of its compounds. Its dose is one-half to one grain two or three times a day.

Auri Oxidum. (*Peroxide of Gold. Auric Acid.*)

Chloride of gold, or the solution of gold in nitromuriatic acid, is treated with magnesia, the precipitate washed with water, and then decomposed by nitric acid; a reddish-yellow powder is obtained, which, on drying, turns brown.

It is somewhat irritating, but has the general properties of powdered gold; in scrofula, syphilis, &c., it has been used in doses of one-tenth to one-half grain twice a day.

Liquor Auri Nitrico-muriatis.

This is merely a solution of six grains chloride of gold in one ounce of nitromuriatic acid, which has been used as a caustic in cancerous affections; it produces a whitish scab.

A stronger solution has been employed for syphilitic and scrofulous ulcers.

Auri Chloridum. (*Perchloride of Gold.*)

It is contained in the solution of gold in nitromuriatic acid, from which it is obtained by evaporation to dryness, and constant stirring towards the end of the process. It is a reddish crystalline powder, very deliquescent; soluble in water, alcohol, and ether. Metals, many metallic salts, and organic compounds, reduce the gold from its solution.

It is very caustic, producing much irritation; when given for some time it is apt to salivate; it is very poisonous. The dose is one-twentieth to one-eighth grain once a day, and very cautiously increased to several doses a day.

Sodii et Auri Chloridum. (*Chloride of Sodium and Gold.*)

This double salt is obtained by preparing from three and a half parts of pure gold the perchloride, dissolving it in water, and mixing therewith one part pure anhydrous chloride of sodium. On evaporating this solution, long four-sided prisms are obtained, which are of a yellow color and unchangeable in the air.

This salt is officinal in some pharmacopœias, most of which, however, direct an excess of chloride of sodium, and to rub the evaporated mass into a fine powder.

Of all the preparations of gold, this double chloride is mostly employed. Its action is similar to that of the perchloride, but much milder. The dose is one-twelfth to one-quarter grain a day of the pure salt.

Auri Iodidum. (*Iodide of Gold.*)

If a solution of perchloride of gold is gradually added to iodide of potassium, the resulting precipitate is at first redissolved on agitation, a soluble double iodide being formed; subsequently the iodide of gold is precipitated, leaving the supernatant liquor free of color.

It is a dark-green powder, easily soluble in hydriodic acid. It must be kept in well-stoppered bottles, as in contact with the air it gradually loses iodine until metallic gold is left behind.

Like other preparations of gold, it is of an alterative effect, but on account of its spontaneous decomposition, it is not very reliable; the dose is about one-sixteenth grain.

Auri Cyanidum. (*Cyanuret of Gold.*)

The cyanuret of gold which has been used in medicine appears to be the protocyanuret. The percyanuret is in white tabular crystals, fusing at 112°, giving off hydrocyanic acid and cyanogen; it is easily soluble in water, alcohol, and ether. That employed medicinally is insoluble in those liquids, but soluble in alkaline cyanurets, ammonia, and sulphuret of ammonium. These properties agree with the protocyanuret of gold, which is prepared by dissolving the fulminating gold, obtained by precipitating a solution of seven parts of gold by ammonia, in a hot solution of six parts of cyanide of potassium, and treating the crystals with muriatic acid in excess, which leaves the proto-cyanuret as a yellow crystalline powder.

It is stated to be one of the mildest compounds of gold, and has been used as an alterative, resolvent, and emmenagogue, in doses of one-twelfth to one-half grain once or twice a day.

All the above preparations of gold are also used externally in ointments, and in cases of syphilis for frictions on the gums and tongue. For the latter purpose, they are generally mixed with twice or three times their weight of some inert powder, and the friction is commenced with about one-sixth grain of the mixture a day, and gradually increased; the milder preparations are used in somewhat larger proportions. The quantity employed in ointments varies with the nature of the complaint, the preparation used, and with the effect which is desired; from two to twenty grains are employed to an ounce of ointment.

Platinum.

This metal is remarkable for its resistance to chemical agents, and for its infusibility. It is soft, of a silver-gray color; very malleable and ductile, though inferior in these respects to gold. Its valuable physical and chemical properties render it indispensable for the preparation of various utensils necessary for a chemical laboratory.

Platinum dissolves in nitromuriatic acid; with oxygen it unites in two proportions, forming an oxide, PtO, and a binoxide, PtO_2; with the halogens and sulphur it forms compounds of a corresponding composition.

Tests for Binoxide of Platinum.—Platinum in solution is recognized by the following behavior towards reagents: Sulphuretted hydrogen and sulphuret of ammonium cause a blackish-brown precipitate of PtS_2, insoluble in muriatic and nitric acid, soluble in alkaline sulphurets and potassa. In the presence of chlorides, or of free muriatic acid, potassa and ammonia produce a crystalline yellow precipitate, soluble in alkalies. Solutions containing free muriatic acid are changed by protochloride of tin to a deep brownish-red color.

Platini Bichloridum, $PtCl_2$.

Bichloride of platinum is obtained by dissolving the metal in aqua regia, and evaporating to dryness. It is a red crystalline mass, turning brown by expelling the water of crystallization; deliquescent; soluble in water and alcohol.

It is poisonous, producing convulsions and death in overdoses. In doses of one-eighth to one-fourth grain, given in mucilaginous liquids, it has been employed like chloride of gold in syphilis, epilepsy, &c., also externally, about fifteen grains to one ounce of ointment.

Sodii et Platini Chloridum, $NaCl+PtCl_2+6HO$.

By mixing bichloride of platinum and chloride of sodium, yellow prisms are obtained by evaporation, which are soluble in water and alcohol.

Its effects are similar to the former, only milder, and it is given in somewhat larger doses.

NOTE ON THE PROGRESS OF PHARMACEUTICAL CHEMISTRY.

In view of the great increase of the variety of chemical substances used in medicine, as shown especially in the second edition of this work, the reflection is suggested, that chemistry and pharmacy are so closely allied as that the progress of the former is inseparably connected with the extension and usefulness of the latter.

Since pharmacy was elevated to a distinct and separate pursuit, it has experienced a steady advance towards the rank of a science.

So far as reliable history goes, the Arabs appear to have been the first nation who had pharmaceutical establishments distinct from the vocation of the physician. In their conquering march westward over the North of Africa and the South of Europe, they exercised an important influence on pharmaceutical regulations. The medicinal preparations of those times were, however, mostly derived from the vegetable and animal kingdoms, and made by the processes of distillation, infusion, decoction, and preserving by sugar and honey.

In the eleventh century, the first apothecary store in Christian Europe was established in Salerno, in Italy, and from that time they have gradually extended among all intelligent nations, till apothecaries are now found in all sections of the world whose inhabitants can lay claim to civilization.

The introduction by Paracelsus of strictly chemical compounds as remedial agents, opened to pharmaceutists the new path for scientific investigation in which they have since done so much, and from that time there have been many devotees to medicine and pharmacy who have distinguished themselves in chemical science.

The names of Scheele, Klaproth, Vauquelin, Proust, Derosne, Serturner, Liebig, and Pelletier attest the zeal of pharmaceutists, while Bœrhaave, Berzelius, Joseph Black, Humphrey Davy, Fourcroy, Berthollet, Wœhler, and many others adorn the roll of the more strictly medical profession.

To the present generation of pharmaceutists, the science is transmitted in greatly improved form. The modern pharmacopœias are robbed of much of their empiricism, and chemicals of definite composition are gradually replacing the crude and unscientific mixtures formerly prescribed.

It remains for us to repay the debt we owe to the past by zealous efforts to add still further to our science for the future.

PART V.

EXTEMPORANEOUS PHARMACY.

CHAPTER I.

ON PRESCRIPTIONS.

In assigning a place in this work to prescriptions, and to the art of prescribing medicines, it is with a full appreciation of its intimate connection with therapeutics, a branch of knowledge with which, as a pharmaceutist, I can lay claim to but little practical acquaintance; and yet this subject has bearings which are peculiarly adapted to arrest the attention of one whose daily avocations place him directly between the physician and the patient, and give him favorable opportunities for judging of the pharmaceutical eligibility of combinations, and not unfrequently of their effects.

The art of prescribing medicines has so intimate a connection with that of preparing and dispensing them, that a treatise on the latter subject, not embracing the former, would be wanting in its most interesting feature to the student of medicine and the physician, and in a work like the present, designed in part for these classes, it seems appropriate to approach the art of dispensing through a brief general treatise on that of prescribing.

If any evidence were needed of the necessity of this kind of instruction, it would be furnished in the acknowledged inaccuracy of extemporaneous prescriptions as generally issued by practitioners. It is a common remark of recent graduates of medicine, that one of their greatest difficulties is in writing prescriptions; lacking the means of systematic instruction in this most important practical duty, they are exceedingly apt to fall into confused and unscientific methods of prescribing, from which no amount of experience entirely rids them.

The art of prescribing is the practical application of the knowledge of therapeutics, chemistry, and pharmacy, to the cure of disease. No department of his duties puts the skill of the physician to a closer test; none calls for the exercise, to a greater extent, of that invaluable quality, whether intuitive or acquired, called *tact;* and yet few departments of medical knowledge are to be acquired with less facility, or are less insisted upon as necessary branches of a medical education.

Although the art of prescribing can only be acquired practically, the general principles pertaining to it are capable of classification, and have been fully discussed.

The celebrated *Pharmacologia* of Dr. Paris, of London, published originally in 1812, and republished in this country in 1844, contains the fullest dissertation in our language upon "the science and art of prescribing." The reader is referred to that elaborate work for a full discussion of the subject. Many of the views taught at that time, however, are now abandoned, and the subject is capable of being much simplified in accordance with modern improvements in pharmacy. The large number of efficient and permanent Galenical preparations make prescribing comparatively simple to the practitioner who has kept pace with the advance of the times, while the publication of *Formularies* in which a variety of preparations of each drug, whether permanent or extemporaneous, are detailed, has to a certain extent substituted an original and extemporaneous system of selection and combination of remedies.

Medicinal preparations which are kept on hand by the apothecary, to be dispensed alone or used in compounding prescriptions, are called *permanent*, while those compounded by direction of the practitioner to meet the indications as they arise, in practice, are called *extemporaneous.*

This distinction, however, is far from being absolute or even well marked. Some of those called permanent are known to deteriorate in a greater or less degree by age, while many classed as extemporaneous will keep an indefinite length of time. For most of the permanent class we have recipes, or prescriptions, either published in *Pharmacopœias*, *Dispensatories*, or *Medical Formularies*, while the extemporaneous are usually the product of the skill and ingenuity of the prescriber at the bedside of his patient. Objections lie against the general use of established prescriptions to the exclusion of those which are dictated by the emergencies of the case, from the impracticability of adapting any set of formulæ to every shade of disease and of idiosyncrasy, and from the impossibility of the practitioner storing securely in his memory their ingredients, proportions, &c.; so that the thorough student has no resource but to acquire a knowledge of the *principles*, to regulate the selection and combination of remedies, and learn the *art* of prescribing *experimentally*. A limited number of prescriptions, framed with a view of illustrating these principles and modes of combination, will, with this object in view, be found highly useful, if not indispensable to the student; but these must be regarded as stepping-stones to a knowledge of the art of prescribing rather than as embodying that knowledge. The vast extent and variety of adaptation of the materia medica preclude the possibility of compressing into any series of prescriptions, a complete view of all the shades of combination and modification which are attainable on enlightened therapeutical and pharmaceutical principles.

In the preparations introduced to view thus far, a prominent distinction has been drawn between those which are officinal in the *U. S. Pharmacopœia*, and those which are not; the use of Italics for the unofficinal, calling attention to their comparatively unimportant position, has been a conspicuous feature in the syllabi intended for the use of the student in committing to memory their names, proportions, properties, and doses. In the part of the work which follows, this distinction is regarded as less important, and most of the formulæ are introduced less with a view to impress them upon the memory, than to illustrate the pharmaceutical principles on which they are based.

The very obvious division of preparations into simple and compound needs no other mention than to explain that the addition of a vehicle or menstruum, not added with a view to its medical effect, does not render a preparation compound, in the sense in which that term is ordinarily applied. *Simple* rhubarb pills contain rhubarb and soap; while *compound* rhubarb pills contain rhubarb, aloes, myrrh, and oil of peppermint; and with a view to furnish distinctions between preparations which have very similar composition, the term compound is sometimes useful. Opium pills contain 1 grain of opium and ½ grain of soap; while *compound* soap pills contain the same ingredients in different proportions.

The Language used in Prescriptions.

In Great Britain and the North of Europe, prescriptions are written in Latin; in France, in the vernacular language. We mostly follow the British custom, although some of our practitioners occasionally depart from the usual style, and follow the *Pharmacopœia* by inditing their prescriptions in plain English. The relative adaptation of Latin and English for the purpose has long been discussed, and is still a mooted point among physicians and pharmaceutists. It is scarcely worth while to dwell upon the arguments advanced on either side, and which seem naturally to suggest themselves. The chief desideratum is to secure accuracy without an unnecessary and cumbersome phraseology, and for this purpose the *officinal names* of all medicines are to be preferred to either of their common and changing synonyms. An extended view of the subject cannot fail to convince one of this. Many medicines are called by very different names in different parts of the country, and the same name is liable to be applied to either of several different drugs.

If snakeroot were ordered, the pharmaceutist might be at a loss whether serpentaria, cimicifuga, asarum, senega, eryngium, or some of the numerous other roots occasionally, or perhaps locally, denominated snakeroots, were desired; while, if the specific English name, as *Virginia*, *Canada*, *black* or *button* snakeroots, was applied, the merit of conciseness would be sacrificed.

If chamomile were ordered, it would be necessary to specify whether Roman, German, or American; while in Latin, anthemis, matricaria, or anthemis cotula would be both short and distinctive.

In the foregoing illustrations, however, we have the least forcible instances. There can be no comparison between the names sugar of lead and plumbi acetas, white vitriol and zinci sulphas, liver of sulphur and potassii sulphuretum, salt of tartar and potassæ carbonas. The name which expresses the chemical composition of a substance is generally, of all that can be devised, the best; and hence, even in common language, most familiar chemical substances are beginning to be called by their chemical names. Although there is little difference between the English and the Latin chemical names, the latter has the advantage for use in prescription: it is easier of abbreviation, or its abbreviations are more familiar; while the omission of the connecting preposition *of*, between the two parts of the name, reduces it to a single compound word, rendering it shorter and more quickly written.

It is often said, and not without truth, that the Latin used in prescription is, for the most part, quite incorrect, and especially when the terminations are attempted; but grammatical errors are certainly far less important than either chemical, pharmaceutical, or therapeutical; and when we consider how few physicians, even among those classically educated, have advantages of keeping up, throughout the busy scenes of their professional career, the knowledge of Latin acquired in their schoolboy days, we can scarcely wonder that many errors of this description occur. Moreover, the language used in prescription, viewed with reference to its abbreviations, signs, and Latinized names of various origin, must be regarded as distinct from the Latin taught in schools, and requires to be studied in connection with scientific nomenclature generally, and, in fact, constitutes a part of the study of materia medica and pharmacy. Every officinal drug and preparation has its particular name given to it authoritatively in the *Pharmacopœia*, and those not there mentioned may be distinguished by their appropriate botanical or chemical designations. The groundwork of a correct writing of prescriptions is a knowledge of these names; and it matters little whether the physician write his prescriptions in Latin or English, if he designates each individual article by its *officinal name*.

The propriety of using the officinal Latinized names in a plain English formula may admit of a doubt, but, if sanctioned by custom and authority, might be adopted, and thus the principal objection to the plain English prescription would be removed.

The officinal name, though framed upon a Latin model, might be separated from the idea of its origin, and used in the prescription as a distinctive pharmaceutical term, following the genius of the language in which it is used: in a Latin prescription, its terminations might be varied as the construction of that language requires; and in an English prescription, might follow the rules for the construction of a correct English sentence. We have very many officinal names that are as commonly incorporated into our language as the English synonyms attached to them, and the objections to considering all the names in the American *Pharmacopœia* as American names are, it appears to me, not such as to overrule a custom which, on so many accounts, is to be desired.

The officinal names are spoken of in detail in the chapter on the *Pharmacopœia*, and the importance of a study of them has been elsewhere referred to; and I repeat, if these were properly mastered by the student, and invariably used to designate the drugs and preparations to which they belong, the garb in which the prescription is clothed would be comparatively of little importance.

There are some cases in which the use of an explanatory synonym in parentheses seems quite necessary, whether the name be Latinized or not; and in such cases it should never be omitted for the sake of elegance or attempted correctness of diction. In prescribing the finer kinds of magnesia, there is no other resource than to say in parentheses (Henry's), (Husband's), or (Ellis's), as the case may be. Liquor aloet. comp. would be quite indefinite without (Mettauer) appended, and tinct. guaiaci comp. would be misunderstood unless accompanied by the added (Dewees) to explain it.

The remarks before made apply to the *names* of substances designated in prescriptions; the other parts of the prescription, which will be referred to more particularly in the sequel, consist chiefly of abbreviations and signs which custom has long sanctioned, and which are considered to pertain particularly to the *Latin* prescription, though, as before stated, occasionally, and without any breach of propriety, used in connection with the English.

In the prescriptions appended to the several chapters which follow, numerous examples are given of both Latin and English prescriptions, and they will be appropriately preceded by the following, taken from Dr. Pereira's *Selecta e Prescriptis.*[1]

Grammatical Explanations of Prescriptions.

(1.) ℞.—Ferri carbonatis, drachmam cum semisse (ʒjss).
(2.) Rhei pulveris, grana quindecim (gr. xv).
(3.) Olei anthemidis, guttas quinque (gtt. v).
(4.) Conservæ rosæ, quantum sufficiat ut fiat massula in pilulas viginti dividenda, quarum sumat æger tres octavis horis.

(1.) Recipe, verb active, imp. mood, 2d pers. sing. agreeing with *Tu*, understood; from *Recipio, ĕre, cepi, ceptum*, 3d conj. act. Governs an accusative.
Drachmam, noun, subst. acc. sing. from *Drachma, æ* f. 1st decl. Governed by *Recipe*.
Cum, preposition. Governing an ablative case.
Semisse, subst. abl. case, from *Semissis, is*, f. 3d decl. Governed by *cum*.
Carbonatis, subst. gen. sing. from *Carbonas, atis*, f. 3d decl. Governed by *Drachmam*.
Ferri, subst. gen. sing. from *Ferrum, i*, n. 2d decl. Governed by *Carbonatis*.

(2.) Recipe, understood.
Grana, subst. acc. pl. from *Granum, i*, n. 2d decl. Governed by *Recipe*, understood.
Quindecim, adj. indeclin.
Pulveris, subst, gen. sing. from *Pulvis, eris*, m. 3d decl. Governed by *Grana*.
Rhei, subst. gen. sing. from *Rheum, i*, n. 2d decl. Governed by *Pulveris*.

(3.) Recipe, understood.
Guttas, subst. acc. pl. from *Gutta, æ*, f. 1st decl. Governed by *Recipe*, understood.
Quinque, adj. indeclin.
Olei, subst. gen. sing. from *Oleum, ei*, n. 2d decl. Governed by *Guttas*.
Anthemidis, subst. gen. sing. from *Anthemis, idis*, f. 3d decl. Governed by *Olei*.

(4.) Recipe, understood.
Quantum, adverb. Governing the genitive case.
Sufficiat, verb impers. potent. mood, pres. tense, from *Sufficio, ĕre, feci, fectum*, neut. and act. 3d conj.

[1] Republished in this country as the *Physician's Prescription Book.*

CONSERVÆ, subst. gen. sing. from *Conserva*, *æ*, f. 1st decl. Governed by *Quantum*.
ROSÆ, subst. gen. sing. from *Rosa*, *æ*, f. 1st decl. Governed by *Conservæ*.
UT, conjunct. Governing a subjunct. mood.
MASSULA, subst. nom. case *a*, *æ*, f. 1st decl.
FIAT, verb. subj. mood, pres. tense, 3d person singular, from *Fio*, *fis*, *factus sum vel fui*, *fieri*, neut. Governed by *Ut*, and agreeing with its nominative case *Massula*.
DIVIDENDA, particip. nom. case fem. gend. from *Dividendus*, *a*, *um* (*à divido*, *i*, *sum*, pass. 3d conj.). Agreeing with *Massula*.
IN, preposition. Governing an accusative case.
PILULAS, subst. acc. pl. from *Pilula*, *æ*, f. 1st decl. Governed by *In*.
VIGINTI, adj. indecl.
QUARUM, relative pronoun, gen. pl. fem. from *Qui*, *quæ*, *quod*. Agreeing with its antecedent *Pilulas* in gender and number. Governed in the gen. case by *Tres*.
ÆGER, adj. mas. gend. nom. *Æger*, *ægra*, *ægrum*. Agreeing with *homo*, understood.
SUMAT, verb, 3d pers. sing. imp. mood, from *Sumo*, *ere*, *psi*, *ptum*, act. 3d conj. Agreeing with *homo*, understood; governing an acc. case.
TRES, ad. acc. pl. fem. from *Tres*, *tres*, *tria*. Agreeing with *Pilulas*, understood, and which is governed by *Sumat*.
HORIS, subst. abl. plural, from *Hora*, *æ*, f. 1st decl.; signifying part of time, and therefore put in the abl. case.
OCTAVIS, adj. abl. plur. fem. from *Octavus*, *a*, *um*. Agreeing with *horis*.

Symbols or Signs used in Prescriptions.

♏. Minim, $\frac{1}{60}$ part of a fluidrachm.
gtt. Gutta, a drop; guttæ, drops.
℈j. Scrupulus vel scrupulum, a scruple=20 grains.
ʒj. drachma, a drachm=60 grains.
fʒj. fluidrachma, a fluid or measured drachm.
℥j. Uncia, an officinal ounce=480 grains.
f℥j. Fluiduncia, a fluid or measured ounce.
℔j. Libra, a pound, understood in prescriptions to apply to an officinal pound of 5,760 grains.
Oj. Octarius, a pint.
gr. Granum, a grain; plural, grana, grains.
ss. Semis, half, affixed to signs as above.

The Latin numerals are employed in prescription—i, ij, iij, iv, v, vi, vij, viij, ix, x, xi, xij, xv, xx, XL, L, C, &c.; and in the directions, when written in Latin, a variety of antiquated terms, explained in Dr. Pereira's little work before mentioned, but requiring too much space for insertion here.

Before leaving the subject of the signs employed in prescription, it seems proper to advert to the errors which frequently occur from their careless use, and which have led some practitioners to advocate their entire abandonment. They are, however, too well established in the actual practice of this country and England, and too convenient to be readily supplanted. The angle and curve ʒ may be made so carelessly as to resemble the ℈ with a flourish at top, and ℥j may look like a ʒj, or may be so completely perverted from its recognized shape as to leave the reader in doubt whether a ℈ or ʒ is intended. Notwithstanding the apparent absurdity of this, there are not a few prescriptions on our files in which the sign intended has been reached only by guessing, or by reasoning upon the known dose of the drug, rather than upon the shape of the sign. A flourishing style of chirography is nowhere less in place than on a physician's prescription. The numerals are equally liable to error if carelessly made, the difference between j and v, and between iv and iij, and between x and v, is often quite obscured by a neglect of the plain and necessary precautions of accuracy and care. It is not easy to illustrate in print what an examination of the chirography of many prescriptions would make apparent, that the *reading* of a prescription frequently requires more skill and judgment than *compounding* it.

Abbreviations.

Mistakes not unfrequently arise from unskilful abbreviations, for, while there can be no objection to shortening many of the long names given to medicines, there is certainly great danger from the inordinate and unskilful exercise of this privilege; the word *cal.* is an occasional and very poor abbreviation for hydrargyri chloridum mite. Through a careless termination of familiar words, serious accidents are liable to occur. Several years have elapsed since I received a prescription for *hydrate potassa* ʒj, to be dissolved in water f℥iij (dose, a teaspoonful), and it was only through a care which has become habitual that I saved a delicate lady in that case from taking large doses of hydrate of (caustic) potassa instead of hydriodate of potassa. There were no directions for use appended, so that I had not the advantage they give in cases of doubt. The abbreviations allowable in prescriptions might fill some pages if tabulated, but it appears to me useless to go into detail on the subject, as no practical advantage would result except to the student who should make them his especial study, while the habit once acquired of writing every word so fully as that it could be mistaken for no other, would quite obviate the evils complained of.

CHAPTER II.

ON THE WRITING OF PRESCRIPTIONS.

The first care to observe in writing a prescription, is to have suitable paper and pencil, or preferably, pen and ink. The habit of some of using the margin of a newspaper, the fly-leaf of a school-book, or any piece of flimsy material at hand, for inditing a prescription, upon which may depend the life of the patient, cannot be too strongly condemned. It indicates a want of care in the physician, which, if carried into other duties, would quite unfit him for the responsibilities of his profession. Many physicians adopt the plan of cutting, from time to time, suitable fragments of good paper, which are carried in a pocket-book or wallet, and are always at hand on emergencies. With a view to economy, the fly-leaves of letters and notices, which would be otherwise wasted, may be pressed out, and appropriated to this object. In Philadelphia, and probably elsewhere, pharmaceutists are in the habit of printing their cards at the head of suitable prescription sheets, and distributing them among physicians with a view to attracting business to their shops; a practice more honored in the breach than in the observance. Some physicians print prescription papers, with their name and address attached, which, however unprofessional some may consider it, is not without one advantage—it enables the apothecary always to trace the prescription readily to its source in case of difficulty.

Having the proper prescription paper, the next step is to write at the top the name of the patient; this precaution, which is very often neglected, is important for several reasons: 1st. It enables the nurse or attendant to distinguish, by a certain and ready means, between prescriptions designed for different patients; and the name being transferred to the label, there is no excuse for a similar mistake in "administering." 2d. It enables the apothecary, in every case, to avoid the mistake so often made in the hurry of business, of dispensing a package of medicine to one of several customers in waiting, which should have been given to another. 3d. It facilitates the recognition of the prescription upon the apothecary's file when its renewal is called for; and, finally, it evinces a care which is commendable on so important an occasion as prescribing for the sick.

The practice of heading a prescription with the generic name of the class of medicines to which it belongs, should be observed when there are two or more in use; as the *Gargle*, the *Liniment*, or the *Fever Mixture*. Frequently, however, this is superseded by giving its designation in the *subscription*, or by proper directions for its use. As a general rule, I would say that all topical remedies should be distinctly marked *For external use*. Some mistakes have originated from neglect of this precaution which would be most ludicrous if the subject was not often too serious for merriment. The administration of an ammoniated liniment, in tablespoonful doses, while a cinchona bark mixture is applied over the seat of rheumatic pain, is a blunder which has occurred, and may again.

It is well, in many cases, to copy on the label the entire prescription. A physician in large practice, unless favored with a very retentive memory, may forget the details of his prescription of the previous day. An aged practitioner of our acquaintance, while in practice for the last few years of his life, made this an invariable rule, with the view of assisting him in the accurate and judicious dispensation of advice from day to day to his patients. The same precaution is important also in travelling. It is often prudent for the physician to direct the apothecary to mark the medicine prescribed *Poison*, or, as is sometimes done, "*Use with care*;" giving, at the same time, the particular instructions for its use.

The prescription may be divided, for the purpose of study, into the following parts, each of which will be separately considered: 1. The superscription. 2. The inscription. 3. The subscription. 4. The signature.

The *Superscription* is of very little importance; divested of its superstitious origin, it consists of a very short abbreviation of the Latin verb *Recipe*, imperative mood of *Recipio*, I take, viz: the letter ℞, which is often printed near the top of the prescription sheets above mentioned. In French, the letter *P* is used for *Prenez*. In English formulas, the ℞ may be substituted by *Take of*.

The *Inscription* is the indication, seriatim, of the names and quantities of the remedies prescribed. The order in which these are written is not a matter of much real importance, as a competent pharmaceutist will, in mixing them, depart from the sequence observed in the prescription, if thought best; while the physician, particularly if not experienced in writing prescriptions, will find it more convenient to follow the order of their therapeutical importance rather than the rotation in which they should be added.

In the sequel I shall refer to the therapeutical classification of ingredients, which, in a well-contrived prescription, would be written in the following order: 1. The basis. 2. The adjuvant. 3. The corrective. 4. The excipient. 5. The diluent.

This is not only the most elegant, but the most natural rotation to be observed.

One of the greatest difficulties to the beginner, in connection with this subject, is in determining, as the prescription proceeds, the appropriate quantity of each ingredient, so as to have each in due proportion, and with its right dose; this becomes easy by the employment of the following

Rule for Apportioning Quantities.—Write down the names of the several ingredients first, without regard to quantity; then having determined upon the quantity of the whole preparation, and the dose to be prescribed, the whole number of doses it will contain will be readily calculated, and the quantity of each ingredient may be affixed.

As doses are, at best, only approximate, we may depart from the precise figures obtained by dividing the whole number of drachms, grains, &c., in the preparation, by the number of doses it will contain, as far as necessary to get even numbers, or convenient fractions of a drachm and ounce.

In directing pills, or powders, we have the means of attaining considerable accuracy, and may readily direct a combination of ingredients to be divided into ten, twenty, or thirty parts, from the very convenient relations of these numbers to the drachm and scruple weights; but it will be found more convenient in dispensing and administering the preparations, to have six, or twelve, or twenty-four parts ordered, as these numbers have relation to the number of grooves in the pill machine, and to the number of hours in a day.

The Table below will assist the beginner in prescribing liquids, and will serve for reference until he becomes accustomed, practically, to this rather difficult part of his duties. Having fixed upon the bulk of his mixture or solution, he will remember that there are *about*

8 wineglassfuls	(each containing	f℥ij) in a pint (Oj, f℥xvj).
30 tablespoonfuls	(" "	f℥ss) in a pint (Oj, f℥xvj).
15 tablespoonfuls	(" "	f℥ss) in half a pint (f℥viij).
12 tablespoonfuls	(" "	f℥ss) in 6 fluidounces (f℥vj).
20 dessertspoonfuls	(" "	fʒij) in 6 fluidounces (f℥vj).
15 dessertspoonfuls	(" "	fʒij) in 4 fluidounces (f℥iv).
30 teaspoonfuls	(" "	fʒj) in 4 fluidounces (f℥iv).
15 teaspoonfuls	(" "	fʒj) in 2 fluidounces (f℥ij).
8 teaspoonfuls	(" "	fʒj) in 1 fluidounce (f℥j).

We have an illustration of this method of division in the officinal liquor morphiæ sulphatis, in which one grain of the salt is dissolved in one fluidounce of water; as there are eight teaspoonfuls in an ounce, one teaspoonful represents one-eighth grain, which is about the usual dose. In the case of liquids to be given by drops, care must be taken to distinguish between aqueous, alcoholic, and oily liquids. By reference to the table, given in the chapter on Metrology, the relative size of drops pertaining to different liquids will appear; in this connection it will be only necessary to refer to that table, and to apply the same general mode of calculation to the apportionment of doses of these.

One cause of fallacy, with the student, in prescribing by drops, arises from confounding the size of drops of one ingredient of a preparation with the size of drops of the whole preparation after it is made. Thus, if a fluidrachm of tincture of belladonna were added to seven fluidrachms of an aqueous solution of morphia, or tartar emetic, we should calculate about sixty drops to each fluidrachm, not one hundred and twenty, which would be proper, were the alcoholic liquid in much the larger proportion.

It will aid the student to acquire facility in the apportionment of quantities, to inquire of himself, or his companion in study, how much of each ingredient is contained in each dose of the various compounds for which prescriptions are given.

The *Subscription* has reference to the manner of mixing and dividing the medicine. In Latin prescriptions, it usually consists of short abbreviations, or signs, which are familiar to pharmaceutists, though in some cases it is written out in full in Latin, and in others in plain English. The verb *misce* (imperative mood of misceo, I mix), or the letter *M.*, designed to represent it, constitutes the most common subscription. Sometimes, where especial skill or care is required in the preparation, *secundum artem*, or *S. A.*, is affixed to it; when omitted, however, this is understood. The verb *solve* (imperative of solvo, I dissolve) is more appropriate where a simple solution is prescribed; or *macera* (imperative of macero), where the process of maceration is directed. Where filtration is necessary, write thereafter *et cola.* When a medicine is directed in very fine powder, the practitioner may make choice of *tere bene* (triturate well), or *fiat pulvis subtilissimus* (make a very fine powder). It is, perhaps, an improvement on the above to direct more specifically the sort of preparation designed; it gives the pharmaceutist a clue, which is sometimes useful to him in compounding, as well as in correcting gross errors. The following terms, with their proper abbreviations and translations, may serve to guide the student in writing his *subscription.* They include the appropriate directions for dividing medicines into powders, pills, lozenges, &c., and will close the notice of this part of the prescription.

Fiat pulvis, Ft. pulv. Make a powder.

Fiant pulveres xij; Ft. pulv. xij.	**Make twelve powders.**
Fiat pulvis et divide in chartulas xij; Ft. pulv. et divid. in chart. xij.	
Fiat pulvis in chartulas xij dividenda; Ft. pulv. in ch. xij div.	
Fiant chartulæ xij; Ft. chart. xij, divid.	

Fiat solutio, Ft. solut. Make a solution.

Fiat injectio, Ft. inject. Make an injection (for urethra.)
Fiat collyrium, Ft. collyr. Make an eye-wash.
Fiat enema, Ft. enema. Make an injection (for rectum.)
Fiat suppositorium, Ft. supposit. Make a suppository.
Fiant suppositoria iv; Ft. suppos. iv. Make 4 suppositories.
Fiat massa, Ft. massa. Make a mass.
Fiant pilulæ xij; Ft. pil. xij. } Make twelve pills.
Fiat massa in pilulas xij dividenda; Ft. mas. in pil. xij div. } Make twelve pills.
Fiat massa et divide in pilulas xij; Ft. mas. div. in pil. xij. } Make twelve pills.
Fiat infusum, Ft. infus. Make an infusion.
Fiat haustus, Ft. haust. Make a draught.
Fiat gargarisma, Ft. garg. Make a gargle.
Fiat mistura, Ft. mist. Make a mixture.
Fiat emulsio, Ft. emuls. Make an emulsion.
Fiat electuarium, Ft. elect. Make an electuary.
Fiat confectio, Ft. confect. Make a confection.
Fiat emplastrum, 6 x 4; Ft. emp. 6 x 4. Make a plaster 6 x 4.
Fiat emp. epispasticum, Ft. emp. epispast. } Make a blister.
Fiat emp. vesicatorium, Ft. emp. vesic. } Make a blister.
Fiat unguentum, Ft. ung. Make an ointment.
Fiat ceratum, Ft. cerat. Make a cerate.
Fiat cataplasma, Ft. cataplas. Make a poultice.
Fiat linimentum, Ft. linim. Make a liniment.
Fiant trochisci xxiv; Ft. troch. xxiv. Make 24 lozenges.
Fiat massa in trochiscos xl dividenda; Ft. mas. in troch. xl div.

The *Signatura* is rarely written in Latin, at least in this country. It comprises the directions as to the dose and mode of administering the medicine, and is especially addressed to the patient, or those in attendance upon him. This should be distinctly written in familiar language. None of the reasons for the employment of a learned, or technical language, in the other portions of the prescription, apply to this; on the contrary, a due regard to the avoidance of mistakes by the apothecary, and by the patient or his attendant, forbids it. It is very common to omit this part of the prescription entirely, and to depend upon a verbal direction as to the use to be made of the medicine. Sometimes two boxes of pills are ordered for the same patient simultaneously, or at short intervals, without any reliable means of distinguishing them, and when they are to be renewed, the apothecary may confound them, in consequence of the patient sending the wrong box, or through a slight error in his own labelling. Of 500 prescriptions taken indiscriminately from the files of three different shops, I find 43 per cent. have no definite directions, and a considerable proportion have no *signatura*. The practice of writing—"To be used as directed"—is equivalent to omitting this part of the prescription, and in labelling, this is adopted by the apothecary in all cases, where the physician has omitted giving any directions.

As an example of the results which may follow from this kind of direction, the following incident has been related by a professional friend: Two vials were in the chamber of a patient, each containing a fluidounce of liquid, and each about the same size; one contained sweet spirit of nitre, and the other blistering collodion. The nitre was to be given in teaspoonful doses occasionally, and the blistering liquid was of course to be applied externally. At twilight, the nurse, not noticing the difference in the color and consistency of the liquids, and finding them both labelled alike, put in the patient's mouth what she should have applied to her chest, thus producing a most distressing inflammation, which deprived the poor patient of her proper food, and doubtless contributed to exhaust her struggling vitality.

The danger of this kind of mistake is lessened by using for any two prescriptions of very different properties, different kinds of vials; thus for a preparation to be taken internally, a fluted flint vial, and for a liniment, one of the plain German flints, or better still, in the one case a round, and in the other an oval vial.

The only remaining part of the prescription to be mentioned, is the addition to the foregoing of the name or initials of the writer, and the date; of these, it may be remarked, that the *name* in full is on every account preferable. In a large city, where there are hundreds of physicians, it is impossible for pharmaceutists, and much less their clerks and assistants, to become familiar with the handwriting and initials of all of them, to say nothing of those instances in which two or more have the same initials. Now if this practice of signing prescriptions has any utility at all, it must be that it should be understood by the apothecary, so that if he suspects an error, or requires any explanations, he may make the necessary inquiries to correct it, without interrogating his customer and exciting alarm. Besides, there are some dangerous substances, especially such as are used for criminal purposes, that the druggist is only justified in vending by the sanction of a responsible name, and this name should, therefore, be clearly and intelligibly written.

The date of the prescription is almost universally written in numerals, at least in Philadelphia; this fashion is probably owing, mainly, to a large number of the most eminent practitioners of the last generation being members of the Society of Friends, and to the wide diffusion of the peculiarities of this sect in the "Quaker City," and from it, as the centre of medical instruction, to other localities;

When the patient is in moderate circumstances, the physician indicates that fact to the apothecary by the letter P, in one of the lower corners of the paper. If very poor, P P is written; from a conscientious apothecary, either of these marks secures a reasonable reduction in the price charged, and its omission by the physician leads to suspicions that the patient is not deserving of charity.

CHAPTER III.

ON THE ART OF SELECTING AND COMBINING MEDICINES.

The study of Materia Medica and Therapeutics is designed to acquaint the student with the uses and powers of remedies, and to prepare him to make a proper selection from these to meet the ever varying phases of disease.

The importance of this kind of knowledge cannot be appreciated until the actual emergencies of practice arise, and the necessity becomes apparent of an extended and a thorough knowledge of the weapons for combating disease.

A full and recent treatise on Materia Medica should always be within reach of the physician, and one or more of the best medical journals should replenish his library with the most recent discoveries and improvements; nowhere can a professional man less afford to economize than in his books.

In this age of active inquiry and unceasing investigation, a very few years suffice to produce important changes, both in the theory and practice of medicine; and the physician who stands still while progress is all around him, can expect no better fate than that of the mechanic, the farmer, or the man of business, who is content with the appliances of the past age in endeavoring to compete with those possessed of the facilities of the present.

While a sound conservatism, a becoming deference to those who have gone before us, and to the great medical authorities in our own time, should prevent a hasty departure from established principles or mode of treatment, there is a wide and profitable range for experiment in the vast extent and variety of the materia medica, and the combinations of which individual remedies are susceptible.

It cannot be denied that many skilful physicians employ a very restricted materia medica; there are hundreds in the United States who carry about with them all the weapons they use for combating the usual forms of disease, in some twenty or thirty vials, inclosed in a pair of saddle-bags; while, for unusual cases, they keep perhaps as many more on their office shelves. Though the frequent success of such cannot be questioned, we can draw no inferences from this fact to disparage the employment of an extended and varied assortment of remedies.

To what purpose has the bounty of nature spread everywhere plants of such varied and unsuspected properties; and why is art from the exhaustless mine of nature ever turning up some new product, endowed with varied and perhaps health-restoring powers, if the physician, into whose special keeping the business of testing their virtues is given, neglects the injunction, "Prove all things; hold fast that which is good?"

In the foregoing remarks, I would not be understood as countenancing a departure from the usual materia medica, except where called for by the requirements of practice, and justified by sound discretion; and much less would I encourage any of those innovations upon well-established principles, which have taken shape in the various *Pathies*, now so prevalent and so lamentably deficient in the indispensable elements of common sense and common honesty.

In the selection of medicines, then, let the physician have before him the whole known materia medica, with a complete knowledge of which he should be equipped from the start. Let him *first* select an individual from its class, with a view to all its properties, as likely to effect the immediate symptoms he is combating, and the general result of the case; and *second*, let him select the best preparation of it with reference tc ciency, to safety, to physical properties, and to all other circumstan— When there is a single medicine, which will fully meet the ir tion, there is no use of mixing it with others, except so far as it :paration in eligible form requires, as in the sequel; when th n officinal preparation, whether simple or compound, which d to the case, it is generally better to prescribe it by its offic.. e, than to attempt a similar original combination; the *pilulæ co s compositæ* are found to answer a common indication in disea ry frequently, that they have almost superseded ex tempora reparations of the same, or nearly the same ingredients; this is t.. though to a less extent, of other officinal preparations. A comm ception is furnished in *pilulæ quiniæ sulphatis*, which are frequ prescribed extemporaneously, in proportions varying from the ., in order t ir being freshly prepared, and still more t ently varied som composition to secure greater solubility c.. .iciency.

Officinal preparations ar ed in emergencies, since they are ready without the delay o nding them, while most forms of extemporaneous prescription req e considerable time for their preparation. Physicians should be s ewhat influenced by economical motives, in prescri of moderate means; preparations which are kept apothecary, are cheaper than those which are mixed e ly. In almost every class of medicines, there are those ry costly; and it is well when they can be substituted b scribing for the poor. Many practitioners are in the h ing for such, the sulphate of cinchonia or chinoidine, inste of a lt of quinia; a plan much resorted to by those residing in remote situations, who have to act as their own apothecaries, and find their practice among the poor a source of expense rather than revenue.

On the Art of Combining Medicines.

Simplicity is an object not to be overlooked in prescribing; notwithstanding the advantage obtained by combining, in a single preparation, the virtues of several medicines, there is, I think, more danger of the inexperienced attempting complications, not sanctioned by sound science, than of his erring on the side of simplicity.

In the remarks which follow, I shall endeavor to treat methodically, and as briefly as possible, the several advantages to be attained by medicinal combinations, and the means by which they may be most readily and safely fulfilled; and in the series of Prescriptions appended, shall endeavor further to illustrate the subject.

In compound prescriptions, we usually recognize one ingredient selected from the materia medica as the most important in a therapeutical point of view. This is designated as the *basis*. Sometimes two or three remedies may be combined to form the basis, but if they have different therapeutical effects, they are considered as *adjuvants*, *correctives*, &c.

Although this classification of ingredients is not absolute, it seems to facilitate the study of the subject, and we proceed to notice—

First. The objects to be obtained by adding to the basis.

a. Dilution.

A great many remedies are too strong to be eligible for use without the addition of a menstruum, to increase the dose and to allow of a more ready division. In giving calomel, in very small alterative doses, it is impossible to apportion it properly without dilution with some suitable substance, such as sugar, as in Prescription No. 63. In using small doses of tartar emetic, sulphate of morphia, or other soluble salts, in the liquid form, it is usual to dilute them with water. In the case of concentrated liquid preparations, as tinctures of aconite root, nux vomica, &c., a less active liquid should generally be added, so as to bring the strength of the preparation to a less dangerous point, especially when prescribed for ignorant or careless persons.

The simple act of dilution may then be regarded as the first, though one of the least important objects in view, in adding to the basis or starting point of the prescription, and the substance so employed, if simply for this end, may be called the *diluent.* Many prescriptions consist merely of the basis and diluent.

b. To heighten, or give Direction to the Effects of the Basis.

It was formerly considered that substances of similar therapeutical powers were mutually increased in energy by admixture. This idea is now generally abandoned, except in so far as the powers of medicines may be heightened by combining them with others capable of rendering the system more susceptible to their action, or of giving them specific direction; thus, aromatic stimulants greatly heighten the effects of tonics, and will be found generally combined with them in tonic preparations. (See *Tonic Tinctures* and *Prescriptions* Nos. 6, 11, 19, and 25.) So rhubarb, by its astringency, modifies the effects of other cathartics, as in Warner's Cordial. We have a further illustration of this in the use of tartar emetic, to give a sedative and diaphoretic direction to saline remedies, as in Prescription No. 51; and of Dover's Powder, to render ext. of colchicum more sedative, as in Prescription No. 34.

Not to multiply illustrations, many of which will naturally occur to the student, it requires to be mentioned that, in some cases, this adjuvant may be best given at a different time from the basis, or rather, that the two may be most profitably separated. Thus, it is customary to purge a patient affected with intermittent before giving quinia; but few practitioners would, unless in unusual cases, combine the cathartic with the tonic dose.

There are sometimes ingredients in a prescription which may be considered either in the light of adjuvants or of vehicles. Thus sulphuric acid in quinia solutions both adds to the effect, as is commonly considered, and affords a means of solution. So extracts, combined with other remedies, may heighten their action, while affording a convenient vehicle for making them into a pilular mass. The adjuvant is, however, rarely introduced, practitioners generally relying upon the independent action of one agent, modified, if required, by another, which is used for the next object.

c. To Correct some objectionable Property in one or both of the other Active Ingredients.

The instances in which this motive for adding to the basis is called into play, are so numerous that it will scarcely be necessary to illustrate, further than to refer to the prescriptions which follow. The combination of opium with calomel, in dysentery, is one of the strongest cases in point. The mercurial is, by this means, made to act as a corrective, in conditions of the system in which, if employed singly in the same dose, might aggravate the symptoms. Certain effects of opium, as a basis, are obviated by many additions. Thus compound spirit of ether is said to diminish its nauseating effect on the stomach, &c.

In administering oil of turpentine, or wormseed oil, as a vermifuge, some corrective is needed which will insure a purgative effect, and prevent its undue absorption.

In the same way oil of turpentine and laudanum are used as correctives to castor oil, diminishing its purgative effects, and preventing griping.

In prescribing senna, the custom is almost universal of adding some aromatic seed to the infusion, to prevent griping. In Prescriptions No. 41, No. 46, No. 53, we have especial instances of the value of correctives.

We may frequently make one substance answer the double purpose of a corrective, and diluent or vehicle. In this connection we find the medicated waters useful for liquid preparations; soap for pills; aromatics for powders; certain stimulating oils in ointments, liniments, &c.

It will be observed that the corrective may be either therapeutical or chemical in its operation, or both. While the effect of adding essential oils or opiates to cathartics, is purely therapeutical, that of combining soap with resins, to correct insolubility, is chemical or pharmaceutical. So, in combining mastich, or other very insoluble resin with aloes, its insolubility is increased or lengthened—an object sometimes of importance, as in Chapman's Dinner Pill.

d. The Proper Incorporation of the Ingredients together.

This object is one of paramount importance in the preparation of medicines. The excipient added for this purpose may be either chemical or mechanical, or both; it may be connected with the therapeutic plan of the prescription, or may be added solely to make it more agreeable to the taste, and more uniform in consistence. This ingredient is more important to the physician, from the fact that, owing to its therapeutic application, the excipient cannot always be left to the choice of the pharmaceutist, whose practical acquaintance with the subject would otherwise qualify him to select the best excipient. The numerous rules that suggest themselves in regard to the proper incorporation of ingredients together can be best brought into view in connection with the next subject to be treated of.

e. On the Different Forms of Medicines.

These are of two principal kinds: those which are adopted to *internal*, and those to *external* use. Or they may be divided into *solid*, *liquid*, and *semifluid* forms; as they are not very numerous, however, and neither classification of them is important, I shall treat of them in the order which experience has shown to be most convenient to the student.

CHAPTER IV.

ON POWDERS AND PILLS.

PULVERES. (POWDERS.)

In the chapter on Drying and Powdering Drugs, &c., some general views are given on the utility of this form of preparation, but it yet remains to point out in a particular manner the uses of powders in extemporaneous prescribing.

1. *The kind of Substances best adapted to this Form of Prescription.*

a. Those medicines which are insoluble; as calomel, phosphate of lime, subnitrate of bismuth, subcarbonate of iron, magnesia, &c.
b. Drugs possessing, in the natural condition, peculiar properties, differing from those which are artificially prepared from them; as cinchona, colomba, digitalis, &c.
c. Those which, in solution, would possess more nauseous or bitter properties than in their undissolved, finely-divided condition; as sulphate of quinia, kino, catechu, &c. They are, for the most part, best suited for making into pills.
d. Those which, combined in a liquid form, would be chemically incompatible.
e. The extracts and blue mass, when dry enough to be reduced to powder.

2. *The kind of Substances unsuited to this Form.*

a. Deliquescent substances; as carb. potassa, unless with special precautions.
b. Substances containing a large amount of water of crystallization (unless dried); as carbonate of soda.
c. Substances, the active principles of which are very volatile; as valerian and assafœtida.

d. Substances physically unsuited to mechanical division; as camphor and guaiacum, unless with certain precautions.

e. Blue mass, and the extracts in their usual condition, although the former and some of the latter are very convenient in the form of powder.

Powders may be prescribed in the form of mixture or draught, always directing the bottle to be shaken before pouring out the dose; or in pill, if their dose is small. They may be prescribed in papers (chartulas), each containing a dose, or in a single large package, the dose being indicated in the directions by some familiar standard of measurement.

These last are the only forms of prescription coming under the present head. Mixtures, pills, &c., will be considered in their appropriate places. Soluble substances, prescribed in powder, may be directed to be dissolved in water, and the solution taken by small doses, so as to save expense to the patient, or to have the medicine in a more portable form, as in travelling. This, however, is an inaccurate way. Seidlitz, soda, and citric fever powders are elegant forms for giving single doses of soluble salts.

When the dose of an insoluble powder is large, as in the case of magnesia, or of phosphate of lime, and it is to be mixed by the patient or attendant, it is well to direct the particular mode of suspending it in water. The directions for magnesia are as follows:—

Put the requisite quantity of clear and cold water (not too much) in a clean glass, and drop into it from the blade of a knife or spoon, the required dose; allow it gradually to mix with the water and subside, after which stir it up and drink immediately. This will be found a more satisfactory way than to pour the water upon the dry powder in the bottom of the glass.

Powders which are viscid and slightly soluble, are, I think, generally more disagreeable than those which are not. Rhubarb is much less pleasant to take in fine powder than when chipped into very small shavings or grated, and suspended through a glass of water.

Some viscid vehicle seems quite necessary to heavy powders like calomel, or mercury with chalk; by sinking to the bottom of the spoon from which administered, these are liable to miss of being swallowed. With medicines prescribed in the form of powders, there is no occasion for the use of excipients, as they are not, strictly speaking, incorporated together; where the dose is small, however, an additional substance may be directed for the purposes of dilution, such as sugar, or a mixture of sugar and gum, or liquorice, or arrowroot fecula. An illustration of this kind of admixture is seen in Prescription No. 54, in which the only utility of the sugar is to give body to the otherwise very small bulk of the powders; also in Castillon's Powders, in which an antacid and astringent, calculated to act as a remedy for the diseased condition, are combined with appropriate nutritious ingredients.

In *Dover's Powder* we have an instance of the diluent being made to subserve an important mechanical end; and I am informed by an intelligent pharmaceutist that, in his vicinity, physicians combine sugar of milk with powders in prescriptions for a like purpose, directing long trituration. Calomel is said by this means to acquire increased efficiency where a rapid constitutional effect is desired; although the assertions of homœopathists, in regard to the virtues of trituration are both extravagant and absurd, yet there is little doubt that, in a case like that of calomel, long attrition with a hard substance, in contact with the atmosphere, is calculated to produce chemical, as well as physical, changes of importance.

The use of adjuvants and correctives is appropriate in the case of powders, equally with other classes of remedies; and, by reference to the prescriptions appended, it will be observed that they are very commonly added. Prescriptions in the form of powders will be associated with those in pilular form in the rotation here observed.

PILULÆ.

Pills are the most popular and convenient of all forms of medicine. In common with powders, they have the advantage of being accurately divided, so that the patient is not dependent upon any of the uncertain means of approximate measurement necessary in administering liquids. They are also more portable. The contact is so slight with the organs of taste, in swallowing, that the most offensive substances can be swallowed in this form with comparatively little inconvenience. There are, however, a few people who cannot swallow them; this is the case, too, with young children, for whom some other form is preferable.

The size of pills is necessarily limited to from four to five grains of vegetable powders, or five to six grains of heavy mineral substances. *including the excipient*, though these quantities are larger than usual.

The kind of Substances best adapted to the Pilular Form.

a. All those suitable to the form of powders, which are given in small doses.
b. The gum resins, balsams, and turpentine.
c. Substances, the operation of which it is desirable to retard; as in certain aperient and alterative pills.
d. Insoluble substances, which are too heavy to give conveniently suspended in water.
e. Very disagreeable and fetid substances.
f. The vegetable extracts.

The kind of Substances unsuited to the Pilular Form.

a. Those which operate only in doses exceeding fifteen or twenty grains, or too large for three or four pills.
b. Deliquescent or efflorescent salts.
c. Bodies of such consistence as to require an undue proportion of dry or viscid material to make a mass, except such as have a very small dose; as croton oil.
d. Very volatile substances; as carbonate of ammonia, except with certain precautions.

e. Deliquescent salts, and those containing a large proportion of water, unless this be suitably absorbed by associated dry powder.
f. Those which are prescribed for immediate effect; as emetics, diffusible stimulants.
g. Essential oil, in quantity exceeding half a drop to each pill.

The formation of a pill mass is sometimes a matter of considerable difficulty; sometimes, from a want of adhesiveness of the ingredients; sometimes, from the difficulty of incorporating them equally together. Under the head of The Art of Dispensing, I shall introduce some hints upon the mode of overcoming difficulties of this kind, and for the present shall confine myself to the mode of *prescribing* pills.

Should the physician indicate the excipient, or leave it optional with the apothecary? In answering this, we necessarily bring into view the therapeutical relations of this ingredient, and shall find that it may be active or inert, according to the choice of the prescriber.

If the basis be a vegetable powder, like rhubarb or aloes, a mass can be readily formed by moisture, without the aid of any adhesive material; if, on the contrary, it be a metallic salt, or an unadhesive vegetable powder, it requires an addition to give it the form of a mass; that addition will add somewhat to the bulk of the ingredients prescribed, and perhaps, if the dose be large, will make the pills too bulky; in this case, it is important that the physician should not overlook the excipient, which he may include among the medicinal ingredients, or make due allowance for, in apportioning the quantity to each pill.

The following rule for prescribing pills will obviate the disadvantage of adding to the size by the use of inert excipients: *when the basis is an unadhesive material, one of the other medicinal ingredients should be an extract or a vegetable powder, which will form a mass by moisture alone.*

To illustrate this, I would refer to prescriptions No. 12 and No. 55, in both of which the adjuvant possesses this quality, while in a large number of cases, the constituent or vehicle is of little or no therapeutic value.

It will be proper in this connection to run over the several substances, added with a view to giving body to pill masses, or adapting medicines to the pilular form, so as to point out the special adaptations of each.

Soap, which is employed in the officinal pills more than any other excipient, is well adapted to combine with resinous substances, the solubility of which it increases, while it acts as an antacid, and perhaps aperient. It has been suggested, that it is incompatible with opium, with which it is prescribed in the officinal *pil. opii*, as the alkali, especially when present in excess, tends to separate the morphia from its native combination. Some experiments made by my assistant, Thomas Weaver, confirm this idea.

Syrup is often used as an excipient, which adds but little to the bulk of a pill mass, and is effectual in some cases, where water alone would not give the requisite tenacity; it does not answer a good purpose, however, with certain metallic salts, which dispose the mass to crumble.

Honey and *molasses*, forms of uncrystallizable sugar, are better adapted to the general purposes of pill making. Masses made with these are not so liable to crumble, and possess the great advantage of remaining moist and soluble for a longer period. On account of the last-named property, honey has been substituted for syrup in the officinal recipe for sulphate of quinia pills, in the last edition of the *Pharmacopœia.*

Gum Arabic is directed to be added, where the requisite adhesiveness will not result from the use of syrup or honey alone; it is not a very good excipient, either added in the form of powder, or of a thick mucilage. Pills made with gum are apt to be very hard. Tragacanth forms a less hard and insoluble mass than acacia. The officinal syrup of gum Arabic is made with a special view to this use.

Alcohol and *essential oils*, by softening down resinous substances, facilitate their incorporation together in mass, and, being held by these with considerable tenacity, prevent their rapidly becoming too hard. Lactucarium may be brought to a pilular consistence by the use of a small proportion of *chloroform*, which rapidly evaporates, leaving the pills of an elegant consistence. Oil of turpentine is well adapted to softening white turpentine, so as to incorporate it with other ingredients, as in Otto's emmenagogue pills. These excipients must be added with care, or they will render the mass quite too soft.

An important use of essential oils in pills, is to prevent mouldiness, and the disagreeable odor which vegetable powders acquire when moistened; they should be added in very small proportion for this purpose, as they rather interfere with than promote the adhesiveness of the mass.

Crumb of bread furnishes a convenient, and when not too dry, a very tenacious vehicle for substances given in small dose, and which require diluting, rather than combining in a small bulk.

Confection of rose is adapted to similar uses, though more moist and less tough in consistence. When made from the rosa gallica, it is astringent, and adapted to combining certain vegetable powders belonging to that class; as usually met with, it contains no tannin, being made from our common varieties of rose. Confection of orange-peel, and aromatic confection, are adapted to similar uses.

The Officinal Pill Masses.—These may be described in this place as preparations well adapted to use as excipients, though very frequently prescribed singly.

Pilulæ Hydrargyri, U.S.

This is the officinal designation of the preparation commonly called blue pill, and directed in the *Pharmacopœia* to be divided into pills of three grains each; as usually kept by physicians and druggists in an undivided state, it is more appropriately called *massa hydrargyri*, mercurial mass. It is usually prepared by drug millers and chemical manufacturers, by triturating together, in appropriate mechanical contrivances, mercury, conserve of rose, liquorice root in powder, and some rather moist viscid material, as powdered althea root, in such proportion that three parts by weight of the mass shall contain one of mercury, thoroughly divided, and partly oxidized.

To my friend and former pupil, Thomas Weaver, the reader is indebted for the suggestion of the following good extemporaneous process for the preparation of this heretofore troublesome mass. It is adapted equally to producing a soft or a pulverulent article, and is so rapid and easy as to supersede the necessity for the use of machinery for small quantities. Its importance as a practical improvement will be appreciated by those who have attempted to prepare blue mass with the pestle and mortar by the officinal process, and by such as have been disappointed in the quality of the manufactured article as met with in commerce.

To make three ounces of Blue Mass extemporaneously.

Take of Mercury	℥j.
Powdered liquorice root	℥ss.
" rose leaves	ʒvj.
Honey	ʒvj.

Triturate the honey, liquorice root, and mercury, rapidly together for three minutes, or until all the globules of mercury disappear, then add the rose leaves, and work the whole into a uniform mass; if it is too stiff, moisten with a little water.

According to James Beatson, late apothecary to the U. S. Naval Hospital, at New York, the same object may be accomplished by triturating the mercury with the honey, until the former is completely extinguished; then adding rose-water, powdered rose leaves, powdered liquorice root, and sugar, to make up the requisite proportion.

W. W. Stoddart triturates the mercury with the powdered liquorice root, kept moist by a little rose-water, and then adds the confection of roses.

To make Powdered Blue Mass.

Take of Mercury	℥j.
Powdered liquorice root	℥j.
" rose leaves	ʒvj.
Simple syrup	f℥ij.

Triturate the mercury, one-fourth of the powdered liquorice root, and the simple syrup rapidly together for three minutes, or until the globules disappear, and then incorporate the powdered rose leaves, and the remainder of the powdered liquorice root, and spread the whole out to dry in a warm place. Reduce this to powder.

Blue mass is, perhaps, the most popular, as it is the mildest form of mercurial preparation; it is well adapted to use in pill or powder, either combined, as in several prescriptions which follow, or singly, in doses of from one to ten grains.

Blue mass, when designed to act on the liver without producing a cathartic effect, may be combined with opium or a pure astringent. It is frequently, however, combined with cathartics, to increase its tendency to operate on the bowels. Perhaps a majority of the mild cathartic pills, prescribed by practitioners and those sold as universal remedies, contain this useful ingredient; and, in fact, blue pills are very commonly known and taken by those who prescribe for themselves for what is popularly known as "biliousness," and various forms of liver complaint.

From specimens of blue mass which have been dried at a moderate heat, a very convenient powder may be prepared, which is well suited for conversion into the pilular form, and into compound powders.

Blue mass was formerly much adulterated, but is now supplied to the trade of reliable quality by several first-rate manufacturers.

Pilulæ Ferri Carbonatis, U.S.

Vallette's Mass is a very mild and soluble preparation of iron, made by incorporating freshly-precipitated protocarbonate of iron with honey, or a mixture of honey and gum tragacanth, or some similar saccharine vehicle which experience has taught the manufacturer to prefer, and by evaporation concentrating into a solid pilular mass. This may be taken by itself, in a dose of from ten to thirty grains, or may be used as an adjuvant or vehicle to other medicinal substances, particularly dry powders, as in those numerous cases where iron, in small doses, is indicated along with bitter tonics.

Pilulæ Copaibæ, U. S.

Copaiba mass, although seldom employed as a vehicle, is not unsuited to this use; it is directed to be made by incorporating one drachm of calcined magnesia with two ounces of copaiva, a recipe which it is very difficult to follow, so as to get a solid mass. The copaiva must be thick and resinoid, and the magnesia recently calcined, or the required thickening will not occur. The introduction of wax, in considerable quantity, to give it consistence, should not be allowed. Its dose is from five to ten grains.

The Extracts.

This class, which is much the best adapted to the pilular form, should not be overlooked in prescribing several ingredients; some one extract can usually be selected which will meet a therapeutical indication, while it serves the purpose of an excipient.

Thus, in sedative or narcotic pills, we have the choice of five or six extracts to incorporate with any unadhesive or other material, so as to gain efficiency without too large a bulk. In directing a tonic remedy in this form, extract of gentian, quassia, cinchona, or nux vomica will come in play. While, as a vehicle, for the mercurials in cutaneous or syphilitic diseases, extract of conium, or of sarsaparilla, may be used. The use of the cathartic extracts, and of extract of taraxacum for similar purposes, is too common to need comment. We also have an illustration of an elegant and efficient compound, made on this principle, in the so-called Dr. Vance's Gout Pills (Prescription No. 28).

The following Tables show, in a general way, the classes of drugs adapted to the form of powder and pill.

Medicines adapted to the Form of Powder.

INSOLUBLE MINERAL SUBSTANCES, VEGETABLE PRODUCTS AND SOME SOLUBLE SUBSTANCES.

INSOLUBLE; TOO LARGE DOSES FOR PILLS.

Carbo ligni.
Magnesia.
Calcis phosph.
Pot. bitart.
Sulphur sublim.
Creta ppt.
Ferri subcarb.
Ferri phosph. and others.
Vegetable Powders:—
Powd. cinchona.
" colomba.
" gentian.
" rhubarb (coarse).
" jalap.
" cubebs,
and others.

IN CERTAIN COMBINATIONS, AND WHEN PILLS ARE OBJECTED TO.

Powd. pil. hydrarg.
" ext. coloc. comp.
" opium.
" digitalis.
" nux vom.
" kino.
" acid, tannic.
" " gallic.
" potas. nit.
Opium alkaloids.
Cinchona "
Subnit. bismuth,
and many others.

Diluents for Substances prescribed in Form of Powders.

Sugar.
Lactin.
Mannite.
Powd. acacia.
" cinnamon,
and others.

Aromatic powder.
Powd. ext. liquorice.
" tragacanth.
" elm bark.

Medicines adapted to Pilular Form.

POWDERS GIVEN IN LESS THAN GR. XV DOSES GUM RESINS EXTRACTS; ALSO OLEO-RESINS AND OILS IN SMALL PROPORTION.

UNADHESIVE MATERIALS.

Calomel.
Pulv. ipecac. et opii.
Bismuth. subnit.
Morphiæ acetas, &c.
Strychnia.
Pulv. digitalis.
" ipecac.
Plumbi acetas.
Ant. et pot. tart.
" sulphuret.
Argenti nitras.
Argenti oxidum.
Ferri pulvis.
" subcarb.
" (other salts).
Potas. iodid.
Camphor, and others.
Difficult to combine, except by Peculiar Treatment:—
Ol. tiglii.
" terebinth.
Ferri iodidum.
Copaiba, and others.

GOOD MEDICINAL EXCIPIENTS.

Extracts.
Pil. hydrarg.
" copaibæ.
" ferri carb.
Terebinthina.
With Moisture:—
Pulv. aloes.
" rhei.
" kino.
" acidi tannici.
" opii.
" scillæ.
Sulph. bebeerinæ.
Ferri citras.
Assafœtida, and others.
With Alcohol:—
Guaiacum, and others.
With Dil. SO_3:—
Quiniæ sulph.
Cinchoniæ sulph.
Quinidiæ sulph.
Quinoidina.

Inert Excipients.

	MUCILAGES.
Pulv. gum Arab.	Syrup of gum.
" tragacanth.	Honey.
Castile soap.	Treacle.
Crumb of bread.	Syrups.
Confections.	

In the following officinal and extemporaneous prescriptions, some of which are extracted from standard works, others from the extensive files of the dispensing establishment over which I preside, and a few which I venture to offer for trial, I have endeavored to point out the most approved methods of compounding medicines in the form of powders and pills.

Examples of Extemporaneous Prescriptions in the form of Powders and Pills, including those in the Pharmacopœia under the heads Pulveres and Pilulæ.

ASTRINGENTS.

No. 1.—*Used in Obstinate Diarrhœa.*

			1 powder.
Take of	Alum	ʒij	20 grs.
	Kino	ʒss	5 grs.

Mix and reduce to a very fine powder, and distribute this into six papers. DOSE, one every two or three hours.

The alum and kino are incompatible in liquid form, and hence, when associated together, should always be prescribed in powder. The dose is too large for the pilular form.

No. 2.—*Adapted to substitute many Simple Vegetable Astringents.*

			Each.
Take of	Tannic acid	gr. xij	1 grain.
	Confection of rose	gr. vj	½ grain.

Make a mass and divide into twelve pills. DOSE, one every two hours.

The above may be made into powders by substituting an aromatic, astringent, or inert powder for the confection.

No. 3.—*Used in Diarrhœa.*

			Each.
Take of	Tannic acid	℈j	2 grs.
	Acetate of morphia	gr. j	$\frac{1}{10}$ gr.
	Sugar	gr. x	1 gr.
	Oil of caraway	♏j	trace.

Triturate together, and distribute into ten papers. DOSE, one every three hours.

Five grains of opium may be substituted for the morphia salt, or by the substitution of sufficient syrup for the sugar, the whole may be made into the pilular form.

No. 4.—*Chalk Powders.*

		Each.
Take of Prepared chalk . .	ʒij	15 grs.
Gum Arabic, in powder		7½ grs.
Sugar, each . .	ʒj	7½ grs.
Powdered cinnamon .	gr. x	1¼ grs.

Triturate together into a uniform powder, and divide into eight doses.

Chalk mixture, No. 71, spoils by keeping in hot weather, and is, moreover, much more bulky than an equal quantity of the ingredients in the above form, which is especially convenient for travellers. Opium, kino, or other remedies adapted to increase or modify its action, may be added in powder, as their Galenical solutions are to the mixture. One of the very best additions for a common form of diarrhœa is that of powdered blue mass, of which gr. xvj to ʒss may be added to the above.

No. 5.—*Powders of Chalk and Opium.*

Take of Precipitated carbonate of lime . .	ʒj.
Tincture of opium	fʒj.
Pulv. pil. hydrarg.	gr. x.

Triturate in a mortar and expose till it is dry, then divide into ten powders. Dose, one every three hours until the symptoms are checked.

No. 6.—*For the Diarrhœa of Young Children.*

		Each.
Take of Acetate of lead	gr. ij	1/6
Opium	gr. ss	1/24
Camphor	gr. j	1/12
Sugar	gr. iij	1/4

Triturate, and divide into twelve papers. Dose, one every two or three hours.

The child should be kept quiet, and fed upon arrowroot, flour boiled in milk, or a mixture of barley-water and cream.

For adults, the whole quantity prescribed may be taken at one dose.

Tonics and Aromatics.

No. 7.—*Anti-Intermittent Powders.*

		Each.
Take of Powdered cinchona . .	℥j	ʒj.
" serpentaria .	ʒij	gr. xv.
Sulphate of quinia . .	gr. viij	gr. j.

Mix and distribute into eight papers. Dose, one every hour, commencing eight hours before the expected paroxysm.

The sulphate of quinia is often omitted, but increases the efficiency of the powder, especially when the bark is not of the finest quality. The serpentaria is often substituted by more powerful stimulants, as cloves, or capsicum, or oil of black pepper; and sometimes to obviate costiveness, a saline cathartic is added.

No. 8.—*Pilulæ Quiniæ Sulphatis*, U. S.

		Reduced.	Each.
Take of Sulphate of quinia . .	℥j	℈ij	1 gr.
Powdered gum Arabic .	ʒij	gr. x	¼ gr.
Honey	q. s.	q. s.	

Make a mass, and divide into 480 pills (reduced quantity, 40), of which the dose in intermittents is one every hour, between the paroxysms.

These officinal pills are less used than formerly, as it is now customary to give larger doses, and less frequently, and they are found less convenient than pills or powders, of three, four, or five grains each.

Sulphate of quinine may be made into pills by the following process, which has been called Parrish's. (See paper by the author, in the *American Journal of Pharmacy*, vol. xxv. p. 291.)

No. 9.—*Pills of the Soluble Sulphate of Quinia.*

		Each.
Take of Sulphate of quinia . .	℈j	gr. v.
Aromatic sulphuric acid .	♏xij	♏iij.

Drop the acid upon the sulphate on a tile or slab, and triturate with a spatula, until it thickens and assumes a pilular consistence, then divide into four pills.

The five grain quinine pill made in this way, is not larger than many pills in common use; they may be conveniently made of two, three, four, or five grains.

The large number of combinations in which sulphate of quinia is associated with other remedies cannot be here noticed; to some of these, as in combining the other alkaloids with it, the elixir of vitriol process is well adapted; in other cases it is inadmissible. If an extract in small quantity, or a vegetable powder, is to be added to the mass, it should be incorporated with the quinia salt, when by trituration on the slab it begins to thicken into a paste.

Persons not accustomed to making quinine pills by this process sometimes allow the sulphate to become too dry and unadhesive to mould into pills. This is from not seizing the proper moment just as the mass has ceased to be too soft, and before it becomes dry; it is then quite plastic, and becomes particularly so by contact with the warmth and moisture of the thumb and fingers. A drop of syrup or honey, which should always be at hand on the counter, by being added at the proper moment will prevent this hardening.

Sulphate of quinia will make a very good pill mass by using one grain of glacial phosphoric acid, or a quarter of a grain of tartaric acid, to each grain of the quinia salt.

No. 10.—*Pills of Sulphate of Cinchonia.*

			Each.
Take of Sulphate of cinchonia	. .	℈j	gr. j.
Powdered tragacanth	. .	gr. ij	gr. $\frac{1}{10}$.

Triturate together, and add sufficient water to make a mass, which divide into twenty pills; these pills are esteemed about equal to those of sulphate of quinia in most cases.

No. 11.—*Pills of Sulphate of Quinidia..*

			Each.
Take of Sulphate of quinidia	. .	℈j	gr. j.
Powdered tragacanth	. .	gr. ij	gr. $\frac{1}{10}$.

Triturate together, and add water sufficient to make a mass, which divide into twenty pills. These are esteemed about equal to sulphate of quinia pills of the same proportion.

The use of tragacanth instead of gum Arabic would be an improvement in the officinal sulphate of quinia pills; it diminishes the size, and keeps them longer moist and soluble.

I have experimented with sulphate of cinchonia and sulphate of quinidia with reference to the formation of pill masses with elixir of vitriol, and find that sulphate of cinchonia requires about one drop to three grains, and sulphate of quinidia three drops to two grains. They thicken into a firm mass with less facility than the quinine salt, and in fact require sometimes an hour or two to become firm enough to roll out; this is remedied by adding a little of some vegetable powder, as gum Arabic or starch, which, however, increases the bulk.

Practitioners are still disposed to examine the relative merits of the cinchona alkaloids as antiperiodics. In the Pennsylvania Hospital, and other of our large charities, the experience of the medical staff is favorable to substituting for the more expensive sulphate of quinia, sulphate of cinchonia, and sulphate of quinidia in the same dose.

A still cheaper form of cinchona preparation is the following:—

No. 12.—*Pills of Chinoidine.*

Take of Chinoidine	. . . . . .	℥j.
Aromatic sulphuric acid	. . . .	♏ v. or q. s.

Soften the chinoidine with the acid, in a mortar, and divide into twenty pills.

Combinations of salts of quinia and iron are much resorted to in anæmia accompanied by want of appetite; of these, two instances are given below.

No. 13.—*Powders of Iron and Quinia.*

			Each.
Take of Subcarbonate of iron	. .	ʒj	5 grs.
Sulphate of quinia	. .	gr. vj	½ gr.
Aromatic powder	. .	gr. xij	1 gr.

Triturate together, and distribute into twelve powders. DOSE, take a powder three times a day before meals.

The proportion of sulphate of quinia should be increased when it is to be employed in convalescence from intermittents.

No. 14.—*Pills of Proto-Carbonate of Iron and Quinia.*

		Each.
Take of Sulphate of quinia . . .	℈j	1 gr.
Mass of carbonate of iron (Vallette's)	ʒj	3 grs.

Mix, and make into twenty pills. DOSE, one twice or three times a day.

In this class of prescription, the sulphates of cinchonia and quinidia, and of bebeerina, may generally be substituted for that of quinia without disadvantage.

No. 15.—*Pulvis Morphiæ Attenuatus.*

℞.—Morphiæ sulphatis	gr. j.
Sacch. lactis	gr. v.

Misce.

One grain is designed to be an equivalent to one grain of opium; it furnishes a convenient form for administering small doses of morphia in prescription.

No. 16.—*Pills of Quevenne's Iron.*

		Each.
Take of Iron in powder	gr. CC	2 grs.
Manna	gr. C	1 gr.

Triturate into a mass and divide into 100 pills.

Manna is an excellent excipient for Ferri pulvis, and will answer in less proportion, if very small pills are desired; when not at hand, it may be substituted by honey and a little gum Arabic, or tragacanth.

In a number of cases it will be desirable to introduce adjuvants; which may be in the form of extract. Extracts of conium, of aconite, cinchona, nux vomica, and quassia, are favorite adjuvants with Quevenne's iron.

No. 17.—*Pulvis Aromaticus,* U. S.

Take of Cinnamon,	
Ginger, of each	℥ij.
Cardamom, deprived of the capsules,	
Nutmeg, grated, of each	℥j.

Rub them together into a very fine powder.

In this preparation, the dry powders of cinnamon and ginger enable us to reduce the oily nutmeg and cardamoms to a fine condition; the whole should be passed through a sieve.

By trituration with honey, syrup of orange-peel, and saffron, this furnishes confectio aromatica.

In compound powders, as in Prescription No. 13, this is a frequent ingredient, and is recommended by an agreeable flavor.

No. 18.—*Dr. Mitchell's Tonic Pills.*

		Each.
Take of Extract of quassia . .	gr. xxxvj	3 grs.
Extract of conium, . .		¼ gr.
Subcarbonate of iron, of each	gr. iij.	¼ gr.

Make into a mass with a few drops of solution of arsenite of potassa (if required); then divide into twelve pills. DOSE, a pill twice or three times daily.

No. 19.—*Tonic and Aromatic Pills.* (Dr. Parrish, Senior.)

		Each.
Take of Sulphate of quinia . .	gr. iij	¼ gr.
Powdered capsicum . .		½ gr.
Mace		½ gr.
Powdered cloves . .		½ gr.
Carbonate of ammonia, each	gr. vj	½ gr.
Oil of caraway . . .	gtt. iij	¼ ♏.
Confection of rose . .	sufficient	q. s.

Form a uniform tenacious mass, and divide into twelve pills.

No. 20.—*Used in Obstinate Intermittents.* (Dr. Chapman.)

		Each.
Take of Sulphate of copper . .	gr. iij	¼ gr.
Powdered opium . .	gr. iv	⅓ gr.
" gum Arabic .	gr. viij	⅔ gr.
Syrup	Sufficient.	

Make a mass, and divide into twelve pills. DOSE, one every three hours.

No. 21.—*Pilulæ Ferri Compositæ*, U.S.

		Each.
Take of Myrrh, in powder . .	ʒij	1½ gr.
Carbonate of soda . .		} FeO,CO_2
Sulphate of iron, of each .	ʒj	} $\frac{5}{16}$ gr.
Syrup	q. s.	q. s.

Rub the myrrh with the carbonate of soda, then add the sulphate of iron, and again rub them; lastly, beat them with the syrup so as to form a mass to be divided into eighty pills.

This pill is similar in composition to Griffith's Iron Mixture. Supposing a reaction to take place between the salts present, proto-carbonate of iron would be produced, which, with the myrrh, forms an admirable remedy in chlorosis, &c. I should greatly prefer the use of a lump of fresh myrrh to the powdered article of commerce.

No. 22.—*Pilulæ Ferri Iodidi*, U. S.

			Each.
℞.—	Sulphate of iron . . .	ʒj	FeI $1\frac{2}{3}$ grs.
	Iodide of potassium . .	℈iv	
	Tragacanth, in powder . .	gr. x	$\frac{1}{4}$ gr.
	Sugar, in powder . . .	ʒss	$\frac{3}{4}$ gr.

Beat them with syrup, so as to form a mass, to be divided into forty pills.

The formation of iodide of iron depends upon the presence of moisture and fluids to produce deliquescence. The mass should be as dry as possible to be plastic, and may then be advantageously kept in a tightly stopped bottle.

No. 23.—*Compound Pills of Iodide of Iron.*

(Prescribed by Dr. Buckler, of Baltimore.)

Take of	Iodide of potassium	ʒij.
	Iodide of iron	ʒj.
	Iodine	gr. vj.
	Extract of conium	ʒj.

Triturate the iodide of potassium, iodide of iron, and iodine together with a few drops of water to the consistence of a soft paste, then add powdered gum Arabic in the proportion of half a grain to each pill, and rub into a smooth paste. Incorporate with the whole the extract of conium, and make into a *soft mass*, with a mixture of equal parts of finely powdered elm bark and liquorice root. Then divide into sixty pills.

The combination of these ingredients is a matter of not a little difficulty by the ordinary method, but this recipe, furnished by Dr. W. S. Thompson, of Baltimore, is very practicable and convenient.

No. 24.—*Pills of Chloride of Iron.* (J. T. Shinn.)

Take of Tincture of muriate of iron . . . . f℥ij.

Evaporate nearly to dryness, and add—

Powdered althea root . . . . . ʒss.

Triturate into a pill mass, and divide into 240 pills, each of which represents about ten drops of the tincture.

They should be kept and dispensed in vials.

No. 25.—*For Chronic Indigestion and Irritability of Stomach.*

			Each.
℞.—	Bismuthi subnitratis . .	ʒj	10 grs.
	Pulveris rhei	ʒss	5 grs.
	" aromatici . .	℈ij	$6\frac{2}{3}$ grs.

Misce et divide in chart. vj. *Signa.*—Take one before each meal.

Nervous Stimulants; Antispasmodics.

No. 26.—*Pilulæ Assafœtidæ*, U. S.

			Reduced.	Each.
Take of	Assafœtida . .	℥iss	gr. xxxvj	gr. iij.
	Soap . . .	℥ss	gr. xij	gr. i.

Beat them with water, so as to form a mass, and divide into 240 pills. (The reduced quantity into 12 pills.) Dose, one to four pills.

No. 27.—*Pilulæ Aloes et Assafœtidæ*, U. S.

			Reduced.	Each.
Take of	Aloes, in powder . .		gr. xvj	gr. 1⅓.
	Assafœtida . . .			gr. 1⅓.
	Soap, each . . .	℥ss		gr. 1⅓.

Beat them with water, so as to form a mass, to be divided into 180 pills. (Reduced, 12 pills.) Dose, one to four pills.

No. 28.—*Pilulæ Galbani Compositæ*, U. S.

			Reduced.	Each.
Take of	Galbanum .			gr. 1½.
	Myrrh, each .	ʒvj	each gr. xviij	gr. 1½.
	Assafœtida .	ʒij	gr. vj	gr. ½.
	Syrup . .	Sufficient	Sufficient	gr. 3½.

Beat them together, so as to form a mass, to be divided into 240 pills. (Reduced, 12 pills.) Dose, one to three pills.

No. 29.—*Dr. Otto's Antispasmodic Powders.*

Take of Black mustard seed,
Powdered sage,
Powdered ginger, equal parts by measure.
Mix thoroughly.

Dose, three teaspoonfuls, for three mornings in succession; discontinue three; then give as before. To be moistened with water or molasses.

This powder is highly recommended, in epilepsy, by several practitioners, and recently by Dr. Charles D. Hendry, of Haddonfield, N. J.

No. 30.—*Pills of Nitrate of Silver.*

Take of	Nitrate of silver	℈j.
	Turpentine (terebinthina, *U. S.*)	ʒj.

Triturate, with the addition of a few drops of oil of turpentine if necessary, to make a uniform pilular mass, which divide into thirty pills. Used in typhoid fever, epilepsy, &c. Dose, one pill every three or four hours.

ARTERIAL STIMULANTS.

No. 31.—*Powders or Pills of Carbonate of Ammonia, &c.*

Take of Muriate of ammonia (granulated),
Dried carbonate of soda, each . . . ℈ij.
Powdered capsicum . . . . . . ℈j.

Triturate into a uniform fine powder, and divide into ten papers, which should be wrapped in tinfoil.

By the aid of moisture, these powders are made to react with each other and develop carbonate of ammonia. To make into pills, add a portion of firm and rather dry conserve of rose. Divide into twenty pills, and keep them in a vial.

A solution of mastich in ether is a good varnish for coating these and similar pills: they should be as dry as possible before using this varnish.

CEREBRAL STIMULANTS, OR NARCOTICS.

No. 32.—*Pilulæ Opii*, U. S.

		Reduced.	Each.
Take of Opium, in powder .	ʒj	gr. xij	gr. j.
Soap	gr. xij	gr. iiss	gr. ⅕.

Beat into a mass with water, and divide into 60 pills. (Reduced, 12.)

The officinal pills of opium have long appeared to me to be defective, and when it is left optional what excipient to employ, I use syrup, or syrup of gum in preference to soap, which is apt to be incompatible with the opium.

Old opium pills are sometimes in request, from their being better retained by an irritable stomach, and from the fact that by their more gradual solution, they affect more favorably the diseases of the lower intestine. The best way to make pills to be kept for this purpose is to select a portion of the solid mass in its natural and plastic condition, and to divide it, without admixture, into the required number of pills; these, as they contract and harden, will become compact and of slow solubility.

No. 33.—*Anodyne Pills.*

		Each.
Take of Acetate of morphia	gr. j	gr. ⅛.
Extract of hyoscyamus . . .	gr. iv	gr. ½.

Triturate into a pill mass, and divide into eight pills. DOSE, one pill, repeated if necessary.

These are very small, and are not astringent in their effects on the bowels.

No. 34.—"*Dr. Vance's Rheumatism and Gout Pills.*"

		Each.
℞.—Extracti colchici acetici . .	ʒss	gr. 1¼.
Pulveris ipecacuanhæ et opii .	ʒiss, gr. vj	gr. iv.

Misce et divide in pilulas xxiv. *Signa.*—Take two at night and one before breakfast and dinner.

This is a most valuable combination, having been found efficacious in a great many cases.

No. 35.—*Lartique's Gout Pills.*

		Each.
℞.—Extracti colocynthidis compositi .	ʒiss, gr. vj	gr. 4.
" colchici acetici . .	gr. x	gr. ⅖.
" digitalis	gr. v	gr. ⅕.

Misce, fiat massa in pilulas xxiv dividenda. *Signa.*—Take two for a dose.

No. 36.—*Pills of Camphor and Opium.*

		Each.
℞.—Camphoræ	gr. xxiv	gr. 2.
Pulveris opii	gr. vj	gr. ½.
Alcoholis	gtt. vj	trace.
Confectionis rosæ	q. s.	q. s.

Misce, et fiant, secundum artem, pilulæ xij. *Signa.*—Dose, from one to two pills.

"Excito-Mótor Stimulants."

No. 37.—*Powders given in Uterine Hemorrhages.*

		Each.
Take of Ergot, freshly powdered . .	ʒj	gr. 10.
Alum, in powder	℈j	gr. 3⅓.

Mix and divide into six equal parts.

Sometimes borax is substituted for alum in similar combinations.

Arterial Sedatives.

No. 38.—*Powders of Nitre and Tartrate of Antimony.*

		Each.
Take of Tartrate of antimony and potassa	gr. j	gr. $\frac{1}{12}$.
Nitrate of potassa		gr. 2½.
Sugar, each	ʒss	gr. 2½.

Triturate into powder, and distribute equally into twelve papers.

Some powders of this class are introduced among the liquid preparations.

EMETICS.

No. 39.—*A Prompt and Efficient Emetic.*

		Each.
℞.—Pulveris ipecacuanhæ . . .	ʒss	gr. xv.
Antimonii et potassæ tartratis . .	gr. ij	gr. j.

Misce et divide in pulveres ij. *Signa.*—Take one in a little molasses, or sugar and water, and follow it by a draught of warm water. If one powder does not produce the effect, the second may be taken soon after.

Sometimes *calomel* is added to emetic powders, and both a purgative and emetic effect are produced. Emetics, as such, are never given in pill.

CATHARTICS AND LAXATIVES.

To this class belong six of the pills, and two of the compound powders of the *Pharmacopœia.*

No. 40.—*Pilulæ Rhei*, U. S.

		Reduced.	Each.
Take of Rhubarb, in powder .	ʒvj.	gr. xxxvj	gr. 3.
Soap . . .	ʒij	gr. xij	gr. 1.

Beat them with water, so as to form a mass, to be divided into 120 pills. (Reduced, into 12 pills.)

The following recipe will make an elegant rhubarb pill without the use of soap, which is objectionable as imparting a disposition to become mouldy, and produce an unpleasant odor when damp.

		Each.
Take of Powdered rhubarb . .	gr. xlviij	gr. iv.
Comp. tincture of cardamom	gtt. xlviij	gtt. iv.

Triturate into a mass, and divide into twelve pills.

No. 41.—*Pilulæ Rhei Compositæ*, U. S.

		Reduced.	Each.
Take of Rhubarb, in powder	℥j	gr. xxiv	gr. 2.
Aloes "	ʒvj	gr. xviij	gr. 1½.
Myrrh "	℥ss	gr. xij	gr. 1.
Oil of peppermint	fʒss	♏ij	♏⅙.

Beat them with water, so as to form a mass, to be divided into 240 pills. (Reduced, into 12 pills.)

No. 42.—*Pilulæ Aloës*, U. S.

		Reduced.	Each.
Take of Aloes, in powder . .			gr. 2.
Soap, each . . .	℥j	℈ij	gr. 2.

Beat them with water, so as to form a mass, to be divided into 240 pills. (Reduced, 20 pills.)

No. 43.—*Pilulæ Hydrargyri Chloridi Mitis*, U. S.

			Each.
Take of Mild chloride of mercury	℥ss	gr. xij	gr. j.
Gum Arabic, in powder	ʒj	gr. iij	gr. ¼.
Syrup	Sufficient quantity.		

Mix together the chloride of mercury and the gum, then beat them with the syrup, so as to form a mass, to be divided into 240 pills. (Reduced, 12 pills.)

These pills are very rarely prescribed, as they contain too large a dose for the slow alterative effects, and are inconveniently small for a cathartic dose. (Compare No. 48 and No. 63.)

No. 44.—*Pilulæ Catharticæ Compositæ*, U. S.

		Reduced.	Each.
Take of Compound extract of colocynth, in powder . . .	℥ss	gr. xvj	1⅓.
Extract of jalap[1] . . .			1 gr.
Mild chloride of mercury, each	ʒiij	gr. xij	1 gr.
Gamboge, in powder . .	℈ij	gr. iiss	⅙.

Mix them together; then with water form a mass, to be divided into 180 pills. (Reduced, twelve pills.)

These well-known and popular pills are very easy to make, if the extracts, both of colocynth and jalap, are powdered before being incorporated with the other ingredients; but if the extract of jalap is of a tough consistence, which it frequently reaches by partial drying, it is almost impossible to incorporate it with the other ingredients. Powdered extract of jalap, as elsewhere stated, is now generally obtainable, and may be kept in a salt mouth bottle like any other powder; a few drops of moisture will form it into a plastic mass. The tough extract should be further dried and powdered, or, if required to be used on an emergency, may be softened by heating and triturating in a capsule with diluted alcohol.

Under the name of *anti-bilious pills*, this preparation is vended in great quantities over the country, and by its admirable combination of cathartic properties, is well adapted to supersede as a popular remedy, the numerous nostrums advertised and sold for similar purposes.

No. 45.—*Pilulæ Aloës et Myrrhæ*, U. S.

		Reduced.	Each.
Take of Aloes, in powder . .	℥ij	gr. xxiv	2 grs.
Myrrh " . .	℥j	gr. xij	1 gr.
Saffron " . .	℥ss	gr. vj	½ gr.
Syrup, sufficient quantity		q. s.	

Beat the whole together so as to form a mass, to be divided into 480 pills. (Reduced, twelve pills.)

[1] Extract of podophyllum might be well substituted in half the quantity, or if in the full proportion, would increase the activity of the pill.

A tonic and emmenagogue cathartic. Saffron may be reduced to powder by heating it in a capsule till it becomes crisp, then triturating it in a mortar.

No. 46.—*Pulvis Aloës et Canellæ*, U.S. (*Hiera Picra.*)

		Reduced.
Take of Aloes	℔j	℥iss.
Canella	℥iij	ʒiij.

Rub them separately into very fine powder, and mix them.

Hiera picra is generally macerated in some kind of spirits, and taken in draughts as a stomachic laxative.

No. 47.—*Pulvis Jalapæ Compositus*, U.S.

Take of Jalap, in powder	℥j.
Bitartrate of potassa	℥ij.

Mix them.

This is a mild laxative, given in doses of gr. xv to ʒss. Sulphur and bitartrate of potassa are much associated in about equal bulks.

No. 48.—*Calomel and Jalap Powder.*

℞.—Hydrargyri chloridi mitis	gr. xv.
Pulveris jalapæ	℈j.

Misce. To be given at a dose.

In the same way rhubarb is very commonly associated with calomel.

No. 49.—*Rhubarb and Magnesia Powder.*

℞.—Pulveris rhei	℈j.
Magnesiæ	℈ij.
Olei menthæ viridis	♏j.

Misce. To be given at a dose.

Charcoal and magnesia constitute another very popular laxative combination.

The weighing and putting up of these powders is very improving practice for the student at the commencement of his novitiate.

No. 50.—*Neutralizing Powder.*

Take of Bicarbonate of soda,
Powdered rhubarb,
" mint (the herb) . . . Equal parts.

Rub the mixed ingredients through a sieve of sixty meshes to the inch.

Dose, a teaspoonful as an antacid remedy in diarrhœa and dyspepsia.

No. 51.—*Mitchell's Aperient Pills.*

		Each.
℞.—Pulveris aloës	gr. xij	1 gr.
" rhei	gr. xxiv	2 grs.
Hydrarg. chlor. mit. . . .	gr. ij	$\frac{1}{6}$ gr.
Antim. et potas. tart. . . .	gr. j	$\frac{1}{12}$ gr.

Misce, fiant pilulæ No. xij.

One acts as an aperient, two or three as a cathartic; they, as well as most of the other aloetic pills, are contraindicated where there is a tendency to hæmorrhoids.

No. 52.—*Epsom Salt and Mannite.*

Take of Sulphate of magnesia . . . . . . ℨj.
Mannite . . . . ℨij.

Triturate into a uniform powder. A good and agreeable cathartic in the above dose.

No. 53.—*Laxative Tonic Pills.* (Dr. Parrish, Sen.)

Take of Powdered Socotrine aloes . . . . ℈ij.
" rhubarb . . . . . ℈iv.
Oil of caraway . . . . . . gtt. xij.
Extract of gentian . . . . . ℈ij.

Make into forty pills. Dose, two before dinner.

No. 54.—*Pills of Alöin and Podophyllin.*

Take of Alöin . . . . gr. xxiv.
Podophyllin . . . . . . gr. xij.
Oleo-resin of ginger . . . . . ♏ iv.

Triturate the solid ingredients into a uniform powder, add the oleoresin or piperoid of ginger, make a mass, and divide into twenty-four pills. Dose, from one to three.

No. 55.—*Dr. Alberty's Small Antibilious Pills.*

		Each.
℞.—Calomelanos	gr. x	$\frac{1}{3}$ gr.
Pulv. gambogiæ	gr. v	$\frac{1}{6}$ gr.

Misce et fiant pilulæ xxx. Dose, two or three pills.

No. 56.—*Pills of Croton Oil.*

		Each.
Take of Croton oil	♏ iv	♏ $\frac{1}{4}$.
Crumb of bread	gr. xvj	gr. j.

Make into sixteen pills.

Croton oil and castor oil are both capable of forming soaps with caustic soda, which, being purified by solution in alcohol, and solidified in moulds, are eligible cathartic preparations.

No. 57.—*Dr. Chapman's Dinner Pills.*

		Reduced.	Each.
Take of Powdered aloes . .			1½ gr.
" mastich, of each	ʒij	gr. xviij	1½ gr.
" ipecac. . .	℈iv	gr. xij	1 gr.
Oil of caraway . .	♏ xij	♏ ij	Trace.

Mix and make into mass with water, and divide into eighty pills. (Reduced quantity, twelve pills.)

These pills are much used in habitual costiveness; the presence of the mastich protracts the solvent action of the fluids upon the aloes, so that one pill, which is a dose, taken before dinner, will produce a gentle operation the next morning.

No. 58.—*Lady Webster Pills.*

Take of Powdered aloes	ʒvj.
" mastich,	
" red roses, each	ʒij.
Syrup	q. s.

Make a mass, and divide into pills of three grains each.

One or two of these taken before a meal, will usually produce an evacuation.

DIURETICS AND EXPECTORANTS.

These classes of medicines are very little given in the form of pill or powder.

No. 59.—*Pilulæ Scillæ Compositæ*, U.S.

		Reduced.	Each.
Take of Squill, in powder . .	ʒj	gr. vj.	½ gr.
Ginger do.			1 gr.
Ammoniac do., each .	ʒij	gr. xij	1 gr.
Soap	ʒiij	gr. xviij	1½ gr.
Syrup, a sufficient quantity		q. s.	

Mix the powders together, then beat them with the soap, and add the syrup so as to form a mass, to be divided into 120 pills. (Twelve pills for the reduced quantity.)

Soap and syrup seem to me as a poor kind of mixture, especially as either would be a sufficient excipient without the other.

No. 60.—*Aromatic Pills.* (*Mütter's.*)

Take of Oil of copaiva,	
" cubebs,	
" turpentine, each	f℥j.
Magnesia	ʒij.

Mix, and form sixty pills.

These are very large, though quite popular in the treatment of gonorrhœa. Some recipes direct gr. iv of powdered opium to this number. They would be improved in a pharmaceutical aspect by substituting copaiva and Venice turpentine for the oils of copaiva and turpentine. The dose is two pills three times a day.

Diaphoretics.

No. 61.—*Pulvis Ipecacuanhæ et Opii*, U. S. (*Dover's Powder.*)

		Reduced.
Take of Ipecacuanha, in powder		gr. j.
Opium, in powder, of each	ʒj	gr. j.
Sulphate of potassa	℥j	gr. viij.

Rub them together into a very fine powder. Dose, ten grains, the reduced quantity in the above recipe.

This valuable preparation is too well known to require much comment; it is used in a great variety of cases in which a sedative diaphoretic is indicated. It should be remembered that the opium is to be dried before being weighed, otherwise the powder may be deficient in strength. It should also be well and thoroughly triturated from containing hard crystals to an almost impalpable powder. It is said to be less liable to nauseate in the form of pills.

Alteratives.

No. 62.—*Compound Pills of Iodide of Mercury.*

		Each.
Take of Iodide of mercury	gr. x	½ gr.
Resin of guaiacum	℈ij	2 gr.
Extract of conium	ʒss	1½ gr.

Triturate the resin of guaiacum into a mass with a little alcohol, then incorporate with it the extract of conium and iodide of mercury, and divide into twenty pills.

These pills are alterative, and may be used in scrofulous and skin diseases. Extract of sarsaparilla may be added to, or substituted for, some of the other ingredients.

No. 63.—*Alterative Powders of Calomel.*

		Each.
℞.—Hydrargyri chloridi mitis	gr. j	$\frac{1}{12}$.
Sacchari	gr. xj	$\frac{11}{12}$.

Misce, fiat pulvis in chartulas xij dividenda.

Signa.—Take one every hour (or two hours), till the gums are touched.

When there is a disposition to undue purging, from gr. ss to gr. ij of powdered opium may be added to the above quantities.

No. 64.—*Plummer's Pills. Pil. Calomelanos Comp.*

Take of Calomel	ʒij.
Precip. sulphuret of antimony	ʒij.
Powd. resin of guaiacum	℥ss.
Molasses	℥ss.

Rub the calomel with the precipitated sulphuret of antimony, then with the guaiacum and molasses to form a mass.

This popular pill is much used, both in this country and in England. The London College directs this to be kept in mass and divided as required, but the Dublin College orders it to be divided into six-grain pills.

Emmenagogues.

No. 65.—*Dr. Otto's Emmenagogue Pills.*

Take of	Calcined sulphate of iron	gr. xlviij.
	Aloes, in powder	gr. xij.
	Turpentine	gr. xxxij.
	Oil of turpentine	gtt. x or q. s.

Make a mass, and divide into thirty pills. Dose, two, three times a day.

Prescribed originally by the late Dr. J. C. Otto, and very frequently by the late Dr. Isaac Parrish; a similar recipe is often directed by Dr. Pepper, in the Pennsylvania Hospital Clinique.

The cautious addition of oil of turpentine insures an adhesive and plastic mass.

Numerous pills containing aloes, myrrh, and iron, given under the head of tonics and cathartics are much used as emmenagogues. (See also *Hooper's Female Pills*, among the patent medicines.)

Coating of Pills.—Pills, though they are the easiest form in which medicine can be taken, are repulsive to some persons, particularly if they contain very bitter or nauseous substances. To overcome this idiosyncrasy, many ways have been devised to render them more attractive and pleasing to the eye, and to hide the nauseous odor of many drugs, which are usually given in this form. Formerly, coatings with silver and gold leaf were much in vogue, but have fallen into merited disuse, with the exception of some base nostrums sold under the name of "golden pills;" if the coating with the metallic leaf is perfect, they are liable to pass through the stomach without being dissolved; and if the coating is imperfect, it does not answer the purpose of hiding taste and smell.

A much better coating is obtained with sugar, the taste and, when freshly prepared, also the smell being entirely covered by it, and of late, sugar-coated pills have, for this reason, come largely into use. There are several ways in which such a coating may be effected at the prescription counter; in all cases, very finely-powdered "dusted" sugar is requisite; some use a mixture of sugar and gum Arabic, which must be intimate and rubbed to the very finest powder. Upon a pill tile, six or eight pills receive a thin covering of mucilage of gum Arabic or tragacanth, by being rolled in it quickly by means of the fingers; they are then immediately transferred to another tile, upon which a thin layer of the saccharine powder has been dusted, and the sugar is made to adhere by giving the pills a rotary motion with the ends of the fingers, slightly pressing on them.

The covering of sugar may also be satisfactorily made by using a box, the inside of which has been turned into a globular form, such as were formerly employed for silvering and gilding pills. Some of the powder is sprinkled into the box, and, after the introduction of the pills previously moistened with mucilage as before, an even coating is effected by giving the box a quick circular movement. The pills are afterwards allowed to dry in a box, and may be made somewhat smoother by rolling them in finely-powdered starch.

If thus treated, a good white coating is obtained, which, however, lacks in elegance if compared with the confectioners' manufacture, but answers all the requisite purposes.

If it appear desirable, the sugar may be previously colored by incorporating a few grains of carmine with it, or rubbing with it some good saffron to a very fine powder, if a yellow color is desired; the latter fades if exposed to the light. The covering with sugar is perfect, and entirely prevents the smell and taste from manifesting themselves for a number of days; but, if freshly-made pills have been thus coated, the evaporating moisture, in penetrating through the sugar, may carry some soluble matter with it and gradually discolor the covering; in a similar way, odorous principles will penetrate to the surface, and finally impart their smell; sugar-coated assafœtida pills though at first free from odor, develope it thus on keeping.

The French use a strong solution of gelatin for effecting a cover to pills, which is probably the best of all, as it is not apt to condense moisture in its pores. The mode of covering with it is very simple; the pills, each of which is stuck upon a long needle, are dipped into the hot concentrated solution, and when cold and not sticky, are removed from the needles and placed in a box to dry perfectly. This coat effectually excludes all deteriorating influences, and pills thus covered may be kept for an indefinite time without losing their medicinal properties; they, moreover, have a very elegant appearance from the hard, glossy, and transparent nature of their surface, which may be colored to suit the fancy, by introducing into the solution of gelatin a sufficient quantity of coloring matter, which is soluble in water.

Sugar pellets or granules, medicated with various substances, are now sometimes called for. They have gained favor in the eyes of many patients on account of their very small size, which makes them to be taken more readily and easily than ordinary pills. Sugar granules are made by the confectioner of white sugar, and are sometimes colored, a matter of mere fancy. They are medicated in the following way: The dose to be contained in each granule is first determined; the medicinal substance is then weighed out in such a quantity as may be evenly divided into the proper doses; it is now dissolved in strong alcohol or ether, sufficient to moisten the requisite quantity of pellets, which are to be constantly agitated in a shallow dish so that the solution may become evenly divided among them, until the solvent has evaporated.

It is evident that, prepared in this way, the globules may slightly vary in the quantity of the absorbed solution, and it is therefore important that the agitation be continued without intermission until no trace of moisture can be detected; the employment of the strongest alcohol or ether is necessary, so that a larger amount of the solvent may be employed without liquefying the sugar. Only such medicines are prepared in this way which are given in very small doses, and the vegetable alkaloids and some neutral principles are particularly adapted to it. Generally, more than one of the granules contain the full dose of the medicine. It has become customary to have them contain the one-hundredth, one-fiftieth, one-twentieth, or the one-sixteenth part of a grain of the medicinal compound.

Trochisci.—Lozenges.

In addition to the description of this class of preparations at page 248, &c., I append the following prescription of Dr. Warrington, as an example of the mode of prescribing them extemporaneously:—

Prescription for Diaphoretic Lozenges.

℞.—Pulv. ipecac. . . . . gr. vj.
Potassæ citrat. . . . . gr. j.
P. ext. glycyrrh.,
Pulv. acaciæ, ā ā . . . . . ʒj, ℈ij.
M.—Ft. trochisci xxiv. Dose, for a child, one every two hours.

The mode of dividing this mass after rolling it into a rectangular sheet may be to cut it equally into six oblong sheets, each of which may be cut into four equal parts by a spatula, the surface being dusted with powdered liquorice or sugar.

Suppositoria.

Suppositories, as a class of medicines, are so seldom prescribed, that I can lay claim to little practical familiarity with their preparation. They are used to insert into the rectum to fulfil several indications; sometimes their action is mechanical, but they usually owe their utility either to a narcotic, astringent, or cathartic ingredient.

The only officinal preparation commonly prescribed in this form, is:—

No. 66.—*Pilulæ Saponis Compositæ*, U. S.

Consisting of opium a half ounce, and soap two ounces, triturated into a mass; this is made into a round or oblong mass of suitable size, say ten grains, and inserted, either by the finger, or by the tube here figured, which is made for the purpose, of wood or ivory.

Fig. 213.

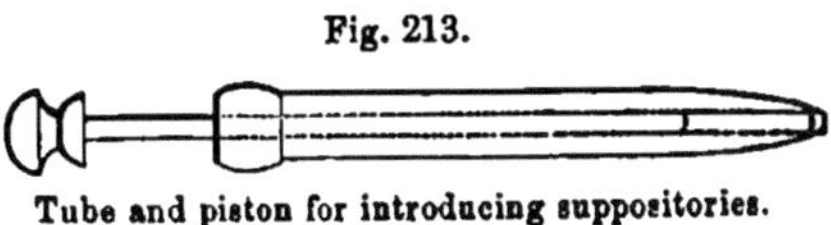

Tube and piston for introducing suppositories.

The suppository is improved by being smeared with some bland fixed oil, which facilitates its introduction. From a paper by Alfred B. Taylor, in the *American Journal of Pharmacy*, vol. xxiv. p. 211, the following recipes are extracted:—

"There is perhaps no substance so well adapted to serve as the vehicle of these applications as the butter of cocoa (oleum cacao), as no combination of suet, spermaceti, or wax, &c., combines in so great a degree the proper hardness or firmness of substance, with the requisite fusibility.

"The following formula is a prescription of Dr. S. W. Mitchell, and has been considerably used.

No. 67.—Take of Cocoa butter . . . . . ℥iss.
Powdered opium . . . . gr. xij.

Mix, and make into twelve suppositories.

"The butter of cocoa is to be melted by a gentle heat. The opium is then to be well rubbed up with a small quantity of the fluid, until thoroughly incorporated, and the remainder of the melted butter gradually added. When cool and slightly thickened, the mass, being well stirred, should then be poured into paper cones.

"If the cocoa butter is too fluid when transferred to the moulds, the opium will settle to the apex of the cone, and not be thoroughly diffused through the substance.

"When perfectly hard, these cones should be pared or scraped at the base until they weigh just one drachm, giving one grain of opium to each suppository.

"Practically, therefore, it will be necessary to make one less than the required number, reserving the parings for another operation."

The following formula has been prescribed by Dr. Pancoast:—

No. 68.—Take of Cocoa butter . . . . . ℥j.
Extract of krameria . . . ℈ij.
Powdered opium . . . . gr. v.

Mix, and make into ten suppositories as above.

"It is stated that cocoa butter is much esteemed in France for its supposed healing qualities, and is a favorite application in cases of piles. With powdered galls or tannic acid, this substance would, therefore, probably, form a useful substitute for the ordinary pile ointment.

"The proportions to be employed would, of course, be regulated entirely by the physician's order.

"In Dorvault's French work on *Practical Pharmacy*, suppositories are described as varying from the size of the little finger to that of the thumb, and weighing from ʒj ¼ to ʒij ½ (five to ten grammes). The author gives as a formula for the vehicle, butter of cocoa melted with an eighth part, by weight, of white wax; or as an inferior substitute, and one less used, common tallow mixed with the same proportion of wax. Soap suppositories are formed by simply cutting soap into convenient shapes. Suppositories are also prepared from honey, by boiling down this substance till it becomes sufficiently hard to retain its shape. There are also formulæ given for anthelmintic, anti-hemorrhoidal, astringent, emmenagogue, laxative, and vaginal suppositories, as well as belladonna, calomel, cicuta, mercurial, and quinine suppositories.

"In Gray's *Supplement to the Pharmacopœia*, there is given the following formula for a suppository, taken from the *Codex Medic. Hamburg.* 1845.

No. 69.—Take of		
	Aloes	ʒvj.
	Common salt	℥iss.
	Spanish soap	℥iss.
	Starch	℥viij.

Mix and make into a mass with honey, and then form into cones of the required size."

No. 70.—*Anthelmintic Suppositories.*

Take of		
	Aloes, in powder	℥ss.
	Chloride of sodium	ʒiij.
	Flour	℥ij.
	Honey	Sufficient.

Form into a firm paste, and make into twelve suppositories. Used in the treatment of ascarides.

CHAPTER V.

LIQUID PREPARATIONS, SOLUTIONS, MIXTURES, &c.

THESE forms include a great variety of preparations. The term mixture is applied strictly to those liquids in which insoluble substances are suspended, but, in a more general sense, to all liquid medicines not included in one of the several classes of solutions, infusions, tinctures, &c. In treating of them here, I shall for convenience include all extemporaneous preparations prescribed in the liquid form, endeavoring to adopt such a classification as will aid the student in acquiring a knowledge of the principles which should guide the practitioner in their composition.

The hints given toward the preparation of ingredients into the form of pills are generally quite reversed in the case of mixtures, which should mostly be composed of substances in part or entirely soluble, or by their lightness readily diffusible in water. In mixtures, the use of excipients is not limited, as in the other case, by the necessity of not exceeding a certain bulk, but they may be freely added with a view to improving the composition physically, pharmaceutically, and therapeutically, and within certain pretty wide bounds, while the range of medical agents prescribed is enlarged by the addition of a great number of fluids, as the fixed and essential oils, ethers, solutions of ammonia, &c. There are reasons, however, which make the art of combining in the liquid, much more difficult than in the solid form. In the presence of the great neutral solvent, the chemical affinities of various saline ingredients are fully brought into play, which, when in a dry or even a plastic condition, are without action upon each other; again, the physical difficulties to be overcome in this form of preparation are greater than in the foregoing, because the variety of materials to be combined is increased. The proper suspension of fixed and essential oils, for instance, is a matter of no little skill, and the division and diffusion of various powders require judgment and skill only attainable by a familiarity with their physical properties.

There is also in the introduction of excipients and adjuvants, great scope for the exercise of ingenuity, to improve not only the flavor, but the appearance of mixtures. (See Prescriptions Nos. 84 and 85, and others.)

Next to a considerable range of practice in the composition of mixtures, I know of no better way to become familiar with the subject, than by a study of a syllabus like that here presented, together with a number of approved formulæ, such as are grouped together in this chapter.

Medicines suited to Liquid Form.

MOST SOLUBLE SALTS, LIGHT INSOLUBLE POWDERS, EXTRACTS, GUM RESINS, FIXED AND ESSENTIAL OILS, AND ALL THE GALENICAL SOLUTIONS.

SOLUBLE.

FORMING ELIGIBLE SOLUTIONS WITH WATER.

Alumen.
Ammon. murias.
Antim. et potass. tart.
Barii chloridum.
Calcii chloridum.
Ferri sulphas.
" et pot. tartras.
Manganesii sulphas.
Magnesiæ sulphas.
Potassæ acetas.
" bicarbonas.
" carbonas.
" citras.
" chloras.
" tartras.
Potassii bromidum.
" iodidum.
Morphiæ acetas.
" murias.
" sulphas.
Sodæ bicarbonas.
" boras.
" carbonas.
" sulphas.
" et pot. tartras.
Sodii chloridum.
Sodæ phosphas.
Acidum citricum.
" tartaricum.
" tannicum.

REQUIRING CERTAIN ADDITIONS TO FORM ELIGIBLE SOLUTIONS.

Quiniæ sulphas.
Cinchoniæ sulphas.
Quinidiæ sulphas.
Chinoidine.
Iodinium.
Hydrarg. iodid. rub.
Requiring viscid substances, as correctives or vehicles.
Ammoniæ carbonas.
Hydrarg. chlorid. corros.
Potassii cyanuretum.
Potassa.

BEST FORMED INTO SOLUTION IN MAKING THE SALTS.

Ammoniæ acetas.
Magnesiæ citras.
Acid. phosphoric.
Potassæ arsenis.
" bitartras.
Arsenici et hyd. iod.
Potassa.
Ferri citras.
" nitras.

INSOLUBLE.

MIXING WITH WATER, BUT NOT FORMING CLEAR SOLUTIONS.

Diffused by Agitation:—
Magnesia.
Potassæ bitart.
Sulphur præcip.
Pulv. cinchonæ.
" ipecac.
Calcis phosphas.
Quiniæ sulph.
Miscible by trituration alone:—
Extractum aconiti.
" belladonnæ.
" conii.
" hyoscyami.
" stramonii.
" taraxaci.
" krameriæ.
" glycyrrhizæ.
Confectiones.
Assafœtida.
Ammoniacum.
Guaiacum.
Myrrha.
Scammonium.
Suspended by the aid of viscid excipients:—
Copaiba.
Ol. amygdalæ.
" ricini.
" olivæ.
" terebinthinæ.
Olea essentia.
Ferri protocarb.

Preparations adapted to Use as Vehicles or Correctives of the unpleasant Taste, and other properties, especially of Saline Substances.

Aquæ medicatæ (generally).	Spt. lavandulæ comp.
Syrupi (generally).	Infusum rosæ comp.
Tinctura cinnamomi.	Saccharum.
" " comp.	Pulv. acaciæ, pulv. sacchari, and with these—
Tinctura cardamomi.	Olea destillata.
" " comp.	Tinct. tolutani.
Tinct. cort. aurant.	" zingiberis.
Mistura amygdalæ.	

Of the most numerous class in the syllabus, those which form eligible solutions without the addition of any chemical or other excipient, it should be remarked that many are so well adapted to combinations with other medicinal or corrective substances as to be rarely prescribed alone. Thus, muriate of ammonia is nearly always prescribed with expectorant remedies in cough mixtures. The bicarbonate and carbonate of potassa, and of soda with prophylactics, as in hooping-cough mixtures; or with stimulants, as in ordinary carminative and antacid remedies, acetate of potassa is much used with other diuretics. Alum and borax are best adapted to gargles and astringent washes, in which other medicines, not incompatible, may be combined. Bromide and iodide of potassium are instances of mineral substances, often combined with vegetable alteratives, which increase their effect and take off at the same time their very unpleasant sensible properties.

In the formulæ which follow, these modes of combination are illustrated as well as those of the less soluble substances displayed in the other groups of the syllabus. The part of this work devoted to pharmaceutical chemistry, contains the mode of preparing those solutions, the medicinal ingredients of which are developed spontaneously in the process of preparation.

Incompatibles.

The subject of incompatibles is, it appears to me, too much of a stumbling-block to the student. A moderate amount of chemical knowledge will serve to guard the practitioner against the use of incompatibles entirely, while the observance of a few simple rules will be sufficient to protect from glaring errors in this respect. In the list of substances incompatible with each other, as published in the older works, perhaps a majority are not likely to be ordered, on account of any fitness they have for each other in their therapeutical relations, while it is well known that some of the most popular of prescriptions are framed with the especial design of producing precipitates, which, being diffused in the resulting liquid, aid its general effect.

Authors have given too absolute a sense to the term incompatible, by giving sanction to the idea that all substances which form insoluble precipitates are incompatible with each other. An insoluble compound is not necessarily inert, but, as experience abundantly proves, is frequently the best and most eligible form for a medicine.

The reactions which occur in the organism are not to be judged of by ordinary chemical laws, as manifested in the laboratory of the chemist. The difference of action between the animal solvents under the influence of the life force, and those employed by the chemist with the mechanical means at his command, are too well known and appreciated to require extended notice. Living beings can dissolve, appropriate, and circulate in their fluids, substances which, to ordinary agencies, are most intractable and insoluble.

Corrosive sublimate, when precipitated by albumen, gluten, and casein, is presented in the most insoluble form possible, and yet this mode of combination is highly recommended by the French as being more easily endured by the stomach, while the alterative effect is both mild and certain. This mode of procedure is stated by Dorvalt to be adapted to a number of mineral salts, such as lead, tin, zinc, copper, silver, platina, gold, &c., all of which form, with albuminous substances, compounds insoluble in water and ordinary solvents, but soluble in the liquids of the alimentary canal, by the aid of which they are placed in condition very suitable for medicinal action.

These facts are applicable to toxicology. When in a case of poisoning from vegetable alkalies, tannin, or an astringent decoction is given; or, after the use of a poisonous dose of arsenious acid, we give hydrated peroxide of iron; or, after corrosive sublimate, albumen; an insoluble compound is formed in each case, and yet it does not follow that these compounds are inert, but only that their immediate effects are destroyed, and their absorption diminished; indeed, it has been proved that, in cases of poisoning, where antidotes had been used successfully, the urine contained both the poison and antidote five or six days after they were taken. The practice of administering purgatives and emetics for the complete evacuation of poisons, even after neutralization, is founded on the fact that they are still capable of slow absorption.

In connection with this subject, it may be well to mention the fact that when active metallic substances, as, for instance, the salts of mercury and of antimony, are taken for some time continuously, they seem to be deposited in the alimentary canal in an insoluble form, so that, by administering a chemical preparation which forms with them soluble salts, they sometimes display their activity to an alarming and even dangerous extent. The rationale of the use of iodide of potassium, after the long-continued use of mercurials, is, that it forms an iodide of mercury, which it dissolves and carries off through the secretions; salivation is sometimes induced, unexpectedly, in this way. It is stated that patients, who have used antimonials, are sometimes nauseated by lemonade made from tartaric acid, owing to the formation of tartar emetic from the undissolved oxide of antimony. These facts are not without interest, in connection with the subject of prescribing.

Considering it necessary, as a general rule, to avoid the association of substances which, by contact, may produce unknown or ill-defined compounds, or compounds different from those intended to be administered, I proceed to state briefly the most important rules relative to incompatibles:—

1. Whenever two salts, in a state of solution can, by the exchange of their bases and acids, form a soluble and an insoluble salt, or two insoluble salts, the decomposition takes place, and the insoluble salt is precipitated, or by combining with the soluble salt, gives birth to a double salt, which is rarely the case.

2. If we mix the solutions of two salts which cannot create a soluble salt, and an insoluble salt, a precipitate will not be formed, and most frequently there will be no decomposition, although this is not invariably the case.

3. In mixing any salt and a strong acid, a decomposition is very apt to take place.

4. Salts with feeble acids, especially carbonic and acetic, are always decomposed by strong acids.

5. Alkalies in contact with the salts of the metals proper, or of the alkaloids, decompose them, precipitating their bases.

6. Metallic oxides, in contact with acids, combine with them and form salts whose properties are sometimes unlike either the acid or the oxides.

7. Vegetable astringents precipitate albumen, gelatin, vegetable alkalies, and numerous metallic oxides, and with salts of iron produce black inky solutions.

8. The condition most favorable to chemical action is a solution of the salts in concentrated form without the intervention of viscid substances, so that when the indications require the employment of two substances which are incompatible, it is well to form a dilute solution of one of them in a mucilaginous or syrupy liquid before adding the other. In this way the decomposition may often be averted.

In the table appended, some preparations are mentioned which, as a general rule, the practitioner should avoid combining with chemical substances; they are best given in simple solution, or some of them, with the addition of the Galenical preparations, or simple saccharine or mucilaginous excipients:—

Acidum hydrocyanicum.
" nitro-muriaticum.
Liquor hydrarg. et arsen. iodid.
" potassæ arsenitis.
" calcis.
" barii chloridi.
" calcii chloridi.
" iodinii compositus.
" potassæ.
" ferri citratis.
" ferri nitratis.
" morphiæ sulphatis.
Tinct. ferri chloridi.
Tinct. iodinii.

Antimonii et potassæ tartras.
Potassii cyanuretum.
" bromidum.
" iodidum.
Ferri et pot. tartras.
Quiniæ sulphas.
Cinchoniæ sulphas.
Quinidiæ sulphas.
Morphiæ sulphas
" murias.
" acetas.
" valerianas.
Zinci acetas.
Potassæ acetas.

In addition to what has been said, it seems proper to notice what will be more particularly brought into view in commenting on the formulas which follow; the intentional use of medicines, in one sense incompatible, for the purpose of producing new and more desirable compounds. The proto-carbonate of iron is in this way produced from the sulphate and a carbonated alkali; the acetate of ammonia by the addition of acetic acid to a solution of the carbonate. In the same way black and yellow wash are extemporaneously prepared by adding to lime-water, calomel and corrosive sublimate, respectively. The association of sulphate of zinc and acetate of lead furnishes a familiar illustration of the same fact; the resulting precipitate of sulphate of lead, occurring as an impalpable powder or magma, is favorable to the therapeutic object in view.

Laudanum is quite incompatible with subacetate of lead; but one of the most popular of lotions contains these ingredients associated, so that it is not correct to say that these substances are incompatible in a medical sense, however, in a purely chemical point of view, they may be considered so.

Pharmaceutical incompatibles are those in which a disturbance of a solution takes place in a way not considered strictly chemical. My observation has satisfied me that these are very commonly associated, though little observed. In speaking of pills, I referred to some pharmaceutical incompatibles, and may now instance others. If we add tincture of Tolu to an aqueous solution, the resin of the Tolu separates almost entirely as a coagulum, and collects on the side of the bottle, thus being lost as a medicinal ingredient of the preparation, besides rendering it very unsightly. The same remark applies to other resinous tinctures.

The admixture of tincture of guaiacum with the spirit of nitric ether is another instance; the resinous tincture gelatinizes into a mass, and is unfit for use. The addition of tincture of cinnamon to infusion of digitalis after filtration, as directed in the *Pharmacopœia*, occasions a precipitate.

List of Pharmaceutical Incompatibles.

Comp. infusion of cinchona, with comp. infusion gentian.
Essential oils with aqueous liquids in quantities exceeding one drop to f℥j. See page 625.
Fixed oils and copaiva, with aqueous liquids, except with excipients.
Spirit of nitric ether with strong mucilages.
Infusions generally with metallic salts.
Compound infusion of gentian with infusion of wild cherry.
Tinctures made with strong alcohol, with those made with weak alcohol.
Tinctures made with strong alcohol, with infusions and aqueous liquids.

Excipients used in Mixtures, &c.

The consideration of excipients will bring into view the best modes of overcoming some of these pharmaceutical incompatibilities.

In the form of mixture we use, in the first place, as diluents—

Water.	Compound infusion of rose.
The medicated waters.	Emulsion of almonds.
Syrups.	Honey of rose.

As excipients or constituents in a stricter sense—

Pow'd acacia, } mixed or singly.	Extracts.
Sugar, } mixed or singly.	Yelk of egg.
Powd. tragacanth.	White of egg.
Confections.	

As flavoring agents with viscid ingredients—

Essential oils of	Cinnamon. Lemon. Aniseed. Caraway, &c.	Tinctures of	Ginger. Tolu. Oil of P. mint " of mint.

As flavoring and coloring agents with or without viscid ingredients—

Tincture of cinnamon.	Comp. tincture of gentian.
Compound tincture of cinnamon.	Fluid extract of vanilla.
Tincture of cardamom.	Ginger syrup.
Compound tincture of cardamom.	Tolu syrup.
Compound spirit of lavender.	Fruit syrups, &c.

The diluents are useful as enabling us to divide the doses of an active medicine to almost any extent; they correspond to the sugar, gum, aromatic powder, &c., prescribed for a similar purpose with powders, and with conserve of rose and some other bulky additions used in pill masses.

The immense utility of excipients, and flavoring agents generally, will be best illustrated by the examples which follow. The skilful employment of these adds greatly to the success of the prescriber.

The necessity of limiting the number of prescriptions given, and the importance of including in them a considerable variety of medicinal agents, will forbid the illustration of all the numerous points in this connection, and much will necessarily be left to be filled up by the ingenuity of the learner.

EXTEMPORANEOUS SOLUTIONS, MIXTURES, &c.

ASTRINGENTS.

No. 71.—*Mistura Cretæ*, U.S. (*Chalk Mixture, or Chalk Julep.*)

Take of Prepared chalk	℥ss.
Sugar,	
Powdered gum Arabic, each	ʒij.
Cinnamon water,	
Water, each	f℥iv.

Rub them together till they are thoroughly mixed.

To this, which is a very popular antacid astringent, the addition is often made of tincture of kino, or some similar vegetable astringent, either with or without tincture of opium. In the absence of cinnamon water, two drops of the oil of cinnamon for each ounce of that water ordered, may be added to the dry ingredients. As the mixture does not keep very well, it is a convenient plan to keep the powders ready mixed, and add the water when required. Chalk mixture is given in an adult dose of ℥ss.

No. 72.—*Parrish's Camphor Mixture.* (Dr. Parrish, Sen.)

℞.—Aquæ camphoræ . . . . f℥iij.
Spiriti lavandulæ compositi . . . . . fʒj.
Sacchari . . . . ʒj.
Misce.

Give a tablespoonful every two hours in diarrhœa and cholera-morbus, adding ten drops of laudanum where there is much pain.

This preparation, which was originally prescribed in 1832, has been found so generally useful and safe that it has become a standard remedy, and is prepared and sold by all druggists in Philadelphia and its vicinity.

No. 73.—*Hope's Camphor Mixture.*

℞.—Aquæ camphoræ . . . . f℥iv.
Acidi nitrosi . . . . ♏ xxx.
Tincturæ opii . . . . ♏ xx vel xl. Misce.

Dose, a tablespoonful every two hours in diarrhœa and dysentery.[1]

No. 74.—*A Remedy used in Uterine Hemorrhages.*

Take of Oil of erigeron . . . . . . fʒj.
Sugar . . . . ʒij.
Gum Arabic . . . . ʒj.
Water . . . . f℥ij, fʒvj.

Triturate the oil with the gum and sugar into a dry powder, then add the water, triturating into a perfect mixture.

Sig.—Take a teaspoonful three times a day.

[1] *Extracted from the Edinburgh Medical and Surgical Journal*, January, 1824. *Observations on the Powerful Effects of a Mixture containing Nitrous Acid and Opium in curing Dysentery, Cholera, and Diarrhœa.* By Thomas Hope, Esq., Surgeon, Chatham.—"More than twenty-six years ago, when attending a case of dysentery in which the usual remedies had been prescribed in vain, the patient determined, on his own accord, to take a medicine I had sent for his nurse, who was worn out with attention to her charge, and complained of excessive thirst. It occurred to me to give an acid to alleviate her complaint, and in order to obviate any unpleasant effects, to join opium with it; I accordingly sent the following: ℞.—Acidi nitrosi ʒij; Ext. opii gr. ij; Aquæ ℥ij.—M. Cap. cochl. minus ter quarterve in die; and the patient with dysentery having taken some of this medicine, the effect produced was so great that it no less surprised him, who, by a continuance of it, recovered, than it did myself.

"The form of the medicine, as I have used it in all the cases referred to, is as under:—

℞.—Acid. nitrosi . . . . . ʒj.
Mist. camphoræ . . . . . ℥viij. Misce et adde
Tinct. opii . . . . . . gtt. xl.

Sig.—One-fourth part to be taken every three or four hours.

"In chronic dysentery, the dose of two ounces three times a day is quite sufficient; the remedy is grateful to the taste; abates thirst; soon removes the intensity of pain; and procures, in general, a speedy and permanent relief. No previous preparation is required for taking it, nor any other care whilst taking it, except the keeping of the hands and feet warm, preserving the body as much as possible from exposure to extreme cold or currents of air, and making use of warm barley-water or thin gruel, and a diet of sago or tapioca.

"It is necessary to mention that the remedy, the good effects of which I now detail, is *nitrous* acid with opium, not *nitric* acid. I have not found nitric acid with opium to produce any good effect, for, having expended my nitrous acid, I sent to a chemist for a fresh supply, who, by mistake, sent me nitric acid, which I used merely by way of trial, but found it not in any way beneficial to my patients."

Dr. E. on and others have had considerable success in the treatment .. .terine hemorrhages with the oil of erigeron; in the doses here prescribed, each f℥ contains gtt. v of the oil.

ALTERATIVES, &c.

No. 75.—*Blue Mass and Chalk Mixture.*

Take of Mercurial mass, in powder . . ʒss.
Prepared chalk . . . . . . ʒj.
Gum Arabic, in powder,
Sugar, do., of each . . ʒss.
Tincture of opium . . . . . ♏xxx.
Aromatic syrup of rhub rb . . f℥j, fʒvj.

Triturate into a uniform mixture.

DOSE, fʒj to stimulate the secretion of bile and check diarrhœa. Tincture of kino or other astringents may be added.

No. 76.—*Creasote Mixture.*

Take of Creasote . . . . gtt. xvj.
Powdered gum Arabic . . . . . ʒj.
Sugar . . . . ʒss.
Water . . . . f℥ij.

Triturate the creasote with and sugar, then gradually add the water and triturate to a un ixture.

DOSE, a teaspoonful contain .. drop of creasote, used in bronchitis, phthisis, &c., and to check vomiting. Creasote is soluble in water to the extent of ♏v to f℥j, and for external use is best made into a suitable solution by shaking up with water.

TONICS.

No. 77.—*Fever and Ague Mixture.*

℞.—Powdered red bark . . . . ʒiij.
Confection of opium,
Lemon-juice . . . . ʒiss.
Port wine . . . . f℥iij.

Mix by trituration in a mortar.

DOSE, three tablespoonfuls morning, noon, and night, the day the fever is off.

Some recipes direct powdered serpentaria in addition to the above.

Though not an elegant, this is a most efficient and valuable combination.

No. 78.—*Solution of Acetate of Chinoidine.*

Take of Chinoidine . . . . One ounce.
Acetic acid . . . . One fluidounce.
Water . . . . Twenty-nine fluidounces.

Make a solution.

Each fluidrachm contains about two grains of chinoidine, and serves as a dose.

This is a cheap form of cinchona preparation, used in the Moyamensing Dispensary, Philadelphia.

No. 79.—*Mistura Ferri Compositi*, U. S. (*Griffith's Myrrh Mixture.*)

Take of Myrrh,
Sugar, of each . . . . . ℨj.
Carbonate of potassa . . . . gr. xxv.
Triturate together into a fine milky mixture with
Rose water . . . . f℥viiss.
Then add Spirit of lavender (simple) . . . f℥ss.
Sulphate of iron, in powder . . . ℈j.

Dose, a tablespoonful according to circumstances, given as a tonic in phthisis, and in anæmic cases generally.

The strict phraseology of the *Pharmacopœia* has been departed from above in the hope of rendering the pharmaceutical points in the preparation more clear.

The sulphate of iron and carbonate of potassa here used, form by double decomposition the sulphate of potassa and protocarbonate of iron, which latter floats in the milky mixture of myrrh and sugar, giving it a green color. This is, however, in very small proportion, so that in each f℥ss dose, there is not more than gr. ss. This preparation is, however, a very useful and an elegant one. (See *Pil. Ferri Carbonatis* and *Pil. Ferri Compositæ.*)

No. 80.—*A good Preparation of Iron and Cinchona.*

(Substitute for Tinctura Cinchonæ Ferrata.—See p. 138.)

℞.—Tinct. cinchonæ et quassiæ comp. . . f℥iv.
Ferri citratis . . . . ℨj.
Acidi citrici . . . . gr. xv.

Triturate the citric acid and citrate of iron together, and dissolve in the tincture of cinchona and quassia. Liq. ferri citratis fℨj (see p. 515) may be used as a substitute for the rather insoluble dry salt. The dose is a teaspoonful, containing two grains of citrate of iron.

The citric acid breaks up any tannate of iron as soon as formed, and it is reproduced on the addition of an alkali. There is a liability to considerable precipitate of cinchonic red, but very little iron is thrown down.

No. 81.—*A Concentrated Solution of Quinia and Iron.*

℞.—Quiniæ sulphatis . . . . . . ℈j.
Tr. ferri chloridi . . . . . . fℨiiss.

Ft. solutio.

One grain of sulph. quinia is contained in every 7½ minims (about 15 drops) of the solution, which is an appropriate dose; it may be made with three times the proportion of quinia salt. To prescribe it in a more diluted form, add water f℥ij, and syrup of orange-peel (or other suitable flavor) f℥iij. The dose will then be a teaspoonful, equivalent to 1 gr. of the quinia salt.

Dr. Gilbert, of Philadelphia, informs me that he finds this a very useful remedy in cases of carbuncle, accompanied by an atonic condition and erysipelatous tendencies.

No. 82.—*A Bitter Tonic for Dyspepsia.*

℞.—Tr. cinchonæ et quassiæ comp. . . . f℥iv.
Tincturæ nucis vomicæ . . . . . f℥j.

Misce.

A teaspoonful three times a day in a little sugar and water.

This is one of the best combinations of its kind; it is much prescribed by Dr. E. Wilson.

No. 83.—*A Mild Antacid for Young Infants.*

℞.—Sodæ bicarb. . . . . ʒss.
Aquæ menthæ . . . . f℥iv.

Ft. solutio.

Prescribed by Dr. Meigs and others. Dose, a teaspoonful, as an innocent substitute for the numerous carminatives.

No. 84.—*Aromatic and Antacid Corrective of Indigestion.*

℞.—Sodæ bicarbonatis . . . . . . ℈iv.
Infus. gentianæ comp. . . . . . f℥iiss.
Aquæ menthæ pip. . . . . . . f℥iij.
Tinct. cardamomi comp. . . . . f℥ss.

Dose, a tablespoonful as required.

The above makes a handsome preparation; it was furnished me by my friend Dr. J. J. Levick.

Arterial Stimulants.

No. 85.—*Carbonate of Ammonia Mixture.*

			Dose contains
Take of	Carbonate of ammonia .		gr. x.
	Powdered gum Arabic .		gr. x.
	Sugar, each	ʒiss	gr. x.
	Comp. spirit of ether, . .		♏xv.
	" tinct. of cardam., each	f℥ij	♏xv.
	Water	f℥iijss	

Make a mixture. Dose, a tablespoonful every two or three hours. A stimulant in low conditions, as in the last stages of disease.

No. 86—*Oil of Turpentine Mixture.*

℞.—Olei terebinthinæ	f℥ij.
Pulv. acaciæ,	
Sacchari, āā	℥iss.
Tinct. opii	♏ L.
Aquæ cinnamomi	f℥vss.

Triturate the gum and sugar with the oil of turpentine, and ℥ij of the cinnamon water, then gradually add the other ingredients. The yolk of an egg may be substituted advantageously for the gum and sugar, and a part of the water. Dose, f℥j, containing about ♏iv of the oil, and ♏j of tincture of opium.

Nervous Stimulants.

No. 87.—*Mistura Assafœtidæ*, U. S. (*Milk of Assafœtida.*)

Take of Assafœtida	℥ij.
Water	Oss.

Rub the assafœtida with the water gradually added until they are thoroughly mixed.

A good extemporaneous way to prepare this very popular antispasmodic, is to form a wine of assafœtida, as directed by Henry N. Rittenhouse, by triturating ℥ss of the gum-resin with f℥x wine. The gum resin should be carefully selected, so as not to require straining; this wine will keep, and is converted into the mixture by adding to water in the proportion of ℥j (by weight) to each f℥j.

James T. Shinn, of this city, proposes the following mode of preparation, which, while it keeps well, enables the practitioner to double the strength of the mixture if desired, or by dilution to furnish it of the officinal strength.

Take of Assafœtida	℥ss.
Diluted acetic acid	f℥ij.
Water	f℥iv.
Sugar	℥iv.

Triturate together into a mixture. To make milk of assafœtida dilute with an equal portion of water.

Milk of assafœtida is much prescribed and extensively used as a domestic remedy. Dose, from f℥j to f℥ss.

No. 88.—"*Chloroform Paregoric*" *of Dr. Henry Hartshorne.*

Take of Chloroform,	
Tincture of opium,	
" of camphor,	
Arom. spt. of ammonia, of each . .	f℥iss.
Oil of cinnamon	gtt. iij.
Brandy	f℥ij.

Dose, f℥ss, or less in spasmodic affections of the stomach, cholera,

&c. Several practitioners have used this preparation with favorable results in severe cases.

NARCOTICS.

No. 89.—*Liquor Morphiæ Sulphatis*, U. S.

		Reduced.
Take of Sulphate of morphia . .	gr. viij	gr. j.
Distilled water . . .	Oss.	f℥j.

Dissolve the morphia in the distilled water. This is an illustration of the most convenient method of giving small doses of soluble substances; here the proportions are so adjusted, that each teaspoonful shall represent ⅛ gr. of morphia, which is a rather small dose.

A favorite prescription for after-pains in obstetric practice, is a solution of sulphate of morphia in camphor water, in the same proportion as the above. DOSE, the same.

ARTERIAL AND NERVOUS SEDATIVES.

No. 90.—*A good Anti-Fever Combination.*

		In each, f℥j.
℞.—Vini antimonii,		♏ viij.
Spt. ætheris nit., āā	f℥ss	♏ viij.
Tinct. digitalis	f℥j	♏ ij.
Syr. acidi citrici	f℥iij	

Misce.

Sig.—Take a teaspoonful every three or four hours.

No. 91.—*Remedy in Pulmonary and Catarrhal Diseases, &c., Unattended by Fever.*

℞.—Acidi hydrocyanici	gtt. xl.
Vini antimonii	f℥ss.
Syrupi tolutani	f℥iss.
Mucil. acaciæ	f℥ij.

M., fiat mistura, capiat cochl. parvum ter quarterve die.

This, with several similar combinations of hydrocyanic acid, is highly recommended by Dr. Horace Green, and published by him among his selections from favorite prescriptions collected from distinguished American physicians, in a scrap-book kept for the purpose. Rendered much more dilute, this is recommended as the best of remedies for hooping-cough.

CATHARTICS.

No. 92.—*Castor Oil Mixture.*

Take of Gum Arabic, in powder,	
Sugar, of each	ʒiij.
Oil of mint	gtt. iv.

Triturate into a uniform powder, and add water f℥vj, or sufficient to bring the mucilage to the consistence of castor oil, then add, by degrees, castor oil f℥j, continuing the trituration till it combines into a perfect emulsion, with a uniform milky appearance; should this fail to appear, add a little more water, or, if the mucilage is evidently too dilute, a little more gum, care being taken to produce the uniform milkiness. Dilute this by adding water sufficient to make f℥iv.

This will make a perfect castor oil emulsion. If oil of turpentine is to be incorporated with it, let it be added to the mixed gum and sugar, before introducing the water and oil, or let it be first perfectly mixed with the castor oil. If laudanum, or some carminative and coloring adjuvant is desirable, it may be added at the time of bottling. In no case should the oil be introduced into the bottle until combined with the other ingredients, as a portion will then adhere to the sides, and be imperfectly incorporated with the gum. Each tablespoonful of this mixture contains f℥j of oil, and may be given every hour till the desired effect is produced.

Several demulcent mixtures—as those of olive oil, almond oil, &c.—may be made upon this model. Copaiva mixture, introduced among the diuretics, may have a similar composition. The proportion of gum and sugar to the oily ingredient (℥iij each, to f℥j) should be remembered, as it applies equally to the other cases named.

Taraxacum and other Mixtures.—By the judicious admixture of the fluid extracts of taraxacum, senna, &c., with saline cathartics, some excellent purgative combinations may be formed.

No. 93.—*A Charcoal and Blue Mass Mixture.*

℞.—Carbo ligni	℥j.
Sodæ bicarb.	℥ss.
Mass. hydrargyri	gr. viij.
Syrupi rhei aromat.	f℥ij.
Aquæ	f℥ij.

Triturate together into a uniform mixture. DOSE, a tablespoonful.

This was furnished by Dr. John D. Griscom, who finds it to meet a very common indication in general practice.

No. 94.—*A Magnesia Mixture for Children.*

Take of Magnesia (Husband's)	℥j.
Powd. gum Arabic	℥ss.

Triturate together, and add

Aromat. syrup of rhubarb	f℥iij.
Fennel-seed water	f℥iss.

A teaspoonful is an appropriate dose. To this mixture may be added, say gr. xv of mercurial mass, which should be triturated with the powder, and, if required, the addition of say ♏viij of laudanum, or f℥j of paregoric. The precaution of shaking up before administering should not be overlooked.

No. 95.—*Extemporaneous Cream of Tartar Draught.*

Take of Tartaric acid . . . . ℨix.
Water . . . . fℨvj.

Make solution, and label No. 1.

Bicarb. potassa . . . . ℨvj.
Water . . . . fℨvj.

Make solution, and label No. 2.

Mix from one to two tablespoonfuls of No. 1 with the same quantity of No. 2, and drink immediately. In this way, the bitartrate of potassa is obtained in solution, although, if the mixture be allowed to stand a few minutes, it will deposit the salt in a white crystalline powder.

The following soluble powders may not inappropriately be introduced here.

No. 96.—*Aperient Seidlitz Powders.*

Take of Bicarbonate of soda . . . . ℈ij.
Tartrate of potassa and soda . . . ℨij.

Mix, and fold in blue paper.

Tartaric acid . . . . . . gr. xxxv.

Fold in white paper.

Directions for use.—Take two glasses, with about a gill of cold water in each; dissolve in one the contents of the blue and in the other of the white paper. Mix, and drink immediately.

DIURETICS.

No. 97.—*Emulsion of Fluid Extract of Cubebs.*

Take of Fluid ext. of cubebs . . . gtt. cxx.
Yolk of egg . . . . One.
Sugar, powdered . . . ℨij.
Mint water sufficient to make a . fℨiij mixture.

Triturate the fluid extract with the powdered sugar and yolk of egg, and then dilute with the water. Direct a teaspoonful four times a day.

This may be made by substituting ℨij powdered gum Arabic, and ℨj sugar, for the yolk of egg. It is a fine stimulant to the mucous surfaces, adapted to catarrhs, &c., as well as to urinary diseases. The dose is fℨj, containing gtt. v of the oleo-resin of cubebs.

No. 98.—*Alkaline Copaiva Mixture.*

℞.—Copaibæ,
Liq. potassæ, āā . . . . . fℨij.
Pulv. acaciæ,
" sacchari, āā . . . . . ℨij.
Aq. menth. virid. . . . . . q. s. ut fiat fℨiv.

Mix the copaiva and solution of potassa, add the water, and triturate with the gum and sugar.

In this prescription, which is prescribed by my friend, Dr. William Hunt, the copaiva is combined into a soap with the alkali, and would be perfectly suspended without the aid of gum and sugar, which are added to obtund the acrid taste. Of course, oil of cubebs, tincture of opium, and other adjuvants, may be added if required. The usual method of suspending copaiva is similar to that given in Prescription No. 92. The dose is a tablespoonful, containing ℳxv of copaiva.

No. 99.—*Extemporaneous Solution of Acetate of Potassa.*

Take of Acetic acid . . . . . f℥vj.
Water . . . . . . f℥iij.
Bicarb. potassa . . . . . ℨiijss, or sufficient to form a neutral solution.

This is designed to obviate the necessity of weighing the very deliquescent acetate of potassa, and will contain, to each fℨj, about ten grains of the salt, which is an appropriate dose. The admixture of fluid extract of taraxacum, or of buchu, or of spirit of nitric ether, will be appropriate in certain cases.

No. 100.—*Scudamore's Mixture for Gout.*

Take of Sulphate of magnesia . . . . . ℥j.
Mint water . . . . f℥x.
Vinegar of colchicum . . . . . f℥j.
Syrup of saffron . . . . . . f℥j.
Magnesia . . . . ℨij, ℈ij.

Mix.

Dose, one to three tablespoonfuls every two hours till four to six evacuations are procured in the twenty-four hours.

No. 101.—*Dewees' Colchicum Mixture.*

Take of Wine of colchicum seed . . . . gtt. xxx.
Denarcotized laudanum . . . . gtt. xxv.
Sugar . . . . gr. xxx.
Water . . . . f℥j.

Mix. To be taken at night in one draught.

No. 102.—*Dr. Atlee's Prescription for Neuralgic and Rheumatic Symptoms.*

Take of Ethereal tincture of guaiacum . . . f℥j.
" " of colchicum . . . fℨvj.
" " of cannabis Ind. . . fℨij.

Mix. Dose, twenty-five to thirty drops every four hours on sugar.

Diaphoretics.

No. 103.—*Liquid Substitute for Dover's Powders.*

℞.—Vin. ipecac. . . . . ℳxvj.
Tinct. opii . . . . ℳxiij.
Spirit. ætheris nit. . . . . f℥j.

Misce.

Sig.—Take at one dose at going to bed.

No. 104.—*Liquor Potassæ Citratis*, U.S. (*Neutral Mixture, or Saline Draught.*)

			Reduced.
Take of Fresh lemon juice	. . . .	Oss	f℥iv.
Bicarbonate of potassa	. . .	q. s.	q. s.

Add the bicarbonate to the lemon-juice till it is perfectly saturated, then filter, or

			Reduced.
Take of Citric acid	. . . . . .	℥ss.	ʒij.
Oil of lemons	. . . . .	♏ij.	♏j.
Water	. . . . . .	Oss.	f℥iv.
Bicarbonate of potassa	. . . .	q. s.	q. s.

Rub the citric acid with the oil of lemon, and afterwards with the water till it is dissolved, then add the bicarbonate gradually till the acid is perfectly saturated; lastly, filter.

The lemon-juice may be obtained by cutting and expressing the lemon either with the fingers or a lemon-squeezer, and the little strainer, Fig. 214, which will set into the top of the graduated mea-

Fig. 214. Fig. 215. Fig. 216.

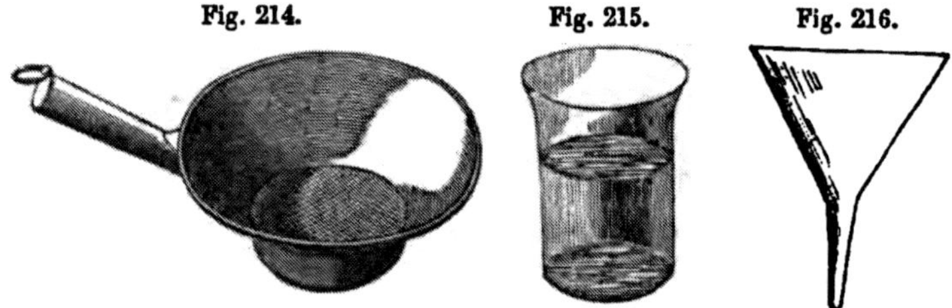

sure, or of a beaker glass, Fig. 215, will serve to separate the seed or any portion of the pulp of the lemon. Care must be taken in adding the bicarbonate to use a glass rod, porcelain spatula, silver spoon, or similar utensil, which will not corrode or impart a metallic taste to the preparation. It will also facilitate the operation of saturating the acid to triturate the crystals of bicarbonate in a dry mortar into a powder before adding it little by little to the liquid. The delay of filtering through paper may be very much obviated by using a fine linen strainer, or by plugging the base of the glass funnel, Fig. 216, with some cotton, and pouring the liquid through it into the containing vial; it is an object to conduct this operation quickly, so as to retain and bottle up as much as possible the carbonic acid gas liberated in the reaction.

There is another point worth attention; in making the solution by the second process with citric acid, it is well to weigh the bicarbonate beforehand, and then the whole amount being added there will be no doubt as to the exact saturation of the acid; this is not practicable in the lemon-juice process, as there is no certainty as to its strength; the proper proportion of bicarbonate, to the ℥ss (240 grs.) of citric acid, is 336 grains; or to the ʒij of acid, 168 grains, or about ʒij, ℈ij;

a proportion which it is well to remember, as it comes in play in all the other processes. It has always been my custom to cease the addition of the alkaline carbonate before it becomes perfectly saturated, or rather to err on the side of acidity than that of alkalinity. A slight excess of alkali may render the solution quite disagreeable, while, on the other hand, the excess of acid should be extremely small. This subject may be concluded by presenting the following additional formulas:—

			Reduced.
No. 105.—Take of	Citrate of potassa	ʒvj	ʒiij.
	Water	Oss	f℥iv.
	Sugar	ʒss	gr. xv.
	Oil of lemon	♏j	gtt. j.

Make a solution.

Here there is no effervescence, and, consequently, no carbonic acid in the solution. In other respects it is the best recipe, because so perfectly neutral and so readily made. The sugar may be omitted or not, at pleasure, but seems to me to improve it. The substitution of carbonic acid water for common water is an improvement in this process.

The following recipe is that of my friend, Ambrose Smith:—

No. 106.—*To Make Effervescing Neutral Mixture Extemporaneously.*

			Reduced.
Take of	Bicarbonate of potassa	℥iij	ʒvj.
	Citric acid	℥ij, ʒiij	℥ss, ℈ij, gr. v.
	Sugar	℥iss	ʒiij.
	Oil of lemon	gtt. xvj	♏iv.

Mix thoroughly and reduce to a uniform powder, and keep in a well-stopped bottle. To make neutral mixture dissolve ʒvj, ℈j in Oss water (ʒiij, gr. x to f℥iv); this proportion, however, is somewhat less than the strength of the lemon-juice saturated with bicarbonate of potassa, and is graduated to suit the views of many practitioners.

No. 107.—*Effervescing Draught.*

Take of	Bicarbonate of potassa	ʒij to ℈ij.
	Water	f℥iv.

Make a solution.

Directions.—Take a tablespoonful of lemon-juice diluted with a tablespoonful of water, and add to it in a tumbler a tablespoonful of this solution, then drink immediately; or thus—

Take of	Bicarbonate of potassa	ʒij, ℈ij.
	Sugar	ʒj.
	Water	f℥iv.

Make a solution and label No. 1; the alkaline solution.

Take of	Citric acid	ʒij.
	Oil of lemon	♏j.
	Water	f℥iv.

Make a solution and label No. 2; the acid solution.

Directions.—To a tablespoonful of No. 1, add a tablespoonful of water, and to the mixture, in a clean tumbler, add a tablespoonful of No. 2; drink immediately.

No. 108.—*Effervescing Fever Powders.*

Take of Citric acid, dried and powdered, ℥v.

Divide into twelve parts wrapped in white writing paper.

Take of Bicarbonate of potassa, dried and powdered, ℥viss.

Divide into twelve parts, wrapped in blue paper.

Inclose these white and blue powders alternately in a tin box.

Directions.—Dissolve the contents of a white paper in a tumbler, one-third full of cold water, then stir in the contents of a blue paper and drink immediately.

A dose is usually given every two or three hours during the prevalence of the fever.

The various forms of citrate of potassa, which are now described, constitute favorite remedies in fever; sometimes spirit of nitric ether, tartar emetic, tincture of digitalis, or other remedies are added to them. The effervescing draught is said to be the best way to give alterative or sedative doses of tartar emetic when the stomach is irritable.

Soda and yeast powders may be introduced here, although not strictly belonging to the class under consideration.

No. 109.—*Carbonated Soda Powders.*

For making a draught of soda water extemporaneously.

Take of Bicarbonate of soda	gr. xxiij.	Fold in a blue paper.
Tartaric acid . .	gr. xx.	Fold in a white paper.

Directions for use.—Dissolve one of the powders contained in the white and blue papers in separate tumblers, each nearly half full of water (spring water is preferable), stir them up for a few seconds, to render the solution complete, then mix their contents and drink immediately. A little syrup may be added to one or both of the glasses before mixing. These are usually put into boxes containing twelve of each kind of powders.

Yeast Powders.

A substitute for yeast in making batter cakes, having the advantage of making the batter perfectly light and ready for baking without delay, and greatly diminishing the liability to become sour. Many dyspeptics, who cannot tolerate fresh light cakes when made with yeast, can eat them with impunity when raised in this way.

Fold in a blue paper Bicarbonate of soda	120 grs.
" in a white paper Tartaric acid	100 grs.

Directions for use.—Put the contents of a white and blue paper into separate teacups filled with water, and stir until perfectly dissolved. Mix a sufficient quantity of batter for six or eight persons a little thicker than usual, to allow for the liquid in which the powders are dissolved; and when ready for baking stir in well the contents of one teacup, then add the other and stir it well, and commence baking immediately.

A more economical way, and sufficiently accurate in view of the harmlessness of the ingredients, is to keep supplies of the bicarbonate of soda and tartaric acid in separate bottles, which will insure their perfect dryness, and then when wanted for use take a small teaspoonful of each, and dissolve as above. The equivalent weights of these ingredients, as given above, have very nearly the same bulk. If bitartrate of potassa is substituted for tartaric acid, it must be used in about twice the quantity, and being insoluble, must be suspended in water and thoroughly stirred in.

Expectorants, &c.

No. 110.—*Mistura Ammoniaci*, U. S. (*Lac Ammoniac.*)

Take of	Ammoniac	ʒij.
	Water	Oss.

Rub the ammoniac with the water, gradually added, until they are thoroughly mixed.

No. 111.—*Mistura Glycyrrhizæ Composita*, U. S. (*Brown Mixture.*)

			Reduced.
Take of	Liquorice, in powder . . .		ʒj.
	Gum Arabic		ʒj.
	Sugar, each	℥ss	ʒj.
	Camph. tincture of opium . .	f℥ij	f℥ss.
	Antimonial wine	f℥j	fʒij.
	Spirit of nitric ether . . .	f℥ss	fʒj.
	Water	f℥xij	f℥iij.

Rub the liquorice, gum Arabic, and sugar with the water, gradually poured upon them; then add the other ingredients, and mix.

The dose of this very popular cough medicine is a tablespoonful, or for children fʒj.

No. 112.—*A Coryza Mixture of Cubebs, &c.*

Take of	Fluid extract of cubebs	fʒj.
	Sulphate of morphia	gr. iss.
	Syrup of senega	
	Syrup of wild-cherry, of each	f℥ij.

Mix.

Dose, a teaspoonful occasionally. Cubebs, by its excellent effects upon the mucous surfaces, is well adapted to the treatment of chronic coughs, coryza, and sore throat.

No. 113.—*Mistura Amygdalæ*, U. S.

Take of Sweet almonds . . . . ℥ss.
Gum Arabic . . . . ʒss.
Sugar . . . . ʒij.
Distilled water . . . . f℥viij.

Macerate the almonds in water, and, having removed their external coat, beat them with the gum Arabic and sugar in a marble mortar till they are thoroughly mixed; then rub the mixture with the distilled water, gradually added, and strain.

This mixture is introduced here, though not belonging appropriately to either of the therapeutical classes. Its chief use is as a vehicle for substances to be used in the liquid form; it may be well substituted by *Syrupus Amygdalæ*, for most purposes.

No. 114.—*A Balsamic Expectorant Mixture.*

℞.—Syrupi tolutani,
" ipecacuanhæ, āā . . . . . f℥j.
Pulv. acaciæ . . . . ʒj.
Tinct. opii camph.,
" lobeliæ, āā . . . . fʒiij.
Aquæ . . . . ℥j.

Triturate the gum and water together, and add the other ingredients in the vial. Dose, a teaspoonful.

This was furnished by Dr. S. W. Butler, of Burlington, N. J., who has used it with great satisfaction.

No. 115.—*Tolu Cough Mixture.*

℞.—Syr. scillæ . . . . f℥j
Pulv. acaciæ,
Sacchari, āā . . . . ʒiij.
Aquæ . . . . f℥vj.
Tinct. tolutani . . . . fʒij.

Misce secundum artem. Dose, fʒj.

No. 116.—*A Mixture of Acetone, Wine of Tar, &c., used in Asthma.*

Take of Acetone . . . . f℥j.
Camph. tinct. of opium,
Antimonial wine, of each . . . . . fʒj.
Wine of tar (Jew's beer) . . . . . f℥ij.

Mix. Dose, a teaspoonful.

Often prescribed by Dr. Washington L. Atlee.

No. 117.—*Spermaceti Mixture.*

Take of Spermaceti . . . . ʒij.
Olive oil . . . . ʒj.
Powd. gum Arabic . . . . . . ℥ss.
Water . . . . f℥iv.

Triturate the spermaceti with the oil, until reduced to a paste, then add the gum, and lastly the water, gradually. Dose, fʒj.

No. 118.—*Hooping-Cough Mixture.*

Take of	Carbonate of potassa	℈j.
	Powdered cochineal	℈ss.
	Sugar	ʒj.
	Water	f℥iv.

Make a mixture. Dose for children, fʒj, every two or three hours. An old and very popular remedy.

No. 119.—*For Hooping-Cough.* (By Golding Bird.)

℞.—Aluminis	gr. xxiv.
Ext. conii	gr. xij.
Aq. anethi (vel fœniculi)	f℥iij.
Syrupi papav.	f℥ij.—M.

Sig.—For an adult, a dessertspoonful every six hours.

No. 120.—*Cod-liver Oil and Biniodide of Mercury.*

Take of	Red iodide of mercury	gr. viij.
	Cod-liver oil	Oj.

Triturate together.

This forms a clear solution, and each tablespoonful dose contains ¼ gr. biniodide of mercury. This is a combination occasionally indicated. Iodine itself is sometimes given in the oil, and from ¼ to ⅛ gr. to f℥j makes a good addition in certain cases.

The mode of administering the fixed oils may here claim attention. None of the modes of compounding these materially improve their taste; but by observing to prevent their contact with the mouth in swallowing, the chief objection to them is obviated. This may be variously accomplished by enveloping them in the froth of fermented liquors, or by pouring them into a glass partially filled with iced water, or an aromatized water, so that no portion of the oil shall touch or adhere to the sides of the glass. When mineral water is convenient, it furnishes, with sarsaparilla syrup, one of the best vehicles for castor or cod-liver oil; there should be but little water drawn, but it should be thrown up as much as possible into froth.

Alteratives.

Alterative preparations are much made by the addition to the various iodine, mercurial, and other alterative salts, of the Galenical preparations of sarsaparilla, conium, &c. As a general rule, these salts are incompatible with each other; those which are insoluble are generally conveniently prescribed with iodide of potassium, which is, in fact, one of their most natural associated solvents. (See *Syrups.*)

ANTHELMINTICS.

No. 121.—*Emulsion of Pumpkin-Seeds.*

Take of Pumpkin-seeds, fresh . . . . . ℥viij.
Sugar . . . . ℥ij.
Gum Arabic, in powder . . . . ℥ss.
Water . . . . Oj.

Blanch the seeds, beat them into a mass with the sugar, then add the gum Arabic, and gradually the water.

Dose, a pint in the course of the day, for *tape-worm*. (See, also, *Oil of Turpentine Mixture*, page 625.)

CHAPTER IV.

EXTERNAL APPLICATIONS.

LOTIONS, COLLYRIA, INJECTIONS, GARGLES, BATHS, INHALATIONS, FUMIGATIONS, CERATES, OINTMENTS, LINIMENTS, AND PLASTERS.

LOTIONS.

THE preparations of this class require no different manipulations from the foregoing; indeed they are, for the most part, simple solutions prepared without any particular skill.

Soluble salts, chiefly of the astringent class, dissolved in distilled water, or in distilled rose-water, designed for external application, constitute *lotions*, or washes; these are to be applied to the surface, usually upon a folded piece of muslin or lint, chiefly for cooling and astringent purposes. Lead-water (page 538) is the only officinal lotion. Vinegar and water, or water alone, is applied for the same purposes. In various chronic skin diseases, lotions containing sulphuret of potassium, chloride of zinc, corrosive chloride of mercury, borax, solution of chlorinated soda, and other chemical agents, are employed. Glycerin, by its solubility in water, and its emollient properties, is well adapted to this form of application. The recipes appended are selected as illustrations of this class; they are all well-known preparations.

No. 122.—*Creasote Lotion.*

℞.—Creasoti . . . . gtt. x.
Aceti . . . . f℈ij.
Aquæ . . . . f℥ij.

Misce.

Applied to phagedenic ulceration, chancres, and a variety of sores.

No. 123.—*Yellow Wash.* (*Aqua Phagedænica.*)

℞.—Hydrargyri chloridi corrosivi . . . . gr. xvj.
Liquoris calcis . . . . f℥viij.

Misce.

The binoxide of mercury is precipitated as a yellow powder, and diffused through the liquid; sometimes the proportion is diminished to gr. j in each f℥. It is a very popular application to certain skin affections and to venereal sores.

No. 124.—*Black Wash.*

℞.—Hydrargyri chloridi mitis	. . . . . .	ʒj.
Liquoris calcis	. . . .	f℥iv.

Misce.

Protoxide of mercury is here thrown down by the lime as a black precipitate, though there is quite an excess of calomel. It has similar applications to the foregoing.

No. 125.—*Granville's Counter-irritant or Antidynous Lotions.*

The mild:—

℞.—Liquoris ammoniæ fortioris	. . . . .	f℥j.
Spiriti rosmarini	. . . .	fʒvj.
Tincturæ camphoræ	. . . .	fʒij.

Misce.

No. 126. The strong:—

℞.—Liquoris ammoniæ fortioris	. . . . .	fʒx.
Spiritus rosmarini	. . . .	fʒiv.
Tincturæ camphoræ	. . . .	fʒij.

Misce.

These preparations will blister in periods varied from two to ten minutes, by saturating with them a piece of linen folded five or six times over a coin, and pressing it upon the part. Over more extended surfaces, a similar method is adopted by protecting the lotion from evaporation.

No. 127.—*Lotion for Chilblains.*

Take of Muriate of ammonia	. . . . .	℥ss.
Water	. . . .	℥iv.
Muriatic acid	. . . .	fʒj.
Alcohol	. . . .	f℥iss.

Apply morning and evening.

No. 128.—*Dr. Thomas's Nipple Wash.*

Take of Alum	. . . .	ʒj.
Tincture of galls	. . . . . .	f℥j.

Triturate together until as nearly dissolved as possible.

No. 129.—*Clemen's Almond Lotion.*

Take of Gum senegal	. . . .	℥iv.
Boiling water	. . . .	Cong. j.

Strain, and when cold add—

Tinct. benzoin	. . . .	fʒij.
Alcohol	. . . .	f℥ij.
Corrosive chloride of mercury	. . . .	ʒj, ℈j.

Dissolve the corrosive chloride in the alcohol, before mixing with the other ingredients.

COLLYRIA.

Collyria [illegible] ptions for application to the eye, called eye-washes. They are [illegible] ly composed of astringent salts, as sulphate or acetate of zinc, su[illegible] of copper, or of iron or nitrate of silver, the proportion seldom [illegible] eding gr. viij to f℥j. A good prescription is appended.

No. 130.—*Thomas's Eye-Water.*

Ta[illegible] lphate of zinc,
[illegible] loride of sodium, each . . . . . ℈j.
[illegible] se-water (distilled) . . . . . f℥j.

Make [illegible] on. and apply, suitably diluted, to inflamed eyes.

The infu[illegible] n of sassafras-pith is a [illegible] d addition to this and similar eye-washes. The aqueous extract, o[illegible] wine of opium, is much used in collyria.

INJECTIONS.

Injections are solutions intended to b[illegible] thrown into the external ear, the urethra, bladder, vagina, &c. [illegible] resemble the foregoing class in composition and in stre[illegible] h. In [illegible] orrhœa, the use of injections of the astringent metallic [illegible] ts is ver[illegible] common, as also of vegetable astringents. It will n[illegible] importa[illegible] this work to give prescriptions for any of [illegible] used for these purposes.

The custom [illegible] r and various bland liquids into the rectum, [illegible] ness, has become exceedingly common of latte[illegible] years, [illegible] f apparatus contrived are numerous and ingenious, constituting a considerable article of trade with druggists and apothecaries.

The forms of self-injection apparatus made by Davidson, Mattson, and others, consisting of a gum-elastic bag designed to be grasped in the hand, and, by alternate contraction and expansion, to draw the fluid from a basin and throw it through a flexible tube and metallic injection-pipe into the rectum or vagina, has almost superseded the old kind which worked with a piston. A French pattern, however, which consists of a cylinder and piston working by a spring, designed to be wound up to its utmost tension, and then, on the opening of a faucet, to throw the whole contents in a continuous stream through the flexible tube and pipe, is preferable to any other in use, having the single objection of expense. The only valve in this instrument is in the piston, and is so simple and durable as to remove one of the most common objections to cylinder injection apparatus.

No. 131.—*Campbell's Injection for Gonorrhœa.*

℞.—Zinci sulph. . . . . ʒss.
Plumbi acet. . . . . ʒj.
Tinct. opii,
" catechu, āā . . . . f℥ij.
Aquæ rosæ . . . . f℥vj.

Misce.

This is an instance in which chemical incompatibles are mixed advisedly so as to produce a very fine precipitate, which being diffused in the liquid and deposited on the mucous membrane of the urethra, favors the therapeutic effect intended.

Gargles.

Gargles and *mouth-washes* are applications much used in the treatment of so-called sore-throat, and in scorbutic affections of the gums, which are exceedingly common, and are popularly treated by counter-irritation, and by the use of astringent and stimulating gargles. Infusions of capsicum, of vegetable astringents, and of sage, with the addition of alum, borax, or sulphate of zinc, and almost invariably honey, are the prevailing remedies of this class. The following recipes may be given.

No. 132.—*For a good Gargle and Mouth-Wash.*

℞.—Sodæ boratis . . . . ʒj.
Aquæ rosæ . . . . f℥ij.
Mellis . . . . f℥j.
Misce et adde
Tincturæ myrrhæ . . . . f℥ss.
" capsici . . . . fʒij.

Sig.—Use as a gargle every two or three hours, diluted with water.

No. 133.—*Gargle of Alum.*

℞.—Aluminis . . . . ℥ss.
Infusi lini . . . . Oss.
Mellis . . . . q. s.
Fiat gargarysma.

Baths.

Baths are either hot, warm, tepid, or cold, or consist in the application of vapor merely. They are variously medicated for the treatment of diseases of the skin, and for producing general or local revulsive effects. They possess little strictly pharmaceutical interest.

Inhalations.

Inhalation has lately been a good deal resorted to as a remedy in chronic catarrhs, bronchitis, incipient phthisis, &c. I have repeatedly prepared the apparatus and furnished the ingredients for the following:—

Prescription for Inhalation.

Into an inhaler of glass put infusum humuli, *U. S.*, f℥iv, at a temperature of about 120° F., and add liq. iodinii compositus, ♏xx. Inhale from five to ten minutes, morning and evening. In acute cases, this is found to give great relief, and by continued application produces most happy restorative effects. In place of Lugol's solution, it has been suggested to use an ethereal or chloroform tincture of iodine, adding a little iodide of potassium to prevent precipitation on adding it to the hop-tea, or other aqueous liquid.

Fig. 217.

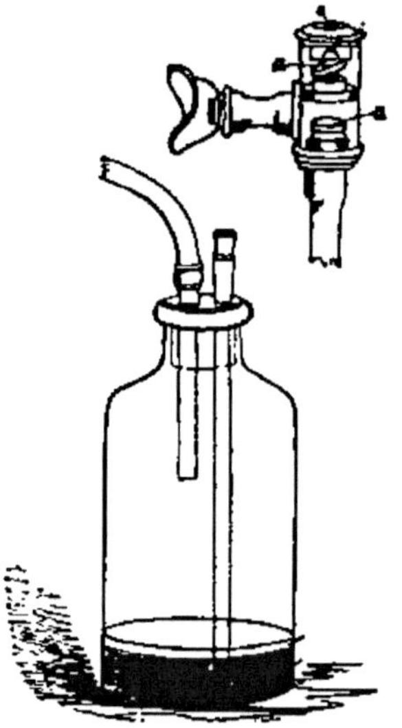

In several cases under my observation in the use of powdered cubebs, a teaspoonful to each charge of warm water, a fresh portion being added each time, inhaled three times every day, has had an excellent effect in removing bronchial affections.

Fig. 217 exhibits two forms of inhaling apparatus; the lower one is adapted to this use. An ordinary wide-mouth packing bottle is fitted with a cork which is perforated by the cork-borer or rat-tail file (see Figs. 181 and 182, page 260), so as to admit of two tubes, the smaller for the ingress of air passing nearly to the bottom of the bottle, while the larger, which is bent to be applied to the mouth, may have its origin just below the bottom of the cork. A little cork may be put into the top of the small tube when not in use. In replenishing the inhaler, before each operation, the cork is removed. The tube may be bent by softening it over the flame of an alcohol lamp or gas-furnace, and holding it in such a position that its own weight will cause it to bend gradually and uniformly to the required curve.

Fumigations.

In various affections it is desirable to have the medicine act on the skin in the form of vapor or gas. For such fumigations, sulphuretted hydrogen is generated by decomposing sulphuret of potassium or calcium with muriatic or nitric acid; nitric acid by nitrate of potassa, or of soda and sulphuric acid; chlorine from chloride of lime by muriatic acid, or by adding to a mixture of three parts chloride of sodium and one of black oxide of manganese two parts of sulphuric acid. These are chiefly used for skin diseases, and for destroying miasms.

Alcoholic fumigations are made by setting fire to half or one ounce of alcohol in an ordinary plate; acetic fumigations, by gradually adding vinegar to a hot brick; ammoniacal fumigations, by throwing carbonate of ammonia upon a hot brick, or adding spirits of hartshorn to boiling hot water; such fumigations are generally applied in rheumatic and similar affections.

Aromatic fumigations are much employed for correcting the bad odor of sick rooms; aromatic resins and balsams are used for this purpose. A good fumigating powder is prepared by the following recipe:—

No. 134.—Take of Frankincense,
Benzoin,
Amber, of each . . Three parts.
Lavender flowers . One part.

Mix.

A good and cheap disinfectant is coffee, which is to be freshly roasted.

Fumigations are applied either to a part or to the whole body; the simplest mode of doing it is to envelop the patient in a blanket, while sitting upon a cane-seat chair, and then prepare them under the chair in the proper manner. The fumes or vapors are then allowed to reach the affected parts of the body. The head is not subjected to this treatment unless in the case of vapor baths designed also to reach the lungs.

Cerates and Ointments.

These classes of preparations are widely separated in the *Pharmacopœia*, where an alphabetical arrangement is adopted, but they so closely resemble each other in a pharmaceutical point of view as to be naturally associated in a work like the present.

The difference between a cerate and an ointment is in their relative firmness and fusibility; the former is designed to be adhesive at the temperature of the body, so as to be applied in the form of a dressing or sort of plaster; the latter is intended to be rubbed upon the surface or applied by inunction; this distinction is, however, not absolute, and the two classes nearly approach each other in properties; the name cerate is derived from cera, wax, and most of the cerates, as also some of the ointments, contain this ingredient.

The medicinal ingredients which enter into these classes of preparations are very numerous; indeed, almost every kind of medicine capable of exercising a topical effect may be prescribed in this form.

The unctuous ingredients used in ointments are chiefly bland and unirritating fats and fixed oils, with more or less wax; the reader is referred, for some account of these, to pages 322—330.

Lard and *suet* resemble each other in most of their properties, except that the latter is more solid and fuses at a higher temperature, while *spermaceti* is still more firm, almost brittle in consistence, and fuses with still less facility; it is recommended by a beautiful pearly whiteness which it imparts, to a certain extent, to its oily combinations. *Wax* is more tough in consistence and still less fusible, its chief use being to give body to cerates and the stiffer ointments.

The uses of *resin* and *turpentine* are twofold, to give body to the cerates into which they enter, and to render them useful as stimulants and fit vehicles for other stimulating substances.

The greatest practical difficulty with ointments arises from their tendency to become rancid by keeping, particularly in warm climates; this is best overcome by observing to free them from unnecessary moisture, and to keep them in well-covered jars. The ointment jar, Fig. 218, is made for the purpose, but as the lid is not air tight, a piece of stout tin foil, or of bladder, or of waxed paper, should be stretched over the top before covering it with the lid.

The introduction of benzoic acid, or of small portions of balsams and essential oils, into the melted ointments, seems to have a favorable effect upon this tendency; and it is observed that the resinous ointments are not liable to it.

Fig. 218.

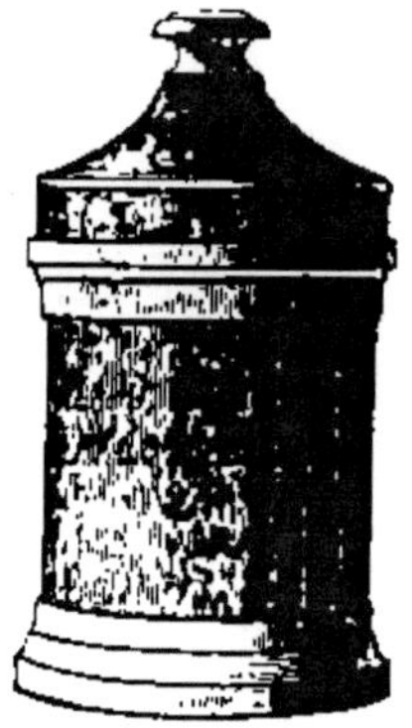

Ointment jar.

For the purposes of study, the cerates and ointments may be thus classified:—

1*st.* Those prepared by the fusion of their ingredients together, and most of them adapted to serve as vehicles for medicinal substances.

2*d.* Those prepared from these first, or from lard alone, by mechanical incorporation of the ingredients with some active medicinal agent.

3*d.* Those in which the unctuous ingredient is decomposed in the process of preparation.

So great a variety of ointments and cerates have been made officinal, that there seems less occasion for departing from the national standard than in the other classes of extemporaneous preparations. Those which are officinal will be presented in syllabi, and a few other remedies, with their mode of preparation, adverted to separately.

FIRST CLASS.—*Cerates and Ointments, much used as Vehicles for Medicinal Substances.*

Ceratum simplex.	1 part white wax, 2 lard.	*Firmest* "healing" dressing.
Ceratum cetacei.	1 part sp. cet., 3 white wax, 6 olive oil.	*Firm* "healing" dressing.
Unguentum simplex.	1 part white wax, 4 lard.	*Softer* "healing" dressing.
Ung. aquæ rosæ.	Almond oil, sp. ceti, white wax, rose-water.	*Softest* "healing" dressing.
Ceratum resinæ (Basilicon).	5 parts resin, 8 parts lard, 2 parts yellow wax.	*Stimulant* dressing.

All these are simple in their mode of preparation; the ingredients are to be placed in a tin cup or a capsule and brought to the melting point, care being taken not to burn them, which may be known by the odor and appearance of smoke given off. When there is a great difference in the fusing points, the least fusible may be placed over the fire first, and the others added afterwards, so as to involve no unnecessary application of heat. Then the whole is to be stirred or triturated together till they have thickened by cooling into a homogeneous soft mass; it may now be set away to harden by further cooling. When rose-water is added, as in the case of cold cream, it is well to warm it a little, otherwise it may chill the spermaceti to its solidifying point and deposit it in a granular condition before the mixed oil or wax are sufficiently stiffened to be homogeneous with it. The first four preparations on the above list are distinguished by different degrees of firmness and fusibility; they are all perfectly bland and unirritating, and are used for their property of protecting the part to which applied from external irritating causes and from the drying action of the air.

Simple cerate is almost exclusively applied to blistered or other raw surfaces as a "healing" dressing; it is not adapted to use as a vehicle for medicinal substances to be applied by inunction, nor can it be conveniently mixed with powders at ordinary temperatures. From overlooking this fact, the mistake is constantly made by physicians of prescribing simple cerate as the vehicle for iodine, the mercurials, &c.; and in view of this, some of the apothecaries make it softer, putting in one-fourth instead of one-third wax; this partially unfits it for the use for which it is mainly designed, to furnish a firm dressing which will not fuse entirely at the temperature of the body.

Simple ointment is designed for the purpose just mentioned as not suited to the cerate, that of furnishing, in warm weather, a good vehicle for medicines in the form of ointment. In the winter, it is frequently substituted by lard when it can be obtained fresh and sweet. It is not unusual to add to simple cerate and simple ointment, when fused in the process of preparing them, a little rose-water, and sometimes a very small portion of borax, which renders them very white without interfering with their remedial qualities.

Spermaceti cerate is intermediate between the foregoing, and has the advantage of being made without the use of lard, which is sometimes difficult to procure of good quality.

Ointment of rose-water, the softest of its class, may be best introduced by giving the following modified recipe, which produces an article superior to that of the *Pharmacopœia*:—

No. 135.—*Unguentum Aquæ Rosæ.* (*Cold Cream.*)

Take of White wax	℥j.
Oil of almonds	f℥iv.
Rose-water	f℥ij.
Borax	ʒss.
Oil of roses	♏v.

Let the wax be melted and dissolved in the oil of almonds by a gentle heat, then dissolve the borax in the rose-water and add the solution to the heated oil, stirring constantly till cool; then add the oil of roses, stirring. It is well to warm the rose-water a little, or to add it to the ointment before it is much cooled, thus preventing any granulation of the wax.

When properly prepared by this, which is the recipe of Dr. L. Turnbull, cold cream is a beautiful, snow white, bland ointment, about the consistence of good lard, and an admirable substitute for that excipient where expense is no object, and especially for applications about the face. It is commonly sold as a lip-salve, and as a healing application to abraded and chapped surfaces generally. The following recipes will produce good substitutes for this, the former of a firmer, and the latter of a more fluid consistence:—

No. 136.—*Rose Lip Salve.*

Take of Oil of almonds	℥iij.
Alkanet	ʒij.

Digest with a gentle heat and strain; then add—

White wax	℥iss.
Spermaceti	℥ss.

Melt with the colored oil and stir it until it begins to thicken, then add—

Oil of rose geranium . . . . . gtt. xxiv.

This may be put into small metallic boxes for the waistcoat pocket.

No. 137.—*Milk of Roses for Chapped Hands.*

Take of Almonds, blanched . . . . . . ℥j.

Beat to a paste, and mix with—

Rose-water . . . . f℥vj.

Heat to about 212° F., and incorporate with—

White wax . . . . ℥j.
Almond oil . . . . ℥ij.
White Castile soap . . . . . . ℥j.

Melt together and thoroughly incorporate, then add—

Honey water . . . . f℥ij.
Cologne water . . . . f℥j.
Oil of bitter almond . . . . . gtt. iv.
Oil of rose geranium . . . . . gtt. v.
Glycerin . . . . f℥ss.

After washing the hands with warm water and Castile or other mild soap, apply the milk of roses, and rub it thoroughly in, then wipe them with a dry towel.

Milk of roses is adapted to being put up in rather wide-mouth vials, and is directed to be applied to chapped hands, or other excoriated parts.

Resin cerate, or *basilicon*, differs from the foregoing in being composed of stimulating substances; it is much used as a dressing to blistered surfaces, with a view to keep up the discharge, and is also a good vehicle for other stimulating substances, as savine, Spanish flies, &c.

No. 138.—*Elemi Ointment.*

Take of Elemi (resin) . . . . ℨij.
Simple cerate . . . . ℥ij.
Resin cerate . . . . ℥ss.
Peruvian balsam . . . . ℥ss.

Fuse together, and mix thoroughly.

This is an elegant substitute for basilicon and Deshler's salve (of the next class). It is much used by Prof. Pancoast, of the Jefferson Medical College.

The London Pharmacopœia contains another formula, which nearly agrees with the following of the Prussian Pharmacopœia:—

No. 139.—Take of Elemi,
Turpentine,
Suet,
Lard, each, equal parts.

Fuse, and mix.

SECOND CLASS.—*Those in which the Medicinal Substance is mechanically mixed with the Unctuous Ingredient.*

	GROUP I.—*Incorporated by Fusion, &c.*	
Cerat. resinæ comp.	Resin, suet, yellow wax, turpentine, flaxseed oil.	Stimulating.
Unguent. picis liq.	Tar and suet equal parts.	Stimulating, antiseptic.
Ceratum cantharidis.	Canth. 12 parts; lard 10 parts; y. wax, resin, each 7 parts.	Epispastic (Blistering Cerate).
	GROUP II.—*Incorporated by Trituration.*	
Cerat. sabinæ.	1 part powdered savin. 6 parts resin cerate.	Stimulating dressing applied to blisters.
Ung. gallæ.	1 part powdered galls. 7 parts lard.	Astringent, used in piles.
Ung. veratri alb.	1 part powdered root. 4 parts lard and oil lemon.	Specific in itch.
Cerat. calaminæ.	℥iij calamine. Lard ℥xij; wax ℥iij.	Mild astringent and desiccant.
Cerat. zinci carb.	1 part ZnO,CO_2. 5 parts simple ointment.	Mild astringent and desiccant.
Ung. zinci oxidi.	1 part ZnO. 6 parts lard.	Mild astringent and desiccant.
Ung. cupri subacet.	1 part $2CuO,\overline{A}c,6HO$. 15 parts simple ointment.	Mild escharotic.
Ung. antimonii.	1 part $KO,SbO_3,2\overline{T}$. 4 parts lard.	Vesicant, producing pustular eruptions.
Ung. hydrargyri.	Equal parts Hg and lard.	Alterative, used to produce mercurial impression.
Ung. hydrar. ammon.	1 part $HgCl,NH_2$. 12 parts simple ointment.	Alterative, desiccant.
Ung. hydr. oxid. rub.	1 part HgO_2. 8 parts simple ointment.	Stimulating, alterative.
Ung. iodinii.	1 part I; ¼ part KI. 24 parts lard.	Discutient, alterative.
Ung. iodinii comp.	1 part I; 2 parts KI. 32 parts lard.	Discutient, alterative.
Ung. potassii iodid.	1 part KI+1 part Aq. 8 parts lard.	Discutient, alterative.
Ung. plumbi carb.	1 part PbO,CO_2. 6 parts simple ointment.	Astringent and desiccant.
Ung. sulphuris.	1 part S. 2 parts lard.	Specific in itch.
Ung. sulphuris comp.	Sulphur ℥j. Ammon. mercury, ʒj. Benz. acid ʒj. Oil bergam. fʒj. Sulph. acid fʒj. Nit. potass. ʒij. Lard ℥vj.	Specific in itch.
Ung. belladonnæ.	1 part extract. 8 parts lard.	Anodyne.
Ung. stramonii.	1 part extract. 8 parts lard.	Anodyne.
Ung. creasoti.	Creasote fʒss. Lard ℥j.	Antiseptic, mild escharotic.

It would extend this chapter beyond the limit laid down, to dwell in detail upon each of these numerous officinal triturated ointments. They may be made in a mortar with the use of the pestle, or on a tile or slab with a spatula. The medicinal ingredient should be invariably in a very fine powder before incorporating it with the ointment; in a few instances it is found necessary to soften the latter beforehand by a moderate heat.

Compound resin cerate, or *Deshler's salve*, is both firmer and more stimulating than basilicon; it is used for similar purposes in burns, scalds, &c.; it is too firm for ready incorporation with dry powders, and is mostly used by itself.

Tar ointment, which is made by melting suet, and, while it is fluid, stirring into it an equal weight of tar until it cools and thickens, is used in scald head and various scaly eruptions with excellent effects.

Blisters and Blistering Cerate.

Ceratum cantharides is conveniently made by melting together in a tin cup, lard, wax, and resin, and sifting into the fused mass powdered Spanish flies, continuing the heat for half an hour, and then removing from the fire and stirring till cool; the active principle of the flies, *cantharidin*, is extracted to a great extent by this digestion in the grease, and the powder itself is also retained and adds to the effect of the preparation. This is sometimes kept in jars, and sometimes, by increasing the proportion of wax and resin a very little, is made firm enough to roll out into rolls like other plasters. Blistering cerate, when ordered in prescription as a cerate to be dispensed by weight and spread at the bedside of the patient, is ordered by its officinal name; when designed to be spread as a plaster, it is called *emplastrum epispasticum*, the size being generally conveyed thus, 3 × 6 (meaning three inches wide by six long), or any other size desired, or a pattern may accompany, giving the shape and size. Sometimes the purpose for which required is expressed, and the precise size and shape are left to the pharmaceutist; at others, it is left optional with the attendant whether to spread the blister himself, or to have it spread at the shop by a prescription like the following: ℞.—Cerati cantharidis q. s., ut fiat emplastrum epispasticum 3 × 6.

The best material for spreading the blister is, I think, adhesive plaster cloth; if a wide margin is left, it is readily made to adhere by warming the margin over a lighted lamp, and pressing it carefully on to the part. It should also be so incised from the edges inward as to be readily adapted to the inequalities of the surface to which applied. Kid or split sheepskin also answers a good purpose, in which case the margin is made very narrow, and three or four strips, about half an inch wide, of adhesive plaster are warmed and drawn over the outside to hold it in its place.

Fig. 219 is a pattern for a pair of blisters to be applied behind the ears; care must be taken to have these the reverse of each other, or, after they are spread, it may be found they both fit the same ear. It is well, in the case of these, to leave the margin much the widest at the part furthest from the ear and below, where the hair will not interfere with its adhesion.

The mode of spreading blisters is too simple to require comment; in cold weather, or when the cerate is very stiff, I use the thumb, which makes a smooth and very neat surface; a spatula slightly warmed answers very well. After the blister is spread, it is well to paint over

Fig. 219.

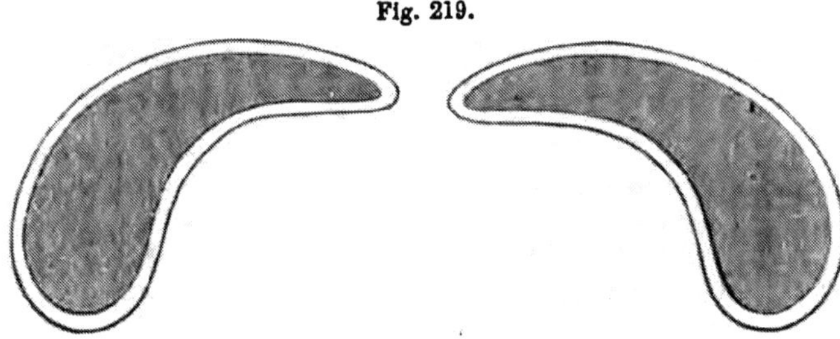

Blisters for temples.

its surface with ethereal tincture of cantharides, which increases its activity, or to lay a piece of tissue paper over its whole surface, and coat this with the ethereal tincture.

It is considered a good precaution to remove the blister as soon as it has thoroughly reddened the skin, and then to apply a cataplasm of bread and milk, elm bark, or ground flaxseed, to raise the skin. A blistering plaster usually requires from six to twelve hours to raise the skin.

No. 140.—*Blistering Collodion.*

Take of Spanish flies, in powder . . .	℥j.
Ether	℥iv, or q. s.
Alcohol	fʒj.
Prepared cotton	q. s.

Treat the flies with the ether by displacement, and having obtained a saturated tincture, or nearly so, evaporate it to f℥ij, and dissolve the cotton in it. Fig. 220 represents the syringe pattern displacer, which is very convenient for this purpose, for small operations; a cork may be fitted, not too tightly, in the top, or it may be covered by a little piece of tinfoil, and inserted in a common vial. Fig. 221 shows the collodion vial, arranged with a camel-hair brush, and well suited to contain this preparation. The great merit of blistering collodion is its applicability to circumscribed surfaces, the fact that it requires no covering of any kind, and that it cannot be improperly removed by the patient, as in cases of insanity, &c. Its action is greatly hastened by repeating the application till the coating is thick, and covering the pellicle before it is dry with a piece of oiled silk or bladder. (For an account of prepared cotton, see pages 275 to 279.)

Fig. 220. Fig. 221.

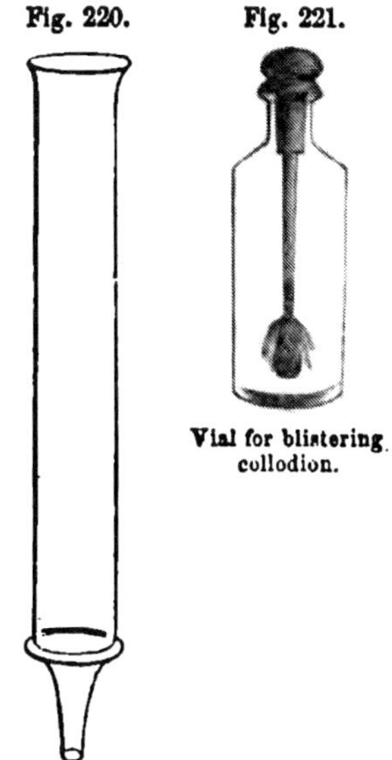

Small syringe pattern displacer.

Vial for blistering collodion.

The different *blistering tissues* are, I believe, all made by extracting cantharidin from the flies with ether or oil of turpentine, and forming it into a plaster, which is then spread on paper, silk, or other suitable fabric. *Brown's cantharidin tissue* is an admirable article, and a most convenient substitute for the old-fashioned blister, though not so well adapted to an extended surface.

For *Savin cerate*, Prof. I. J. Grahame has proposed a new formula, which yields a more elegant preparation, by dispensing with the use of the powdered savin. He first prepares an alcoholic fluid extract, which in one fluidounce contains the virtues of one ounce of English savin; the following is his proposed formula for the cerate:—

No. 141.—Take of		
	Lard	℥vijss.
	Resin	℥iss.
	Yellow wax . . .	℥iij.
	Fluid extract of savin .	f℥ij.

Melt the first three articles together, and when nearly cool, add the fluid extract, and confine the stirring to completion.

Ointment of galls may be well substituted by an ointment of tannic acid, in the proportion of about ℈j to ℥j; having the advantage of containing no ligneous particles, which, when the unctuous ingredients are absorbed, remain as a source of irritation to the part.

The following is recommended as a compound adapted to treating hæmorrhoids.

No. 142.—*Pile Ointment.*

Take of		
	Tannic acid	ʒss.
	Liniment of subacetate of lead . .	fʒss[1]
	Simple ointment	ʒvij.

Triturate the tannic acid first with the liniment, and then incorporate with the ointment.

Cerate of calamine is a modification of *Turner's cerate*, an old and highly approved astringent and desiccant, used especially in treating burns and scalds; its preparation is easy, but its principal ingredient being very inferior, as generally met with, it has been almost entirely superseded by the *cerate of precipitated carbonate of zinc*, and the *ointment of oxide of zinc* which follow it; the latter is much softer in consistence than either of the former, which are designed to be applied on a piece of lint or old linen.

Red precipitate ointment (ung. hydr. oxid. rub.) is a very important preparation, being most extensively used as an eye-salve and the basis of almost all the popular medicines of that description. By trituration, the oxide becomes changed to an *orange-colored* powder, which imparts a similar hue to the ointment (see *page* 562); it is variously diluted to meet the case for which prescribed; when it becomes rancid it assumes a red color, or changes to blue, and should be thrown away.

Mercurial ointment requires special mention from its mode of preparation; it is directed to be made by long trituration of mercury one

[1] See page 494, Prescription No. 121.

part, with mixed lard and suet one part; it is, however, a very slow process unless facilitated by appropriate machinery, and even then the temptation is strong to sacrifice its bland and pure alterative effect to the convenience of using a portion of rancid grease to reduce the mercury, thus producing intentionally the very condition which in ointments it is desirable to avoid. This ointment is usually made of one part of mercury to two or three of the unctuous ingredients. When ordering it, the physician should specify "*one-half mercury.*" Its uses are numerous, one of the chief of which is that of inducing the mercurial impression by its application to the thighs, armpits, &c. The numerous curious synonyms applied to this ointment it would be interesting to collect.

The *ointments containing iodine* are much prescribed, and by the introduction of sufficient iodide of potassium and water to the iodine before adding the lard, form homogeneous and perfect ointments.

The use of the *narcotic extracts* in the preparation of ointments is a recent improvement, and may be extended to all medicines of that class, including opium, which in aqueous extract, possesses advantages over the powdered drug.

Belladonna and *stramonium* ointments, as shown in the syllabus, are made by trituration from the extracts, taking care to soften the extract by triturating with water before adding the simple ointment or lard.

Aconite ointment is made in the same way and in the same proportion, ʒj to ℥j.

The following unofficinal ointment is of use in neuralgia, a piece the size of a pea being applied over the part three or four times a day.

No. 143.—*Aconitia Ointment.*

Take of Aconitia . . . . gr. xvj.
Olive oil . . . . ʒss.
Triturate together, and then incorporate with
Lard . . . . ℥j.

A good substitute for this very expensive preparation, will be found among the liniments.

No. 144.—*Tetter Ointment prescribed by the late Dr. S. G. Morton.*

Take of Calomel,
Alum (dried), in powder,
Carbonate of lead,
Oil of turpentine, each . . . . ʒij.
Simple ointment . . . . . ℥iss.

Triturate the powders together till they are impalpable and thoroughly mixed, then incorporate them with the oil and cerate.

This is one of the very best ointments of its class, as proved by trials during a series of years.

The mode of using it is to apply it at night, wash off with pure Castile soap in the morning, wipe dry, and dust with pure starch.

No. 145.—*Tetter Ointment prescribed by Dr. Physic.*

℞.—Hydrarg. ammoniat.	℈j.
Hydrarg. chlor. corros.	gr. x.
Alcoholis	f℥j.
Plumbi acetatis	ʒss.
Adipis	℥j.

Triturate the corrosive chloride with the alcohol, add the white precipitate and sugar of lead, and make an ointment, to be applied twice daily.

No. 146.—*A Salve resembling "Becker's Eye Balsam."*

Take of Calamine,	
Tutty, of each	ʒiss.
Red oxide of mercury	ʒvj.
Camphor, in powder	ʒj.
Almond oil	ʒj.
White wax	℥iss.
Fresh butter	℥viij.

Reduce the mineral substances to a very fine powder, and incorporate with the oil in which the camphor has been dissolved with the wax and butter previously melted together. The butter must be deprived of salt, if it contains it, by washing with warm water. The reputation of Becker's Eye Balsam is widely extended.

No. 147.—*Compound Iron Ointment.*

Take of Common iron rust	℥iijss.
Powdered red oxide of mercury . .	℥j, ʒj.
Make into an impalpable powder, and add to	
Washed lard	℥ij.

For the cure of chronic inflammation of the eyelid (conjunctiva), particularly of a scrofulous character, eruptions on the face and body of young children, &c.

No. 148.—*Ointment of Cod-liver Oil.*

Take of Fresh cod-liver oil	7 parts.
White wax,	
Spermaceti, of each	1 part.

Melt together, stirring as it cools.

This is used in ophthalmia and opacity of the cornea, either alone or combined with a little citrine ointment, also as a friction or dressing for scrofulous indurations and sores, in rheumatism, stiff joints, and several skin diseases. It is said to have been used in porrigo or scald head when other remedies have failed.

No. 149.—*Ointment of Croton Oil.*

Take of Croton oil . . . . . ♏xxx.
Lard (softened) . . . . . ℥j.

Mix well.

Rubefacient and counter-irritant in rheumatic and other diseases. When rubbed repeatedly on a part it produces redness and a pustular eruption.

No. 150.—*Hufeland's Stimulating Ointment.*

Take of Beef gall . . . . ʒiij.
White soap . . . . . . ʒiij.
Althea ointment . . . . . ℥j.
Petroleum . . . . . . ʒij.

Mix by the aid of heat, and as it cools add

Powd. carbonate of ammonia . . ʒss.
" camphor . . . . . ʒj.

Triturate together.

Althea ointment is still officinal in most European Pharmacopœias; but some have discontinued it for the use of the mucilaginous decoctions of marshmallow root and flaxseed. The Bavarian and Greek Pharmacopœias order, instead of it, an ointment of yellow wax and lard, colored by turmeric. The following embraces the directions of the French Codex of 1839:—

No. 151.—Take of Powdered fœnugreek . 2 parts
Olive oil . . . 32 "

Digest for six hours, strain and add—

Yellow wax . . . 8 parts.
Burgundy pitch . . 4 "
Turpentine . . . 4 "

Strain, and stir until cool.

THIRD CLASS.—*Officinal Ointments made by digesting the Medicinal Ingredient in Lard.*

Ung. tabaci, ℥j leaves to ℔j lard. Narcotic.
Ung. mezerei, ℥iv bark to lard ℥xiv, wax ℥ij. Stimulating.
Ung. cantharidis (with boiling water), ℥ij to ℥viij resin cerate. Stimulating.

The members of this class are made by the action of lard at an elevated temperature upon medicinal substances. As long as moisture is extracted from the leaf or bark, it is shown by escaping as steam through the fused grease; when it becomes perfectly placid, it is decanted and strained. The vegetable structure is now found to have become crisp, dry, and inert, and the lard is impregnated with its properties. This plan was formerly more in vogue; the use of extracts, as in the case of Ung. belladonnæ and Ung. stramonii, is a much shorter and equally good way.

No. 152.—*Improved Tobacco Ointment.*

Take of	Tobacco leaves	℥v.
	Vinegar	Oij.

Digest the leaves in the vinegar till evaporated to Oss; strain and express the liquid, then evaporate by moderate heat to about f℥iij; triturate this with

	Extract of belladonna	℥j.
Then take	Camphor, in powder	ʒviss.
	Resin cerate	℥viss.

Mix these by fusion at a moderate heat, and incorporate them with the mixed extracts of tobacco and belladonna. This is a very superior stimulating and anodyne application, first published by Wm. J. Allinson, of Burlington, N. J.

No. 153.—*Garlic Ointment.*

Take of	Fresh garlic	2 or 3 cloves.
	Lard	℥j.

Digest at a moderate heat for half an hour and strain; a useful application to the chest in croup.

Ung. cantharidis is not made as described for this class, though not classifiable elsewhere. Boiling water is here the solvent used, and the aqueous extract is incorporated with the resin cerate, which, as in the case of savine ointment in the last group, is used as a vehicle. These two ointments are chiefly used for the same purpose. (See *Pharmacopœia* for this and the other recipes.)

Care must be taken to distinguish, in prescriptions, between the cerate and ointment of cantharides; the former being blistering cerate, and the latter only a stimulating dressing for blisters.

FOURTH CLASS.—*In which the Unctuous Ingredient is Chemically changed.*

Ung. hydrarg. nit. A powerful stimulant and alterative; citrine ointment.
Ceratum saponis. A bland and soothing dressing.
Cerat. plumbi S. acet. A cooling and mild application; Goulard's cerate.

Citrine ointment is made by mixing f℥ix hot oil (the officinal recipe orders neat's foot, but lard oil does very well),[1] and ℥iij lard, with an acid nitrate of mercury; prepared by dissolving ℥j mercury in fʒxiv nitric acid, which should be of full officinal strength, a brisk effervescence occurs, nitric oxide is given off, and the olein of the fat is converted into elaidin; by stirring with a wooden spatula till it cools, a beautiful citrine colored soft ointment will generally be obtained. It is a very variable preparation, however.

Soap cerate is made by boiling solution of subacetate of lead with soap; the oil acids of the soap being liberated, combine with the oxide of lead of the subacetate, and the acetic acid is saturated by the alkali of the soap; by the addition of olive oil and white wax, a beau-

[1] Dr. A. Hewson recommends cod-liver oil for this purpose.

tiful and very stiff cerate is formed, which forms a connecting link between the cerates and the plasters.

Goulard's Cerate.

This preparation contains subacetate of lead combined with olive oil, white wax, and camphor; it should be made in small quantities so as to be used before it becomes rancid, which is shown by its odor and white color on the surface exposed to the air.

The following extemporaneous recipe makes a good substitute for Goulard's cerate.

℞.—Liq. plumbi subacetatis . . . . f℥ijss.
Linimenti camphoræ . . . . . ℥ss.
Cerati simplicis . . . . . . ℥xij.

Mix together on a tile.

An excellent combination of this, attributed to Dr. Parrish, Senior, is as follows:—

No. 154.—*Compound Cerate of Lead.*

℞.—Cerat. plumbi subacet.,
Cerat. simp., āā . . . . . . ℥ss.
Hydrarg. chlor. mit.,
Pulveris opii, āā . . . . . . ʒj.

Mix.

Used in cutaneous eruptions of a local character.

EMPLASTRA, *U. S.* (PLASTERS.)

These are external applications of a consistence thicker than cerates, and of such tenacity and adhesiveness at the temperature of the body that when warmed and applied they will adhere firmly. They are used for two principal objects: 1st, to furnish mechanical support and to protect the part from the air; and, 2d, to convey medicinal effects, especially of a stimulant and discutient character.

In the chapter on Fixed Oils, page 324, the subject of the preparation and properties of lead plaster, oleo-margarate of lead, is fully presented. This preparation is the basis of most plasters, though a considerable number are made from resinous substances which were treated of under that head on pages 350 to 355.

Lead plaster associated with soap is rendered less adhesive and more bland in its characters, furnishing an emollient preparation often confounded with soap cerate. By mixing with resin, lead plaster is rendered more adhesive, and somewhat more irritating. This is its most common preparation, and, when spread on cotton cloth, constitutes *adhesive plaster* cloth. Some elegant plaster cloths are now imported from England in which this excellent "body" is incorporated with mercury, belladonna, opium, &c., and spread upon cotton, linen, or silk fabrics. The anodyne plasters of this description leave nothing to desire.

These should be kept in tin cans, and when adhesive plaster especially is disposed to crackle, it should be held to the fire till fused on the surface, and then laid away to cool thoroughly before being again rolled up. In applying adhesive plaster, it should be warmed from the unspread side, to insure its being softened throughout.

The skilful association of the medicinal substances prescribed in the officinal plasters, is accomplished mainly by fusion and stirring together; in the case of *opium plaster*, water is added to lessen the liability to injury from the heat employed. *Belladonna plaster* is made by incorporating the extract with resin and lead plaster, the extract being softened and added as the plaster thickens by cooling.

In *mercurial plaster*, and plaster of *ammoniac* and *mercury*, a little sulphur and oil are used to extinguish the mercury before associating it with the plaster.

Ammoniac plaster is peculiar in its mode of preparation; it consists of the pure gum-resin as dissolved in vinegar, strained and evaporated.

EMPLASTRA.—*Syllabus of Officinal Plasters.*

Emp. plumbi.	(See page 324.)	Diachylon plaster.
Emp. resinæ.	1 part p. resin. 6 parts lead plaster.	Adhesive plaster.
Emp. saponis.	1 part soap. 9 parts lead plaster.	Very mild and less adhesive.
Emp. belladonnæ.	1 part extract. 2 parts emp. resinæ.	Anodyne in neuralgia, &c.
Emp. ferri.	1 part. $F2O_3+FeO,CO_2$. 8 parts lead plaster. 2 parts B. pitch.	Red strengthening roborant plaster.
Emp. hydrargyri.	3 parts mercury. 1 part olive oil. 1 part resin. 6 parts lead plaster.	Discutient; alterative.
Emp. opii.	1 part opium. 1½ parts B. pitch. 6 parts lead plaster.	Anodyne.
Emp. ammoniaci.	G. resin, purified by dil. acet. acid.	Stimulant; resolvent.
Em. ammoniaci cum hydrarg.	Ammoniac ℔j. Mercury ℥iij. Olive oil f℥j. Sulphur gr. viij.	Discutient; stimulant.
Emp. assafœtidæ.	Assafœtida ℔j. Lead plaster ℔j. Galbanum ℔ss. Yellow wax ℔ss.	Antispasmodic.
Emp. picis Burgundicæ.	12 parts B. pitch. 1 part y. wax.	"Strengthening plaster."
Emp. picis cum canth.	7 parts B. pitch. 1 part. cerat. canth.	Warming plaster.

Several unofficinal plasters are worthy of insertion here, though it is not designed to devote much space to the subject of the preparation of plasters, that being a branch of pharmacy little practised by the physician or dispensing pharmaceutist.

No. 155.—*Emplastrum Universalis.*

A plaster is officinal in several of the European *Pharmacopœias* under different names, which appears to be identical with Keyser's

Universal plaster, which is sold extensively in this country as a trum.

The following is the formula of the Prussian *Pharmacopœia;* proportions are by weight:—

Take of Red lead, in very fine powder . . . ℥viij.
Olive oil . . . . ℥xvj.

Boil them in a proper vessel with constant agitation until the w has assumed a blackish-brown color, then add—

Yellow wax . . . . ℥iv.

And after this has been melted and well mixed,

Camphor . . . . ʒij.

Previously dissolved in a little olive oil.

Now pour it out into suitable boxes, or into paper capsules, t cut into square cakes when cold.

No. 156.—*Dewees's Breast Plaster.* (*A Modified Formula.*)

Take of Lead plaster . . . . ℥iij.
Ammoniac plaster . . . . . . ℥ss.
Logan's plaster . . . . ℥iss.
Spermaceti,
Camphor, of each . . . . . . ʒij.

Melt the plasters together, then add the spermaceti and camp and remove from the fire.

No. 157.—*Logan's Plaster.*

Take of Litharge,
Carbonate of lead, of each . . . ℔j. com.
Castile soap . . . . . . 12 oz. com.
Fresh butter . . . . . . 4 oz.
Olive oil . . . . . . $2\frac{1}{2}$ pints.
Powdered gum mastich . . . . 2 drachms.

Mix the soap, oil, and butter together; then add the lead and it gently over a slow fire for an hour and a half, or until it has a brown color, stirring constantly; the heat may then be increased the boiling continued, till a portion of the melted plaster b dropped on a smooth board is found not to adhere, then remov from the fire and add the powdered gum mastich.

No. 158.—*Pancoast's Sedative Plaster.*

Take of Extract of belladonna,
Mercurial plaster,
Lead plaster . . . . . . Equal parts.

Mix by fusion and trituration.

No. 159.—*Arnica Plaster.*

Among the remedies of this class, introduced within a few y this is one of the most popular, being used as a strengthening pla and as a stimulating application to sprains. The following formula is by Prof. Procter:—

Take of Arnica flowers	1 lb. offic.
Alcohol	3 pints.
Water	1 pint.
Adhesive plaster	22 oz. offic.

Mix the alcohol and the water together, and pour two pints of the mixture over the arnica previously bruised finely; allow it to stand for forty-eight hours, pack it in a percolator and pour on slowly the remainder of the alcohol, until three pints of tincture are obtained. Evaporate this in a water bath till reduced to a soft resinous extract (weighing about two and a quarter ounces), and incorporate it by stirring with the adhesive plaster previously melted, and form into rolls. If spread upon sheep-skin, this plaster will be found to be an excellent and adhesive stimulating strengthening plaster.

The spreading of plasters, which was formerly an important part of the business of the apothecary, has now, like many other operations of his art, been monopolized by manufacturers who bring machinery to their aid, so that it will scarcely require a detailed description in a work of the design and scope of the present.

Figs. 222 and 223 show plaster irons of the kinds adapted to different sizes and kinds of plasters, the larger size being suitable to spread a large plaster of slowly fusible material. The heat necessary to melt

Fig. 222.

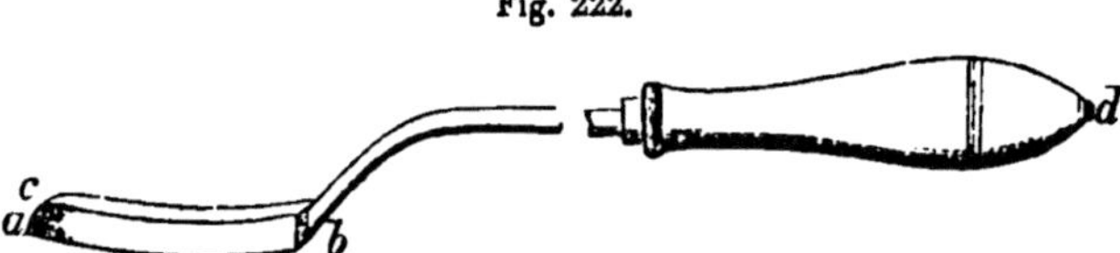

the plaster is derived from the iron, which should be first warmed to such temperature as that, while it will occasion the plaster to flow, it will not scorch it. The iron should also retain sufficient heat till the operation is complete, to impart a smooth surface to the stiffened plaster. The small iron will do well to spread a warming plaster, belladonna plaster, or the similar easily fusible kinds.

Fig. 223.

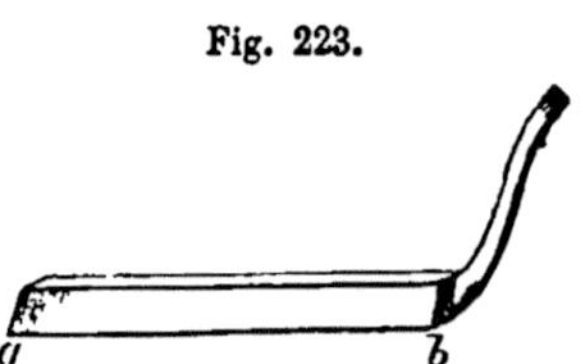

The material on which plasters are spread, may be varied according to their use. Resinous plasters and warming plasters to be applied to the back or breast, as counter-irritants and mechanical supports, are spread on thick sheepskin, while opium and belladonna plasters, which are generally smaller and frequently applied about the face, may be spread on kid, split skin, or cotton cloth, as in the case of those imported from England; these have precisely the consistence proper for this kind of application, and are less cumbrous and disagreeable than those spread on kid. I have found advantage in spreading the large lead plasters and others to be applied over the breast of the female on the kind of skin called "*chamois*," which is made more flexible and yielding, though equally durable with the differently dressed "sheepskin."

Machine-spread Strengthening Plasters.

These are immensely popular outside the profession for a great variety of ailments, and they are undoubtedly better adapted to meet the public demand for cough remedies, "pain eradicators," &c., than the great majority of the "pectoral syrups," and "hot drops," &c., so extensively vended. Recently, the manufacturers have prepared specific kinds of plasters, and sold them under appropriate names, as Burgundy pitch, hemlock, and warming plasters, so as to put them within the range of physicians' prescriptions. Some of them should make the series of officinal plasters in appropriate sizes and compounded according to the *Pharmacopœia*, and there would certainly be a demand for them, as apothecaries seldom covet the labor of preparing them extemporaneously.

Annular Corn-Plasters.

Under this name I have prepared a very convenient application to corns. Adhesive plaster is spread on *thick buckskin*, and then with a punch cut into small round plasters, about $\frac{3}{8}$ inch in diameter, then with another punch a small hole is cut in the middle. Applied over a sore corn, it protects from the pressure of the shoe and gives great relief.

White felt and *amidou plasters* imported from England, have the same shape and general character of these; they consist of a gelatinous preparation, similar to that used in making court plaster, spread upon peculiar thick material of great softness and elasticity.

CATAPLASMS.

The following is introduced as a specimen of the unofficinal class of cataplasms, of which mustard plaster and the numerous varieties of poultices are examples.

No. 160.—*Spice Plaster.* (Dr. Parrish, Sen.)

Take of Powd. capsicum,
" cinnamon,
" cloves, each . . . . 2 ounces.
Rye meal,
Spirits,
Honey, of each . . . . Sufficient.

To be made into a cataplasm by trituration on a plate, and spreading upon a close fabric. It should be made up when required.

Linimenta, *U. S.* (Liniments.)

These are fluid or semifluid preparations designed to be smeared upon the surface, and either covered by lint or rubbed on until partially absorbed. The officinal members of this class are displayed in the following syllabus.

The Officinal Liniments.

Class 1.—*In which the Oily Ingredient is saponified.*

Linimentum ammoniæ (Volatile liniment.)	Liq. ammonia, 1 part. Olive oil, 2 parts.	Stimulating, rubefacient.
Linimentum calcis	Lime-water, Flaxseed oil, equal parts.	"Healing," or demulcent.

Class 2.—*Oils charged with Stimulating Ingredients.*

Linim. cantharidis.	Cantharis ℥j. Oil turpentine Oj.	Digested and strained.
" camphoræ.	Camphor 1 p. Olive oil 4 p.	Triturated in a mortar.

Cass 3.—*Semifluid Mixtures, made with Heat.*

Linim. terebinthinæ. (Kentish's ointment.)	Resin cerate ℔j. Oil turpentine Oss.	A useful stimulant in burns and scalds.
Linim. saponis camphorata (Opodeldoc.)	*Common* soap ℥iij. Camphor ℥j. Oil rosemary f℥j. " origanum f℥j. Alcohol Oj.	The soap dissolved in alcohol by heat, and the stimulants added. Soft solid.

Remarks on the Liniments.

The first class contains two very opposite therapeutical agents.

Volatile liniment is a powerful stimulant, much used as a counter-irritant in sore throats, and also in rheumatism.

Lime liniment is applied with the most happy effects to recent scalds and burns; it is one of the most useful of preparations in the apothecaries' daily routine of minor surgery.

Liniment of Spanish flies is capable of use as a vesicant, being applied on lint, and covered to confine its vapor.

Camphor liniment is well adapted as a vehicle of many substances applied in the form of stimulating liniment; it is well combined with liq. ammoniæ, as in Prescription No. 161.

Kentish's ointment, though so different from lime liniment, is used in the same cases; it is applied to recent burns, until the peculiar inflammation, called "the fire," subsides.

Opodeldoc is much used as an application to sprains, rheumatic pains, &c.; it is always put up in small wide-mouth vials, into which the finger is inserted, to soften and extract it. It differs from camphorated tincture of soap, chiefly in being made from animal oil soap, which thickens into a soft mass when it cools.

No. 161.—*Linimentum Ammoniæ Camphorata.*

Take of Camphor liniment . . . . . 2 parts.
Water of ammonia . . . . . 1 part.

Mix.

An improvement on volatile liniment, as above.

No. 162.—*Liniment prescribed in Catarrhal Croup.* (Dr. J. L. Parrish, Ala.)

Take of Camphor . . . . ʒij, ℈ij.
Oil of turpentine (recent) . . . f℥j.

Make a solution.

No. 163.—*Astringent Liniment.*

Take of Tannic acid . . . . . . ℥j.
Glycerin . . . . f℥j.

Make a solution.

This is adapted to the treatment of sore nipples and engorgements of the neck of the uterus; it may be diluted with water at pleasure.

No. 164.—*Linimentum Plumbi Subacetatis.*

Take of Solution of subacetate of lead,
Glycerin, of each . . . . . . f℥j.

This is designed to enable the physician to apply subacetate of lead in a concentrated form, and to facilitate its dilution with neutral liquids, without its becoming so readily decomposed.

No. 165.—*Linimentum Aconiti Radicis.* (Prof. Procter.)

Take of Aconite root, in powder . . . ℥iv.
Glycerin . . . . fʒij.
Alcohol . . . . q. s.

Macerate the aconite with half a pint of alcohol for 24 hours, then pack it in a small displacer, and add alcohol gradually, until a pint of tincture has passed.

Distil off f℥xij, and evaporate to fʒxij; to this add alcohol ʒij and the glycerin.

This is intended to substitute ointment of aconitia as an external anæsthetic application. Cut a piece of lint of the required size, and saturate it with the liniment; when applied, it should be covered with oiled silk, should be used with great care, and never on an abraded surface.

No. 166.—*Linimentum Hyperici.* (*Red Oil.*)

Take of Flowers of hypericum (fresh), a convenient quantity.
Olive oil, sufficient to cover it.

Macerate in the sun for fourteen days, express and strain.

A well-known popular application to recent bruises and sprains.

The flowers of hypericum (St. John's wort) are also used internally in the form of tincture and infusion.

No. 167.—*Arnica Liniment.* (*Glycerole of Arnica.*)

Take of	Arnica flowers, bruised	4 ounces.
	Glycerin	1 pound.

Digest at a moderate temperature on a water-bath, express and strain, or preferably, with Smith's steam displacer, displace the glycerin by steam pressure. For this preparation, the cheap impure glycerin of commerce answers an excellent purpose.

No. 168.—*Glycerin Lotion.*

Take of	Rose water	1 pint.
	Quince seed	2 drachms.

Macerate, strain, and add—

	Glycerin	1℔.

This is an elegant application to chapped hands, and may do very well for a hair dressing. Rose-water may be substituted by orange-flower water, or other aqueous perfumes.

No. 169.—*Liniment of Iodide of Potassium.*

Take of	Common soap (U.S.P.)	℥j, ʒvj.
	Alcohol, 95°	f℥viiiss.
	Iodide of potassium	℥iss.
	Water	f℥iss.
	Oil of Garden lavender	ʒss.

Dissolve the soap in the alcohol by the means of a gentle heat, and filter, if it is not perfectly transparent; then add the oil of lavender and the iodide of potassium dissolved in the water, mix, and bottle while warm. The strength of this liniment is about one drachm to the ounce.

No. 170.—*Gelatinized Chloroform.*

Take of	Chloroform,	
	White of egg, of each	fʒvj.

Put them into a wide-mouth, two ounce vial, shake it, and allow it to stand for three hours.

This is applied as a local anæsthetic with remarkable success.

CHAPTER V.

ON THE ART OF DISPENSING MEDICINES.

THIS very extensive subject constitutes the most difficult practical branch of pharmacy, for, in addition to the variety and extent of knowledge required for the performance of the various duties involved in it, a salesman and dispenser of medicines must possess rare personal qualities to render him popular and successful in his calling.

Neatness, agility, and readiness of manner, combined with uniform watchfulness and care in all the important manipulations required of him, will always inspire confidence, and secure patronage; while slothfulness, negligence, and indifference to what may seem petty details, will invariably inure to the disadvantage of their possessor. It is not designed, in this *Introduction to Practical Pharmacy*, to devote much space to this subject; it is too important a matter to be superficially treated, and yet it would require more space to systematize its various details, than would comport with the general plan of this work.

In the hints which are here offered, I shall have chiefly in view the country practitioner, whose necessities compel him to undertake the business of dispensing, and the *student* of medicine and pharmacy, who would seek to obtain from books the leading topics on which to found his practical and experimental routine of studies.

In the first preliminary chapter, most of the forms of apparatus required by the country practitioner in dispensing were described and fully illustrated, and in the succeeding parts of the work, many useful implements, chiefly employed in manufacturing processes, have been introduced in connection with their uses and modes of construction, a few will be illustrated along with the manipulations yet to be treated upon. It will be observed that many of these forms of apparatus are by no means indispensable, and that all the processes described throughout the work can be performed with but few and cheap implements.

The Furniture of the Office or Shop.

The *dispensing office or shop* should have a counter of size proportioned to its anticipated use, with a closet in it, and a few drawers; it should be placed very near to the bottles containing the medicines. The physician will require no more than a table of perhaps six or eight feet long, unless his dispensing business exceeds the requirements of his own medical and surgical practice, but this should be made of about three feet in height, solid, and with a heavy top of hard wood, or otherwise covered with oil cloth.

Fig. 224 exhibits the back view of the dispensing counter in my

Fig. 224.

DISPENSING COUNTER.

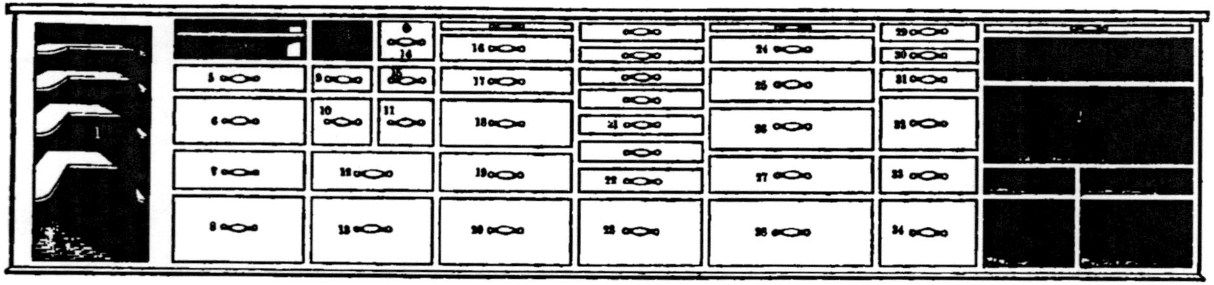

1. Closet 20 in. wide by 14 deep, containing extracts and ointments in 4 oz. and ℔ss jars; the arrangement of the shelves on each side and across the back of the case allows of 60 jars; this is protected by a door not shown in the drawing.
2. Open shelves for mortars and pestles, ointment slabs, adhesive plaster, plaster irons, &c.
3. Slide consisting of two shelves, into which the paste-pot is secured.
4. Open space for towels.

5, 6, 7, 8. Drawers for prescription vials from f℥ij to f℥xij, separated by partitions across the drawers up to the shoulders of the vials.

9, 10, 11. Cork drawers, with partitions so as to contain a variety of sizes.

12, 13. Syringes and gum-elastic wares.

14. The till, conveniently arranged to hold the sales book, the petty cash book, &c.

15. The drawer for postage and dispatch stamps. (To this point the two top drawers are made short to allow of the show case which is set in to the depth of 7 inches on the front of the counter.)

16. Cut paper for packages.

17. Capping and fancy papers.

18, 19. Sheepskins, chamois, &c.

20. Sand paper and syringes.
The series containing 21, 22 and 23, are drawers for cut and uncut labels.

24, 25, 26, 27. Pill, powder, and ointment boxes, and jars, assorted.

28. Large uncut paper.

29, 30. Two pill machines.

31. Pill tiles.

32. Tool drawer.

33, 34. Uncut castile soap.

Over 2, 24, and 16, are slides of oak and cherry, for folding powders and larger packages.

own shop—it is fourteen feet long, thirty-two and a half inches wide, and three feet high. The top is covered in part with marble and in part with oil cloth; a large glass show case occupies part of the top, but not the whole width, the bottom being inches below the top level of the counter. The whole structure is movable, being in three parts, so accurately fitted together as not to show a seam or crack at the junction. A sink and hydrant are fitted to the left hand end, which joins the curved mineral water counter, its chief use is in connection with this branch of the business. The washing of bottles, implements, &c., being accomplished in a large sink on the operating counter back.

In prescription stores, a few rows of f℥iv and f℥ij ground stoppered bottles and extract jars are frequently placed in a case on the counter, within reach of the operator when using the scales; these are filled with all the medicines most called for in small quantities, and entering into usual extemporaneous prescriptions.

The following list embraces most of those articles eligible for this position:—

IN 4OZ. BOTTLES.

Potass. iodid.
" bicarb.
" chloras.
Quin. sulph.
Cinchon. sulph.
Quinidiæ sulph.
Acid. tannic.
Acid. gallic. pulv. rhei
" aloes.
" acaciæ.
" sacchari.
" ext. glycyrrhizæ.
" glycyrrhizæ.
" saponis.
" aromatic.
" cort. aurant.
" althææ.
Plumbi acetas.
Magnesia (Husband's).
Calc. carb. præcip.
Creta præparat.
Pulv. ammon. muriat.
" ipecac. et opii.
" ipecacuanhæ.
" gambogiæ.

IN 2OZ. BOTTLES.

Antim. et pot. tart.
" sulphuret. præcip.
Iodinium.
Hydrarg. chlor. mit.
" cum creta.
Pulv. pil. hydrarg.
" ext. jalapæ.
" " coloc. comp.
Ferri pulvis.
" citras.
" et quiniæ citras.
" " strychniæ citras.
" valerianas.
Argenti nitras.
Cupri sulphas.
Zinci sulphas.
" valerianas.
" acetas.
Pulv. digitalis.
" scillæ.
" camphoræ.
" opii.
" hydrarg. oxid. rub.
" bismuthi subnitratis.
" " subcarbonatis.
" Potassii bromidi, &c.

The poisonous articles, such as hydrocyanic acid, strychnia, the salts of morphia, and strychnia, aconitia, atropia, and emetia, may be kept on a small shelf inside the scale case, or in a separate case not so easily accessible. Small labels will be found in the physician's books of labels which are adapted to this part of the counter or shop furniture.

The counter should contain the large scales (see Fig. 26, p. 42), and the prescription scales and case (Fig. 23. p. 40), which, however, should be so placed as not to be jarred by the contusion of substances with the pestle and mortar, and may very appropriately be placed on an adjacent shelf or table appropriated exclusively to them, and quite within reach in manipulating at the counter. A closet or shelves under the counter may be appropriated to mortars and pestles, funnel, displacement apparatus, infusion mug, evaporating dishes, &c.; one shallow drawer with divisions should be appropriated to papers, cut for dispensing, as below described; another to labels, pill boxes, powder boxes, corks, scissors, &c., each in a separate apartment; another may contain the pill machine and tile, the spatulas, and plaster iron; a place must be appropriated to a towel and a tank, or, preferably, a hydrant with a sink should be near at hand; a few deep drawers will be found useful for containing the drugs bought in packages, and for which no bottles are provided. On the top of the counter, which may be covered with oil-cloth, the cork presser, the twine reel, and the alcohol lamp and graduated measure, may be appropriate ornaments. If practicable to have another counter for small manufacturing operations, it would be well to avoid cumbering the dispensing counter with a gas furnace, but otherwise the arrangements described in pp. 163 and 164 will be convenient; it may be led by a ground burner from the pendant or side-light nearest at hand, and will be very convenient for heating purposes. The remarks on p. 159, in regard to the office stove, should not be overlooked.

Among the little conveniences, it is well not to overlook a cork-screw, Fig. 226, which should be hung on a tack, in an accessible place. With an eye to convenience and to furnishing a manipulating counter, a *spritz*, Fig. 225, may be suitably disposed on it; much will depend on the size of the top, and care must be taken not to crowd the space to be used in manipulation. A retort stand, Fig. 227, or the improved Wiegand's pattern, Fig. 164, p. 176, should be on the counter

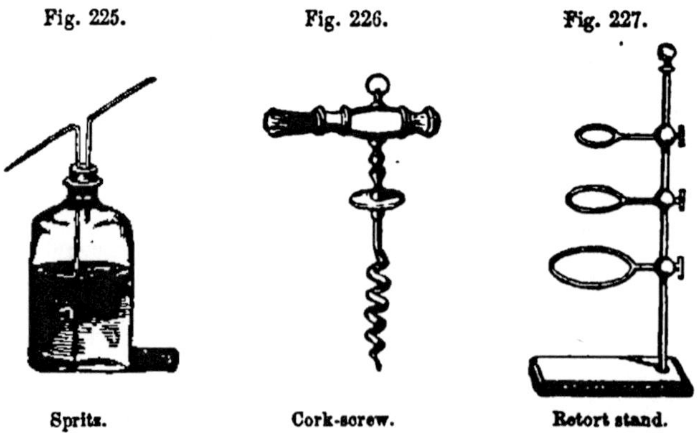

Fig. 225. Spritz. Fig. 226. Cork-screw. Fig. 227. Retort stand.

or at hand, to be used for filtering, displacement, &c.; although for such purposes, it seems quite important that a table or shelf should be especially appropriated. The little mill, Fig. 41, p. 48, can be screwed on to the end of the working counter, and removed at pleasure. It is well to have immediately under the top of the dispensing counter, two slides, on which most of the manipulations are performed; one of these should be kept exclusively for powders, and the other used indiscriminately, to save the top from being soiled.

The stock of medicines should be arranged in a case, or on plain shelves, within a few feet of the counter. In the appendix will be found the dimensions necessary for the outfits there published. The shelves should be somewhat more extended than the actual dimensions required at first, to allow for additions from time to time, and care should be taken in making these additions to have the glass ware correspond with the original stock. In the first preliminary chapter, the whole subject of glass ware is fully displayed.

The best kind of vessel for keeping herbs and aromatic seeds, indeed all plants and parts of plants, is a *tin-can*, such as is shown in Fig. 228. These are procurable ready painted or japanned, at prices little exceeding those of bottles, and besides being less liable to break, are found to preserve the greenness and aroma of the drugs much better than the transparent glass bottles. The lids are large enough to slip easily on to the can, which is slightly tapering toward the top, and the weight of which causes it to drop on to the counter, when the lid is evenly raised. The lid should, of course, have its edge protected by a seam to prevent its becoming bruised by frequent use.

Fig. 228.

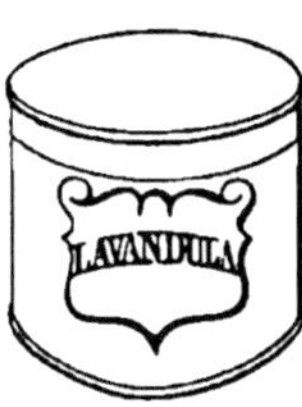

Tin can for keeping herbs.

The books of reference, which should be ample—and if the proprietor himself, and those under his instructions, would keep pace with the advance of the times, should contain the *American Journal of Pharmacy*, and *American Druggist's Circular*, bound from year to year—should be in a neighboring case; this might be advantageously arranged to contain also a skeleton, and the surgical, dental, and obstetric instruments, bandages, splints, &c.

The bougies and catheters should be in a tin case, so also the adhesive plaster, blistering tissue, gum-elastic bougies, nipple shields, &c. It is to be regretted that the proper arrangement and garnishing of the dispensing office should be generally considered of so little importance by practitioners at the commencement of their career; it is apt to have more effect upon the future success of the physician than he can appreciate in advance. (See directions to accompany outfit, Appendix.)

Folding of Powders.

The first manipulation taught students in the school of practical pharmacy is this very elementary pursuit. There are, however, thousands who have felt the want of such instruction all their lives. The paper usually purchased for folding packages of medicine is called "white druggists' wrapping paper;" its size is called double medium, each sheet being about 38 × 24½ inches. This sheet cut into 2 sheets

24½ × 19 = the *medium* size. The medium sheet is thus conveniently divided for dispensing purposes:—

Into 4 sheets	12 × 9½	inches	= ½ ℔	papers.
6 "	9½ × 8	"	= ¼ ℔	papers.
12 "	6¼ × 6¼	"	= 1 oz.	papers.

Fig. 229 shows a ½ ℔ paper. To fold a package, this is laid upon the scale plate and filled with an appropriate quantity; of a moderately heavy article, like Epsom salts or cream of tartar, this will be 4 oz. (com.); of a light article, like senna or chamomile, say 1 oz. (com.). The paper is placed before the operator in the direction here shown; a little crease is made on the nearest end so as to form a flap into which the furthest edge is fitted, and the whole turned over upon the containing substance so as to form a crease when laid evenly down upon it, at the midde or near the furthest side, according as a wide or narrow bundle is desired.

Fig. 229.

Paper for package.

The cylinder is now loosely closed up at one end by turning it over, and is held up with the crease toward the operator, the thumb pressing it firmly to prevent its bulging. Now, with the forefinger, the upper end of the cylinder is pressed in against the containing substance, and the two sides of the paper being rolled into the position they naturally take, the whole upper flap is laid down immediately above the containing substance and pressed into a firm and even crease. The package is now inverted, the other end is opened out, rolled in, and folded over in like manner.

The next operation is to label the package; this requires very little paste, only sufficient to prevent its slipping about; the label is put immediately in line with the crease, unless this is too low down, and then it connects the crease with the part below. The next operation is to tie the package, which is done by laying it on the flat or labelled side and passing the string first across it and then lengthwise, securing it by a bow-knot at the edge where it was first creased. When the package is large or quite oblong, the string is made to pass twice across it and once lengthwise. The string used should be thin and free from fuzz; linen is the best material. The ball of tying string may be put into a small apartment of the drawer and gradually unwound as required, or it may be used from a reel. Fig. 231 shows a new upright reel, made by Wiegand, possessing several advantages over the horizontal form; the twine can be drawn from it in every direction with equal facility, and by means of a rim of brass surrounding the lower head of the spool, all possibility of the twine tangling upon the spindle is effectually precluded; a cutter is fixed upon the top, which proves very convenient for cutting the string;

Fig. 230. Fig. 231.

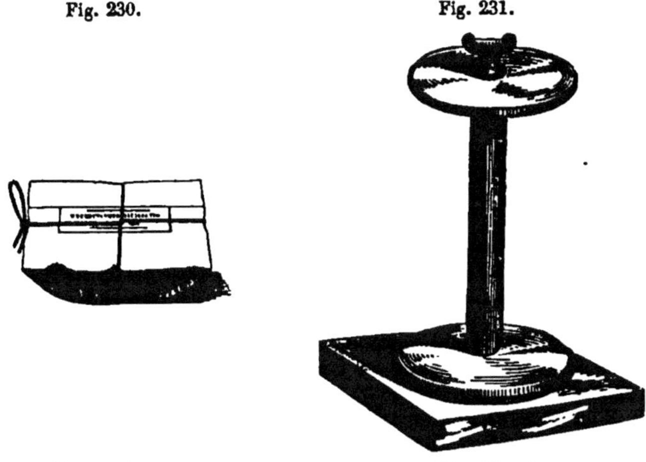

Paper package. Upright reel.

the reel is made of brass, handsomely finished, and set upon a polished Italian marble base.

Small powders for containing but a single dose of medicines should be put up in glazed writing paper. The kind called *flat-cap* is economical and adapted to the purpose. A sheet of flat-cap will furnish sixteen of the most common size, or nine of the larger or Seidlitz powder size. Fig. 232 represents the shape of these. A little crease

Fig. 232. Fig. 233. Fig. 234.

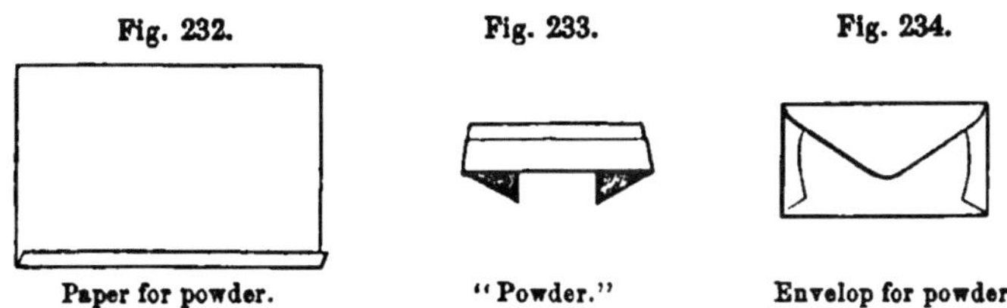

Paper for powder. "Powder." Envelop for powder.

is made along the long side into which the opposite edge is laid, and the paper being folded over is laid down in the crease just beyond the middle, or *at* the middle, according to the width desired. The ends are now folded over a spatula so as to make flaps of equal length, and the package or powder, as it is called, is complete. In dispensing simple powders, I use a small envelop, Fig. 234, which is just the right size, and leaves nothing to desire.

Powders are often directed in considerable numbers, frequently, as in Prescription 65, twelve at once; in this case, it is important to have the powders all of one length, so as to fit in a little box, called a powder-box or lozenge-box.

Figs. 235 and 236 represent gauges for folding powders; their use is twofold—to regulate the length of the powder, and to facilitate the folding with a folder; the two end creases are made by simply pressing the paper over the blades between the thumb and finger.

Fig. 235. Fig. 236.

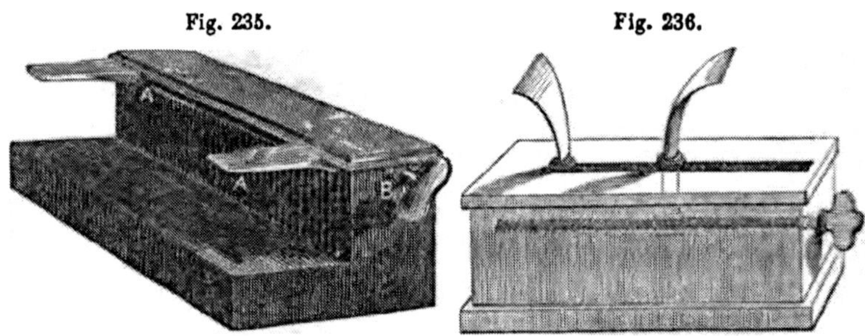

Wiegand's powder folder. Powder folder.

Fig. 235 is a recent improvement of S. Lloyd Wiegand, of this city; the blades A A are less liable to become unsteady, and are of better shape than those of the old kind. The screw regulates their distance apart. The expense of these is saved by cutting a piece of tin of the required width, and tacking it on to one corner of the slide appropriated to powders. With a penknife, the board may be cut out to the thickness of the tin, so that the paper will slip readily on to the tin, and be turned over by the thumb and finger; this is substituted on the counter shown in Fig. 224 by a small wooden powder folder, screwed on to the face of the slide appropriated to dispensing powders; a great many powders can be put up in a few minutes by this plan.

Preparation and Dispensing of Pills.

The preparation of pills can only be learned by practice, and I am not about to attempt to explain it in detail.

The ingredients in the form of powder being weighed, are placed in a mortar, or on a tile, and thoroughly mixed; two spatulas being at hand, a small addition of some excipient, as already pointed out, is to be made, care being taken not to add an excess, which the inexperienced are apt to do. The little bottle, Fig. 237, is made for the use of the analytical chemist in moistening substances with a single drop of a reagent; it will be useful to contain water for the purpose named. The drop guide, Fig. 238, or a similar extemporaneous contrivance, will answer the same purpose. Many pill masses are spoiled by getting a few drops too much water accidentally into them; they should always be very thoroughly triturated before the addition of fresh portions of liquid.

Fig. 237. Fig. 238.

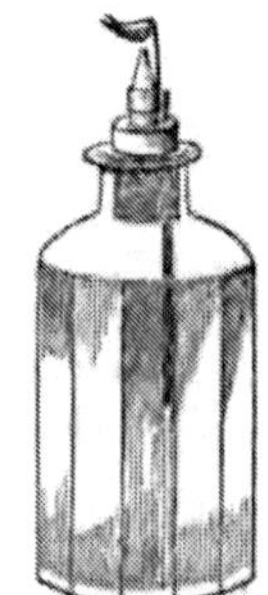

Bottle for moistening pill masses. Bottle with drop machine.

The use of extracts in making pills has already been treated of, as also the whole subject of the selection of ingredients and excipients, and we proceed to a few hints on the mode of mixing, dividing, and preserving them.

The aid of heat may be called in with considerable advantage when the extracts are tough and unmanageable; the mortar being warmed upon a stove will enable the operator to soften the extracts by trituration, and they may thus be thoroughly incorporated together. The warmth, moisture, and flexibility of the hand may frequently be brought into requisition with materials that refuse to soften and adhere, though generally it is desirable to avoid working the mass in the hands, in presence of the customer; when the materials are readily miscible, the whole process may be conveniently performed in the mortar, and the removal of the mass completely effected by the use of the pestle and spatulas.

Pills may be divided with a spatula, by the eye, or by the aid of a graduated tile; a great many pharmaceutists use this altogether, but it has always appeared to me it must be from ignorance of the

Fig. 239.

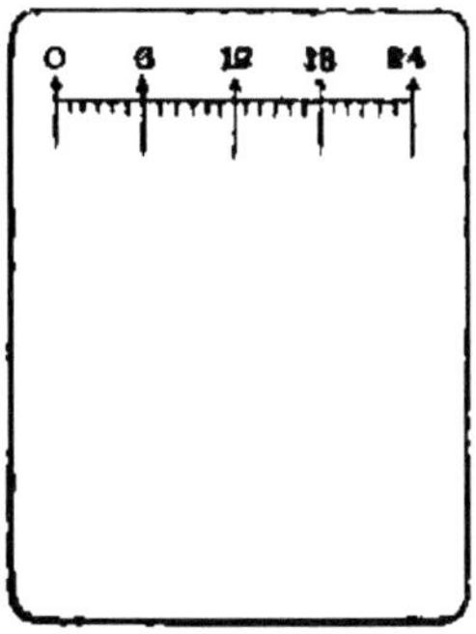

Graduated pill tile.

Fig. 240.

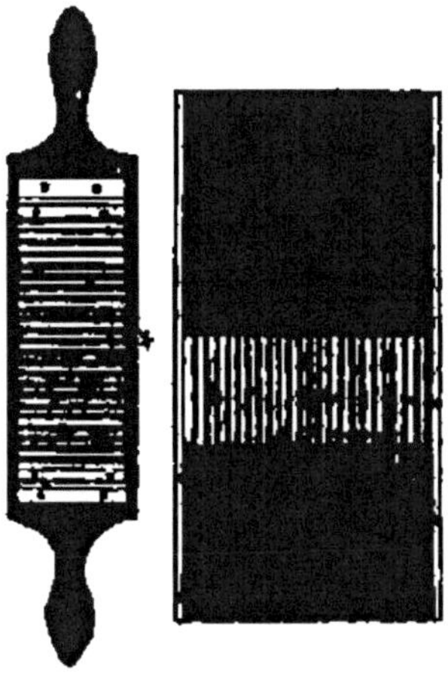

Pill machine.

proper use of the pill machine, Fig. 240. If the mass is plastic, it may be rolled between the two smooth surfaces into a perfect cylinder equally thick at both ends, and by then adjusting the cutting surfaces, the whole mass will be immediately turned into the appropriate number of pills, which, if about the size appropriate to the machine, will be so round as to require no further rolling. In large dispensing establishments, several machines are sometimes kept adapted to different sizes, one for pills of opium or Quevenne's iron, another for compound cathartic or aloetic pill, and another for compound rhubarb and other large pills. There is a practical hint in relation to the use of the pill machine which should be mentioned in this connection: it is, that the cutting surfaces will only work on each other perfectly in one way; every roller is, therefore, marked with a star, a little brass tack, a number, or some other designation, and a corresponding one is made on the machine, indicating in which direction the roller is to be worked on the machine in cutting. In Fig. 240, this is shown by two stars. From not being aware of this precaution, many abandon the use of a machine, which is one of the greatest of conveniences in pharmacy.

Fig. 241.

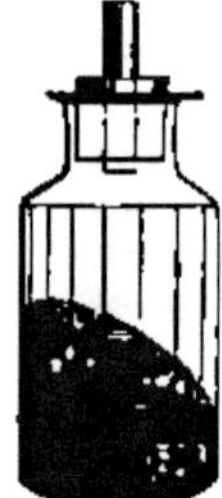

Dusting bottle.

Pills, when kept on hand, should be kept in bottles, into which they should not be put until well dried on an open box lid, or paper folded at the edges for the purpose. There are three kinds of pill boxes described on page 53. Pills containing volatile ingredients should be dispensed in a small wide-mouth vial. Such are made for this purpose.

Fig. 241 shows a bottle arranged to contain lycopodium, powdered liquorice root, or sifted arrowroot, one or more of which may be kept at hand in dispensing pills, both for the dusting of the pill machine, and for filling boxes in which they are dispensed. One of these bottles may have powdered gum Arabic also, so as to add that ingredient conveniently to pill masses in process of their manufacture. The mode of construction will scarcely need a remark; a perforated cork, short piece of tube, and ℥j or ℥ij vial, constitute the apparatus.

The Dispensing of Liquids.

Here the graduated measure will at once come into play. We draw from the tincture bottle both for dispensing directly and mixing in prescription, and the habit should be fixed, which is easily established, of holding the stopper by the little finger, while holding the measure with the thumb and forefinger. The measure must be held opposite the eye to measure the quantity with accuracy, and, after it has been done, the stopper is immediately to be replaced and the bottle set back on the shelf. The whole process is well shown in Fig. 242. The liability to mistakes in compounding is greatly increased by the accumulation of bottles on the counter; and it should be the habit to replace each bottle immediately, and to note the label as it is taken down and as it is put back; if a drop of liquid remains on the lip after decanting, it should be collected on the point of the stopper before putting it in again, and thus prevented from running down the side.

By attention to the liability of liquids to ferment, or to part with volatile active principles, or to deteriorate by exposure to atmospheric influence, the pharmaceutist will learn that advantages almost invariably result from the selection of small, well-stoppered bottles for the dispensing shelves. These bottles are necessarily frequently opened, admitting air, and they are exposed to bright light, which is one of the most potent causes of chemical change. Small bottles are also much more convenient to handle than large ones, and by having suitable funnels at hand, may be replenished as often as required from stock bottles kept in the cellar or other appropriate depository.

Under the head of solution, in the second part of this work, and of the liquid forms of medicines in the fifth part, and, indeed, throughout all the practical parts, I have endeavored to impress such facts connected with the preparation and use of this class of medicines as would be most useful to the student, and I may conclude the subject here by reference to the selection of vials, corking, labelling, &c., on

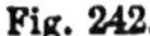

Fig. 242.

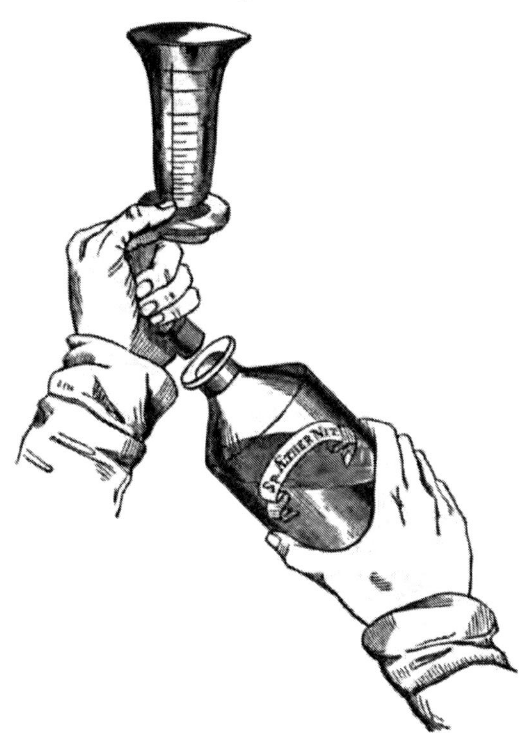

which a few hints may be given. Of the several varieties of vials shown on page 35, the kind best adapted to the purposes of the country physician is the German flint, Fig. 243; it has the advantage over the flint vial of being cheaper, and, as is generally believed, stronger; while it is far better than the common quality of green glass. The manufacturers of green glass have recently made many of their vials without lips, from the fact that dealers in handling and repacking the lipped vials suffer loss from these being much broken about the lip. A vial is, however, of little use for many of the purposes of the physician without a good, rather broad, and thin lip, which will allow of the pouring of the liquid from it without its running back and down the sides of the vial. This is especially true of small vials from which drops are to be administered.

There is no economy in procuring cheap corks, as prices are pretty exactly according to quality, and of the inferior qualities a large number are quite unfit for use. The cork presser, Fig. 244, is now so common and well known as scarcely to require mention; in using it, care should be taken to press the whole length of the cork, other-

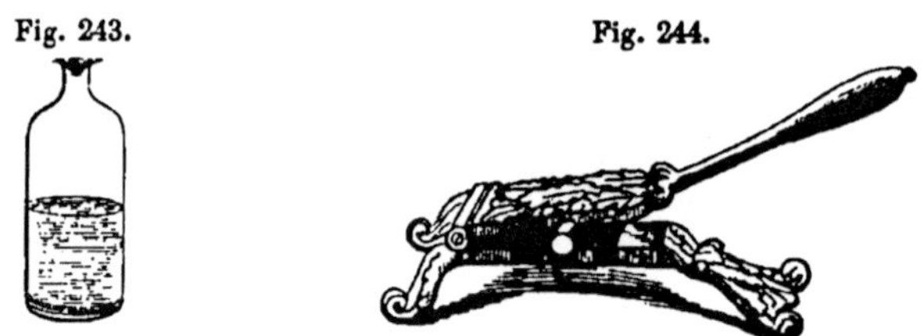

Fig. 243. Fig. 244.

wise, if it is rather dry, it may be cracked at the point where the pressure of the machine ceases, and hence will break off in attempting to remove it from the bottle.

The cork drawer should not be too near the fire, as they are deteriorated by long-continued drying. The cork should always be adjusted to the bottle before putting the liquid into it, so that if it should not fit, it may not be injured by contact with the liquid, and may be thrown in with the corks again.

The neat appearance depends chiefly on its being clean and having a clear fresh surface at top; this may generally be attained by the use of a sharp knife, care being taken not to cut off so short as to be inconvenient to extract again. The practice of capping over the cork with a piece of fancy paper or damp kid gives a handsome finish to the preparation, and secures it from being opened by children or others who may be sent for the medicine; but in small sales it scarcely repays for the time consumed.

The fashion of stamping the cork at top with a dye upon sealing-wax has lately become quite general. Heavy and good quality tin foil is a beautiful capping for corks, and may be applied without a string to secure it; it will take the impression of a stamp with considerable distinctness. With a view of capping operations, a small pair of scissors, different from those adapted to the general purposes of the counter, will be almost indispensable.

Labelling medicinal preparations is very much neglected by country practitioners, frequently for want of facilities; it is, however, too important a matter to be overlooked in any well-ordered dispensary. A small sheet of blank labels may be procured for a trifling sum, adapted exactly to the wants of the particular individual, or the druggist should have them printed for his customers. I have for several years sold from a set somewhat like the following, which by filling up the blanks serve most the purposes of the physician :—

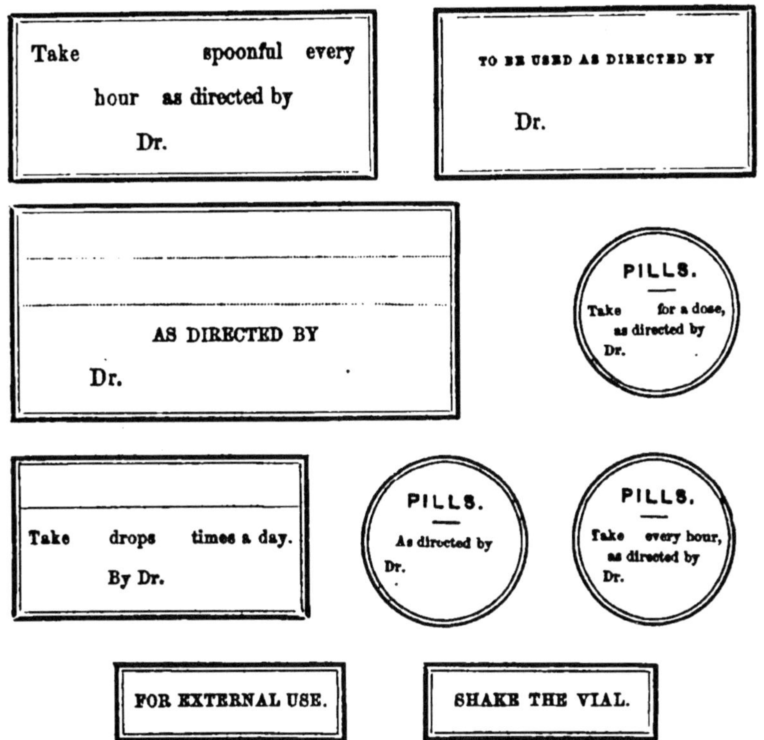

The apothecary will of course have, besides his ordinary printed slip labels, suitable prescription labels, with his business card and an appropriate space for filling up with the names of drugs, or with directions and the number and date of the prescription, for future reference. Nothing adds more to the reputation of the apothecary for neatness, than a careful and elegant style of writing on these labels, and this is much promoted by having a smooth surface to write upon, a desk at a convenient elevation, a free-flowing writing fluid and good pen, all conveniences readily attainable.

The next facility for labelling is a good paste bottle, and paste. Fig. 245 shows a convenient little wide mouth bottle, which may be of f℥ij or f℥iv capacity, with a perforated cork into which a plug is inserted, extending half an inch below the cork, on to which is fitted a camel-hair brush, always dipping into the paste; this little vial may be supplied with paste from another and larger bottle. The paste may be made by either of the following processes:—

Fig. 245.

Paste bottle and brush.

Glycem —Recommended by Dr. Goddard as suitable for fixing paper to ... id other surfaces, and as keeping very well:—

Tak	ʒum Arabic	One ounce.
	Boiling water	Two fluidounces.
	ʒlycerin	Two fluidrachms.

Make a ... on.

Paste preserved with Acetic Acid.

Take of	Powdered gum Arabic,	
	Powdered tragacanth, of each .	ʒss.
	Water	℥iss or sufficient.
	Acetic acid	♏ xx.

Mix them.

The application of paste to a series of labels may be accomplished by laying the labels successively upo a small piece of soft paper, which must be renewed as soon as it ecomes somewhat daubed, or by laying them on a piece of smooth d hard wood, which should be cleaned and dried once every day. ien the label is applied to the glass, it should be cover r a niece paper somewhat larger than itself, and tightly and ur r till quite smooth; it is a mistake to put a thick c the paper, as it then spreads on to the andin , soiling them, and in drying shrinks a inkles filled and properly corked, the vial d wrapped in a piece of white paper. is s ole for a f℥iv vial.

A good pen, with a point, suitai e for filling up the blanks on the labels, and a desk, should be within convenient reach; also a blank book or file on which to preserve the prescription for future reference, the day book or blotter, the book of "wants" in which each article is to be entered for purchase or preparation, before it is entirely out, and a note book of facts and experiences, which, if diligently kept, will, by lapse of time, become a valuable heirloom of the office or shop.

Management and Discipline of the Shop.

Much of the success of the pharmaceutical store will be dependent upon the discipline maintained among those to whom the details of the business are necessarily intrusted, and the difficulties surrounding the proper management of the business will increase as it extends and involves the employment of more numerous apprentices or other employees, unless the general duties of all are specifically laid down, and the particular duties of each well defined and insisted upon.

The rules which follow were prepared by a gentleman of considerable experience, and unusual success in business; they were designed for a store employing three apprentices, and as originally prepared were so admirable that I have inserted them almost entire. Although, of course, they require modifications to suit the circumstances of different establishments, their general tenor is adopted to all, and the high tone of professional and moral rectitude they require, renders them worthy the acceptance of every apprentice, who would deserve the approval of his employer, and of every employer who desires the best interests of his apprentice.

RULES OF A PHARMACEUTICAL STORE.

Specific Duties of the Senior Apprentice.

First.—To see that the specific duties of his Juniors are promptly and well performed.

Second.—To wait on the counter in the morning before breakfast, that they may not be hindered in the performance of their duties.

Third.—In case of the absence of either of his Juniors, to take the place of his first Junior.

Fourth.—He is to take charge of the books.

Fifth.—To take knowledge of, and properly note any articles that may be needed for the store, including goods to be purchased, and preparations to be made.

Sixth.—To see that the furniture of the store is well supplied with such articles as are kept on hand in quantity.

Seventh.—To keep a note book of what is necessary to be done in the ordinary business of the store, and to designate employment for his Juniors.

Eighth.—In the absence of the Proprietor, to take entire charge of the store, and to be alone responsible for its business.

Specific Duties of the First Junior Apprentice.

First.—It will be his duty to dust the counters and desks thoroughly every morning. This service must be performed before breakfast, and repeated as often through the day as necessary.

Second.—In case of the absence of the second Junior apprentice he is to perform his duties.

Third.—He is to paste the prescriptions in the book kept for that purpose or to file them, once every week.

Fourth.—He will copy the bills into the bill-book once every week.

Fifth.—It will be his duty to keep the drawers well supplied with paper for wrapping purposes, including what is necessary to be cut.

Sixth.—It will be his duty to clean the scales, large and small, once every week, and oftener, if necessary.

Specific Duties of the Second Junior Apprentice.

First.—He is to open the store in the morning, make the fire, and attend to it through the day, sweep out the store, wash the mortars,

&c., keep the mineral water counter clean, and the syrup bottles filled. These duties are to be performed in part before breakfast.

Second.—It will be his duty to take entire charge of the labels, keeping a register of those needed, and having the drawers always well supplied with those trimmed for use; also, to have the proper drawers well provided with clean vials and with boxes.

Third.—It will be required of him to do such errands as the business of the store may demand, and to close the store at night.

General Regulations of the Store.

First.—Business hours will include the time between breakfast and 6 o'clock P. M., except when special duty may require it otherwise.

Second.—During business hours all hands must be on their feet, and must be employed either in waiting on the counter or at some regular store duty.

Third.—As waiting on the counter is a duty which requires most knowledge and experience, the Senior apprentice must always serve where there is one customer; when two, the first Junior apprentice will assist, and when three the second Junior will aid.

Fourth.—The Senior apprentice must always take that part of the duty which requires most knowledge and skill. This order of duty must never be deviated from if circumstances will at all admit of it.

Fifth.—Never put up an article without you are certain it is right.

Sixth.—In every instance, customers must be waited on with promptitude, and in case one only is present and several articles are wanting, or a prescription, or in any instance where assistance will expedite, the first Junior, and the second, if necessary, will aid.

Seventh.—Every other duty must give way to that of waiting on the counter, except when serious detriment would be the consequence.

Eighth.—Every person entering the store, whether pauper or president, infant or adult, white or colored, must be treated with courtesy and kindness.

Ninth.—Boisterous mirth and a sullen temper are to be equally avoided as productive of neither business nor business character. The acquisition of a uniformly cheerful temperament is an attainment worth far beyond the price it usually costs.

Tenth.—There are to be no masters and no servants. Each one is to feel conscious of the fact that the performance of the duties assigned to him are just as necessary and as important as what pertains to any other hand in the store. All useful employment is honorable. Indolence is a disgrace.

Eleventh.—An afternoon of every week will be devoted to cleaning the store, in which all must share as occasion offers.

Twelfth.—As neatness, order, cleanliness and accuracy are necessary and not mere accomplishments in a Pharmaceutist, all are required to practise them constantly.

Thirteenth.—Every apprentice will be expected to become a graduate of the College of Pharmacy, and will be furnished with tickets for the lectures of the College and every opportunity for availing himself of the honor of the degree of that Institution.

Fourteenth.—To deserve this degree, will require a severe economy of leisure hours, and their application to the study of those books which relate to the theoretical and practical knowledge necessary to make an accomplished Pharmaceutist.

Fifteenth.—Apprentices need but few social acquaintances, and they should be very select. While the occasional visit of a well behaved young friend will be countenanced, lounging in the store will not be tolerated.

Sixteenth.—Each apprentice will have at his disposal an afternoon and evening every week, and every other Sunday. The afternoon will comprise the time between 12 o'clock, at noon, and 6 o'clock P. M., and the evening between 6 o'clock P. M., and the closing of the store. These privileges will not be interfered with unnecessarily.

Seventeenth.—No apprentice residing in the house, will be allowed to be absent at night after the closing of the store without special permission.

Eighteenth.—A vacation of two weeks, every year, will be allowed each apprentice.

Nineteenth.—It is not the wish of the proprietor of the store that any of his apprentices should extol an article beyond its merit to advance his pecuniary interest, or to say or do aught in the performance of his duty that he would not be willing that others should say or do to him under the same circumstances.

Twentieth.—As all are presumed to be members of the proprietor's family, their intercourse will be characterized with the courtesy becoming young gentlemen.

Twenty-first.—No bond of apprenticeship will be required except the honor of the individual.

Twenty-second.—Should the party wishing to leave before the allotted time expires have a good reason for so doing, the proprietor will not probably object, and should his cause be a bad one, and be persisted in, the proprietor will certainly not offer a hindrance to his going.

Twenty-third.—A cheerful compliance with the foregoing rules is confidently expected, and the repeated infraction of a known regulation of the store will be cause for a dismissal.

APPENDIX.

ON THE MANAGEMENT OF A SICK CHAMBER.

THE following excellent hints on the management of the sick chamber are chiefly from the pen of a lady of intelligence and experience. Although addressed especially to nurses, they should be carefully studied by practitioners of medicine, upon whom the responsibility of giving direction to the conduct of the sick chamber mainly devolves.

Ventilation.

Few persons who are in the habit of visiting the sick, can have failed to notice the great difference in the state of the air, in those chambers where cleanliness and good management have been in exercise, and those wherein the value and importance of neatness, and the careful admission of a free current of fresh air have been overlooked. If, then, temporary visitors are sensible of the difference, how much more deeply interested must the suffering patient be in the attainment of a free and healthy atmosphere.

Cleanliness.

Since it is often very difficult to get a sick room swept, it may be desirable, if it can be done unheard, to get at least a part of the carpeting away now and then, that it may be well shaken. A few tea-leaves may be thrown over a part of the room at a time, and very quietly taken up with a hand-brush. And in those cases which are not at all critical, and where anything damp can be admitted into the room with impunity, a mop, which, after being dipped in water, has been *well trundled*, may be just used for a few minutes to remove the flue from under the bed; or it may be very carefully passed over a carpet, if nailed down.

Change of Posture.

It is scarcely to be believed, until experienced, the relief from suffering which a change of posture produces; neither is it generally thought of, how much alleviation would be known in many instances, even by the fresh cording of the sacking of the bed, and a general attention to a level position; a hard bed or hard mattress, for a suffering invalid is far from recommended, but an arrangement for a level position will often afford great comfort. The sacking first tightly corded (but splines instead of sacking are much better), then a straw palliasse, which, if not newly made, ought to be raised by a fresh supply of straw in the *middle, where* a heavy pressure may have rendered it very uneven; over this, a good feather bed, which ought to be gently pressed and made level, then a mattress, composed first of a thick bed of horsehair, and well overlaid with excellent long wool; it ought to have room for the bed-post at each of its four corners, so that it may not only be turned *daily* from *side* to *side*, but also from the *head* to the *feet*; indeed, it is better, as it regards even the straw palliasse, to adopt such a plan as may admit of the turning of it, and, as it is heavy and unyielding, it is better to have the corners cut out at each of its two parts, making a small oblong of the same material and height, to tie on in the middle; or an inconvenient aperture might be made there. The proper arrangement of pillows is of no small importance, and in cases of high fever a change of pillows is very desirable; this, too, furnishes an opportunity for putting on fresh pillow-cases.

Cleanliness of the Person.

Washing, refreshing, whenever able, also brushing the teeth and hair—the latter may be rubbed with bay rum, lavender water, cologne, &c. All this, subject to the strength of the patient, and the permission of the medical attendant. It may, by some, be deemed needless to give the above hint, but it cannot be doubted that by t se the full enjoyment and benefit of a thorough attention to th the person.

Washin Glasses.

An appropriate table, not liable to injur is a great convenience in a sick room; so is a small wicker basket, with c ipartments to hold the different bottles of medicine and articles of diet. t may be also useful to have a couple of baskets with compartments to l ld glasses or cups, one of these being sent out with the things which need ashing, and always ready to be exchanged.

I

In our hot summers, one of the ractical difficulties in nursing is the spoiling of articles of food prep he sick or for infants, and which must be kept at hand for use, especially during the night; it is also a desideratum to have ice at hand for cooling drinks, &c. A good contrivance for this purpose is made by I. S. Williams, of Philadelphia. It consists of a double can, the inside of galvanized iron, and the outside of tin, with an air-chamber between; near the bottom is a diaphragm, below which a piece of ice is placed, and a bowl or other utensil is arranged to set upon this, and to be conveniently lifted out by a wire handle. This answers a good purpose.

Change of Linen.

A frequent change of linen is a great comfort and benefit, in most cases. Let the bed linen be frequently changed (when suitable), and, in serious cases of fever, it may be useful to untuck the bottom of the bed and gently shake the upper clothes, so as to let the warm and impure air pass away. Let the sheets and blankets be of full size, that they may be *tucked thoroughly* under the mattress, or *whatever* is at the top. It is a comfort to the patient to have all straight and smooth under him, and nurses are recommended to attend to this more than once in a day.

Change of Room.

In some particular cases of long and depressing sickness, a change of room, conducted with great prudence, may be found a powerful auxiliary in the aid towards recovery.

Avoidance of Noises.

Much conversation is often injurious, and WHISPERING OFFENSIVE. Place a pan covered with sand underneath the fire, to receive the cinders, and have a second ready to make an exchange when taken up; also use a wooden poker. Let the number of the visitors in the room be chiefly confined to those whose services are effective, and let all wear shoes with list or cloth soles or slippers. The rustling of silk gowns may prove an annoyance to those who are in a very weak state, also the rattling of cups, stirring the fire, &c.

Sitting up.

Let the linen-horse be timely placed before the fire, with every article likely to be needed; and, if the clothes are to be put on and washing included, let the hot water and all be ready, so as to avoid the least bustle. Spread a blanket on the floor for the patient to walk over.

Neatness.

An increased delicacy of the stomach and sense of nicety, are the concomitants of disease, and, therefore, the nurse and all around should be particularly careful, not only as to the neatness of their own persons, but that every dose of medicine, and all food, be presented in the most tempting, clean, and delicate way. To promote this, it may be desirable, in long illnesses, to have at hand a variety of small vessels of different sizes.

Avoidance of Exciting Subjects.

Those only who have suffered from severe illness, can well judge of the importance of preserving a quiet mental atmosphere; *how little* those suffering with languor and pain are competent to sustain the pressure which a tale of woe may impose. The subjects of conversation should be much guarded, while a cheerful demeanor, and innocently lively manner, may help to assuage or lessen the sense of distress.

Protection from Light, and from the Blaze of Fire and Candle.

Diseases are so variable in their effects, that no minute plan is suggested for any particular case. However cheering the light of the sun in many instances, there are affections where a judicious nurse would be called upon to screen the invalid from the blaze of day. She should remember that, by a little arrangement of shutters and curtains, a room may still be made cheerful by a sort of subdued light; while in some distressing affections of the head, &c., from severe fever, the patient can hardly be too much indulged by the darkening of the room. In such a case, the blaze of the fire must greatly augment suffering. Screens ought to be at hand, as well for that as for the candle.

Important that the Nurse be taken care of.

Any nurse who is much engaged in night service, ought to be very carefully spared in the day. She must have rest, or she cannot long hold out. When sitting up at night, some strong coffee or tea, ready made, should be prepared, that it be warmed and taken without the least disturbance to the sick person. Some nurses make a great noise with the clattering of tea-things, which ought to be avoided.

Temperature.

On removing the patient into another room, this ought, if in the spring, autumn, or winter, and even in part of the summer, to be very carefully prepared with not only a good fire, but an attention to the doors and windows, that all be shut, and the temperature brought up to the state of the room about to be left. When at any time a patient's room be aired, the curtains should be drawn closely round the bed. Just raising the window for an inch or two will be useful, if it be for a short time; but, rather than run any risk to the invalid, throw on an additional blanket. It is most important to keep the air of the room in a fresh and wholesome state.

To prevent Pressure on any particular part.

Make circular cushions, in the form of a ring, of old linen and stuffed with bran. A patient, obliged by disease to lie continually on one side, will find great relief to the *ear* or prominent *bones* by these "ring cushions."

Leeches.

On taking off leeches, plunge them into *quite* warm beer; they will, in most cases, immediately disgorge themselves. Apply a succession of warm poultices made of bread and milk, or linseed meal. The linseed meal should be stirred *quickly* while *boiling* water is poured upon it.

Gentleness and Kindness.

All who surround the patient should be kind, and meek, and gentle, and patient; not a sound of harshness, or evidence of discord should reach his ear. Any discussion of the nearest relatives or friends, as to whether *this* or *that* be best, should be avoided in his presence. Some persons, with the greatest desire to do right, do *too much*, and, without intending it, interrupt a sufferer by unimportant questions and inquiries, and by moving about the room, when they would often do a much greater service by sitting quietly beside the bed, attending to requests emanating from the patient, whose feelings and preferences should always be consulted and accorded with, if not in any way interfering either with medical directions, or being in themselves palpably improper and injurious. There is, perhaps, scarcely any situation in which the call is greater upon the Christian virtues than in a sick chamber, for it very often happens that disease makes a great impression upon the nervous system, and pain and suffering disturb the accustomed placidity of the invalid; who, with every desire to bend patiently under the affliction, may now and then seem scarcely able to appreciate the kindest efforts to minister to his need.

To avoid Unseasonable Interruption.

Particularly guard the sufferer who has just fallen asleep. The person having the chief responsibility should be instructed to pass the feathery end of a quill through the keyhole, whenever sleep or any other cause renders interruption unsuitable; and this sign should be strictly regarded. It is far better than risking disturbance to the patient by trying a locked door. Tie the quill to the handle of the door, that it be not lost.

A Dying-bed.

Let no one annoy the patient by sitting on the bed, or indulging in earnest expressions of surprise or grief. All around ought to be still; no calling out "Oh, he's dying," &c.

It should be carefully ascertained that the body be placed in the easiest posture. The bed-curtains should be, in most cases, gently undrawn, and the least possible interruption given to the admission of fresh air. All but those who are fanning the patient, or perhaps moistening the parched mouth, or otherwise promoting his comfort, should be careful to keep at a distance from the bed, and be quietly seated. It is believed that few can tell the suffering often inflicted on the dying by the thoughtless bustle of attendants and *even friends*. The speaking in a loud tone, the setting down of even a glass or phial, may often cause distress. No sound should disturb, beyond an occasional and necessary whisper, the solemn period of dissolution.

PREPARATIONS USED AS ARTICLES OF DIET FOR THE SICK AND CONVALESCENT.

Arrowroot Pap.

Take of arrowroot one large tablespoonful; water, one pint. First mix the arrowroot well into a paste with a little of the cold water; bring the remainder of the water to a boiling heat; then stir in the arrowroot; let it boil a few minutes; sweeten it with loaf sugar.

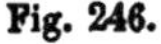
Fig. 246.

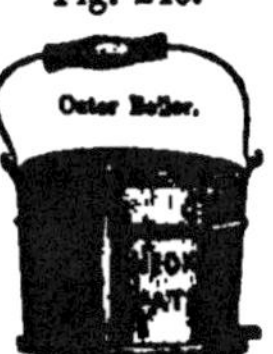

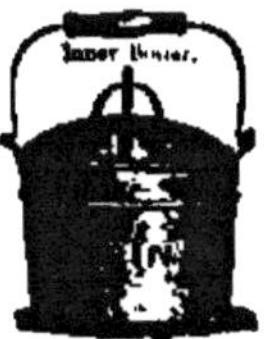

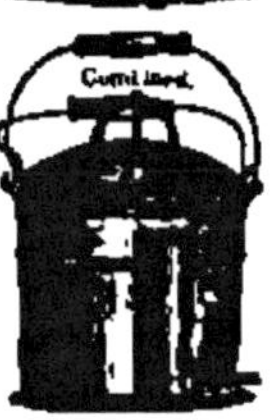

The preparation of arrowroot pap with milk renders it richer and more nutritious, though sometimes not allowable.

The application of direct heat to preparations of this description, always involves the danger of scorching them, and the intervention of a water bath is found to prevent the accident. The apparatus here figured is made for the purpose, and is a useful utensil in any family. The drawing explains itself.

Arrowroot Pap, with Milk.

Put in a saucepan, to boil, one pint of milk; stir very smoothly, into a cup of cold milk, a dessertspoonful of arrowroot; when the milk boils, stir in the arrowroot; continue to stir until it is cooked, which will be in five or ten minutes; then remove it from the fire, and sweeten to the taste.

Toast Water.

Cut a slice of stale bread half an inch thick, a finger length long; cut off the crust, and toast it quite brown, but not scorched; while hot, put it into a half pint pitcher; pour over half a pint of boiling water; cover it tightly, and when cool pour it off and strain.

Mulled Wine.

Put cinnamon or allspice (to the taste) into a cup of hot water to steep; add three eggs, well beaten, with sugar; heat to a boil a pint of wine; then put in the spice and eggs, while boiling, and stir them until done, which will be in three minutes.

Jelly for Invalids.

Cut a penny roll into thin slices; toast them to a light brown; then boil gently in a quart of water until it jellies; strain it upon a few shavings of lemon-peel; sweeten, and add, if liked, a little wine and nutmeg.

Eggnog.

Take the yelks of eight eggs; beat them with six large spoonfuls of pul-

grate ... sugar; when this is a cream, add the third part of a nutmeg; to this stir one tumblerful of good brandy, and one wineglass of good ... wine; mix them well together; have ready the whites of the eggs, beat to a stiff froth, and beat them into the mixture; when all are well mixed, add three pints of rich milk.

Panada.

Cut two slices of stale bread half an inch in thickness; cut off the crust; toast them a nice brown; cut them into squares of two inches in size; lay them in a bowl, sprinkle a little salt over them, and pour on a pint of boiling water; grate a little nutmeg.

Tapioca.

Soak two tablespoonfuls of very clean tapioca in two teacups of cold water over night; in the morning, add a little salt, one pint of milk, or water if milk cannot be taken; si ... quite soft; stir well while cooling; when done, pour into a bow... all ...ved, add sugar, a spoonful of wine, and a little nutmeg.

Rice Jelly.

Take of rice, one-quarter of a pound white sugar, half a pound; water, one quart. Boil these well together, carefully stirring them till the whole becomes a glutinous mass. Strain off into a dish or form. When cool, it is fit for use. This preparation may be flavored with rose-water, orange-flower water, or lemon-juice, as may best suit t[he] palate of the patient, or as directed by the physician.

... Jelly.

Take of Iceland moss, two ... water, one quart. First wash the moss in some cold water; ... the quart of water, and boil slowly till very thick, adding wh... ... [suf]ficiently sweet, then strain through a cloth. When cold, it will be fit for use, and may be eaten with spices, if allowed. Irish moss jelly may be prepared in the same way.

Sago Jelly.

Take four tablespoonfuls of sago, one quart of water, juice and rind of one lemon; sweeten to the taste. Mix all the ingredients well together; let it stand for half an hour; then put it on to boil, till the particles are entirely dissolved; it should be constantly stirred. It is very much improved by the addition of wine.

Calves' Feet Jelly.

Boil two calves' feet in one gallon of water, down to a quart; then strain it, and, when cold, skim off all the fat; take up all the clear jelly. Put the jelly into a saucepan, with a pint of wine, half a pound of loaf sugar, the juice of four lemons, the white of six or eight eggs beaten into a froth. Mix all well together. Set the saucepan upon a clear fire, and stir the jelly till it boils. When it has boiled ten minutes, pour it through a flannel bag till it runs clear.

Essence of Beef.

This is prepared from lean meat, by cutting it into small pieces, adding a little salt, then introducing into a wide-mouth bottle, corked tightly, and heating it gradually by immersing in a kettle of water, to which heat is applied till it boils. After a few hours digesting in this way, the juice is drawn off, and constitutes the most concentrated form of nourishment.

Beef Tea.

Take of lean beef one-quarter of a pound, a pint and a half of water, salt sufficient to season it. When it begins to boil, skim it five minutes; then add two blades of mace; continue the boiling ten minutes longer, when it will be ready for use.

Chicken Broth.

Clean half a chicken; on it pour one quart of cold water, and a little salt; put in a spoonful of rice; boil two hours very slowly, and tightly covered; skim it well; just before using it, put in a little chopped parsley.

Chicken Jelly.

Cut up a chicken; put it into a stone jar; break all the bones; cover very closely; set the jar into boiling water; keep it boiling three hours and a half; strain off the liquor; season with salt and a very little mace.

Rice Jelly.

Boil a quarter of a pound of the best rice flour, with half a pound of loaf sugar, in a quart of water, until the whole becomes one glutinous mass; strain off the jelly, and let it stand to cool. This is nutritious and light.

Slippery Elm Bark Jelly.

Four large spoonfuls of the bark, chipped; pour on it one quart of cold water; let it stand all night; stir it, and let it settle; the next morning pour off the water; slice the rind of a lemon very thinly, and, with the juice, put it in the water strained; let it simmer, very gently, fifteen minutes; then sweeten, and pour in a mould to cool and harden; take out the rind before putting in the mould.

Wine Whey.

Boil a pint of new milk; add to it a glass or two of white wine; put it on the fire until it just boils again; then set it aside till the curd settles; pour off the clean whey; sweeten to the taste; cider is as good as wine to curdle, if it is good country cider.

Corn Meal, or Oatmeal Gruel.

Put in a clean saucepan one pint of water to boil; when boiling, mix of oatmeal two large spoonfuls, in a half pint of milk, and a little salt; stir this into the boiling water; stir it well; let it simmer thirty minutes; then strain it through a hair-sieve; if the patient can bear it, a large spoonful of the best brandy stirred in after it is strained and sweetened, and a little grated nutmeg; if corn meal is used, stir the dry corn meal into the boiling water; two large spoonfuls to a pint of boiling water, and a half new milk; season as the other.

Vegetable Soup.

Take two white potatoes, one onion, a piece of well-baked bread. Put these into a clean stewpan, in one quart of water; boil them down to a pint; throw into the vessel some parsley or celery; cover the vessel closely; remove it from the fire, and allow the herbs to steep, while the liquor is cooling, under cover; season to the taste.

Castillon's Powders.

Take of Powdered tragacanth,
Powdered sago,
Powdered salep,
Sugar, each, one ounce;
Prepared oyster-shell, two drachms.
Mix them thoroughly, and fold into papers containing each one drachm.

Directions.—Mix a powder with four tablespoonfuls of cold milk in a bowl. Then transfer it to a milk-pan, and, while stirring, pour upon it gradually one pint of boiling milk, and boil for a quarter of an hour. Sugar may be added, to the taste.

PHYSICIANS' OUTFITS.

Catalogue of One Hundred and Twenty-five Medicines and Pharmaceutical Preparations which can be put up in the best ground glass stoppered bottles, and substantial white-ware jars, uniformly and correctly labelled, and furnished ready packed for transportation for SEVENTY-FIVE DOLLARS, *(exclusive of implements and apparatus).*

1 ℔ Acacia.
½ ℔ " pulvis.
1 pint Alcohol.
½ pint Acidum aceticum.
1 oz. " benzoicum.
4 oz. " citricum.
1 oz. " hydrocyanicum dil.
4 oz. " muriaticum.
4 oz. " nitricum.
½ pint " sulphuric aromat.
1 oz. " tannicum.
4 oz. Aloes pulvis (Soc.).
8 oz Alumen.
4 oz. Ammoniæ carbonas.
1 pint " liquor.
4 oz. " murias.
½ pint " spiritus arom.
4 oz. Antim. et potass. tartras.
½ oz. Argenti nitras cryst.
½ oz. " " fusum.
4 oz. Assafœtida.
1 oz. Bismuthi subnitras.
8 oz. Camphora.
2 oz. Cardamomum.
6 oz. Creta præparata.
4 oz. Calc. carb. præcip.
6 oz. Chloroformum.
8 oz. Cinchona rub. pulv.
1 oz. Cinchoniæ sulphas.
1 oz. Creasotum.
8 oz. Ceratum cantharides.
8 oz. " resinæ.
8 oz. " simplex.
½ pint Copaiba,
1 ℔ Cubebæ pulv.
2 oz. Collodium.
1 oz. " cantharidal.
4 oz. Ergota (whole or in powder).
1 ℔ Æther (letheon).
1 oz. Extractum aconiti.
1 oz. " belladonnæ.
1 oz. " conii.
1 oz. " hyoscyami.
2 oz. " coloc. comp. pulv.
2 oz. " jalapæ pulv.
1 oz. " nucis vomicæ.
1 oz. " quassiæ.
8 oz. " taraxaci.
1 ℔ " sennæ fluidum.
1 ℔ " spigeliæ et sennæ fluidum.
½ pint " valerianæ fluidum.
4 oz. Ferri carb. massa (Vallette).
8 oz. " subcarb.
1 oz. " citras.
1 oz. " pulvis.
½ pint " sesqui sulph. solut. (with directions for preparing hydrated peroxide when required.)
8 oz. Fœniculum.
1 oz. Gambogiæ pulv.
1 ℔ Gentiana contus.
4 oz. Glycyrrhiza ext. pulv.
4 oz. " rad. pulv.
2 oz. Glycerin.
½ ℔ Hydrarg. massa.
½ ℔ " chlor. mit.
1 oz. " cum. creta.
2 oz. " oxid. rub.
½ oz. " prot. iodid.
1 oz. Iodinium.
4 oz. Ipecacuanhæ pulvis.
4 oz. Jalapæ pulvis.
8 oz. Juniperus.
2 oz. Kino.
4 oz. Liquor iodinii comp.

4 oz. Liquor ferri iodid.
½ pint " hydrarg. et arsen. iodid.
½ pint " potassæ arsenitis.
1 ℔ bot. Magnesia.
½ ℔ Magnesia carb.
5 ℔ " sulphas.
6 oz. Manna.
⅛ oz. Morphiæ sulphas.
⅛ oz. " acetas.
⅛ oz. " murias.
4 oz. Myrrha.
1 oz. Oleum anisi.
1 oz. " cinnamomi
1 oz. " limonis.
1 oz. " menthæ pip.
1 bot. " olivæ.
1 pint " ricini.
1 pint " terebinthinæ.
1 oz. " tiglii.
2 oz. Opii pulvis.
8 oz. Plumbi acetas.
2 oz. " carbonas.
2 oz. Potassa (caustic).
4 oz. " bicarbonas.
¾ ℔ " bitartras.
4 oz. " citras.
4 oz. " nitras.
8 oz. " sulphas.
2 oz. Potassii iodidum.
3 oz. Pulvis ipecac. et opii.
8 oz. Quassia.
1 oz. Quiniæ sulphas.
6 oz. Rheum (E. Ind.).
4 oz. Rhei pulvis.
4 oz. Sapo (Castil.).
9 oz. Sarsaparilla.
2 oz. Scilla pulv.
8 oz. Senna (Alex.).
8 oz. Senega.
8 oz. Serpentaria.
℔iss Sodæ bicarbonas.
4 oz. " boras pulv.
8 oz. " et potass. tart.
4 oz. " phosphas.
8 oz. Spigelia.
⅛ oz. Strychnia.
4 oz. Sulphur præcip.
¾ ℔ " sublim.
½ pint Spt. ammon. arom.
½ pint " ætheris comp.
1 pint " " nitrici.
½ pint " lavand. comp.
½ pint Syrupus ipecacuanhæ.
1 pint " pruni virg.
1 pint " rhei aromat.
1 pint " scillæ.
½ pint " senegæ.
4 oz. Tinctura aconiti rad.
1 pint " cinchonæ C.
½ pint " digitalis.
½ pint " ferri chloridi.
1 pint " opii.
1 pint " " camph.
1 pint " zingiberis.
½ ℔ Unguentum hydrargyri.
½ ℔ " " nitratis.
½ ℔ " simplex.
½ ℔ Uva ursi.
½ ℔ Valeriana.
1 pint Vinum antimonii.
½ pint " ergotæ.
½ pint " colchici rad.
⅛ oz. Veratria.
4 oz. Zinci oxidum P.
8 oz. " sulphas.

The necessary implements can be purchased for twenty-five dollars, making, with the foregoing, an aggregate expense of *one hundred dollars.*

The following list embraces the number and character of the bottles used in this collection:—

12 Oij SM. Bottles or tin cans.
11 Oj " "
13 Oj Tr. Bottles.
15 Oss SM. Bottles.
18 ℥iv SM. Bottles.
24 f℥j and f℥ij SM. and Tr. Bottles.
12 Covered Jars.
6 Packing Bottles.

A case made to contain the above collection should be five feet high, exclusive of cornice, and four feet wide. It should contain shelves arranged as follows:—

1. For ointment, and extract jars and implements.
2. " (narrow) two dozen 2oz. and 1oz. ground stoppered bottles.
3. " 12 quart salt-mouth bottles.
4. " 13 pint " "
5. " 13 pint tincture bottles.
6. " 15 half-pint salt-mouth bottles.
7. " 15 " tincture bottles.
8. " 18 4oz. tincture and salt-mouth bottles.

An under case and several drawers might be appropriated to additional apparatus and implements.

FIFTY DOLLAR OUTFIT.

The following list of One Hundred Medicines and Preparations can be put up in substantial Ground Stoppered Bottles, neatly and uniformly labelled, so as to form a convenient and compact Cabinet of Materia Medica, for Forty-Three Dollars, and with the Apparatus and Implements attached for Fifty Dollars.

8 oz. Acacia.
½ pint Acidum aceticum.
8 oz. " citricum.
2 oz. " muriaticum.
3 oz. " nitricum.
½ pint " sulph. arom.
1 oz. " tannicum.
2 pints Alcohol.
4 oz. Alumen.
4 oz. Ammoniæ carbonas.
4 oz. " murias.
1 pint " liquor.
½ pint " spiritus arom.
1 oz. Antim et potass. tart.
¼ oz. Argenti nitras cryst. }
½ oz. " " fus. }
4 oz. Assafœtida.
8 oz. Camphora.
2 oz. Cardamomum.
4 oz. Ceratum cantharidis.
3 oz. Chloroformum.
2 oz. Collodium.
½ pint Copaiba.
1 oz. Creasotum.
6 oz. Creta præparata, or }
4 oz. Calcis carb. præcip. }
4 oz. Cupri sulphas.
2 oz. Ergota (whole or powdered).
½ pint Æther (Letheon).
1 oz. Extractum aconitii.
1 oz. " belladonnæ "
1 oz. " colocynth. comp. pulv.
1 oz. " conii
2 oz. " gentianæ
1 oz. " hyoscyami
1 oz. " jalapæ pulv.
8 oz. " valerianæ fl'd.
8 oz. Ferri subcarbonas.
1 oz. " pulvis (per hydrogen).
½ pint " chloridi tinct.
4 oz. Fœniculum.
8 oz. Gentiana contus.
4 oz. Hydrarg. massa.
6 oz. " chlorid mit.
2 oz. " oxid. Rub.
2 oz. " cum. creta.
1 oz. Iodinium.
½ pint Liquor hydrarg. et arsen. iod.
½ pint " potassæ arsenitis.
8 oz. Magnesia.
3 lb " sulphas.
⅛ oz. Morphiæ sulphas.
2 oz. Myrrha.
½ oz. Oleum cinnamomi.
½ oz. " limonis.
½ oz. " menthæ pip.
1 pint " ricini.
1 pint " terebinthinæ.
½ oz. " tiglii.
6 oz. Plumbi acetas.
3 oz. Potassæ bicarb.
12 oz. " bitartras.
3 oz. " citras.
6 oz. " nitras.
2 oz. Potassii iodidum.
6 oz. Pulvis acaciæ.
3 oz. " aloes, Soc.
1 oz. " digitalis.
4 oz. " ext. glycyrrhizæ.
1 oz. " gambogiæ.
1 oz. " ipecacuanhæ.
3 oz. " " et opii.
4 oz. " jalapæ.
1 oz. " opii.
4 oz. " rhei (E. Ind.).
2 oz. " scillæ.
6 oz. " sodæ boras.
8 oz. Quassia.
1 oz. Quiniæ sulphas.
4 oz. Rheum.
6 oz. Sapo (castil. alb.).
6 oz. Sarsaparilla.
4 oz. Senega.
4 oz. Serpentaria.
1 lb Sodæ bicarb.
4 oz. Spigelia.
8 oz. Sulphur sublim.
1 pint Spiritus ætheris nit.
½ pint " " comp.
1 pint " lavand. comp.
½ pint Syrupus ipecacuanhæ.
½ pint " scillæ.
½ pint " rhei arom.
1 pint Tinctura cinchonæ comp.
1 pint " opii.
1 pint " " camph.
4 oz. Unguentum hydrarg. (½ mercury).
4 oz. " " nitratis.
4 oz. Uva ursi.
½ pint Vin. colchici rad.
2 oz. Zinci oxidum.
6 oz. " sulphas.
4 oz. Zingiberis.

IMPLEMENTS.

Scales and weights.		½ doz. ℥viij.	1 Funnel.
℥iv. Grad. Meas.		½ doz. ℥vj.	1 qr. Wrap'g & filtering paper.
1 Mortar and pestle.	½ gross vials.	1 doz. ℥iv.	1 gr. Vial corks.
1 Pill tile.	German flint.	1½ doz. ℥ij.	2 papers pill boxes.
2 Spatulas.		1½ doz. ℥j.	2 yds. Adhesive plaster in tin case.
		1 doz. ℥ss.	

The Medicines contained in the Fifty Dollar Outfit are differently arranged as follows:—

12 pint Salts and Tinctures.

Oj Liquor ammoniæ.	Oj Tinct. opii.	8 oz. Camphora.
Oj. Spt. æther. nit.	8 oz. Acacia.	3 oz. Magnesia.
8 oz. Sulphur sublim.	Oj Tinct. opii camph.	12 oz. Pot. bitart.
Oj. Spt. Lavand. comp.	Oj " cinchonæ comp.	℔j Sodæ bicarb.

14 eight oz. Tinct. Bottles.

½ pint. Acidum aceticum.	½ pint Syrup. ipecac.	½ pint Tinct. ferri chlor.
½ pint Acid. sulph. arom.	½ pint Copaiba.	½ pint Syrupus rhei arom.
½ pint Fowler's solution.	½ pint Vin. colchici.	½ pint Donovan's solution.
½ pint Æther.	½ pint Syrup. scillæ.	½ pint Ext. valerian. fluid.
½ pint Spt. ammon. arom.	½ pint Spt. æther. comp.	

14 eight oz. Salt-mouth Bottles.

6 oz. Pulv. acacia.	6 oz. Potass. nit.	4 oz. Assafœtida.
4 oz. Pul. ext. glycyrrhizæ.	6 oz. Pulv. sodæ boras.	4 oz. Ammon. murias.
6 oz. Plumbi acet.	6 oz. Zinci sulph.	6 oz. Creta præparata.
4 oz. Jalapæ pulv.	4 oz. Alumen.	8 oz. Ferri subcarb.
4 oz. Pulv. rhei.	4 oz. Ammon. carb.	

17 four oz. Salt-mouth and Tinct. Bottles.

3 oz. Acid citricum.	2 oz. Zinci oxidum.	3 oz. Potass. citras.
1 oz. " tannicum.	2 oz. Acid. muriat.	2 oz. " iodid.
1 oz. Quiniæ sulph.	6 oz. Hydr. chlor. mit.	3 oz. Pulv. aloes, Soc.
3 oz. Chloroform.	2 oz. Myrrha.	3 oz. " ipecac. et opii.
4 oz. Cupri sulph.	3 oz. Acid. nitric.	3 oz. " scillæ.
2 oz. Ergot.	3 oz. Potassæ bicarb.	

20 two oz. Salt-mouth and Tinct. Bottles.

1 oz. Antim. et pot. tart.	1 oz. Creasotum.	1 oz. Pulv. digitalis.
¼ et ½ Argent. nit. (cr's f'd).	2 oz. Hydr. ox. rub.	½ oz. Ol. limon.
1 oz. Ext. colocynth. comp.	2 oz. " cum creta.	1 oz. Pulv. gambogia.
½ oz. Ol. tiglii.	½ oz. Ol. cinnamomi.	1 oz. " ipecac.
1 oz. Ext. jalapæ.	1 oz. Iodinium.	2 oz. Collodium.
1 oz. Ferri pulvis.	⅛ oz. Morphiæ sulph.	½ oz. Ol. menth. pip.

EXTRACTS AND OINTMENTS, ETC.

4 oz. Cerat. Canth.	4 oz. Pil. hydrarg.	1 oz. Ext. conii.
4 oz. Ung. hydrag.	1 oz. Ext. aconit.	2 oz. " gentianæ.
4 oz. " " nit.	1 oz. " belladonna.	1 oz. " hyoscyami.

44

PACKAGES, ETC.

Oj Alcohol, Oj Ol. ricini, Oj Ol. terebinth. } in pint packers.	4 oz. Zingiber.	4 oz. Serpentaria.
6 oz. Sarsaparilla.	3 oz. Fœniculum.	4 oz. Uva ursi.
4 oz. Senega.	2 ℔ Mag. sulph.	2 oz. Cardamom.
4 oz. Spigelia.	4 oz. Rheum.	8 oz. Gentiana contus.
	8 oz. Quassia.	4 oz. Cinchona.
	6 oz. Sapo.	

This collection will conveniently fill a case three feet six inches wide and four feet high, containing six shelves, and two or more drawers to contain packages, &c.

Advice to the Young Physician on the Commencement of Practice, to accompany the Fifty Dollar Outfit.

After opening your box of medicines, &c., the bottles are to be carefully wiped, and the paper or kid tied over the stoppers removed, place them on the shelves thus:—

1st, pints; 2d, half pint salt mouths; 3d, half pint tinctures; 4th, ℥iv salt mouths. The 2 ounce bottles should be placed below the pints, on a small and narrow shelf, so as to be more readily seen and more conveniently reached than on the top.

The shelves should be long enough to admit of one or two additional bottles on each.

About three feet from the floor, and next below the smallest bottles, should be a wider shelf, at least two feet wide, with a slide drawing out from it, if there is no separate counter. This is to manipulate upon: here are kept the ointment jars, and the implements generally. If there are drawers below, it would be well to keep the vials in one, the corks in another, the pill boxes in a third, and then the paper packages separately or together in drawers.

The serpentaria, valerian, fennel, and cardamom, are best put in tin cans, or separate drawers from the others.

The quire of wrapping paper should be cut into appropriate sized pieces, 6 in. square, for ℥j, 8 by 10 in. for ℥iv packages, and 3 by 4 in. of this or a better quality of glazed writing paper, for folding up smaller packages. (See *Dispensing Powders.*)

The ℥iv and ℥j papers thus cut, may be put in a drawer, or strung upon a string passed through one corner, and hung by a tack, at a convenient point easy of access.

The next thing is to procure two or more towels, and a place to keep them—out of sight, but not out of mind.

If you carry medicines in a pocket case, saddle-bags, or medicine chest, you should fix a time, at regular intervals, to replenish the bottles, and to put up in the small-sized papers single doses of Dover's powder, calomel, tartar emetic, &c., which may be carried in the pocket of your pocket case, or the tray of your saddle-bags.

It is well to put up occasionally and label, single doses of Dover's powder, calomel, alone or in its various combinations, or any favorite remedies in suitable forms for use.

By having combinations of this kind, found to be, by experience, the most useful, in the class of cases met with in the neighborhood, already put up, during moments of leisure, it will facilitate the business of prescribing: at the same time care should be taken not to get into a routine method of prescribing.

When at leisure, it will be well to prepare from the ingredients in the outfit, which will be found all in a suitable condition (the extracts being dried and powdered), 180 *compound cathartic pills*. These may be put up in little paper pill boxes, containing four, and labelled with one of the blank labels, stating the dose at *three*; when dispensed, tell the patient to take the additional one in six hours, if three do not operate.

Pills of opium may be made by the *Pharmacopœia* process, say 24 to begin with; part of these may be made without the soap, and put away in a little box for a year or two, to become old, for use in dysentery.

Pills of quinine may be made by either of the processes given in this work of such size as may best suit your views, in relation to the dose; 5 grain pills are the largest that can be conveniently taken.

A good laxative pill will be desired in many instances, particularly in dyspeptic cases, accompanied by costiveness. Chapman's dinner pill will be found very useful; two pills being taken immediately before or after dinner, will pass through the alimentary canal with the food, and operate the next morning.

For prescribing iron, one may choose between subcarbonate, which is well adapted to children, and may be given alone or mixed with sugar (DOSE, 5 to 10 grains), tincture of chloride of iron, which is usually given in 10 to 20 drop doses, and ferri pulvis, which may be most conveniently given in pill combined with one of the extracts, as extract of gentian for a pure tonic, or extract of conium as a sedative, alterative, and tonic, or extract of aconite or belladonnæ, as a narcotic and tonic; where there is a disposition to indigestion, subcarbonate would suit best.

Of vegetable tonics there are extract of gentian, compound tincture of cinchona, sulphate of quinia, gentian root, serpentaria, quassia, cimicifuga, used in chorea, uva ursi, used in affections of the urinary organs as both tonic and astringent; also chimaphila not unlike the last in medical properties, and believed to be a good alterative to combine with sarsaparilla in skin diseases. I have also added cinchona bark; bruise this in the iron mortar and place ℥j in the funnel, supporting it by a little plugget of carded cotton; then add a few ounces of water, and f℥j of elixir of vitriol; after it has passed, return it till it comes through clear, and add the remainder of the water to make Oj infus. cinchonæ, U. S. P.

Astringents are perhaps most used in the treatment of bowel complaints, particularly among children; sometimes they are combined with mercurials, as for instance blue mass, thus:—

℞.—Pil. hydrargyri,
Acid. tannici, āā . . . . gr. xij.
Ol. cinnamomi . . . . gtt. j.

M. ft. pil. xij.

Perhaps opium is most employed in these cases, as in the very common prescription.

℞.—Hydrarg. chlor. mit.,
Pulv. opii, āā . . . . . gr. xij.
Plumbi acetas . . . . . gr. xxiv.

M. ft. pil. xxiv.

Sulphate of copper, nitrate of silver, sulphate of zinc, and acetate of lead, are the most common remedies of this class for external use, as in eye-waters, gonorrhœa injections, and gargles for sore throat; they are found efficient in quite dilute solutions, as for instance, from two grains to ten grains, to f℥j of water. Gargles are improved by the addition of honey.

Cathartics.—Beside magnesia and its sulphate, and the well known castor oil, you have choice of either comp. cathartic pills, before mentioned, blue mass in 5 to 10 grain doses for adults, 2 to 5 for children. In giving blue mass to children it is very convenient to have it in the liquid form. Try the following:—

℞.—Pil. hydrarg. . . . . . . gr. iv.
Sacchari . . . . . . ℈j.
Syr. rhei arom. . . . . . f℥j.

Triturate the blue mass and sugar into a powder, and this with the syrup.

There are generally about 8 teaspoonfuls in an ounce, hence a teaspoonful dose would contain ½ grain. Hydrarg. cum creta is best given in powders with a little sugar, sometimes with powd. opium or Dover's powder.

Powd. rhubarb is generally given with calomel as a sort of corrective, acting on the bowels as a tonic, and by its after effects as rather an astringent. Powd. jalap or gamboge is combined with calomel for a different purpose, the latter being very drastic. Croton oil, if ever used internally, should be diluted largely with castor oil, or mucilage, or made into pill with crumb of bread.

Senna is usually given thus:—

℞.—Sennæ . . . . ℥ss.
Mannæ . . . . ʒij.
Fœniculi . . . . . . ʒj.

M. *Sig.*—Make an infusion and give at one dose.

Sometimes ʒij or ℥ss of Epsom salts, or of bitartrate of potassa, may be added.

Sometimes a half pint of the infusion is directed (a pint to be simmered down to Oss). Dose, a wineglassful every three hours till it operates.

Of Narcotics.—Opium, of course, is the chief; it is contained in the outfit in the following forms: Powder (in ℥ij salt mouth) tincture, camphorated tincture, sulphate of morphia, and in combination with ipecac in Dover's powder.

Powdered opium is used in pills and powders, in all sorts of combinations, it is the best for use in either of these forms, the quantity though small will last a long time. Laudanum is of great utility internally and externally, alone and in combination; it is incompatible with alkalies, including ammonia; these throw down the morphia as a precipitate. Paregoric is the best form for use in expectorant mixtures, and in diarrhœa remedies, sulphate of morphia is generally prescribed in solution (see liq. morph. sulph., U. S. P.). Sometimes 8 grs. are dissolved in f℥j water, to make a solution of the strength of laudanum or rather stronger. Dose, 10 to 20 drops. If this is made, it should be colored and carefully distinguished from the officinal solution; it is convenient to carry in pocket case or saddle-bags.

Dover's powder put up in 5 gr. and 10 gr. papers will be found extremely convenient and very useful.

Extracts of conium, belladonna, and aconite, will frequently be preferable to opium. These as made by Tildens may be relied on; average dose of each about ½ grain to begin with, increased to 1 gr.

Camphor may be given in pill, combined with other medicines. It is made by incorporating an extract or a little crumb of bread with the camphor first powdered by adding a few drops of alcohol and triturating.

Aqua camphoræ, U. S. P., is a good form for giving it, also, Parrish's camphor mixture.

℞.—Aq. camphoræ . . . . . f℥iij.
Spt. lav. comp. . . . . . f℥j.
Sacchari . . . . . . ʒj.—M.

Dose, a tablespoonful occasionally in diarrhœa, 20 drops of laudanum added when there is pain. For external use, and sometimes internally, in small doses, say 5 to 10 drops on sugar use, the following

℞.—Camphor . . ʒj.		or	℞.—Camphor . ʒij.
Chloroform . . f℥j.			Chloroform . f℥j.
Make solution.			Make solution.

Assafœtida is very useful in diseases of children in the form of mist. assafœtidæ. (See also pil. assafœtidæ and pil. aloes et assafœtidæ.)

Comp. spt. of ether will mix with aqueous or alcoholic solutions, and is frequently added to them; the ether in the outfit is for use in inhalation, or as a cooling external application.

Digitalis is a most powerful nervous sedative; the tincture is put up in the outfit under the impression that it is the most eligible preparation; it keeps well. Use it cautiously.

Of Antacids.—Make choice between bicarbonate of potassa, the most powerful, bicarb. soda the most agreeable, and aromatic spirit of ammonia, the most gratefully stimulant. The two latter are much prescribed together in cases of flatulence and of sick headaches from indigestion. They are given in solution, quite dilute, and are said to act like a charm. Magnesia is much employed to meet similar indications and especially when a laxative is required. Prepared chalk is adapted to similar cases, conjoined with a tendency to diarrhœa (see ℞. for mist. cretæ, U. S. P.) Instead of cinnamon water in this preparation, oil of cinnamon may be dropped into the solid ingredients in the mortar in the proportion of 2 drops for each f℥j of cinnamon water.

If copaiba should be called for, the following recipe will be found a good one:—

℞.—Copaibæ . . . . . . ℥j.

Measure this in the graduate, then make a mucilage as follows:—

Pulv. acaciæ,
Sacchari, āā . . . . . . ʒiij.
Aquæ . . . . ℥j.

Add the copaiba, and triturate until a milky thick compound is produced, dilute this with additional water, and add whatever other ingredients may be desired, as for instance, oil of cubebs, oil of cinnamon, comp. spt. lavender, spt. nitric ether, or laudanum. This being brought to the measure of f℥viij and put up in a vial, is labelled. Dose, a tablespoonful three times a day, and charged at not less than 50 cents.

Finally, it remains to speak of *fever mixtures*, used chiefly for their effect on the skin as diaphoretics.

The formulæ are much used in which citrate of potassa is the base; these are given in considerable detail in this work.

A grain of tartar emetic adds to the effect of a 4 ounce vial of neutral mixture, when it would not sicken too much. Spt. nitric ether is often added, but gives this otherwise pleasant mixture an ethereal taste. Morphia is not incompatible with it. Wine of colchicum, added, adapts it to cases with a gouty tendency.

Of ointments and cerates little need be said. Ung. hydrargyri is very useful in its way. Ung. hydrarg. nit. will often require diluting with lard; for tetter or ringworms, it is an admirable mild caustic application; the spatula should not be put into it if it can be avoided.

Blistering cerate will be much in demand. Blisters may be spread upon strong glazed paper with very narrow margin. I often use my thumb in spreading them, which softens the cerate so as to [illegible] uniformly on the surface. Adhesive plaster cloth [illegible] spreading blisters on; by leaving a wide margin [illegible] may be made to adhere to the part without any extra [illegible] Blisters to go behind the ears should have a wide [illegible] only. The drawing in the chapter on plasters is rather [illegible]

Finally, prepare ung. hydrarg. oxid. rub., taking the [illegible] der the oxide into a very fine orange-colored powder) [illegible] lard, for inflamed eyelids, &c.

TWENTY-FIVE DOLLAR OUTFIT.

The following Sixty-One articles can be put up in handsome [illegible] pered Bottles, and Queensware Jars, neatly labelled, [illegible] portation, for Twenty Dollars, and the list of Implements [illegible] Dollars.

2 oz. Acidum citricum.
4 oz. " sulph. arom.
8 oz. Alcohol.
½ oz. Argenti nitras.
2 oz. Camphora.
4 oz. Ceratum cantharidis.
3 oz. Chloroformum.
2 oz. Collodium.
4 oz. Copaiba.
3 oz. Creta præparata, or
2 oz. Calcis carb. præcip.
3 oz. Cupri sulph.
8 oz. Æther (Letheon).
1 oz. Extract. aconiti.
1 oz. " belladonnæ.
1 oz. " coloc. c. pulv.
1 oz. " gentianæ.
1 oz. " hyoscyami.
1 oz. " jalapæ pulv.
8 oz. " sennæ fl'd.
8 oz. " valerianæ fl'd.
3 oz. Ferri subcarb.
1 oz. " pulvis.
8 oz. " chlor. tinct.
4 oz. Hydrarg. massa.
3 oz. " chlorid. mit.
1 oz. " oxid. rub.
8 oz. Liquor ammoniæ.
4 oz. " iodinii comp.
4 oz. " hydr. et arsen. iod.
8 oz. " potassæ arsenitis.
½ oz. Morphiæ sulph.
2 oz. Myrrha.
½ oz. Oleum limonis.
½ oz. " cinnamomi.
½ oz. Pil. cathart. comp.
3 oz. Plumbi acetas.
2 oz. Potassæ bicarb.
3 oz. " citras.
3 oz. Pulvis acaciæ.
3 oz. " aloes, Soc.
2 oz. " ext. glycyrrhizæ [illegible]
1 oz. " ipecacuanhæ.
2 oz. " " [illegible]
1 oz. " opii.
2 oz. " rhei.
½ oz. Quiniæ sulphas.
2 oz. Sapo, Castil. [illegible]
4 oz. Sodæ bicarb.
8 oz. Spt. æther. nit.
4 oz. " ammon. arom.
4 oz. " æther. comp.
8 oz. " lavand. comp.
4 oz. Syrup. ipecac.
8 oz. " rhei ar.
8 oz. " scillæ.
8 oz. Tinct. opii.
8 oz. " zingiberis.
4 oz. Ung. hydrarg. [illegible]
8 oz. Vin. antimon.
4 oz. Vin. colchici [illegible]
3 oz. Zinci sulph.

IMPLEMENTS.

Scales and weights.
4 oz. Grad. measure.
1 Mortar and pestle.
1 doz. 1 oz. Vials.
1 doz. ½ oz. "
½ doz. 2 oz. "
½ doz. 4 oz. Vials.
2 Spatulas.
2 papers Pill boxes.
½ gross Vial corks.
1 case Adhesive plaster.
1 Funnel. 1 [illegible]

This collection will conveniently fill a case twenty-[illegible] four feet high, having seven shelves, to be filled as follows:

1st with Ointment [illegible] and Implements.
2d " 7 8 oz. Tinct. Bottles.
3d " [illegible] "
4th " 9 4 oz. S.M. Bottles.
5th for 9 4 oz. S.M. [illegible]
6th " 9 4 oz. Tinct. [illegible]
7th " 11 2 oz. G.S. [illegible]

LIST OF PLANTS GROWING IN PHILADELPHIA CITY LIMITS,

AND THE

ADJACENT PARTS OF NEW JERSEY,

WITH THEIR HABITAT, TIME OF FLOWERING, PROPER TIME FOR COLLECTION, ETC.

[*The nomenclature is chiefly that of Gray, late edition; the months expressed in numerals.*]

Botanical name.	Common name.	Flowers.	Collect.	When.	Habitat and Remarks.
Achillea millefolium	Yarrow, milfoil	6—9	Herb	6—9	All fields.
Acorus calamus	Sweet flag	5—6	Rhizome	Late in autumn or early spring	Swamps.
Actea alba	Baneberry	5	Root		[illegible]. Rocky woods.
Adiantum pedatum	Maiden hair		Leaves		Beautiful fern. Moist woods.
Æsculus hippocastanum	Horsechestnut		Young bark	Spring	
Agrimonia Eupatoria	Agrimony	6, 7	Herb & root		Borders of woods.
Aletus farinosa	Stargrass		Root		Woods and hills.
Alisma plantago	Water plantain		Leaves		Swamps.
Ambrina anthelminticum	Wormseed	7, 8	Fruit	10	Said to grow in South Camden. Difficult to distinguish from A. ambrosioides; the odor stronger, which is retained when dried.
Ambrina ambrosioides		7, 8	Fruit	10	Odor same as preceding.
Ambrina botrys	Jerusalem oak	7, 8	Fruit	10	Odor dissipated in drying.
Anagallis arvensis	Scarlet pimpernel	6, 7			Fields.
Andromeda mariana	Stagger-bush	5			North of Camden; abundant.
Anemone nemorosa	Wind flower	4			Moist woodlands and clearings.
Anthemis arvensis	Wild chamomile	6 and after	Heads	6, 7	Cultivated grounds; sub. for A. nobilis.
Apocynum androsæmifolium	Dog's bane	6	Root	Autumn	Copses and fence rows; flowers delicate pink.
Apocynum cannabinum	Indian hemp	6	Root	Autumn	Copses and fence rows; flowers white.
Aquilegia Canadensis	Wild columbine	5, 6			Rocky woods, near streams.
Aralia nudicaulis	False sarsaparilla	6	Root	Autumn	Rocky woods.
Aralia racemosa	Wild spikenard	7			Rich woods and fence rows.
Archangelica atropurpurea	Purple angelica	5	Root and herb		Meadows; sub. for Angelica archangelica of Europe.
Arum triphyllum	Indian turnip	5	Dried cormus	8, 9	Damp woods and meadows.
Arctostaphylos uva ursi	Bearberry		Leaves	Autumn	New Jersey woods.
Aristolochia serpentaria	Virginia snakeroot	5	Root	Autumn	Moist woods.
Asarum Canadense	Wild ginger	5, 6	Root	Autumn	Moist, rich woodlands.
Asclepias incarnata	Flesh-colored asclepias	6, 7, 8	Root		Meadows; along streams.

List of Plants—Continued.

Botanical name.	Common name.	Flowers.	Collect.	When.	Habitat and Remarks.
Asclepias syriaca (or A. cornuti)	Wild cotton	6, 7, 8	Root	Autumn	Meadows; along streams.
Asclepias tuberosa	Pleurisy root	7	Root	Autumn	Sandy old fields: juice *not* milky; orange-colored flowers.
Aspidium filix mas	Male fern		Rhizome	Summer	
Berberis vulgaris	Barberry	7, 8	Berries		
Baptisia tinctoria	Wild indigo	7	Root and all		Woods.
Cassia Marilandica	Wild senna	7, 8	Leaves	8—9	Near streams; common N. of Camden.
Catalpa cordifolia	Catawba tree	6	Seeds		
Ceanothus Americanus	New Jersey tea	6	Root and leaves	Summer	Woods.
Celastrus scandens	Climbing staff-tree	6	Bark		Thickets and fence rows.
Chamælirium tuteum		6			Clearings and woods.
Chelidonium majus	Celandine	5	All	Autumn	Near old settlements.
Chimaphila umbellata	Pipsissewa	6	Leaves and stem	Autumn	Common in woods of N. exposure.
Chimaphila maculata	Spotted wintergreen	6		Autumn	Common in woods of N. exposure
Cicuta maculata	Water hemlock	7		7, 8	Along swampy rivulets.
Cichorium intybus	Succory, chickory	9	Dried root		Fields near Wissahickon.
Cimicifuga racemosa	Black snakeroot	6, 7	Root	Autumn	Common in rich, moist woods.
Clematis Virginica	Virgin's bower	7, 8	Leaves		Moist thickets; sub. for C. erecta.
Collinsonia Canadensis	Heal-all	7, 8, 9			Rich woods.
Comptonia asplenifolium	Sweet fern	4	All		Slaty woods and hillsides.
Conium maculatum	Hemlock	6, 7	Leaves and fruit	7, 8	Old settlements and waste places; an active poison; when partially dry the odor is remarkably like that of mice.
Convallaria polygonatum	Solomon's seal	5	Root	Autumn	Rich woods, and fence rows.
Convolvulus panduratus	Wild potato	6, 7, 8	Root	Autumn	West of Schuylkill.
Cornus Florida	Dogwood	5	Bark	Spring	Woods, everywhere.
Cornus sericea	Swamp dogwood	6, 7	Bark	Spring	Swamps; same properties as preceding.
Cunila mariana	Dittany	6, 7	Herb	6, 7	Slaty hills.
Cynoglossum officinale	Hound's tongue		Root		Rich woods.
Cypripedium acaule	Stemless lad. slip.	5, 6			Swamps: common near Camden.
Cytisus scoparius	Broom	6, 7	Tops	6, 7	Fairmount Park.
Datura stramonium	Jamestown weed	6, 7	Leaves, root, and seed	7—8 8—9	A rank weed.
Daucus carota	Wild carrot	6, 7	Root and seed	7, 8	A common nuisance among farmers.
Diospyros Virginiana	Persimmon	5, 6	Fruit and bark	10	Abundant near Camden and elsewhere.
Dirca palustris	Leatherwood	4	Bark		
Erigeron Canadense	Canada fleabane	7, 8	All	7, 8	Old fields (thoroughw't).
Erigeron Philadelphicum	Philadelphia fleabane (scabious)	6, 7	All	6, 7	Fields everywhere.
Erigeron Heterophyllum	Various-leaved fleabane	6, 7	All	6, 7	Fields everywhere.
Eryngium Virginianum	Button snakeroot	8	Root	Autumn	Swamps near Camden.
Erythronium Americanum	Dogtooth violet	5	Bulb		Swampy woods near streams.

List of Plants—Continued.

Botanical name.	Common name.	Flowers.	Collect.	When.	Habitat and Remarks.
Epiphegus Virginianus	Cancer root	8, 9			Under beech trees.
Epigæa repens	Trailing arbutus	4	Leaves	Summer	Near Camden woods; common.
Euonymus Americanus	Burning bush	9	Bark & seeds		Near Wissahickon.
Eupatorium perfoliatum	Bone-set	8, 9	All	8, 9	Meadows.
Euphorbia corollata	Large flowering spurge	7, 8	Root	Autumn	Dry soil near Camden.
Euphorbia ipecacuanha	Ipecac. spurge	5, 8	Root	Autumn	Sandy shores near Camden, N. J.
Fumaria officinalis	Fumitory	5, 8	Leaves		
Galium Aparine	Goosegrass	5	Herb		Fence rows and hedges.
Gaultheria procumbens	Teaberry	7	Leaves	Autumn	Moist grounds near Redbank.
Gentiana andrewsii	Closed gentian	8, 9			Confounded with G. catesbæi.
Geranium maculatum	Crow-foot	5, 7	Root	Autumn	Moist fields and fence rows.
Geum rivale	Purple avens	5, 6	Root	Autumn	Wet meadows; rare near Philadelphia.
Gillenia trifoliata	Indian physic	6, 7	Root	Sept.	Rocky woods and hillsides.
Hamamelis Virginica	Witch hazel	10	Bark & leaves		Woods, near streams.
Hedeoma pulegioides	Pennyroyal	7	All	7	Sterile fields.
Helenium autumnale	Sneezeweed	8	Leaves, flowers	8	Along the Delaware.
Helianthemum Canadense	Frostwort	6	All	6	Dry sandy soil, near Camden, N. J.
Hepatica triloba	Liverwort	4, 5	Leaves	Summer	Woods.
Heracleum lanatum	Cow parsnips	5	Root		Meadows; when dried very fragrant.
Heuchera Americana	Alum root	6, 7	Root	Autumn	Rocky hill-sides; shady places.
Humulus lupulus	Hop	7	Ripe strobiles	7, 8	Cultivated; indigenous along streams.
Hydrangea arborescens	Wild hydrangea	7	Root	Spring	West bank of Schuylkill, above Manayunk.
Hydrastis Canadensis	Yellow root	5	Root and bark	Autumn	Schuylkill opposite Manayunk; rich woods.
Hypericum perforatum	St. John's wort	7	Summits	7	A common weed in fields.
Ilex opaca	American holly	6	Leaves and seed		Moist woodlands.
Inula helenium	Elecampane	7, 8	Root	Autumn	Low meadows.
Impatiens fulva	Touch-me-not	7, 8			Low grounds. Rills.
Iris versicolor	Blue flag	6	Rhizome		Meadows.
Juglans cinerea	Butternut	5	Inn'r b'k of root	5, 6	Rich woods.
Juniperus communis	Juniper	4	Fruit and tops		Collect in the year after flowering.
Juniperus Virginiana	Red cedar	4	Leaves and tops		
Kalmia latefolia	Laurel	6	Leaves	Summer	Hilly woods.
Lactuca elongata	Wild lettuce	7	Herb	7	Virtue resides in milky juice.
Laurus benzoin	Spice-wood	4	Bark	Spring	Moist woods.
Lappa major	Burdock		Root		Collect in Spring.
Liatris spicata	Gay feather	7	Root		Moist woods. (Button snakeroot.)
Ligustrum vulgare	Privet	5, 6	Leaves, flowers		Used for hedges.
Linaria vulgaris	Toad-flax	6—9	Herb	In flower	
Liquidambar styraciflua	Sweet gum		Bark		Meadows and swamps, near tide-water.

List of Plants—Continued.

Botanical name.	Common name.	Flowers.	Collect.	When	Habitat and Remarks.
Liriodendron tulipifera	Tulip tree	5	Bark		Forests.
Lithospermum officinale	Stone-weed, common gromwell	5, 6			Waste grounds.
Lobelia inflata	Indian tobacco	7, 8, 9	Root and tops	8, 9	Fields and roadsides; common.
Lobelia cardinalis	Cardinal flower	7, 10			Low grounds.
Lycopodium clavatum	Club moss		Pollen		Thickets.
Lycopus Virginicus	Bugle weed, pilewort	8	Herb	8	Swamps and meadows.
Lycopus sinuatus	Water horehound	7			Swamps.
Magnolia glauca	Magnolia	6, 7	Bark	Spring	Swamps; abundant near Camden.
Malva rotundifolia	Running mallows	5	Herb		Substitute for M. Sylvestris of Europe.
Marrubium vulgare	Horehound	7, 8	All	7, 8	Very abundant
Maruta cotula	Dog's fennel, May weed	6—9	Flowers	6—9	Roadsides and yards; inferior sub. for Anthemis nobilis.
Melissa officinalis	Balm	7, 8	Leaves	6, 7	Gardens.
Melissa clinopodioid.	Wild basil	8, 9			Fence rows.
Menispermum Canadense	Moonseed	7	Root		Along Wissahickon.
Mentha piperita	Peppermint	8	All	8	Escaped from gardens
Mentha viridis	Spearmint	8	All	8	
Monarda punctata	Horsemint	6—9	Herb	Summer	Near Camden.
Monarda fistulosa	Wild bergamot	7			Along streams.
Medeola Virginica	Indian cucumber	6	Root		Moist woods.
Nepeta Cataria	Catmint	6	All	Summer	A common weed on farms.
Nepeta glechoma	Ground ivy	5	Herb	5, 6	Old settlements.
Nymphæa odorata	Water lily	7	Root		Rare; in ditches south of Camden.
Œnothera biennis	Primrose	7, 8			Common everywhere.
Origanum vulgare	Marjoram	6—10	Herb	Summer	Dry soil; near Columbia Railroad bridge.
Oxalis acetosella	Wood sorrel	6	All	6	Very common.
Panax quinquefolium	Ginseng	7	Root	Autumn	Found, but very rare, near Philadelphia
Phytolacca decandra	Poke	7	Berries and root	9 10	Common clearings and fence rows.
Plantago major	Plantain		Leaves		Common in fields and yards.
Podophyllum peltatum	May apple	5	Rhizome	10	Moist woods.
Polygala senega	Seneka snakeroot	5	Root	9, 10	Rare: rich, hilly woodlands.
Prinos verticillatus	Black alder	6	Bark	10—4	Swamps.
Populus tremuloides	Aspen	4	Bark	9—4	
Prunella vulgaris	All-heal	6	Herb	6, 7	Waysides; common.
Prunus Virginiana (cerasus serotina)	Wild cherry	5	Bark		Common in fields and forests.
Pulmonaria Virginica	Lungwort				Near Wissahickon.
Quercus alba	White oak		Bark	Spring	Woods.
Quercus tinctoria	Black oak		Bark	Spring	Woods.
Ranunculus bulbosus	Buttercup	5, 6	All	5, 6	Common everywhere.
Rhus glabrum	Sumach	7	Fruit	9, 10	Old fields; &c.
Rhus radicans	Poison vine	6, 7			Fences.
Rhus toxicodendron	Poison oak	6, 7	Leaves		Woods.
Rhus vernix	Swamp sumach		Leaves		Swamps; powerful poison.
Rubus trivialis	Dewberry	5	Root	Autumn	
Rubus villosus	Blackberry	5	Root	Autumn	
Rumex obtusifolius	Dock	6, 7	Root	Autumn	Common in fields and yards.
Rumex acetosella	Sorrel	5, 6	Leaves	Summer	Common pest in fields and yards.

List of Plants—Continued.

Botanical name.	Common name.	Flowers.	Collect.	When.	Habitat and Remarks.
Rumex crispus	Curled or sour dock	5	Root		
Sabbatia angularis	Wild centaury	7, 8	All	8	A common, showy plant.
Salix alba	White willow	4, 5	Bark		
Sambucus Canadensis	Elder	5, 6	Flowers	5, 6	
Sanguinaria Canadensis	Bloodroot	4	Rhizome	Autumn	Clearings.
Sanicula Marilandica	Sanicle	7			Woods.
Saponaria officinalis	Soapwort				Old settlements.
Sarracenia purpurea	Fly-trap	7			Rare; swamps south of Camden.
Sassafras officinale	Sassafras	5	Bark of root	9—4	Fence rows.
Scutellaria lateriflora	Skullcap	7			Moist places.
Sisymbrium officinale	Hedge mustard	5			Waste places.
Solanum dulcamara	Bittersweet	7, 8		Autumn	About houses.
Solidago odora	Sweet golden rod	8, 9		8, 9	Abundant north of Camden.
Symplocarpus fœtidus	Skunk cabbage	3, 4		9—3	Swamps.
Tanacetum vulgare	Tansy	7—9			Escaped from gardens.
Taraxacum Dens-leonis (Leontodon Taraxacum)	Dandelion	4—5	Root	8, 9	A common weed.
Trillium cernuum	Three-leaved nightshade	5			Moist woods.
Tephrosia Virginiana	Goat's rue				Near Camden.
Triosteum perfoliatum	Fever root	6			Moist fields, near lime stone.
Ulmus fulva	Slippery elm	4	Bark		Rare.
Urtica dioica	Nettle				Too common.
Veratrum viride	Amer. hellebore	6	Root	Autumn	Shady swamps.
Verbascum thapsus	Mullein				Very common.
Veronica officinalis	Speedwell	6			Fields.
Veronica Virginica	Neckweed				Meadows.
Viola pedata	Violet	5			North of Camden; very abundant.

RECIPES FOR SOME OF THE MORE IMPORTANT POPULAR MEDICINES.

Dalby's Carminative.

The published recipes for this, as found in the formularies, are not those used generally by druggists. Some of the ingredients in the original recipes are procurable with difficulty, and add so much to the expense of the preparation, that by common consent they are left out. The formula, as given by the College of Pharmacy, is nearly identical with that which I have used for a number of years, and I give it below.

Take of	Carbonate of Magnesia	℥vj	75.
	Carbonate of potassa	ʒij	3.125
	Sugar	℥xvj	200.
	Tincture of opium	f℥iij	op. 37.5
	Water	Ov	1000.
	Oils of caraway,		
	Fennel, and peppermint, of each	♏x.	

(To the above may be added—

French brandy	f℥iv.
Prepared chalk	℥ij.)

Triturate together the essential oils, sugar, magnesia (and prepared chalk, if added), then add the water, and afterwards the remainder.

Dalby's carminative contains one grain of opium to about an ounce.

Dewees' Carminative.

Take of	Carbonate of magnesia	℥jss.
	Sugar	℥iij.
	Tincture of assafœtida	f℥iij.
	Tincture of opium	f℥j.
	Water	Oiss.

Triturate together until they are mixed.

Bateman's Pectoral Drops.

			Parts.
Take of	Diluted alcohol	Cong. j	1000.
	[1]Red sanders, rasped	℥ss	31.25

Digest for twenty four hours, filter, and add—

Opium, in powder	℥ss	31.25
Catechu, in powder	℥ss	31.25
Camphor	℥ss	31.25
Oil of anise	fʒj	7.81

Digest for ten days.

This preparation contains about one grain each of opium, catechu, and camphor, to the f℥ss, corresponding in strength with tinctura opii camphorata, *U. S.*

[1] Substituted by Caramel ℥iij.

Godfrey's Cordial.

			Parts.
Take of Tincture of opium . .	f℥vj	op. 34.5	1000.
Molasses (sugar-house) . .	Oiv	367.8	
Alcohol	f℥viij	46.	
Water	Oviss	551.7	
Carbonate of potassa . .	ʒv		57.5
Oil of sassafras. . . .	fʒj		11.

Dissolve the carbonate of potassa in the water, add the molasses, and heat over a gentle fire till they simmer, remove the scum which rises, and add the laudanum and oil of sassafras, having previously mixed them well together.

This preparation contains a little over one grain of opium to the ounce, and is about half the strength of the foregoing.

Balsam of Honey.

Take of Balsam tolu . . . . ℥j.
Benzoic acid . . . . ʒiss.
Honey . . . . ℥vj.
Opium (powd.) . . . . ʒij.
Cochineal . . . . ʒj.
French brandy . . . . Oiij.

Mix, and digest together for a few days, then filter.

Composition Powders. (Thompsonian.)

Take of Powd. bayberry root . . . . ℔j.
" ginger . . . . ℔ss.
" cayenne . . . . ℥j.
" cloves . . . . ℥j.

Mix, by passing through a sieve.

No. 6. Hot Drops. (Thompsonian.)

Take of Capsicum (powd.) . . . . . ℥j.
Myrrh (contus.) . . . . . ℥iv.
Alcohol . . . . Oij. Displace.

Haarlem Oil.

℞.—Ol. sulphurat. . . . . Oiij.
Petrol. Barbadens . . . . Oj.
Ol. succin. (crude) . . . . Oiss.
Ol. terebinth. . . . . Oviij.
Ol. lini . . . . Oiv.—Mix.

Turlington's Balsam of Life.

The officinal tinctura benzoini composita is sold under this name, but the druggists who put it up in the peculiar and very odd shaped vials, in which it was originally vended in wrappers descriptive of its virtues, use various recipes for making it. The following is that published by the Philadelphia College of Pharmacy, and used in many of the best establishments. The original recipe for this, as filed in the office of rolls in London, contained twenty-eight ingredients.

Take of Alcohol	. . . .	Oiv.
Benzoin	. . . .	℥vj.
Liquid storax	. . . .	℥ij.
Socotrine aloes	. . . .	℥ss.
Peruvian balsam	. . . .	℥j.
Myrrh	. . . .	℥ss.
Angelica	. . . .	ʒij.
Balsam tolu	. . . .	℥ij.
Extract of liquorice	. . . .	℥ij.

Digest for ten days and strain.

British Oil.

Take of Oil of turpentine	. . . .	f℥iv.
" flaxseed	. . . .	Oiij.
" amber	. . . .	Oj.
" juniper	. . . .	f℥ss.
Petroleum (Barbadoes)	. . . .	℥ij.
" (American)	. . . .	℥ij.

Mix them well together.

Whitehead's Essence of Mustard.

℞.—Ol. terebinth.	. . . . . .	Oxij.
Camphor	. . . . . .	1½ lbs. com.
Ol succin. rectif.	. . . . .	f℥iv.
Sem. sinapis, pulv. (Flava)	. . . .	16 oz. com.

Digest for seven days, filter, and add—

Tr. curcuma	. . . . . .	q. s.—Add color.

Hooper's Female Pills.

Take of Aloes	℥viij	400 parts.
Dried sulphate of iron, .	℥ij, ʒiss	200 "
or Crystallized sulphate of iron .	℥iv	
Extract of black hellebore .	℥ij	100 "
Myrrh	℥ij	100 "
Soap	℥ij	100 "
Powd. canella	℥j	50 "
" ginger	℥j	50 "
		1000 parts.

Beat them well together into a mass with syrup, or water, and divide into pills, each containing two and a half grains.

Richard's Chalk Mixture.

Take of Precip. carbonate of lime,		
Sugar,		
Comp. spt. lavender,		
Tinct. kino, of each	. . . . . .	1 ounce.
Essence of cinnamon	. . . . . .	15 drops.
Water	. . . .	3 ounces.
Tincture of opium	. . . . . .	1 drachm.

Mix.

Marshall's Pills.

Take of Comp. extract of colocynth,
Mercurial mass,
Powdered aloes,
" Castile soap,
" rhubarb, of each . . . . . 1 drachm.

Make into five grain pills.

Anderson's Scots' Pills.

Take of Aloes	℥xxiv	787
Soap	℥iv	131
Colocynth	℥j	33
Gamboge	℥j	33
Oil of anise	f℥ss	16
		1000 parts.

Let the aloes, colocynth, and gamboge, be reduced to a very fine powder, then beat them and the soap with water into a mass of a proper consistence, to divide into pills, each containing three grains.

Worm Tea.

Take of Senna,	
Manna,	
Spigelia, of each	℥ss.
Fennel seed	ʒj.
Worm seed	ʒss.
Savine	℈ij.
Bitartrate of potassa	℈ij.

Make into one package.

Directions.—Pour into this a quart of boiling water, and let it digest for ten or fifteen minutes; of the clear liquid sweetened, give to children two years old and upwards, a small teacupful *warm*, morning, noon, and night, on an empty stomach. It may be given three or four days successively, if necessary.

The fluid extract of pink root and senna, *U. S. P.*, may be substituted for this, and has the advantage of being ready for use without the trouble of extemporaneous preparation.

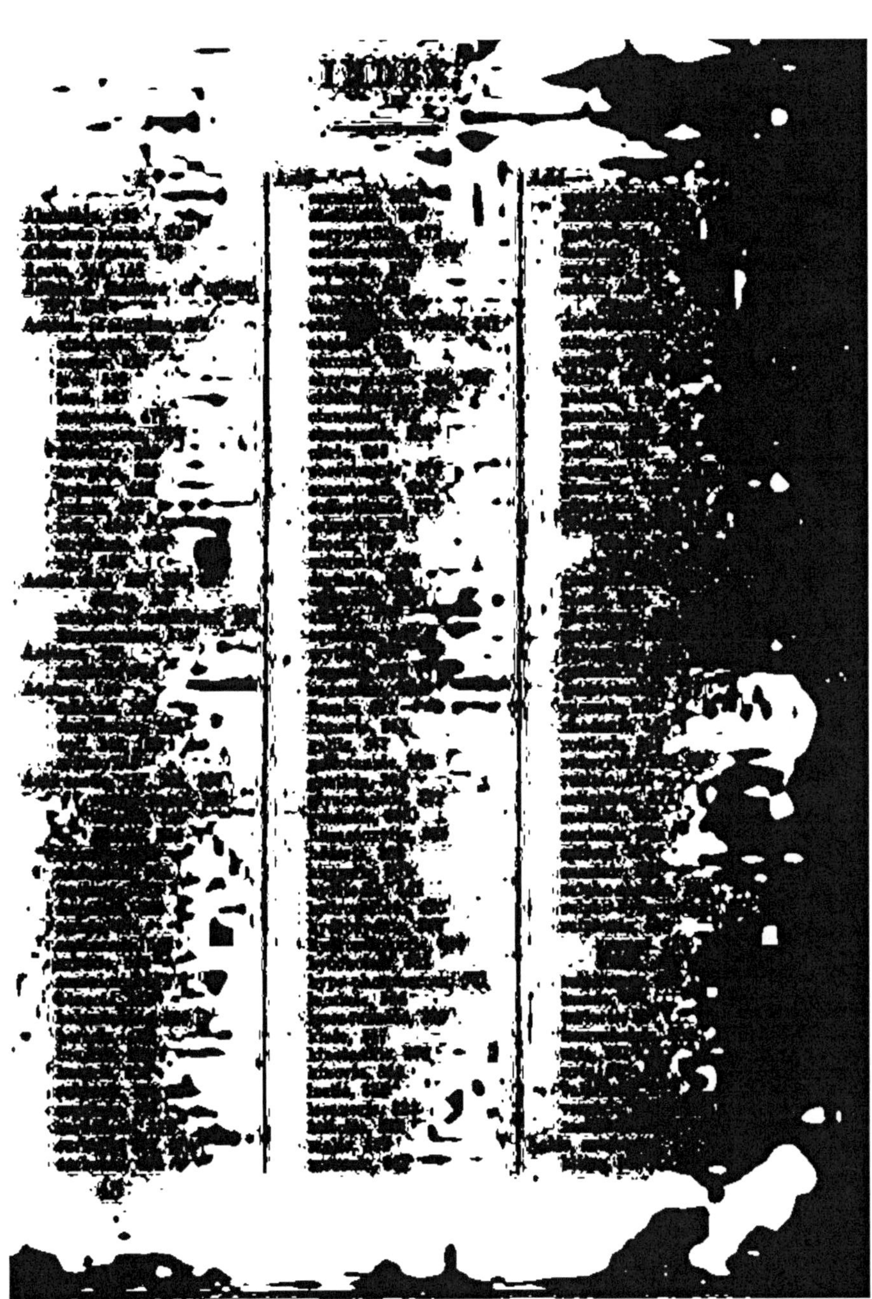

B

C

D

E

Hos.

N

O

P

THE END.

BLANCHARD & LEA'S
MEDICAL AND SURGICAL PUBLICATIONS.

TO THE MEDICAL PROFESSION.

The prices on the present catalogue are those at which our books can generally be furnished by booksellers throughout the United States, who can readily procure any which they may not have on hand. To physicians who have not convenient access to bookstores, we will forward them by mail, at these prices, *free of postage* (as long as the existing facilities are afforded by the post-office), for any distance under 3,000 miles. As we open accounts only with booksellers, the amount must in every case, without exception, accompany the order, and we assume no risks of the mail, either on the money or on the books; and as we deal only in our own publications, we can supply no others. Gentlemen desirous of purchasing will, therefore, find it more advantageous to deal with the nearest booksellers whenever practicable.

BLANCHARD & LEA.

PHILADELPHIA, September, 1860.

*** We have just issued a new edition of our ILLUSTRATED CATALOGUE of Medical and Scientific Publications, forming an octavo pamphlet of 80 large pages, containing specimens of illustrations, notices of the medical press, &c. &c. It has been prepared without regard to expense, and will be found one of the handsomest specimens of typographical execution as yet presented in this country. Copies will be sent to any address, by mail, free of postage, on receipt of nine cents in stamps.

Catalogues of our numerous publications in miscellaneous and educational literature forwarded on application.

☞ The attention of physicians is especially solicited to the following important new works and new editions, just issued or nearly ready:—

TWO MEDICAL PERIODICALS, FREE OF POSTAGE,

Containing over Fifteen Hundred large octavo pages,

FOR FIVE DOLLARS PER ANNUM.

THE AMERICAN JOURNAL OF THE MEDICAL SCIENCES, subject to postage, when not paid for in advance, - - - - - - - - - $5 00

THE MEDICAL NEWS AND LIBRARY, invariably in advance, - - 1 00

or, BOTH PERIODICALS mailed, FREE OF POSTAGE, for Five Dollars remitted in advance.

THE AMERICAN JOURNAL OF THE MEDICAL SCIENCES,

EDITED BY ISAAC HAYS, M. D.,

is published Quarterly, on the first of January, April, July, and October. Each number contains at least two hundred and eighty large octavo pages, handsomely and appropriately illustrated, wherever necessary. It has now been issued regularly for nearly FORTY years, and it has been

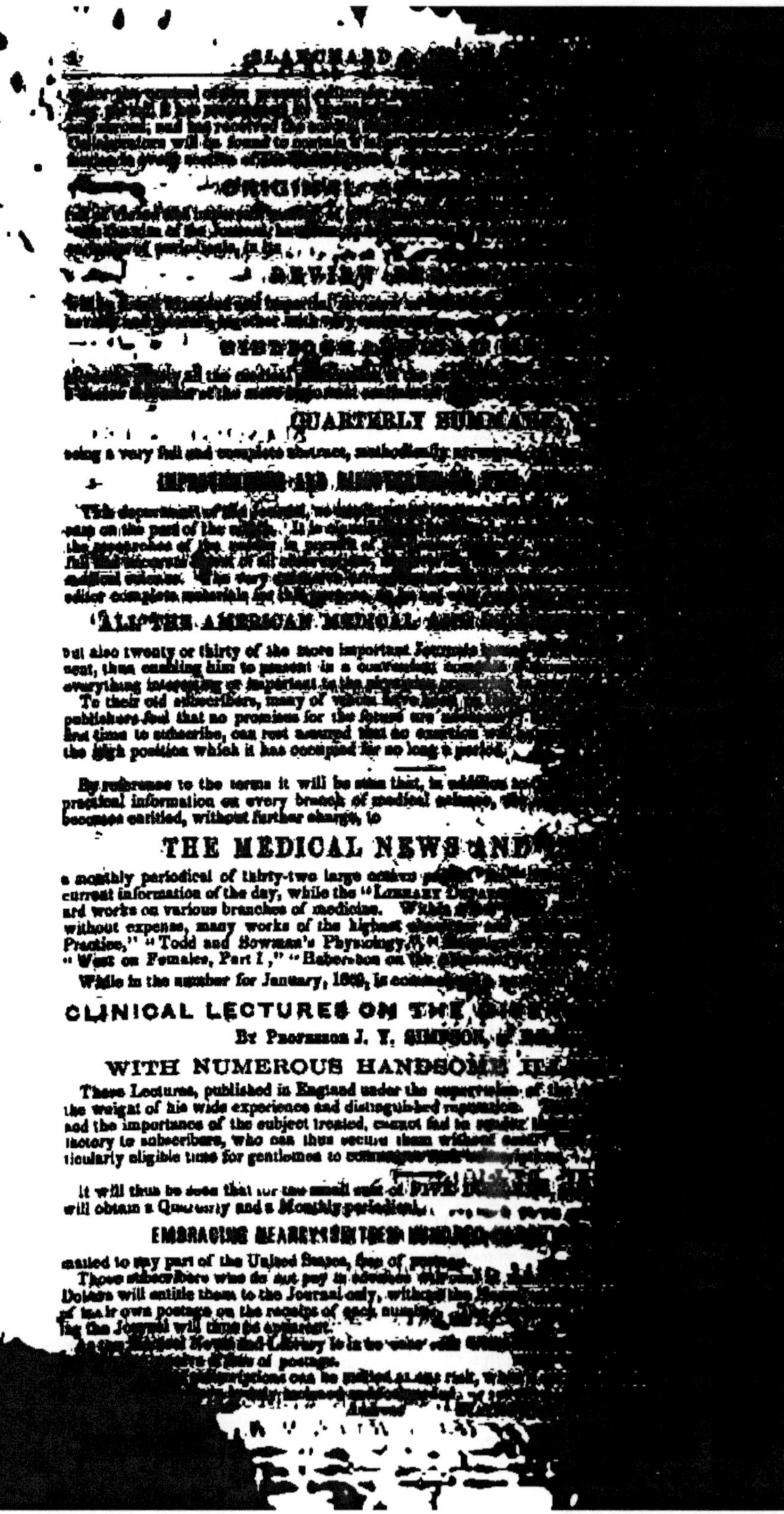

QUARTERLY SUMMA[illegible]

being a very full and complete abstract, methodically [illegible]

[illegible]

ALL THE AMERICAN MEDICAL [illegible]

but also twenty or thirty of the more important Journals [illegible]
ment, thus enabling him to present in a convenient [illegible]
everything interesting or important to the [illegible]
To their old subscribers, many of whom have [illegible]
publishers feel that no promises for the future are [illegible]
first time to subscribe, can rest assured that no exertion [illegible]
the high position which it has occupied for so long a period.

By reference to the terms it will be seen that, in addition [illegible]
practical information on every branch of medical science, [illegible]
becomes entitled, without further charge, to

THE MEDICAL NEWS AND [illegible]

a monthly periodical of thirty-two large octavo pages [illegible]
current information of the day, while the "Library Depa[illegible]
ard works on various branches of medicine. With[illegible]
without expense, many works of the highest [illegible]
Practice," "Todd and Bowman's Physiology," "[illegible]
"West on Females, Part I," "Habershon on the [illegible]
While in the number for January, 1860, is comm[illegible]

CLINICAL LECTURES ON THE [illegible]

By Professor J. Y. SIMPSON, [illegible]

WITH NUMEROUS HANDSOM[illegible]

These Lectures, published in England under the supervision of th[illegible]
the weight of his wide experience and distinguished reputation. [illegible]
and the importance of the subject treated, cannot fail to render [illegible]
factory to subscribers, who can thus secure them without [illegible]
ticularly eligible time for gentlemen to [illegible]

It will thus be seen that for the small sum of FIVE D[illegible]
will obtain a Quarterly and a Monthly periodical, [illegible]

EMBRACING NEARLY [illegible]

mailed to any part of the United States, free of postage.
Those subscribers who do not pay in advance [illegible]
Dollars will entitle them to the Journal only, without the [illegible]
of their own postage on the receipt of each number. [illegible]
for the Journal will thus be apparent.
As the Medical News and Library is in the [illegible]
[illegible] free of postage.

ASHTON (T. J.),
Surgeon to the Blenheim Dispensary, &c.

ON THE DISEASES, INJURIES, AND MALFORMATIONS OF THE RECTUM AND ANUS; with remarks on Habitual Constipation.
From the third and enlarged London edition. With handsome illustrations. In one very beautifully printed octavo volume, of about 300 pages. (*Now Ready.*) $3 00.

INTRODUCTION. CHAPTER I. Irritation and Itching of the Anus. II. Inflammation and Excoriation of the Anus. III. Excrescences of the Anal Region. IV. Contraction of the Anus. V. Fissure of the Anus and lower part of the Rectum. VI. Neuralgia of the Anus and extremity of the Rectum. VII. Inflammation of the Rectum. VIII. Ulceration of the Rectum. IX. Hemorrhoidal Affections. X. Enlargement of Hemorrhoidal Veins. XI. Prolapsus of the Rectum. XII. Abscess near the Rectum. XIII. Fistula in Ano. XIV. Polypi of the Rectum. XV. Stricture of the Rectum. XVI. Malignant Diseases of the Rectum. XVII. Injuries of the Rectum. XVIII. Foreign Bodies in the Rectum. XIX. Malformations of the Rectum. XX. Habitual Constipation.

The most complete one we possess on the subject.—*Medico-Chirurgical Review.*

Its merits as a practical instructor, well arranged, abundantly furnished with illustrative cases, and clearly and comprehensively, albeit too diffusely, written, are incontestable. They have been sufficiently endorsed by the verdict of his countrymen in the rapid exhaustion of the first edition, and they would certainly meet with a similar reward in the United States were the volume placed within the reach of American practitioners. We are satisfied after a careful examination of the volume, and a comparison of its contents with those of its leading predecessors and contemporaries, that the best way for the reader to avail himself of the excellent advice given in the concluding paragraph above, would be to provide himself with a copy of the book from which it has been taken, and diligently to con its instructive pages. They may secure to him many a triumph and fervent blessing.—*Am. Journal Med. Sciences*, April, 1868.

ALLEN (J. M.), M. D.,
Professor of Anatomy in the Pennsylvania Medical College, &c.

THE PRACTICAL ANATOMIST; or, The Student's Guide in the Dissecting-ROOM.
With 266 illustrations. In one handsome royal 12mo. volume, of over 600 pages, leather. $2 25.

However valuable may be the "Dissector's Guides" which we, of late, have had occasion to notice, we feel confident that the work of Dr. Allen is superior to any of them. We believe with the author, that none is so fully illustrated as this, and the arrangement of the work is such as to facilitate the labors of the student in acquiring a thorough practical knowledge of Anatomy. We most cordially recommend it to their attention.—*Western Lancet.*

We believe it to be one of the most useful works upon the subject ever written. It is handsomely illustrated, well printed, and will be found of convenient size for use in the dissecting-room.—*Med. Examiner.*

ANATOMICAL ATLAS.

By Professors H. H. SMITH and W. E. HORNER, of the University of Pennsylvania. 1 vol. 8vo., extra cloth, with nearly 650 illustrations. ☞ See SMITH, p. 27.

ABEL (F. A.), F. C. S. AND C. L. BLOXAM.

HANDBOOK OF CHEMISTRY, Theoretical, Practical, and Technical; with a Recommendatory Preface by Dr. HOFMANN.
In one large octavo volume, extra cloth, of 662 pages, with illustrations. $3 25.

ASHWELL (SAMUEL), M. D.,
Obstetric Physician and Lecturer to Guy's Hospital, London.

A PRACTICAL TREATISE ON THE DISEASES PECULIAR TO WOMEN.
Illustrated by Cases derived from Hospital and Private Practice. Third American, from the Third and revised London edition. In one octavo volume, extra cloth, of 528 pages. $3 00.

The most useful practical work on the subject in the English language.—*Boston Med. and Surg. Journal.*

The most able, and certainly the most standard and practical, work on female diseases that we have yet seen.—*Medico-Chirurgical Review.*

ARNOTT (NEILL), M. D.

ELEMENTS OF PHYSICS; or Natural Philosophy, General and Medical.
Written for universal use, in plain or non-technical language. A new edition, by ISAAC HAYS, M. D. Complete in one octavo volume, leather, of 484 pages, with about two hundred illustrations. $2 50.

BIRD (GOLDING), A. M., M. D., &c.

URINARY DEPOSITS: THEIR DIAGNOSIS, PATHOLOGY, AND THERAPEUTICAL INDICATIONS.
Edited by EDMUND LLOYD BIRKETT, M. D. A new American, from the fifth and enlarged London edition. With eighty illustrations on wood. In one handsome octavo volume, of about 400 pages, extra cloth. $2 00. (*Just Issued.*)

The death of Dr. Bird has rendered it necessary to entrust the revision of the present edition to other hands, and in his performance of the duty thus devolving on him, Dr. Birkett has sedulously endeavored to carry out the author's plan by introducing such new matter and modifications of the text as the progress of science has called for. Notwithstanding the utmost care to keep the work within a reasonable compass, these additions have resulted in a considerable enlargement. It is, therefore, hoped that it will be found fully up to the present condition of the subject, and that the reputation of the volume as a clear, complete, and compendious manual, will be fully maintained.

BUDD (GEORGE), M. D., F. R. S.,
Professor of Medicine in King's College, London.

ON DISEASES OF THE LIVER. Third American, from the third and enlarged London edition. In one very handsome octavo volume, extra cloth, with four beautifully colored plates, and numerous wood-cuts. pp. 500. $3 00.

Has fairly established for itself a place among the classical medical literature of England.—*British and Foreign Medico-Chir. Review*, July, 1857.

Dr. Budd's Treatise on Diseases of the Liver is now a standard work in Medical literature, and during the intervals which have elapsed between the successive editions, the author has incorporated into the text the most striking novelties which have characterized the recent progress of hepatic physiology and pathology; so that although the size of the book is not perceptibly changed, the history of liver diseases is made more complete, and is kept upon a level with the progress of modern science. It is the best work on Diseases of the Liver in any language.—*London Med. Times and Gazette*, June 27, 1857.

This work, now the standard book of reference on the diseases of which it treats, has been carefully revised, and many new illustrations of the views of the learned author added in the present edition.—*Dublin Quarterly Journal*, Aug. 1857.

BY THE SAME AUTHOR.

ON THE ORGANIC DISEASES AND FUNCTIONAL DISORDERS OF THE STOMACH. In one neat octavo volume, extra cloth. $1 50.

BUCKNILL (J. C.), M. D.,
Medical Superintendent of the Devon County Lunatic Asylum; and
DANIEL H. TUKE, M. D.,
Visiting Medical Officer to the York Retreat.

A MANUAL OF PSYCHOLOGICAL MEDICINE; containing the History, Nosology, Description, Statistics, Diagnosis, Pathology, and Treatment of INSANITY. With a Plate. In one handsome octavo volume, of 536 pages. $3 00.

The increase of mental disease in its various forms, and the difficult questions to which it is constantly giving rise, render the subject one of daily enhanced interest, requiring on the part of the physician a constantly greater familiarity with this, the most perplexing branch of his profession. At the same time there has been for some years no work accessible in this country, presenting the results of recent investigations in the Diagnosis and Prognosis of Insanity, and the greatly improved methods of treatment which have done so much in alleviating the condition or restoring the health of the insane. To fill this vacancy the publishers present this volume, assured that the distinguished reputation and experience of the authors will entitle it at once to the confidence of both student and practitioner. Its scope may be gathered from the declaration of the authors that "their aim has been to supply a text-book which may serve as a guide in the acquisition of such knowledge, sufficiently elementary to be adapted to the wants of the student, and sufficiently modern in its views and explicit in its teaching to suffice for the demands of the practitioner."

BENNETT (J. HUGHES), M. D., F. R. S. E.,
Professor of Clinical Medicine in the University of Edinburgh, &c.

THE PATHOLOGY AND TREATMENT OF PULMONARY TUBERCULOSIS, and on the Local Medication of Pharyngeal and Laryngeal Diseases frequently mistaken for or associated with, Phthisis. One vol. 8vo., extra cloth, with wood-cuts. pp. 130. $1 25.

BENNETT (HENRY), M. D.

A PRACTICAL TREATISE ON INFLAMMATION OF THE UTERUS, ITS CERVIX AND APPENDAGES, and on its connection with Uterine Disease. To which is added, a Review of the present state of Uterine Pathology. Fifth American, from the third English edition. In one octavo volume, of about 500 pages, extra cloth. $2 00. (*Now Ready.*)

The ill health of the author having prevented the promised revision of this work, the present edition is a reprint of the last, without alteration. As the volume has been for some time out of print, gentlemen desiring copies can now procure them.

BOWMAN (JOHN E.), M. D.

PRACTICAL HANDBOOK OF MEDICAL CHEMISTRY. Second American, from the third and revised English Edition. In one neat volume, royal 12mo., extra cloth, with numerous illustrations. pp. 288. $1 25.

BY THE SAME AUTHOR.

INTRODUCTION TO PRACTICAL CHEMISTRY, INCLUDING ANALYSIS. Second American, from the second and revised London edition. With numerous illustrations. In one neat vol., royal 12mo., extra cloth. pp. 350. $1 25.

BEALE ON THE LAWS OF HEALTH IN RELATION TO MIND AND BODY. A Series of Letters from an old Practitioner to a Patient. In one volume, royal 12mo., extra cloth. pp. 296. 80 cents.

BUSHNAN'S PHYSIOLOGY OF ANIMAL AND VEGETABLE LIFE; a Popular Treatise on the Functions and Phenomena of Organic Life. In one handsome royal 12mo. volume, extra cloth, with over 100 illustrations. pp. 234. 80 cents.

BUCKLER ON THE ETIOLOGY, PATHOLOGY, AND TREATMENT OF FIBRO-BRONCHITIS AND RHEUMATIC PNEUMONIA. In one 8vo. volume, extra cloth. pp. 150. $1 25.

BLOOD AND URINE (MANUALS ON). BY JOHN WILLIAM GRIFFITH, G. OWEN REESE, AND ALFRED MARKWICK. One thick volume, royal 12mo., extra cloth, with plates. pp. 460. $1 25.

BRODIE'S CLINICAL LECTURES ON SURGERY. 1 vol. 8vo. cloth. 350 pp. $1 25.

BARCLAY (A. W.), M. D.,

Assistant Physician to St. George's Hospital, &c.

A MANUAL OF MEDICAL DIAGNOSIS; being an Analysis of the Signs and Symptoms of Disease. In one neat octavo volume, extra cloth, of 424 pages. $2 00. (*Lately issued.*)

Of works exclusively devoted to this important branch, our profession has at command, comparatively, but few, and, therefore, in the publication of the present work, Messrs. Blanchard & Lea have conferred a great favor upon us. Dr. Barclay, from having occupied, for a long period, the position of Medical Registrar at St. George's Hospital, possessed advantages for correct observation and reliable conclusions, as to the significance of symptoms, which have fallen to the lot of but few, either in his own or any other country. He has carefully systematized the results of his observation of over twelve thousand patients, and by his diligence and judicious classification, the profession has been presented with the most convenient and reliable work on the subject of Diagnosis that it has been our good fortune ever to examine; we can, therefore, say of Dr. Barclay's work, that, from his systematic manner of arrangement, his work is one of the best works "for reference" in the daily emergencies of the practitioner, with which we are acquainted; but, at the same time, we would recommend our readers, especially the younger ones, to read thoroughly and study diligently the *whole* work, and the "emergencies" will not occur so often.—*Southern Med. and Surg. Journ.*, March, 1858.

To give this information, to supply this admitted deficiency, is the object of Dr. Barclay's Manual. The task of composing such a work is neither an easy nor a light one; but Dr. Barclay has performed it in a manner which meets our most unqualified approbation. He is no mere theorist; he knows his work thoroughly, and in attempting to perform it, has not exceeded his powers.—*British Med. Journal*, Dec. 5, 1857.

We venture to predict that the work will be deservedly popular, and soon become, like Watson's Practice, an indispensable necessity to the practitioner.—*N. A. Med. Journal*, April, 1858.

An inestimable work of reference for the young practitioner and student.—*Nashville Med. Journal*, May, 1858.

We hope the volume will have an extensive circulation, not among students of medicine only, but practitioners also. They will never regret a faithful study of its pages.—*Cincinnati Lancet*, Mar. '58.

An important acquisition to medical literature. It is a work of high merit, both from the vast importance of the subject upon which it treats, and also from the real ability displayed in its elaboration. In conclusion, let us bespeak for this volume that attention of every student of our art which it so richly deserves—that place in every medical library which it can so well adorn.—*Peninsular Medical Journal*, Sept. 1858.

BARLOW (GEORGE H.), M. D.

Physician to Guy's Hospital, London, &c.

A MANUAL OF THE PRACTICE OF MEDICINE. With Additions by D. F. Condie, M. D., author of "A Practical Treatise on Diseases of Children," &c. In one handsome octavo volume, leather, of over 600 pages. $2 75.

We recommend Dr. Barlow's Manual in the warmest manner as a most valuable vade-mecum. We have had frequent occasion to consult it, and have found it clear, concise, practical, and sound. It is eminently a practical work, containing all that is essential, and avoiding useless theoretical discussion. The work supplies what has been for some time wanting, a manual of practice based upon modern discoveries in pathology and rational views of treatment of disease. It is especially intended for the use of students and junior practitioners, but it will be found hardly less useful to the experienced physician. The American editor has added to the work three chapters—on Cholera Infantum, Yellow Fever, and Cerebro-spinal Meningitis. These additions, the two first of which are indispensable to a work on practice destined for the profession in this country, are executed with great judgment and fidelity, by Dr. Condie, who has also [illegible] happily in imitating the conciseness and [illegible] of style which are such agreeable characteristics of the original book.—*Boston Med. and Surg. Journal*.

BARTLETT (ELISHA), M. D.

THE HISTORY, DIAGNOSIS, AND TREATMENT OF THE FEVERS OF THE UNITED STATES. A new and revised edition. By Alonzo Clark, M. D., Prof. of Pathology and Practical Medicine in the N. Y. College of Physicians and Surgeons, &c. In one octavo volume, of six hundred pages, extra cloth. Price $3 00.

It is the best work on fevers which has emanated from the American press, and the present editor has carefully availed himself of all information existing upon the subject in the Old and New World, so that the doctrines advanced are brought down to the latest date in the progress of this department of Medical Science.—*London Med. Times and Gazette*, May 2, 1857.

This excellent monograph on febrile disease, has stood deservedly high since its first publication. It will be seen that it has now reached its fourth edition under the supervision of Prof. A. Clark, a gentleman who, from the nature of his studies and pursuits, is well calculated to appreciate and discuss the many intricate and difficult questions in pathology. His annotations add much to the interest of the work, and have brought it well up to the condition of the science as it exists at the present day in regard to this class of diseases.—*Southern Med. and Surg. Journal*, Mar. 1857.

It is a work of great practical value and interest, containing much that is new relative to the several diseases of which it treats, and, with the additions of the editor, is fully up to the times. The distinctive features of the different forms of fever are plainly and forcibly portrayed, and the lines of demarcation carefully and accurately drawn, and to the American practitioner is a more valuable and safe guide than any work on fever extant.—*Ohio Med. and Surg. Journal*, May, 1857.

BROWN (ISAAC BAKER),

Surgeon-Accoucheur to St. Mary's Hospital, &c.

ON SOME DISEASES OF WOMEN ADMITTING OF SURGICAL TREATMENT. With handsome illustrations. One vol. 8vo., extra cloth, pp. 276. $1 60.

Mr. Brown has earned for himself a high reputation in the operative treatment of sundry diseases and injuries to which females are peculiarly subject. We can truly say of his work that it is an important addition to obstetrical literature. The operative suggestions and contrivances which Mr. Brown describes, exhibit much practical sagacity and skill, and merit the careful attention of every surgeon-accoucheur.—*Association Journal*.

We have no hesitation in recommending this book to the careful attention of all [illegible] who make female complaints a part of their study and practice.—*Dublin Quarterly Journal*.

CARPENTER (WILLIAM B.), M.D., F.R.S., &c.,

Examiner in Physiology and Comparative Anatomy in the University of London.

PRINCIPLES OF HUMAN PHYSIOLOGY; with their chief applications to Psychology, Pathology, Therapeutics, Hygiène, and Forensic Medicine. A new American from the last and revised London edition. With nearly three hundred illustrations. Edited, with additions, by Francis Gurney Smith, M.D., Professor of the Institutes of Medicine in the Pennsylvania Medical College, &c. In one very large and beautiful octavo volume, of [illegible] large pages, handsomely printed and strongly bound in leather, with raised bands. [illegible]

In the preparation of this new edition, the author has spared no labor to render it [illegible] a complete and lucid exposition of the most advanced condition of its [illegible] amount of the additions required to effect this object thoroughly [illegible] the volume, preventing objections arising from the unwieldy bulk of the [illegible] those portions not bearing directly upon Human Physiology, designing to [illegible] his forthcoming Treatise on General Physiology. As a full and accurate [illegible] siology of Man, the work in its present condition therefore presents even greater [illegible] the student and physician than those which have heretofore won for it the [illegible] guished favor which it has so long enjoyed. The additions of Prof. Smith [illegible] whatever may have been wanting to the American student, while the introduction of [illegible] illustrations, and the most careful mechanical execution, render the volume one of the [illegible] tractive as yet issued.

For upwards of thirteen years Dr. Carpenter's work has been considered by the profession generally, both in this country and England, as the most valuable compendium on the subject of physiology in our language. This distinction it owes to the high attainments and unwearied industry of its accomplished author. The present edition (which, like the last American one, was prepared by the author himself), is the result of such extensive revision, that it may almost be considered a new work. We need hardly say, in concluding this brief notice, that while the work is indispensable to every student of medicine in this country, it will amply repay the practitioner for its perusal by the interest and value of its contents.—*Boston Med. and Surg. Journal.*

This is a standard work—the text-book used by all medical students who read the English language. It has passed through several editions in order to keep pace with the rapidly growing science of Physiology. Nothing need be said in its praise, for its merits are universally known; we have nothing to say of its defects, for they only appear where the science of which it treats is incomplete.—*Western Lancet.*

The most complete exposition of physiology which any language can at present give.—*Brit. and For. Med.-Chirurg. Review.*

The greatest, the most reliable, and the best book on the subject which we know of in the English language.—*Stethoscope.*

To eulogize this great work would be [illegible] We should observe, however, that [illegible] the author has remodelled a large [illegible] former, and the editor has added [illegible] terest, especially in the form of [illegible] may confidently recommend it as the [illegible] work on Human Physiology in our [illegible]—*Southern Med. and Surg. Journal.*

The most complete work on the [illegible] language.—*Am. Med. Journal.*

The most complete work now extant in our language.—*N. O. Med. Register.*

The best text-book in the language on this extensive subject.—*London Med.* [illegible]

A complete cyclopedia of this [illegible]—*N. Y. Med. Times.*

The profession of this country, [illegible] of Europe, have anxiously [illegible] the announcement of this new [illegible] Human Physiology. The [illegible] many years been unable [illegible] siology in all our medical [illegible] tion among the profession [illegible] any work in any department [illegible]

It is quite unnecessary [illegible] work as its merits [illegible] announcement of its [illegible] pleasure to every [illegible] perusal will be of infinite service [illegible] physiological science.—*Ohio Med. and Surg. Journal.*

BY THE SAME AUTHOR.

PRINCIPLES OF COMPARATIVE PHYSIOLOGY. New American, from the Fourth and Revised London edition. In one large and handsome octavo volume, with over three hundred beautiful illustrations. pp. 752. Extra cloth, $4.80; leather, [illegible]

The delay which has existed in the appearance of this work has been caused by the [illegible] revision and remodelling which it has undergone at the hands of the author, and [illegible] of new illustrations which have been prepared for it. It will, therefore, be [illegible] work, and fully up to the day in every department of the subject, rendering it [illegible] for all students engaged in this branch of science. Every effort has been made to [illegible] graphical finish and mechanical execution worthy of its exalted reputation [illegible] mechanical arts of this country.

This book should not only be read but thoroughly studied by every member of the profession. None are too wise or old, to be benefited thereby. But especially to the younger class would we cordially commend it as best fitted of any work in the English language to qualify them for the reception and comprehension of those truths which are daily being developed in physiology.—*Medical Counsellor.*

Without pretending to it, it is an encyclopedia of the subject, accurate and complete in all respects—a truthful reflection of the advanced state at which the science has now arrived.—*Dublin Quarterly Journal of Medical Science.*

A truly magnificent work—in itself a perfect physiological study.—*Ranking's Abstract.*

This work stands without its fellow. It is one few men in Europe could have undertaken; it is one no man, we believe, could [illegible] cessful an issue as Dr. Carpenter [illegible] its production a physiological [illegible] the labors of others, [illegible] critical, and unprejudiced [illegible] of combining the varied, heterogeneous [illegible] his disposal, so as to form an harmonious [illegible] We feel that this abstract [illegible] imperfect idea of the [illegible] idea of its unity, of [illegible] material has been [illegible] sources, to condense [illegible] ity of the reasoning [illegible] of language in which [illegible] profession only, but [illegible] must feel deeply [illegible] great work. It [illegible] his high reputation.—[illegible]

CARPENTER (WILLIAM B.), M. D., F. R. S.,

Examiner in Physiology and Comparative Anatomy in the University of London.

THE MICROSCOPE AND ITS REVELATIONS. With an Appendix containing the Applications of the Microscope to Clinical Medicine, &c. By F. G. SMITH, M. D. Illustrated by four hundred and thirty-four beautiful engravings on wood. In one large and very handsome octavo volume, of 724 pages, extra cloth, $4 00; leather, $4 50.

Dr. Carpenter's position as a microscopist and physiologist, and his great experience as a teacher, eminently qualify him to produce what has long been wanted—a good text-book on the practical use of the microscope. In the present volume his object has been, as stated in his Preface, "to combine, within a moderate compass, that information with regard to the use of his 'tools,' which is most essential to the working microscopist, with such an account of the objects best fitted for his study, as might qualify him to comprehend what he observes, and might thus prepare him to benefit science, whilst expanding and refreshing his own mind." That he has succeeded in accomplishing this, no one acquainted with his previous labors can doubt.

The great importance of the microscope as a means of diagnosis, and the number of microscopists who are also physicians, have induced the American publishers, with the author's approval, to add an Appendix, carefully prepared by Professor Smith, on the applications of the instrument to clinical medicine, together with an account of American Microscopes, their modifications and accessories. This portion of the work is illustrated with nearly one hundred wood-cuts, and, it is hoped, will adapt the volume more particularly to the use of the American student.

Every care has been taken in the mechanical execution of the work, which is confidently presented as in no respect inferior to the choicest productions of the London press.

The mode in which the author has executed his intentions may be gathered from the following condensed synopsis of the

CONTENTS.

Those who are acquainted with Dr. Carpenter's previous writings on Animal and Vegetable Physiology, will fully understand how vast a store of knowledge he is able to bring to bear upon so comprehensive a subject as the revelations of the microscope; and even those who have no previous acquaintance with the construction or uses of this instrument, will find abundance of information conveyed in clear and simple language.—*Med. Times and Gazette.*

Although originally not intended as a strictly medical work, the additions by Prof. Smith give it a positive claim upon the profession, for which we doubt not he will receive their sincere thanks. Indeed, we know not where the student of medicine will find such a complete and satisfactory collection of microscopic facts bearing upon physiology and practical medicine as is contained in Prof. Smith's appendix; and this of itself, it seems to us, is fully worth the cost of the volume.—*Louisville Medical Review*, Nov. 1856.

BY THE SAME AUTHOR.

ELEMENTS (OR MANUAL) OF PHYSIOLOGY, INCLUDING PHYSIOLOGICAL ANATOMY. Second American, from a new and revised London edition. With one hundred and ninety illustrations. In one very handsome octavo volume, leather. pp. 566. $3 00.

In publishing the first edition of this work, its title was altered from that of the London volume, by the substitution of the word "Elements" for that of "Manual," and with the author's sanction the title of "Elements" is still retained as being more expressive of the scope of the treatise.

To say that it is the best manual of Physiology now before the public, would not do sufficient justice to the author.—*Buffalo Medical Journal.*

In his former works it would seem that he had exhausted the subject of Physiology. In the present, he gives the essence, as it were, of the whole.—*N. Y. Journal of Medicine.*

Those who have occasion for an elementary treatise on Physiology, cannot do better than to possess themselves of the manual of Dr. Carpenter.—*Medical Examiner.*

The best and most complete exposé of modern Physiology, in one volume, extant in the English language.—*St. Louis Medical Journal.*

BY THE SAME AUTHOR. (*Preparing.*)

PRINCIPLES OF GENERAL PHYSIOLOGY, INCLUDING ORGANIC CHEMISTRY AND HISTOLOGY. With a General Sketch of the Vegetable and Animal Kingdom. In one large and very handsome octavo volume, with several hundred illustrations.

The subject of general physiology having been omitted in the last editions of the author's "Comparative Physiology" and "Human Physiology," he has undertaken to prepare a volume which shall present it more thoroughly and fully than has yet been attempted, and which may be regarded as an introduction to his other works.

BY THE SAME AUTHOR.

A PRIZE ESSAY ON THE USE OF ALCOHOLIC LIQUORS IN HEALTH AND DISEASE. New edition, with a Preface by D. F. CONDIE, M. D., and explanations of scientific words. In one neat 12mo. volume, extra cloth. pp. 178. 50 cents.

CONDIE (D. F.), M.D., &c.

A PRACTICAL TREATISE ON THE DISEASES OF CHILDREN. Fifth edition, revised and augmented. In one large volume, 8vo., leather, [illegible] (*Just Issued*, 1859.)

In presenting a new and revised edition of this favorite work, the publishers [illegible] that the author has endeavored to render it in every respect "a complete and [illegible] of the pathology and therapeutics of the maladies incident to the earlier stages of [illegible] and exact account of the diseases of infancy and childhood." To accomplish this [illegible] the whole work to a careful and thorough revision, rewriting a considerable [illegible] several new chapters. In this manner it is hoped that any deficiencies which [illegible] existed have been supplied, that the recent labors of practitioners and [illegible] roughly incorporated, and that in every point the work will be found [illegible] it has enjoyed as a complete and thoroughly practical book of reference [illegible]

A few notices of previous editions are subjoined.

Dr. Condie's scholarship, acumen, industry, and practical sense are manifested in this, as in all his numerous contributions to science.—*Dr. Holmes's Report to the American Medical Association.*

Taken as a whole, in our judgment, Dr. Condie's Treatise is the one from the perusal of which the practitioner in this country will rise with the greatest satisfaction.—*Western Journal of Medicine and Surgery.*

One of the best works upon the Diseases of Children in the English language.—*Western Lancet.*

We feel assured from actual experience that no physician's library can be complete without a copy of this work.—*N. Y. Journal of Medicine.*

A veritable pediatric encyclopædia, and an honor to American medical literature.—*Ohio Medical and Surgical Journal.*

We feel persuaded that the American medical profession will soon regard it not only as a very good, but as the VERY BEST "Practical Treatise on the Diseases of Children."—*American Medical Journal.*

In the department of infantile therapeutics, the work of Dr. Condie is considered one of the best which has been published in the English language. —*The Stethoscope.*

We pronounced the first edition [illegible] work on the diseases of [illegible] language, and, notwithstanding [illegible] published, we still regard it [illegible] *Examiner.*

The value of works by [illegible] cases which the physician is [illegible] will be appreciated by [illegible] die has gained for [illegible] for students, and a [illegible] those engaged in [illegible]

This is the fourth edition [illegible] lar treatise. During the [illegible] tion, it has been subjected to a thorough [illegible] by the author; and all [illegible] pathology and therapeutics [illegible] included in the present volume [illegible] we do not know of a better [illegible] dren, and to a large part [illegible] yield as [illegible] *Journal.*

Perhaps the most [illegible] fore the profession [illegible] may say in the [illegible] rior to most of [illegible] *Journal.*

CHRISTISON (ROBERT), M. D., V. P. R. [illegible]

A DISPENSATORY; or, Commentary on the Pharmacopœias [illegible] and the United States; comprising the Natural History, Description, [illegible] tions, Uses, and Doses of the Articles of the Materia Medica. Second [illegible] proved, with a Supplement containing the most important New Remedies [illegible] tions, and two hundred and thirteen large wood-engravings. By R. [illegible] In one very large and handsome octavo volume, leather, raised bands, of [illegible]

COOPER (BRANSBY B.), F. R. S.

LECTURES ON THE PRINCIPLES AND PRACTICE OF SURGERY. In one very large octavo volume, extra cloth, of 750 pages. $3 00.

COOPER ON DISLOCATIONS AND FRACTURES OF THE JOINTS.—Edited by BRANSBY B. COOPER, F. R. S., &c. With additional Observations by Prof. J. C. WARREN. A new American edition. In one handsome octavo volume, extra cloth, of about 500 pages, with numerous illustrations on wood. $3 25.

COOPER ON THE ANATOMY AND DISEASES OF THE BREAST, with twenty-five Miscellaneous and Surgical Papers. One large volume, imperial 8vo., extra cloth, with 252 figures, on 36 plates. $2 50.

COOPER ON THE STRUCTURE AND DISEASES OF THE TESTIS, AND ON THE THYMUS GLAND. One vol. imperial 8vo., extra cloth, with 177 figures on 29 plates. $2 00.

COPLAND ON THE [illegible] TREATMENT OF PALSY AND [illegible] In one volume, royal [illegible] 80 cents.

CLYMER ON FEVERS [illegible] PATHOLOGY, AND [illegible] octavo volume, leather, [illegible]

COLOMBAT DE L'ISERE [illegible] OF FEMALES, and [illegible] their Sex. Translated [illegible] ditions, by C. D. M[illegible] revised and improved. [illegible] tavo, leather, with numerous [illegible] $3 50.

CARSON (JOSEPH), M. D.,

Professor of Materia Medica and Pharmacy in the University of [illegible]

SYNOPSIS OF THE COURSE OF LECTURES ON MATERIA [illegible] AND PHARMACY, delivered in the University of Pennsylvania. [illegible] tion. In one very neat octavo volume, extra cloth, of 208 pages. [illegible]

CURLING (T. B.), F. R. S.,

Surgeon to the London Hospital, President of the Hunterian [illegible]

A PRACTICAL TREATISE ON DISEASES OF THE [illegible] TIC CORD, AND SCROTUM. Second American, from the [illegible] tion. In one handsome octavo volume, extra cloth, with numerous [illegible]

CHURCHILL (FLEETWOOD), M. D., M. R. I. A.

ON THE THEORY AND PRACTICE OF MIDWIFERY. A new American from the fourth revised and enlarged London edition. With Notes and Additions, by D. FRANCIS CONDIE, M. D., author of a "Practical Treatise on the Diseases of Children," &c. With 194 illustrations. In one very handsome octavo volume, leather, of nearly 700 large pages. $3 50. (*Now Ready*, Sept. 1860)

This work has been so long an established favorite, both as a text-book for the learner and as a reliable aid in consultation for the practitioner, that in presenting a new edition it is only necessary to call attention to the very extended improvements which it has received. Having had the benefit of two revisions by the author since the last American reprint, it has been materially enlarged, and Dr. Churchill's well-known conscientious industry is a guarantee that every portion has been thoroughly brought up with the latest results of European investigation in all departments of the science and art of obstetrics. The recent date of the last Dublin edition has not left much of novelty for the American editor to introduce, but he has endeavored to insert whatever has since appeared, together with such matters as his experience has shown him would be desirable for the American student, including a large number of illustrations. With the sanction of the author he has added in the form of an appendix, some chapters from a little "Manual for Midwives and Nurses," recently issued by Dr. Churchill, believing that the details there presented can hardly fail to prove of advantage to the junior practitioner. The result of all these additions is that the work now contains fully one-half more matter than the last American edition, with nearly one-half more illustrations, so that notwithstanding the use of a smaller type, the volume contains almost two hundred pages more than before.

No effort has been spared to secure an improvement in the mechanical execution of the work equal to that which the text has received, and the volume is confidently presented as one of the handsomest that has thus far been laid before the American profession; while the very low price at which it is offered should secure for it a place in every lecture-room and on every office table.

A better book in which to learn these important points we have not met than Dr. Churchill's. Every page of it is full of instruction; the opinion of all writers of authority is given on questions of difficulty, as well as the directions and advice of the learned author himself, to which he adds the result of statistical inquiry, putting statistics in their proper place and giving them their due weight, and no more. We have never read a book more free from professional jealousy than Dr. Churchill's. It appears to be written with the true design of a book on medicine, viz: to give all that is known on the subject of which he treats, both theoretically and practically, and to advance such opinions of his own as he believes will benefit medical science, and insure the safety of the patient. We have said enough to convey to the profession that this book of Dr. Churchill's is admirably suited for a book of reference for the practitioner, as well as a text-book for the student, and we hope it may be extensively purchased amongst our readers. To them we most strongly recommend it.—*Dublin Medical Press*, June 20, 1860.

To bestow praise on a book that has received such marked approbation would be superfluous. We need only say, therefore, that if the first edition was thought worthy of a favorable reception by the medical public, we can confidently affirm that this will be found much more so. The lecturer, the practitioner, and the student, may all have recourse to its pages, and derive from their perusal much interest and instruction in everything relating to theoretical and practical midwifery.—*Dublin Quarterly Journal of Medical Science.*

A work of very great merit, and such as we can confidently recommend to the study of every obstetric practitioner.—*London Medical Gazette.*

This is certainly the most perfect system extant. It is the best adapted for the purposes of a textbook, and that which he whose necessities confine him to one book, should select in preference to all others.—*Southern Medical and Surgical Journal.*

The most popular work on midwifery ever issued from the American press.—*Charleston Med. Journal.*

Were we reduced to the necessity of having but one work on midwifery, and permitted to choose, we would unhesitatingly take Churchill.—*Western Med. and Surg. Journal.*

It is impossible to conceive a more useful and elegant manual than Dr. Churchill's Practice of Midwifery.—*Provincial Medical Journal.*

Certainly, in our opinion, the very best work on the subject which exists.—*N. Y. Annalist.*

No work holds a higher position, or is more deserving of being placed in the hands of the tyro, the advanced student, or the practitioner.—*Medical Examiner.*

Previous editions, under the editorial supervision of Prof. R. M. Huston, have been received with marked favor, and they deserved it; but this, reprinted from a very late Dublin edition, carefully revised and brought up by the author to the present time, does present an unusually accurate and able exposition of every important particular embraced in the department of midwifery. * * The clearness, directness, and precision of its teachings, together with the great amount of statistical research which its text exhibits, have served to place it already in the foremost rank of works in this department of remedial science.—*N. O. Med. and Surg. Journal.*

In our opinion, it forms one of the best if not the very best text-book and epitome of obstetric science which we at present possess in the English language.—*Monthly Journal of Medical Science.*

The clearness and precision of style in which it is written, and the great amount of statistical research which it contains, have served to place it in the first rank of works in this department of medical science.—*N. Y. Journal of Medicine.*

Few treatises will be found better adapted as a text-book for the student, or as a manual for the frequent consultation of the young practitioner.—*American Medical Journal.*

BY THE SAME AUTHOR. (*Lately Published.*)

ON THE DISEASES OF INFANTS AND CHILDREN. Second American Edition, revised and enlarged by the author. Edited, with Notes, by W. V. KEATING, M. D. In one large and handsome volume, extra cloth, of over 700 pages. $3 00, or in leather, $3 25.

In preparing this work a second time for the American profession, the author has spared no labor in giving it a very thorough revision, introducing several new chapters, and rewriting others, while every portion of the volume has been subjected to a severe scrutiny. The efforts of the American editor have been directed to supplying such information relative to matters peculiar to this country as might have escaped the attention of the author, and the whole may, therefore, be safely pronounced one of the most complete works on the subject accessible to the American Profession. By an alteration in the size of the page, these very extensive additions have been accommodated without unduly increasing the size of the work.

BY THE SAME AUTHOR.

ESSAYS ON THE PUERPERAL FEVER, AND OTHER DISEASES PE-CULIAR TO WOMEN. Selected from the writings of British Authors previous to the close of the Eighteenth Century. In one neat octavo volume, extra cloth, of about 450 pages.

CHURCHILL (FLEETWOOD), M. D., M. R. [illegible]

ON THE DISEASES OF WOMEN; including those of [illegible] bed. A new American edition, revised by the Author. With Notes and [illegible] on Condie, M. D., author of "A Practical Treatise on the Diseases of Children," [illegible] rous illustrations. In one large and handsome octavo volume, leather, of [illegible]

This edition of Dr. Churchill's very popular treatise may almost be [illegible] thoroughly has he revised it in every portion. It will be found greatly enlarged, [illegible] brought up to the most recent condition of the subject, while the very [illegible] them introduced, representing such pathological conditions as can be [illegible] a novel feature, and afford valuable assistance to the young practitioner. [illegible] peared desirable for the American student have been made by the editor, Dr. [illegible] marked improvement in the mechanical execution keeps pace with the [illegible] which the volume has undergone, while the price has been kept at the former [illegible]

It comprises, unquestionably, one of the most exact and comprehensive expositions of the present state of medical knowledge in respect to the diseases of women that has yet been published.—*Am. Journ. Med. Sciences*, July, 1857.

This work is the most reliable which we possess on this subject; and is deservedly popular with the profession.—*Charleston Med. Journal*, July, 1857.

We know of no author who deserves that approbation, on "the diseases of females," to the same extent that Dr. Churchill does. [illegible] only thorough treatise we [illegible] and it may be consulted [illegible] dents as a masterpiece [illegible] —*The Western Journal of* [illegible]

As a comprehensive [illegible] work of reference for practitioners, [illegible] other that has ever issued on the [illegible] the British press.—*Dublin* [illegible]

DICKSON (S. H.), M. D.,

Professor of Practice of Medicine in the Jefferson Medical College, Philadelphia.

ELEMENTS OF MEDICINE; a Compendious View of Pathology [illegible] peutics, or the History and Treatment of Diseases. Second edition, revised. [illegible] handsome octavo volume, of 750 pages, leather. $3 75. (*Just Issued.*)

The steady demand which has so soon exhausted the first edition of this work [illegible] that the author was not mistaken in supposing that a volume of this character [illegible] elementary manual of practice, which should present the leading principles [illegible] practical results, in a condensed and perspicuous manner. Disencumbered of [illegible] and fruitless speculations, it embodies what is most requisite for the student, [illegible] same time what the active practitioner wants when obliged, in the daily calls of his [illegible] refresh his memory on special points. The clear and attractive style of the author [illegible] whole easy of comprehension, while his long experience gives to his teachings an [illegible] where acknowledged. Few physicians, indeed, have had wider opportunities [illegible] experience, and few, perhaps, have used them to better purpose. As the [illegible] voted to study and practice, the present edition, revised and brought up to the [illegible] will doubtless maintain the reputation already acquired as a condensed and [illegible] text-book on the Practice of Medicine.

DRUITT (ROBERT), M. R. C. S., &c.

THE PRINCIPLES AND PRACTICE OF MODERN SURGERY. [illegible] and revised American from the eighth enlarged and improved London edition. Illustrated [illegible] four hundred and thirty-two wood-engravings. In one very handsomely printed [illegible] leather, of nearly 700 large pages. $3 50. (*Now Ready*, Sept. 1859.)

A work which like DRUITT'S SURGERY has for so many years maintained the [illegible] ing favorite with all classes of the profession, needs no special recommendation [illegible] to a revised edition. It is only necessary to state that the author has spared [illegible] work up to its well earned reputation of presenting in a small and convenient [illegible] condition of every department of surgery, considered both as a science and as [illegible] services of a competent American editor have been employed to introduce [illegible] have escaped the author's attention, or may prove of service to the American [illegible] several editions have appeared in London since the issue of the last American [illegible] has had the benefit of repeated revisions by the author, resulting in a very [illegible] improvement. The extent of these additions may be estimated from the [illegible] about one-third more matter than the previous American edition, and [illegible] adoption of a smaller type, the pages have been increased by about one hundred, [illegible] hundred and fifty wood-cuts have been added to the former list of illustrations. [illegible]

A marked improvement will also be perceived in the mechanical [illegible] work, which, printed in the best style, on new type, and fine paper, [illegible] regards external finish; while at the very low price affixed it will be [illegible] volumes accessible to the profession.

This popular volume, now a most comprehensive work on surgery, has undergone many corrections, improvements, and additions, and the principles and the practice of the art have been brought down to the latest record and observation. Of the operations in surgery it is impossible to speak too highly. The descriptions are so clear and concise, and the illustrations so accurate and numerous, that the student can have no difficulty, with instrument in hand, and book by his side, over the dead body, in obtaining a proper knowledge and sufficient tact in this much neglected department of medical education.—*British and Foreign Medico-Chirurg. Review*, Jan. 1860.

In the present edition the author has entirely rewritten many of the chapters, and has incorporated the various improvements and additions in modern surgery. On carefully going over it, we find that nothing of real practical [illegible] ted; it presents a faithful [illegible] lating to surgery up to the [illegible] servedly a popular manual, [illegible] and practitioner.—*London* [illegible]

In closing this brief [illegible] dially as ever this most [illegible] hand-book. It must [illegible] only to the student of surgery, [illegible] practitioner who may [illegible] himself to the study of [illegible] *London Med. Times and* [illegible]

In a word, this [illegible] Manual of Surgery [illegible] or practitioner [illegible] *Journal of Med. Science* [illegible]

DALTON, JR. (J. C.), M. D.

Professor of Physiology in the College of Physicians, New York.

A TREATISE ON HUMAN PHYSIOLOGY, designed for the use of Students and Practitioners of Medicine.

With two hundred and fifty-four illustrations on wood. In one very beautiful octavo volume, of over 600 pages, extra cloth, $4 00; leather, raised bands, $4 25. (*Just Issued.*)

This system of Physiology, both from the excellence of the arrangement studiously observed throughout every page, and the clear, lucid, and instructive manner in which each subject is treated, promises to form one of the most generally received class-books in the English language. It is, in fact, a most admirable epitome of all the really important discoveries that have always been received as incontestable truths, as well as of those which have been recently added to our stock of knowledge on this subject. We will, however, proceed to give a few extracts from the book itself, as a specimen of its style and composition, and this, we conceive, will be quite sufficient to awaken a general interest in a work which is immeasurably superior in its details to the majority of those of the same class to which it belongs. In its purity of style and elegance of composition it may safely take its place with the very best of our English classics; while in accuracy of description it is impossible that it could be surpassed. In every line is beautifully shadowed forth the emanations of the polished scholar, whose reflections are clothed in a garb as interesting as they are impressive; with the one predominant feeling appearing to pervade the whole—an anxious desire to please and at the same time to instruct.—*Dublin Quarterly Journ. of Med. Sciences*, Nov. 1859.

The work before us, however, in our humble judgment, is precisely what it purports to be, and will answer admirably the purpose for which it is intended. It is *par excellence*, a text-book; and the best text-book in this department that we have ever seen. We have carefully read the book, and speak of its merits from a more than cursory perusal. Looking back upon the work we have just finished, we must say a word concerning the excellence of its illustrations. No department is so dependent upon good illustrations, and those which keep pace with our knowledge of the subject, as that of physiology. The wood-cuts in the work before us are the best we have ever seen, and, being original, serve to illustrate precisely what is desired.—*Buffalo Med. Journal*, March, 1859.

A book of genuine merit like this deserves hearty praise before subjecting it to any minute criticism. We are not prepared to find any fault with its design until we have had more time to appreciate its merits as a manual for daily consultation, and to weigh its statements and conclusions more deliberately. Its excellences we are sure of; its defects we have yet to discover. It is a work highly honorable to its author; to his talents, his industry, his training; to the institution with which he is connected, and to American science.—*Boston Med. and Surgical Journal*, Feb. 24, 1859.

A new book and a first rate one; an original book, and one which cannot be too highly appreciated, and which we are proud to see emanating from our country's press. It is by an author who, though young, is considerably famous for physiological research, and who in this work has erected for himself an enduring monument, a token at once of his labor and his success.—*Nashville Medical Journal*, March, 1859.

Throughout the entire work, the definitions are clear and precise, the arrangement admirable, the argument briefly and well stated, and the style nervous, simple, and concise. Section third, treating of Reproduction, is a monograph of unapproached excellence upon this subject, in the English tongue. For precision, elegance and force of style, exhaustive method and extent of treatment, fulness of illustration and weight of personal research, we know of no American contribution to medical science which surpasses it, and the day is far distant when its claims to the respectful attention of even the best informed scholars will not be cheerfully conceded by all acquainted with its range and depth.—*Charleston Med. Journal*, May, 1859.

A new elementary work on Human Physiology lifting up its voice in the presence of late and sturdy editions of Kirke's, Carpenter's, Todd and Bowman's, to say nothing of Dunglison's and Draper's, should have something superior in the matter or the manner of its utterance in order to win for itself deserved attention and a name. That matter and that manner, after a candid perusal, we think distinguish this work, and we are proud to welcome it not merely for its nativity's sake, but for its own intrinsic excellence. Its language we find to be plain, direct, unambitious, and falling with a just conciseness on hypothetical or unsettled questions, and yet with sufficient fulness on those living topics already understood, or the path to whose solution is definitely marked out. It does not speak exhaustively upon every subject that it notices, but it does speak suggestively, experimentally, and to their main utilities. Into the subject of Reproduction our author plunges with a kind of loving spirit. Throughout this interesting and obscure department he is a clear and admirable teacher, sometimes a brilliant leader.—*Am. Med. Monthly*, May, 1859.

DUNGLISON, FORBES, TWEEDIE, AND CONOLLY.

THE CYCLOPÆDIA OF PRACTICAL MEDICINE: comprising Treatises on the Nature and Treatment of Diseases, Materia Medica, and Therapeutics, Diseases of Women and Children, Medical Jurisprudence, &c. &c.

In four large super-royal octavo volumes, of 3254 double-columned pages, strongly and handsomely bound, with raised bands. $12 00.

_ This work contains no less than four hundred and eighteen distinct treatises, contributed by sixty-eight distinguished physicians, rendering it a complete library of reference for the country practitioner.

The most complete work on Practical Medicine extant; or, at least, in our language.—*Buffalo Medical and Surgical Journal*.

For reference, it is above all price to every practitioner.—*Western Lancet*.

One of the most valuable medical publications of the day—as a work of reference it is invaluable.—*Western Journal of Medicine and Surgery*.

It has been to us, both as learner and teacher, a work for ready and frequent reference, one in which modern English medicine is exhibited in the most advantageous light.—*Medical Examiner*.

We rejoice that this work is to be placed within the reach of the profession in this country, it being unquestionably one of very great value to the practitioner. This estimate of it has not been formed from a hasty examination, but after an intimate acquaintance derived from frequent consultation of it during the past nine or ten years. The editors are practitioners of established reputation, and the list of contributors embraces many of the most eminent professors and teachers of London, Edinburgh, Dublin, and Glasgow. It is, indeed, the great merit of this work that the principal articles have been furnished by practitioners who have not only devoted especial attention to the diseases about which they have written, but have also enjoyed opportunities for an extensive practical acquaintance with them, and whose reputation carries the assurance of their competency justly to appreciate the opinions of others, while it stamps their own doctrines with high and just authority.—*American Medical Journ.*

DEWEES'S COMPREHENSIVE SYSTEM OF MIDWIFERY. Illustrated by occasional cases and many engravings. Twelfth edition, with the author's last improvements and corrections. In one octavo volume, extra cloth, of 600 pages. $3 20.

DEWEES'S TREATISE ON THE PHYSICAL AND MEDICAL TREATMENT OF CHILDREN. The last edition. In one volume, octavo, extra cloth, 548 pages. $2 80

DEWEES'S TREATISE ON THE DISEASES OF FEMALES. Tenth edition. In one volume, octavo, extra cloth, 532 pages, with plates. [illegible]

DUNGLISON (ROBLEY), M.D.,

Professor of Institutes of Medicine in the Jefferson Medical College, Philadelphia.

NEW AND ENLARGED EDITION.

MEDICAL LEXICON; a Dictionary of Medical Science; containing [illegible] Explanation of the various Subjects and Terms of Anatomy, Physiology, Pathology, [illegible] Therapeutics, Pharmacology, Pharmacy, Surgery, Obstetrics, Medical Jurisprudence, [illegible] &c. Notices of Climate and of Mineral Waters; Formulæ for Officinal, Empirical, and [illegible] Preparations, &c. With French and other Synonymes. Fifteenth edition, revised, [illegible] greatly enlarged. In one very large and handsome octavo volume, of [illegible] in small type; strongly bound in leather, with raised bands. Price $4 [illegible]

Especial care has been devoted in the preparation of this edition to render it [illegible] worthy a continuance of the very remarkable favor which it has hitherto [illegible] sale of Fifteen large editions, and the constantly increasing demand, [illegible] the profession as the standard authority. Stimulated by this fact, the author has [illegible] present revision to introduce whatever might be necessary "to make it a [illegible] ble—if not indispensable—lexicon, in which the student may search [illegible] every term that has been legitimated in the nomenclature of the science." [illegible] large additions have been found requisite, and the extent of the author's labors [illegible] from the fact that about Six Thousand subjects and terms have been introduced [illegible] dering the whole number of definitions about Sixty Thousand, to accommodate [illegible] ber of pages has been increased by nearly a hundred, notwithstanding [illegible] of the page. The medical press, both in this country and in England, has [illegible] dispensable to all medical students and practitioners, and the present improved [illegible] that enviable reputation.

The publishers have endeavored to render the mechanical execution worthy of [illegible] universal use in daily reference. The greatest care has been exercised to obtain the [illegible] accuracy so necessary in a work of the kind. By the small but exceedingly [illegible] an immense amount of matter is condensed in its thousand ample pages, while [illegible] found strong and durable. With all these improvements and enlargements, the [illegible] at the former very moderate rate, placing it within the reach of all.

This work, the appearance of the fifteenth edition of which, it has become our duty and pleasure to announce, is perhaps the most stupendous monument of labor and erudition in medical literature. One would hardly suppose after constant use of the preceding editions, where we have never failed to find a sufficiently full explanation of every medical term, that in this edition "*about six thousand subjects and terms have been added*," with a careful revision and correction of the entire work. It is only necessary to announce the advent of this edition to make it occupy the place of the preceding one on the table of every medical man, as it is without doubt the best and most comprehensive work of the kind which has ever appeared.—*Buffalo Med. Journ.*, Jan. 1858.

The work is a monument of patient research, skilful judgment, and vast physical labor, that will perpetuate the name of the author more effectually than any possible device of stone or metal. Dr. Dunglison deserves the thanks not only of the American profession, but of the whole medical world.—*North Am. Medico-Chir. Review*, Jan. 1858.

A Medical Dictionary better adapted for the wants of the profession than any other with which we are acquainted, and of a character which places it far above comparison and competition.—*Am. Journ. Med. Sciences*, Jan. 1858.

We need only say, that the addition of 6,000 new terms, with their accompanying definitions, may be said to constitute a new work, by itself. We have examined the Dictionary attentively, and are most happy to pronounce it unrivalled of its kind. The erudition displayed, and the extraordinary industry which must have been demanded, in its preparation and perfection, redound to the lasting credit of its author, and have furnished us with a volume *indispensable* at the present day, to all who would find themselves *au niveau* with the highest standards of medical information.—*Boston Medical and Surgical Journal*, Dec. 31, 1857.

Good lexicons and encyclopedic works generally, are the most labor-saving contrivances which literary men enjoy; and the labor which is required to produce them in the perfect manner of this example is something appalling to contemplate. The author tells us in his preface [illegible] thousand terms and subjects [illegible] before, was considered [illegible] of the kind in any language. [illegible] March, 1858.

He has raised [illegible] tions, and remodelled [illegible] pils. No less than [illegible] and terms are [illegible] edition, swelling the [illegible] sixty thousand! [illegible] sion a complete and [illegible] terminology, without rival [illegible] —*Nashville Journ. of Med.* [illegible]

It is universally [illegible] this work is incomparably [illegible] plete Medical Lexicon [illegible] The amount of labor which [illegible] has bestowed upon it is truly [illegible] learning and research [illegible] are equally remarkable. [illegible] tion are unnecessary, [illegible] thinks of purchasing [illegible] than this.—*St. Louis* [illegible] 1858.

It is the foundation [illegible] ry, and should always [illegible] books purchased by [illegible] *Monthly*, Jan. 1858.

A very perfect work of [illegible] most perfect in the English [illegible] *Surg. Reporter*, Jan. [illegible]

It is now emphatically [illegible] the English language [illegible] tate.—*N. H. Med. Journ.* [illegible]

It is scarcely [illegible] cal library wanting a [illegible] must be imperfect.—[illegible]

We have ever considered [illegible] lished, and the present [illegible] no equal in the world [illegible] Jan. 1858.

The most complete [illegible] found in any language.—[illegible]

BY THE SAME AUTHOR.

THE PRACTICE OF MEDICINE. A Treatise on Special [illegible] rapeutics. Third Edition. In two large octavo volumes, leather, [illegible]

DUNGLISON (ROBLEY), M. D.,

Professor of Institutes of Medicine in the Jefferson Medical College, Philadelphia.

HUMAN PHYSIOLOGY. Eighth edition. Thoroughly revised and extensively modified and enlarged, with five hundred and thirty-two illustrations. In two large and handsomely printed octavo volumes, leather, of about 1500 pages. $[illegible] 00.

In revising this work for its eighth appearance, the author has spared no labor to render it worthy a continuance of the very great favor which has been extended to it by the profession. The whole contents have been rearranged, and to a great extent remodelled; the investigations which of late years have been so numerous and so important, have been carefully examined and incorporated, and the work in every respect has been brought up to a level with the present state of the subject. The object of the author has been to render it a concise but comprehensive treatise, containing the whole body of physiological science, to which the student and man of science can at all times refer with the certainty of finding whatever they are in search of, fully presented in all its aspects; and on no former edition has the author bestowed more labor to secure this result.

We believe that it can truly be said, no more complete repertory of facts upon the subject treated, can anywhere be found. The author has, moreover, that enviable tact at description and that facility and ease of expression which render him peculiarly acceptable to the casual, or the studious reader. This faculty, so requisite in setting forth many graver and less attractive subjects, lends additional charms to one always fascinating.—*Boston Med. and Surg. Journal*, Sept. 1856.

The most complete and satisfactory system of Physiology in the English language.—*Amer. Med. Journal.*

The best work of the kind in the English language.—*Silliman's Journal.*

The present edition the author has made a perfect mirror of the science as it is at the present hour. As a work upon physiology proper, the science of the functions performed by the body, the student will find it all he wishes.—*Nashville Journ. of Med.*, Sept. 1856.

That he has succeeded, most admirably succeeded in his purpose, is apparent from the appearance of an eighth edition. It is now the great encyclopædia on the subject, and worthy of a place in every physician's library.—*Western Lancet*, Sept. 1856.

BY THE SAME AUTHOR. (*A new edition.*)

GENERAL THERAPEUTICS AND MATERIA MEDICA; adapted for a Medical Text-book. With Indexes of Remedies and of Diseases and their Remedies. Sixth Edition, revised and improved. With one hundred and ninety-three illustrations. In two large and handsomely printed octavo vols., leather, of about 1100 pages. $6 00.

In announcing a new edition of Dr. Dunglison's General Therapeutics and Materia Medica, we have no words of commendation to bestow upon a work whose merits have been heretofore so often and so justly extolled. It must not be supposed, however, that the present is a mere reprint of the previous edition; the character of the author for laborious research, judicious analysis, and clearness of expression, is fully sustained by the numerous additions he has made to the work, and the careful revision to which he has subjected the whole.—*N. A. Medico-Chir. Review*, Jan. 1858.

The work will, we have little doubt, be bought and read by the majority of medical students; its size, arrangement, and reliability recommend it to all; no one, we venture to predict, will study it without profit, and there are few to whom it will not be in some measure useful as a work of reference. The young practitioner, more especially, will find the copious indexes appended to this edition of great assistance in the selection and preparation of suitable formulæ.—*Charleston Med. Journ. and Review*, Jan. 1858.

BY THE SAME AUTHOR. (*A new Edition.*)

NEW REMEDIES, WITH FORMULÆ FOR THEIR PREPARATION AND ADMINISTRATION. Seventh edition, with extensive Additions. In one very large octavo volume, leather, of 770 pages. $3 75.

Another edition of the "New Remedies" having been called for, the author has endeavored to add everything of moment that has appeared since the publication of the last edition.

The articles treated of in the former editions will be found to have undergone considerable expansion in this, in order that the author might be enabled to introduce, as far as practicable, the results of the subsequent experience of others, as well as of his own observation and reflection; and to make the work still more deserving of the extended circulation with which the preceding editions have been favored by the profession. By an enlargement of the page, the numerous additions have been incorporated without greatly increasing the bulk of the volume.—*Preface.*

One of the most useful of the author's works.—*Southern Medical and Surgical Journal.*

This elaborate and useful volume should be found in every medical library, for as a book of reference, for physicians, it is unsurpassed by any other work in existence, and the double index for diseases and for remedies, will be found greatly to enhance its value.—*New York Med. Gazette.*

The great learning of the author, and his remarkable industry in pushing his researches into every source whence information is derivable, have enabled him to throw together an extensive mass of facts and statements, accompanied by full reference to authorities; which last feature renders the work practically valuable to investigators who desire to examine the original papers.—*The American Journal of Pharmacy.*

ELLIS (BENJAMIN), M. D.

THE MEDICAL FORMULARY: being a Collection of Prescriptions, derived from the writings and practice of many of the most eminent physicians of America and Europe. Together with the usual Dietetic Preparations and Antidotes for Poisons. To which is added an Appendix, on the Endermic use of Medicines, and on the use of Ether and Chloroform. The whole accompanied with a few brief Pharmaceutic and Medical Observations. Tenth edition, revised and much extended by Robert P. Thomas, M. D., Professor of Materia Medica in the Philadelphia College of Pharmacy. In one neat octavo volume, extra cloth, of [illegible] pages. $[illegible]

ERICHSEN (JOHN),

Professor of Surgery in University College, London, &c.

THE SCIENCE AND ART OF SURGERY; BEING A TREATISE ON SURGICAL INJURIES, DISEASES, AND OPERATIONS.

New and improved American, [illegible] and carefully revised English edition. Illustrated with over [illegible]. In one large and handsome octavo volume, of one thousand [illegible], raised bands. $4 50. (Just Issued.)

The very distinguished favor with which this work has been received [illegible] has stimulated the author to render it even more worthy of the [illegible] attained as a standard authority. Every portion has been carefully [illegible] have been made, and the most watchful care has been exercised [illegible] of the most advanced condition of surgical science. In this manner the work has [illegible] about a hundred pages, while the series of engravings has been [illegible] rendering it one of the most thoroughly illustrated volumes before the profession. [illegible] the author having rendered unnecessary much of the notes of the former American [illegible] has been added in this country; some few notes and occasional illustrations have [illegible] introduced to elucidate American modes of practice.

It is, in our humble judgment, decidedly the best book of the kind in the English language. Strange that just such books are not oftener produced by public teachers of surgery in this country and Great Britain. Indeed, it is a matter of great astonishment, but no less true than astonishing, that of the many works on surgery republished in this country within the last fifteen or twenty years as text-books for medical students, this is the only one that even approximates to the fulfilment of the peculiar wants of young men just entering upon the study of this branch of the profession.—Western Jour. of Med. and Surgery.

Its value is greatly enhanced by a very copious well-arranged index. We regard this as one of the most valuable contributions to modern surgery. To one entering his novitiate of practice, we regard it the most serviceable guide which he can consult. He will find a fulness of detail leading him through every step of the [illegible] first lesson of [illegible]

[illegible]

Prof. Erichsen's work, [illegible] surpassed; his nine hundred [illegible] finely illustrated, are rich in [illegible] and [illegible] for information [illegible] hour of peril.—N. O. [illegible]

FLINT (AUSTIN), M. D.,

Professor of the Theory and Practice of Medicine in the University of [illegible]

PHYSICAL EXPLORATION AND DIAGNOSIS OF DISEASES [illegible]ING THE RESPIRATORY ORGANS.

In one large [illegible] cloth, 636 pages. $3 00.

We regard it, in point both of arrangement and of the marked ability of its treatment of the subjects, as destined to take the first rank in works of this class. So far as our information extends, it has at present no equal. To the practitioner, as well as the student, it will be invaluable in clearing up the diagnosis of doubtful cases, and in shedding light upon difficult phenomena.—Buffalo Med. Journal.

A work of original [illegible] We recommend the treatise [illegible] to become a [illegible] large extent upon [illegible] carries the evidence of [illegible] tion upon every page. It [illegible] and, through them, to the profession [illegible] It is, what we cannot [illegible]

BY THE SAME AUTHOR. (Now Ready.)

A PRACTICAL TREATISE ON THE DIAGNOSIS, PATHOLOGY, AND TREATMENT OF DISEASES OF THE HEART.

In one [illegible] 500 pages, extra cloth. $2 75.

We do not know that Dr. Flint has written anything which is not first rate; but this, his latest contribution to medical literature, in our opinion, surpasses all the others. The work is most comprehensive in its scope, and most sound in the views it enunciates. The descriptions are clear and methodical; the statements are substantiated by facts, and are made with such simplicity and sincerity, that without them they would carry conviction. The style is admirably clear, direct, and free from dryness. With Dr. Walshe's excellent treatise before us, we have no hesitation in saying that Dr. Flint's book is the best work on the heart in the English language.—Boston Med. and Surg. Journal, Dec. 15, 1859.

We have thus endeavored to present our readers with a fair analysis of this remarkable work. Preferring to employ the very words of the distinguished author, wherever it was possible, we have essayed to condense into the briefest space the general views of his observations and suggestions, and to direct the attention of our brethren to the abounding stores of valuable matter here collected and arranged for their use and instruction. No medical library will hereafter be considered complete without this volume; and we trust it will promptly find its way into the hands of every American student and physician.—N. Am. Med. Chir. Review, Jan. 1860.

This last work of Prof. Flint will add much to his previous well-earned celebrity, as a writer of great force and beauty, and, with his previous work, places him at the head of American writers upon diseases of the chest. [illegible] upon the heart as a [illegible] more valuable [illegible] kind that has yet [illegible] Dec. 1859.

With more than [illegible] this work, for it [illegible] books for our schools [illegible] the most valuable practical [illegible] Med. [illegible], Nov. 1859.

In regard to the [illegible] hesitation in [illegible] diciness. [illegible] such a work [illegible] hands of every practitioner.—[illegible] April, 1860.

But these are very trivial [illegible] present no [illegible] of the author's ability [illegible] ence.—Dublin [illegible] Feb. 1860.

He has achieved [illegible] and his place [illegible] is becoming [illegible] whose skill is [illegible] degree. Our [illegible] analysis, and [illegible] commending it [illegible] readers in the profession.—[illegible] Feb. 1860.

FOWNES (GEORGE), PH. D., &c.

A MANUAL OF ELEMENTARY CHEMISTRY; Theoretical and Practical.

From the seventh revised and corrected London edition. With one hundred and ninety-seven illustrations. Edited by ROBERT BRIDGES, M. D. In one large royal 12mo. volume, of 600 pages. In leather, $1 65; extra cloth, $1 50. (*Just Issued.*)

The death of the author having placed the editorial care of this work in the practised hands of Drs. Bence Jones and A. W. Hoffman, everything has been done in its revision which experience could suggest to keep it on a level with the rapid advance of chemical science. The additions requisite to this purpose have necessitated an enlargement of the page, notwithstanding which the work has been increased by about fifty pages. At the same time every care has been used to maintain its distinctive character as a condensed manual for the student, divested of all unnecessary detail or mere theoretical speculation. The additions have, of course, been mainly in the department of Organic Chemistry, which has made such rapid progress within the last few years, but yet equal attention has been bestowed on the other branches of the subject—Chemical Physics and Inorganic Chemistry—to present all investigations and discoveries of importance, and to keep up the reputation of the volume as a complete manual of the whole science, admirably adapted for the learner. By the use of a small but exceedingly clear type the matter of a large octavo is compressed within the convenient and portable limits of a moderate sized duodecimo, and at the very low price affixed, it is offered as one of the cheapest volumes before the profession.

Dr. Fownes' excellent work has been universally recognized everywhere in his own and this country, as the best elementary treatise on chemistry in the English tongue, and is very generally adopted, we believe, as the standard text book in all our colleges, both literary and scientific.—*Charleston Med. Journ. and Review*, Sept. 1858.

A standard manual, which has long enjoyed the reputation of embodying much knowledge in a small space. The author has achieved the difficult task of condensation with masterly tact. His book is concise without being dry, and brief without being too dogmatical or general.—*Virginia Med. and Surgical Journal.*

The work of Dr. Fownes has long been before the public, and its merits have been fully appreciated as the best text-book on chemistry now in existence. We do not, of course, place it in a rank superior to the works of Brande, Graham, Turner, Gregory, or Gmelin, but we say that, as a work for students, it is preferable to any of them.—*London Journal of Medicine.*

A work well adapted to the wants of the student It is an excellent exposition of the chief doctrines and facts of modern chemistry. The size of the work, and still more the condensed yet perspicuous style in which it is written, absolve it from the charges very properly urged against most manuals termed popular.—*Edinburgh Journal of Medical Science.*

FISKE FUND PRIZE ESSAYS — THE EFFECTS OF CLIMATE ON TUBERCULOUS DISEASE. By EDWIN LEE, M.R.C.S., London, and THE INFLUENCE OF PREGNANCY ON THE DEVELOPMENT OF TUBERCLES. By EDWARD WARREN, M.D., of Edenton, N.C. Together in one neat 8vo. volume, extra cloth. $1 00.

FRICK ON RENAL AFFECTIONS; their Diagnosis and Pathology. With illustrations. One volume, royal 12mo., extra cloth. 75 cents.

FERGUSSON (WILLIAM), F. R. S.,

Professor of Surgery in King's College, London, &c.

A SYSTEM OF PRACTICAL SURGERY. Fourth American, from the third

and enlarged London edition. In one large and beautifully printed octavo volume, of about 700 pages, with 393 handsome illustrations, leather. $3 00.

GRAHAM (THOMAS), F. R. S.

THE ELEMENTS OF INORGANIC CHEMISTRY, including the Applica-

tions of the Science in the Arts. New and much enlarged edition, by HENRY WATTS and ROBERT BRIDGES, M. D. Complete in one large and handsome octavo volume, of over 800 very large pages, with two hundred and thirty-two wood-cuts, extra cloth. $4 00.

*** Part II., completing the work from p. 431 to end, with Index, Title Matter, &c., may be had separate, cloth backs and paper sides. Price $2 50.

From Prof. E. N. Horsford, Harvard College.

It has, in its earlier and less perfect editions, been familiar to me, and the excellence of its plan and the clearness and completeness of its discussions, have long been my admiration.

No reader of English works on this science can afford to be without this edition of Prof. Graham's Elements.—*Silliman's Journal*, March, 1858.

From Prof. Wolcott Gibbs, N. Y. Free Academy.

The work is an admirable one in all respects, and its republication here cannot fail to exert a positive influence upon the progress of science in this country.

GRIFFITH (ROBERT E.), M. D., &c.

A UNIVERSAL FORMULARY, containing the methods of Preparing and Ad-

ministering Officinal and other Medicines. The whole adapted to Physicians and Pharmaceutists. SECOND EDITION, thoroughly revised, with numerous additions, by ROBERT P. THOMAS, M. D., Professor of Materia Medica in the Philadelphia College of Pharmacy. In one large and handsome octavo volume, extra cloth, of 650 pages, double columns. $3 00; or in sheep, $3 25.

It was a work requiring much perseverance, and when published was looked upon as by far the best work of its kind that had issued from the American press. Prof Thomas has certainly "improved," as well as added to this Formulary, and has rendered it additionally deserving of the confidence of pharmaceutists and physicians.—*Am Journal of Pharmacy.*

We are happy to announce a new and improved edition of this, one of the most valuable and useful works that have emanated from an American pen. It would do credit to any country, and will be found of daily usefulness to practitioners of medicine; it is better adapted to their purposes than the dispensatories.—*Southern Med. and Surg. Journal.*

It is one of the most useful books a country practitioner can possibly have.—*Medical Chronicle.*

This is a work of six hundred and fifty-one pages, embracing all on the subject of preparing and administering medicines that can be desired by the physician and pharmaceutist.—*Western Lancet.*

The amount of useful, every-day matter, for a practicing physician, is really immense.—*Boston Med. and Surg. Journal.*

This edition has been greatly improved by the revision and ample additions of Dr Thomas, and is now, we believe, one of the most complete works of its kind in any language. The additions amount to about seventy pages, and no effort has been spared to include in them all the recent improvements [illegible] work of this kind appears to us indispensable [illegible] physician, and there is none we can more [illegible] recommend.—*N. Y. Journal of Medicine.*

[illegible]

A SYSTEM OF [illegible]

[illegible] Illustrated by [illegible] octavo volumes, [illegible] Price [illegible]

[illegible]

"The objects of this work [illegible] practice of surgery, [illegible] faithful and available guide [illegible] writers [illegible] department of [illegible] at undue length, [illegible] from other sources, [illegible] has been to embrace the whole domain of surgery, [illegible] to notice [illegible] the great family of [illegible] plished, it is not for [illegible] to determine. [illegible] properly appertaining to surgery, [illegible] in these volumes. If a larger space than [illegible] inflammation and its results, [illegible] grounded upon long and close observation, [illegible] general practitioner. Special attention [illegible] and an elaborate chapter has been introduced [illegible]

That these intentions have been carried out [illegible] shown by the great extent of the work, and the length [illegible] concentrating on the task his studies and his [illegible] years of lecturing on surgical topics have given, [illegible]

Of Dr. Gross's treatise on Surgery we can say no more than that it is the most elaborate and complete work on this branch of the healing art which has ever been published in any country. A systematic work, it admits of no analytical review; but, did our space permit, we should gladly give some extracts from it, to enable our readers to judge of the classical style of the author, and the exhausting way in which each subject is treated.—*Dublin Quarterly Journal of Med. Science*, Nov. 1859.

The work is so superior to its predecessors in matter and extent, as well as in illustrations and style of publication, that we can honestly recommend it as the best work of the kind to be taken home by the young practitioner.—*Am. Med. Journ.*, Jan. 1860.

The treatise of Prof. Gross is not, therefore, a mere text-book for undergraduates, but a systematic record of more than thirty years' experience, reading, and reflection by a man of observation, sound judgment, and rare practical tact, and as such deserves to take rank with the renowned productions of a similar character, by Vidal and Boyer, of France, or those of Chelius, Blasius, and Langenbeck, of Germany. Hence, we do not hesitate to express the opinion that it will speedily take the same elevated position in regard to surgery that has been given by common consent to the masterly work of Pereira in Materia Medica, or to Todd and Bowman in Physiology.—*N. O. Med. and Surg. Journal*, Jan. 1860.

[illegible] behalf.—[illegible] *Journal*, Oct. [illegible]

BY THE SAME AUTHOR.

ELEMENTS OF PATHOLOGICAL ANATOMY. [illegible]

revised and greatly improved. In one large and very [illegible] hundred and fifty beautiful illustrations, of [illegible] Price in extra cloth, $4 75; leather, raised bands, [illegible]

The very rapid advances in the Science of Pathological [illegible] rendered essential a thorough modification of this work, [illegible] ment of the present state of the subject. The very [illegible] executed, and the amount of alteration which it has [illegible] "with the many changes and improvements now [illegible] a new treatise," while the efforts of the author have [illegible] execution of the volume, rendering it one of the [illegible]

We most sincerely congratulate the author on the successful manner in which he has accomplished his proposed object. His book is most admirably calculated to fill up a blank which has long been felt to exist in this department of medical literature, and as such must become very widely circulated amongst all classes of the profession.—*Dublin Quarterly Journ. of Med. Science*, Nov. 1857.

We [illegible] *Charleston* [illegible]

BY THE SAME AUTHOR.

A PRACTICAL TREATISE ON FOREIGN BOD[illegible]

[illegible] In one handsome octavo volume, extra cloth, with [illegible]

GROSS (SAMUEL D.), M. D.,

Professor of Surgery in the Jefferson Medical College of Philadelphia, &c.

A PRACTICAL TREATISE ON THE DISEASES, INJURIES, AND MALFORMATIONS OF THE URINARY BLADDER, THE PROSTATE GLAND, AND THE URETHRA.

Second Edition, revised and much enlarged, with one hundred and eighty-four illustrations. In one large and very handsome octavo volume, of over nine hundred pages. In leather, raised bands, $5 25; extra cloth, $4 75.

Philosophical in its design, methodical in its arrangement, ample and sound in its practical details, it may in truth be said to leave scarcely anything to be desired on so important a subject.—*Boston Med. and Surg. Journal.*

Whoever will peruse the vast amount of valuable practical information it contains, will, we think, agree with us, that there is no work in the English language which can make any just pretensions to be its equal.—*N. Y. Journal of Medicine.*

A volume replete with truths and principles of the utmost value in the investigation of these diseases.—*American Medical Journal.*

GRAY (HENRY), F. R. S.,

Lecturer on Anatomy at St. George's Hospital, London, &c.

ANATOMY, DESCRIPTIVE AND SURGICAL.

The Drawings by H. V. Carter, M. D., late Demonstrator on Anatomy at St. George's Hospital; the Dissections jointly by the Author and Dr. Carter. In one magnificent imperial octavo volume, of nearly 800 pages, with 363 large and elaborate engravings on wood. Price in extra cloth, $6 25; leather raised bands, $7 00. *(Just Issued.)*

The author has endeavored in this work to cover a more extended range of subjects than is customary in the ordinary text-books, by giving not only the details necessary for the student, but also the application of those details in the practice of medicine and surgery, thus rendering it both a guide for the learner, and an admirable work of reference for the active practitioner. The engravings form a special feature in the work, many of them being the size of nature, nearly all original, and having the names of the various parts printed on the body of the cut, in place of figures of reference with descriptions at the foot. They thus form a complete and splendid series, which will greatly assist the student in obtaining a clear idea of Anatomy, and will also serve to refresh the memory of those who may find in the exigencies of practice the necessity of recalling the details of the dissecting room; while combining, as it does, a complete Atlas of Anatomy, with a thorough treatise on systematic, descriptive, and applied Anatomy, the work will be found of essential use to all physicians who receive students in their offices, relieving both preceptor and pupil of much labor in laying the groundwork of a thorough medical education.

The work before us is one entitled to the highest praise, and we accordingly welcome it as a valuable addition to medical literature. Intermediate in fulness of detail between the treatises of Sharpey and of Wilson, its characteristic merit lies in the number and excellence of the engravings it contains. Most of these are original, of much larger than ordinary size, and admirably executed. The various parts are also lettered after the plan adopted in Holden's Osteology. It would be difficult to over-estimate the advantages offered by this mode of pictorial illustration. Bones, ligaments, muscles, bloodvessels, and nerves are each in turn figured, and marked with their appropriate names; thus enabling the student to comprehend, at a glance, what would otherwise often be ignored, or at any rate, acquired only by prolonged and irksome application. In conclusion, we heartily commend the work of Mr. Gray to the attention of the medical profession, feeling certain that it should be regarded as one of the most valuable contributions ever made to educational literature.—*N. Y. Monthly Review*, Dec. 1859.

In this view, we regard the work of Mr. Gray as far better adapted to the wants of the profession, and especially of the student, than any treatise on anatomy yet published in this country. It is destined, we believe, to supersede all others, both as a manual of dissections, and a standard of reference to the student of general or relative anatomy.—*N. Y. Journal of Medicine*, Nov. 1859.

This is by all comparison the most excellent work on Anatomy extant. It is just the thing that has been long desired by the profession. With such a guide as this, the student of anatomy, the practitioner of medicine, and the surgical devotee have all a newer, clearer, and more radiant light thrown upon the intricacies and mysteries of this wonderful science, and are thus enabled to accomplish results which hitherto seemed possible only by the specialist. The plates, which are copied from recent dissections, are so well executed, that the most superficial observer cannot fail to perceive the positions, relations, and distinctive features of the various parts, and to take in more of anatomy at a glance, than by many long hours of diligent study over the most erudite treatise, or, perhaps, at the dissecting table itself.—*Med. Journ. of N Carolina*, Oct. 1859.

For this truly admirable work the profession is indebted to the distinguished author of "Gray on the Spleen." The vacancy it fills has been long felt to exist in this country. Mr. Gray writes throughout with both branches of his subject in view. His description of each particular part is followed by a notice of its relations to the parts with which it is connected, and this, too, sufficiently ample for all the purposes of the operative surgeon. After describing the bones and muscles, he gives a concise statement of the fractures to which the bones of the extremities are most liable, together with the amount and direction of the displacement to which the fragments are subjected by muscular action. The section on arteries is remarkably full and accurate. Not only is the surgical anatomy given to every important vessel, with directions for its ligation, but at the end of the description of each arterial trunk we have a useful summary of the irregularities which may occur in its origin, course, and termination.—*N. A. Med. Chir. Review*, Mar. 1859.

Mr. Gray's book, in excellency of arrangement and completeness of execution, exceeds any work on anatomy hitherto published in the English language, affording a complete view of the structure of the human body, with especial reference to practical surgery. Thus the volume constitutes a perfect book of reference for the practitioner, demanding a place in even the most limited library of the physician or surgeon, and a work of necessity for the student to fix in his mind what he has learned by the dissecting knife from the book of nature.—*The Dublin Quarterly Journal of Med. Sciences*, Nov. 1858.

In our judgment, the mode of illustration adopted in the present volume cannot but present many advantages to the student of anatomy. To the zealous disciple of Vesalius, earnestly desirous of real improvement, the book will certainly be of immense value; but, at the same time, we must also confess that to those simply desirous of "cramming" it will be an undoubted godsend. The peculiar value of Mr. Gray's mode of illustration is nowhere more markedly evident than in the chapter on osteology, and especially in those portions which treat of the bones of the head and of their development. The study of these parts is thus made one of comparative ease, if not of positive pleasure; and those bugbears of the student, the temporal and sphenoid bones, are shorn of half their terrors. It is, in our estimation, an admirable and complete text-book for the student, and a useful work of reference for the practitioner; its pictorial character forming a novel [illegible] which we have already sufficiently [illegible] [illegible] *Med. Sci.*, July, 1859.

GIBSON'S INSTITUTES AND PRACTICE OF SURGERY. Eighth edition, improved and altered. With thirty-four plates. In two handsome octavo volumes, containing about 1,000 pages, leather, raised bands. $6 50.

GARDNER'S MEDICAL CHEMISTRY, for the use of Students and the Profession. In one royal 12mo. vol., cloth, pp. 396, with wood-cuts. $1.

GLUGE'S ATLAS OF PATHOLOGICAL HISTOLOGY. Translated, with Notes and Additions by Joseph Leidy, M. D. In one volume, very large imperial quarto, extra cloth, with 320 copper-plate figures, plain and colored. [illegible]

HUGHES' INTRODUCTION TO THE PRACTICE OF AUSCULTATION AND OTHER MODES OF PHYSICAL DIAGNOSIS IN DISEASES OF THE LUNGS AND HEART. Second edition. 1 vol. royal 12mo. [illegible] 304. $1 00.

HAMILTON (FRANK H.), M. D.,

Professor of Surgery in the University of Buffalo, &c.

A PRACTICAL TREATISE ON FRACTURES AND DISLOCATIONS. [illegible]

one large and handsome octavo volume, of over 750 pages, with 289 illustrations. [illegible] Ready, January, 1860.)

This is a valuable contribution to the surgery of most important affections, and is the more welcome, inasmuch as at the present time we do not possess a single complete treatise on Fractures and Dislocations in the English language. It has remained for our American brother to produce a complete treatise upon the subject, and bring together in a convenient form those alterations and improvements that have been made from time to time in the treatment of these affections. One great and valuable feature in the work before us is the fact that it comprises all the improvements introduced into the practice of both English and American surgery, and though far from omitting mention of our continental neighbors, the author by no means encourages the notion—but too prevalent in some quarters—that nothing is good unless imported from France or Germany. The latter half of the work is devoted to the consideration of the various dislocations and their appropriate treatment, and its merit is fully equal to that of the preceding portion.—*The London Lancet*, May 5, 1860.

It is emphatically *the* book upon the subjects of which it treats, and we cannot doubt that it will continue so to be for an indefinite period of time. When we say, however, that we believe it will at once take its place as the best book for consultation by the practitioner; and that it will form the most complete, available, and reliable guide in emergencies of every nature connected with its subjects; and also that the student of surgery may make it his text-book with entire confidence, and with pleasure also, from its agreeable and easy style—we think our own opinion may be gathered as to its value.—*Boston Medical and Surgical Journal*, March 1, 1860.

The work is concise, judicious, and accurate, and adapted to the wants of the student, practitioner, and investigator, honorable to the author and to the profession.—*Chicago Med. Journal*, March, 1860.

We venture to say that this is not alone the only complete treatise on the subject in the language, but the best and most practical we have ever read. The arrangement is simple and systematic, the diction clear and graphic, and the illustrations numerous and remarkable for accuracy of delineation. The various mechanical appliances are faithfully illustrated, which will be a desideratum [illegible] practitioners who cannot conveniently [illegible] daily applied.—*New York Med. Press*, [illegible]

We turned this work to [illegible] author, but to the profession [illegible] we to review it thoroughly, [illegible] the mind of the reader [illegible] opinion expressed in the [illegible] best book of its kind [illegible] in surgery will [illegible] he who does not, will [illegible] *Medical News*, March, 1860.

Now that it is before us, [illegible] much as was expected [illegible] the undertaking, it has [illegible] achieved more than was [illegible] its title does not express [illegible] contents. On the whole, [illegible] work than of any [illegible] from the American medical [illegible] tainly be very largely [illegible] pate its attention [illegible] *ville Medical Record*, Mar. [illegible]

Every surgeon, young and [illegible] himself of it, and give it a [illegible] which he will be richly [illegible] and Surg. Journal, March, [illegible]

Dr. Hamilton is fortunate [illegible] filling the void, we long felt, [illegible] to be at once acknowledged [illegible] requests, and a work of [illegible] sincerely congratulate the [illegible] States on the appearance of [illegible] one of their number. We [illegible] of it as an original work, [illegible] entific point of view, and [illegible] guide in a most difficult and [illegible] study and practice. On every [illegible] we hope that it may [illegible] as an evidence of [illegible] the Atlantic, and [illegible] widely known at home [illegible] from which every one may [illegible] affording an example of [illegible] untiring industry in authorship [illegible] may emulate.—*Am. Med. Journal*, [illegible]

HOBLYN (RICHARD D.), M. D.

A DICTIONARY OF THE TERMS USED IN MEDICINE [illegible]

COLLATERAL SCIENCES. A new American edition. Revised, with [illegible] by Isaac Hays, M. D., editor of the "American Journal of the Medical Sciences." [illegible] royal 12mo. volume, leather, of over 500 double columned pages. [illegible]

To both practitioner and student, we recommend this dictionary as being convenient in size, accurate in definition, and sufficiently full and complete for ordinary consultation.—*Charleston Med. Journ.*

We know of no dictionary better arranged and adapted. It is not encumbered with the obsolete terms of a bygone age, but it contains all that are now in use; embracing every [illegible] down to the very [illegible]

Hoblyn's Dictionary has [illegible] us. It is the best [illegible] ought always to be [illegible] *Southern Med. and Surg. Journal*.

HOLLAND'S MEDICAL NOTES AND REFLECTIONS. From the third London edition. In one handsome octavo volume, extra cloth. $3.

HORNER'S SPECIAL ANATOMY AND HISTOLOGY. Eighth edition, [illegible] and modified. In two large [illegible] extra cloth, of more than [illegible] illustrations. $6 00.

HABERSHON (S. O.), M. D.,

Assistant Physician to and Lecturer on Materia Medica and Therapeutics [illegible]

PATHOLOGICAL AND PRACTICAL OBSERVATIONS [illegible]

OF THE ALIMENTARY CANAL, ŒSOPHAGUS, STOMACH, [illegible] TINES. With illustrations on wood. In one handsome octavo volume, [illegible] cloth. $1 75. (*Now Ready*.)

JONES (T. WHARTON), F. R. S.,

Professor of Ophthalmic Medicine and Surgery in University College, London, &c.

THE PRINCIPLES AND PRACTICE OF OPHTHALMIC MEDICINE AND SURGERY.

With one hundred and ten illustrations. Second American from the second and revised London edition, with additions by EDWARD HARTSHORNE, M. D., Surgeon to Wills' Hospital, &c. In one large, handsome royal 12mo. volume, extra cloth, of 500 pages. $1 50.

The work sustains, in every point, the already high reputation of the author as an ophthalmic surgeon as well as a physiologist and pathologist. We entertain little doubt that this book will become what its author hoped it might become, a manual for daily reference and consultation by the student and the general practitioner. The work is marked by that correctness, clearness, and precision of style which distinguish all the productions of the learned author.—*British and For. Med. Review.*

JONES (C. HANDFIELD), F. R. S., & EDWARD H. SIEVEKING, M.D.,

Assistant Physicians and Lecturers in St. Mary's Hospital, London.

A MANUAL OF PATHOLOGICAL ANATOMY.

First American Edition, Revised. With three hundred and ninety-seven handsome wood engravings. In one large and beautiful octavo volume of nearly 750 pages, leather. $3 75.

As a concise text-book, containing, in a condensed form, a complete outline of what is known in the domain of Pathological Anatomy, it is perhaps the best work in the English language. Its great merit consists in its completeness and brevity, and in this respect it supplies a great desideratum in our literature. Heretofore the student of pathology was obliged to glean from a great number of monographs, and the field was so extensive that but few cultivated it with any degree of success. As a simple work of reference, therefore, it is of great value to the student of pathological anatomy, and should be in every physician's library.—*Western Lancet.*

KIRKES (WILLIAM SENHOUSE), M. D.,

Demonstrator of Morbid Anatomy at St. Bartholomew's Hospital, &c.

A MANUAL OF PHYSIOLOGY.

A new American, from the third and improved London edition. With two hundred illustrations. In one large and handsome royal 12mo. volume, leather. pp. 586. $2 00. (*Lately Published.*)

This is a new and very much improved edition of Dr. Kirkes' well-known Handbook of Physiology. It combines conciseness with completeness, and is, therefore, admirably adapted for consultation by the busy practitioner.—*Dublin Quarterly Journal.*

Its excellence is in its compactness, its clearness, and its carefully cited authorities. It is the most convenient of text-books. These gentlemen, Messrs. Kirkes and Paget, have really an immense talent for silence, which is not so common or so cheap as prating people fancy. They have the gift of telling us what we want to know, without thinking it necessary to tell us all they know.—*Boston Med. and Surg. Journal.*

One of the very best handbooks of Physiology we possess—presenting just such an outline of the science as the student requires during his attendance upon a course of lectures, or for reference whilst preparing for examination.—*Am. Medical Journal.*

For the student beginning this study, and the practitioner who has but leisure to refresh his memory, this book is invaluable, as it contains all that it is important to know, without special details, which are read with interest only by those who would make a specialty, or desire to possess critical knowledge of the subject.—*Charleston Med. Journal.*

KNAPP'S TECHNOLOGY; or, Chemistry applied to the Arts and to Manufactures. Edited by Dr. RONALDS, Dr. RICHARDSON, and Prof. W. R. JOHNSON. In two handsome 8vo. vols., with about 500 wood engravings. $6 00.

LAYCOCK'S LECTURES ON THE PRINCIPLES AND METHODS OF MEDICAL OBSERVATION AND RESEARCH. For the Use of Advanced Students and Junior Practitioners. In one royal 12mo. volume, extra cloth. Price $1.

LUDLOW (J. L.), M. D.

A MANUAL OF EXAMINATIONS

upon Anatomy, Physiology, Surgery, Practice of Medicine, Obstetrics, Materia Medica, Chemistry, Pharmacy, and Therapeutics. To which is added a Medical Formulary. Third edition, thoroughly revised and greatly extended and enlarged. With 370 illustrations. In one handsome royal 12mo. volume, leather, of 816 large pages $2 50.

The great popularity of this volume, and the numerous demands for it during the two years in which it has been out of print, have induced the author in its revision to spare no pains to render it a correct and accurate digest of the most recent condition of all the branches of medical science. In many respects it may, therefore, be regarded rather as a new book than a new edition, an entire section on Physiology having been added, as also one on Organic Chemistry, and many portions having been rewritten. A very complete series of illustrations has been introduced, and every care has been taken in the mechanical execution to render it a convenient and satisfactory book for study or reference. The arrangement of the volume in the form of question and answer renders it especially suited for the office examination of students and for those preparing for graduation.

We know of no better companion for the student during the hours spent in the lecture room, or to refresh, at a glance, his memory of the various topics crammed into his head by the various professors to whom he is compelled to listen.—*Western Lancet*, May, 1857.

LAWRENCE (W.), F. R. S., &c.

A TREATISE ON DISEASES OF THE EYE.

A new edition, edited, with numerous additions, and 243 illustrations, by ISAAC HAYS, M. D., Surgeon to Will's Hospital, &c. In one very large and handsome octavo volume, of 950 pages, strongly bound in leather with raised bands. $5 00.

LALLEMAND AND WILSON.

A PRACTICAL TREATISE ON THE CAUSES, SYMPTOMS, AND TREATMENT OF SPERMATORRHŒA.

By M. LALLEMAND. Translated and edited by HENRY J. McDOUGALL. Third American edition. To which is added —— ON DISEASES OF THE VESICULÆ SEMINALES; AND THEIR ASSOCIATED ORGANS. With special reference to the Morbid Secretions of the Prostatic and Urethral Mucous Membrane. By [illegible] WILSON, M. D. In one neat octavo volume, of about 400 pp., extra cloth. $2 00. [illegible]

LA ROCHE (R.), M. D., &c.

YELLOW FEVER, considered in its Historical, Pathological, [illegible] Therapeutical Relations. Including a Sketch of the Disease as it has occurred [illegible] from 1699 to 1854, with an examination of the connection between it and the [illegible] the same name in other parts of temperate as well as in tropical regions. [illegible] handsome octavo volumes of nearly 1500 pages, extra cloth. $7 00.

From Professor S. H. Dickson, Charleston, S. C., September 18, 1855.

A monument of intelligent and well applied research, almost without example. It is, indeed, in itself, a large library, and is destined to constitute the special resort as a book of reference, in the subject of which it treats, to all future time.

We have not time at present, engaged as we are, by day and by night, in the work of combating this very disease, now prevailing in our city, to do more than give this cursory notice of what we consider as undoubtedly the most able and erudite medical publication our country has yet produced. But in view of the startling fact, that this, the most malignant and unmanageable disease of modern times, has for several years been prevailing in our country to a greater extent than ever before; that it is no longer confined to either large or small cities, but penetrates country villages, plantations, and farm-houses; that it is treated with scarcely better success now than thirty or forty years ago; that there is vast mischief done by ignorant pretenders to knowledge in regard to the disease, and in view of the probability that a majority of southern physicians will be called upon to treat the disease, we trust that this able and comprehensive treatise will be very generally read in the south.—*Memphis Med. Recorder.*

This is decidedly the great American medical work of the day—a full, complete, and systematic treatise, unequalled by any other upon the all-important subject of Yellow Fever. The laborious, indefatigable, and learned author has devoted to it many years of arduous research and careful study [illegible] is such as will reflect the highest [illegible] author and our country.—[illegible] *Journal.*

The genius and [illegible] could not have been better employed [illegible] erudition of this [illegible] and to the glory of [illegible] country. It is [illegible] rity upon the subject of Yellow Fever [illegible] and physician will [illegible] of the vast total of [illegible] the awful scourge which [illegible] The style is so [illegible] vigorate the mind [illegible] the gifted author, [illegible] ceeded in bringing [illegible] harmony with the [illegible] Take it all in all, it [illegible] of, but dreamed not that it would [illegible] waiting eye and tangible reality.—[illegible] *of Medicine.*

We deem it fortunate that [illegible] Dr. La Roche should have been [illegible] at this particular time. [illegible] gest of all that is known [illegible] malady has long been felt [illegible] met in the work before us. [illegible] praise to say that Dr. La Roche [illegible] presenting the [illegible] monograph, one [illegible] well ordered library.—[illegible]

BY THE SAME AUTHOR.

PNEUMONIA; its Supposed Connection, Pathological and [illegible] tumnal Fevers, including an Inquiry into the Existence and Morbid Agency of [illegible] handsome octavo volume, extra cloth, of 500 pages. $3 00.

LEHMANN (C. G.)

PHYSIOLOGICAL CHEMISTRY. Translated from the second [illegible] George E. Day, M. D., F. R. S., &c., edited by R. E. Rogers, M. D., [illegible] in the Medical Department of the University of Pennsylvania, with [illegible] Funke's Atlas of Physiological Chemistry, and an Appendix of plates. [illegible] and handsome octavo volumes, extra cloth, containing 1200 pages, with nearly [illegible] trations. $6 00.

This great work, universally acknowledged as the most complete and authoritative [illegible] the principles and details of Zoochemistry, in its passage through the press [illegible] Professor Rogers such care as was necessary to present it in a correct and [illegible] is, therefore, presented as in every way worthy the attention of all who [illegible] the modern facts and doctrines of *Physiological Science.*

The most important contribution as yet made to Physiological Chemistry.—*Am. Journal Med. Sciences,* Jan. 1856.

The present volumes belong to the small class of medical literature which comprises elaborate works of the highest order of merit.—*Montreal Med. Chronicle,* Jan. 1856.

The work of Lehmann stands unrivalled as the most comprehensive book of reference and information extant on every branch of the subject on which it treats.—*Edinburgh Monthly* [illegible] *Science.*

Already well known [illegible] tific world, Professor Lehmann [illegible] quires no laudatory [illegible] It is now presented to [illegible] command would [illegible] portion of the [illegible] *Journal,* Dec. 1855.

BY THE SAME AUTHOR. (*Lately Published.*)

MANUAL OF CHEMICAL PHYSIOLOGY. Translated [illegible] with Notes and Additions, by J. Cheston Morris, M. D., with an Introductory [illegible] *Force,* by Professor Samuel Jackson, M. D., of the University of Pennsylvania [illegible] trations on wood. In one very handsome octavo volume, extra cloth, of 336 pages [illegible]

From Prof. Jackson's Introductory Essay.

In adopting the handbook of Dr. Lehmann as a manual of Organic Chemistry [illegible] students of the University, and in recommending his original work of Physiological [illegible] for their more mature studies, the high value of his researches, and the great [illegible] rity in that important department of medical science are fully recognized. [illegible]

MAYNE'S DISPENSATORY AND THERAPEUTICAL REMEMBRANCER. Comprising the entire lists of Materia Medica, with every Practical Formula contained in the three British Pharmacopœias. Edited, with the addition of the Formulæ of the U. S. Pharmacopœia, by R. E. Griffith, M. D. 1 12mo. vol. ex. cl., 300 pp. 75 c.

MALGAIGNE'S OPERATIVE [illegible] on Normal and Pathological [illegible] lated from the French [illegible] A. B., M. D. [illegible] In one handsome [illegible] nearly six hundred [illegible]

MEIGS (CHARLES D.), M. D.,

Professor of Obstetrics, &c. in the Jefferson Medical College, Philadelphia.

OBSTETRICS: THE SCIENCE AND THE ART. Third edition, revised and improved. With one hundred and twenty-nine illustrations. In one beautifully printed octavo volume, leather, of seven hundred and fifty-two large pages. $3 75.

The rapid demand for another edition of this work is a sufficient expression of the favorable verdict of the profession. In thus preparing it a third time for the press, the author has endeavored to render it in every respect worthy of the favor which it has received. To accomplish this he has thoroughly revised it in every part. Some portions have been rewritten, others added, new illustrations have been in many instances substituted for such as were not deemed satisfactory, while, by an alteration in the typographical arrangement, the size of the work has not been increased, and the price remains unaltered. In its present improved form, it is, therefore, hoped that the work will continue to meet the wants of the American profession as a sound, practical, and extended SYSTEM OF MIDWIFERY.

Though the work has received only five pages of enlargement, its chapters throughout wear the impress of careful revision. Expunging and rewriting, remodelling its sentences, with occasional new material, all evince a lively desire that it shall deserve to be regarded as improved in *manner* as well as *matter*. In the *matter*, every stroke of the pen has increased the value of the book, both in expungings and additions.—*Western Lancet*, Jan. 1857.

The best American work on Midwifery that is accessible to the student and practitioner.—*N. W. Med. and Surg. Journal*, Jan. 1857.

This is a standard work by a great American Obstetrician. It is the third and last edition, and, in the language of the preface, the author has "brought the subject up to the latest dates of real improvement in our art and Science."—*Nashville Journ. of Med. and Surg.*, May, 1857.

BY THE SAME AUTHOR. *(Just Issued.)*

WOMAN: HER DISEASES AND THEIR REMEDIES. A Series of Lectures to his Class. Fourth and Improved edition. In one large and beautifully printed octavo volume, leather, of over 700 pages. $3 60.

The gratifying appreciation of his labors, as evinced by the exhaustion of three large impressions of this work has not been lost upon the author, who has endeavored in every way to render it worthy of the favor with which it has been received. The opportunity thus afforded for another revision has been improved, and the work is now presented as in every way superior to its predecessors, additions and alterations having been made whenever the advance of science has rendered them desirable. The typographical execution of the work will also be found to have undergone a similar improvement, and the volume, it is hoped, will be found in all respects worthy to maintain its position as the standard American text-book on the Diseases of Females.

A few notices of the previous editions are appended.

In other respects, in our estimation, too much cannot be said in praise of this work. It abounds with beautiful passages, and for conciseness, for originality, and for all that is commendable in a work on the diseases of females, it is not excelled, and probably not equalled in the English language. On the whole, we know of no work on the diseases of women which we can so cordially commend to the student and practitioner as the one before us.—*Ohio Med. and Surg. Journal.*

The body of the book is worthy of attentive consideration, and is evidently the production of a clever, thoughtful, and sagacious physician. Dr. Meigs's letters on the diseases of the external organs, contain many interesting and rare cases, and many instructive observations. We take our leave of Dr. Meigs, with a high opinion of his talents and originality.—*The British and Foreign Medico-Chirurgical Review.*

Every chapter is replete with practical instruction, and bears the impress of being the composition of an acute and experienced mind. There is a terseness, and at the same time an accuracy in his description of symptoms, and in the rules for diagnosis, which cannot fail to recommend the volume to the attention of the reader.—*Ranking's Abstract.*

It contains a vast amount of practical knowledge, by one who has accurately observed and retained the experience of many years, and who tells the result in a free, familiar, and pleasant manner.—*Dublin Quarterly Journal.*

Full of important matter, conveyed in a ready and agreeable manner.—*St. Louis Med. and Surg. Jour.*

There is an off-hand fervor, a glow, and a warm-heartedness infecting the effort of Dr. Meigs, which is entirely captivating, and which absolutely hurries the reader through from beginning to end. Besides, the book teems with solid instruction, and it shows the very highest evidence of ability, viz., the clearness with which the information is presented. We know of no better test of one's understanding a subject than the evidence of the power of lucidly explaining it. The most elementary, as well as the obscurest subjects, under the pencil of Prof. Meigs, are isolated and made to stand out in such bold relief, as to produce distinct impressions upon the mind and memory of the reader.—*The Charleston Med. Journal.*

Professor Meigs has enlarged and amended this great work, for such it unquestionably is, having passed the ordeal of criticism at home and abroad, but been improved thereby; for in this new edition the author has introduced real improvements, and increased the value and utility of the book immeasurably. It presents so many novel, bright, and sparkling thoughts; such an exuberance of new ideas on almost every page, that we confess ourselves to have become enamored with the book and its author; and cannot withhold our congratulations from our Philadelphia confreres, that such a teacher is in their service.—*N. Y. Med. Gazette.*

BY THE SAME AUTHOR.

ON THE NATURE, SIGNS, AND TREATMENT OF CHILDBED FEVER. In a Series of Letters addressed to the Students of his Class. In one handsome octavo volume, extra cloth, of 365 pages. $2 60.

The instructive and interesting author of this work, whose previous labors in the department of medicine which he so sedulously cultivates, have placed his countrymen under deep and abiding obligations, again challenges their admiration in the fresh and vigorous, attractive and racy pages before us. It is a delectable book. * * * This treatise upon child-bed fevers will have an extensive sale, being destined, as it deserves, to find a place in the library of every practitioner who scorns to lag in the rear.—*Nashville Journal of Medicine and Surgery.*

BY THE SAME AUTHOR; WITH COLORED PLATES.

A TREATISE ON ACUTE AND CHRONIC DISEASES OF THE NECK OF THE UTERUS. With numerous plates, drawn and colored from nature in the highest style of art. In one handsome octavo volume, extra cloth. $4 50.

MACLISE (JOSEPH), SURGEON.

SURGICAL ANATOMY. Forming one volume, very large [illegible] With sixty-eight large and splendid Plates, drawn in the best style [illegible] taining one hundred and ninety Figures, many of them the size of life, [illegible] and explanatory letter-press. Strongly and handsomely bound in extra cloth, [illegible] cheapest and best executed Surgical works as yet issued in this country. $11 [illegible]

*** The size of this work prevents its transmission through the post-office [illegible] who desire to have copies forwarded by mail, can receive them in five parts, [illegible] wrappers. Price $9 00.

One of the greatest artistic triumphs of the age in Surgical Anatomy.—*British American Medical Journal.*

No practitioner whose means will admit should fail to possess it.—*Ranking's Abstract.*

Too much cannot be said in its praise; indeed, we have not language to do it justice.—*Ohio Medical and Surgical Journal.*

The most accurately engraved and beautifully colored plates we have ever seen in an American book—one of the best and cheapest surgical works ever published.—*Buffalo Medical Journal.*

It is very rare that so elegantly printed, so well illustrated, and so useful a work, is offered at so moderate a price.—*Charleston Medical Journal.*

Its plates can boast a superiority which places them almost beyond the reach of competition.—*Medical Examiner.*

Country practitioners will find these plates of immense value.—*N. Y. Medical Gazette.*

A work which has no parallel [illegible] racy and cheapness in the English [illegible] *Journal of Medicine.*

We are extremely gratified [illegible] profession the completion of [illegible] work, which, as a whole, [illegible] valled, both for accuracy [illegible] coloring, and [illegible] subject in hand.—[illegible] *Surgical Journal.*

This is by far the ablest work [illegible] many that has come [illegible] know of no other work [illegible] dent, in any degree, for neglect of [illegible] tion. In those sudden emergencies [illegible] arise, and which require the [illegible] of minute [illegible] keeps the details of [illegible] fresh in the memory.—[illegible] *cine and Surgery.*

MILLER (HENRY), M. D.,

Professor of Obstetrics and Diseases of Women and Children in the University [illegible]

PRINCIPLES AND PRACTICE OF OBSTETRICS, &c.; Including [illegible] ment of Chronic Inflammation of the Cervix and Body of the Uterus, considered [illegible] cause of Abortion. With about one hundred illustrations on wood. In one very [illegible] tavo volume, of over 600 pages. (*Lately Published.*) $3 75.

The reputation of Dr. Miller as an obstetrician is too widely spread to require [illegible] of the profession to be specially called to a volume containing the experience of his long [illegible] practice. The very favorable reception accorded to his "Treatise on Human [illegible] some years since, is an earnest that the present work will fulfil the author's [illegible] within a moderate compass a complete and trustworthy text-book for the student [illegible] ference for the practitioner.

We congratulate the author that the task is done. We congratulate him that he has given to the medical public a work which will secure for him a high and permanent position among the standard authorities on the principles and practice of obstetrics. Congratulations are not less due to the medical profession of this country, on the acquisition of a treatise embodying the results of the studies, reflections, and experience of Prof. Miller. Few men, if any, in this country, are more competent than he to write on this department of medicine. Engaged for thirty-five years in an extended practice of obstetrics, for many years a teacher of this branch of instruction in one of the largest of our institutions, a diligent student as well as a careful observer, an original and independent thinker, wedded to no hobbies, ever ready to consider without prejudice new views, and to adopt innovations if they are really improvements, and withal a clear, agreeable writer, a practical treatise from his pen could not fail to possess great value.—*Buffalo Med. Journal*, Mar. 1858.

In fact, this volume must take its place among the standard systematic treatises on obstetrics; a position to which its merits justly [illegible] is such that the [illegible] ject is discussed and [illegible] its practical bearings, [illegible] acceptable and valuable to [illegible] titioners. We cannot [illegible] notice, without [illegible] profession on the [illegible] treatise. The author [illegible] feel proud, and we [illegible] will find [illegible] obstetrics is taught and [illegible] art.—*The Cincinnati Lancet* [illegible]

A most [illegible] home medical [illegible] alike on the author and [illegible] is attached. The [illegible] most useful guide to [illegible] titioner, ready in [illegible] pages a fair résumé of the [illegible] science; and we hope [illegible] tion generally [illegible] *Med. Journal*, [illegible]

MACKENZIE (W.), M. D.,

Surgeon Oculist in Scotland in ordinary to Her Majesty, &c. &c.

A PRACTICAL TREATISE ON DISEASES AND INJURIES [illegible] **EYE.** To which is prefixed an Anatomical Introduction explanatory of [illegible] the Human Eyeball, by Thomas Wharton Jones, F. R. S. From the Fourth [illegible] larged London Edition. With Notes and Additions by Addinell Hewson [illegible] Wills Hospital, &c. &c. In one very large and handsome octavo volume, [illegible] plates and numerous wood-cuts. $5 25.

The treatise of Dr. Mackenzie indisputably holds the first place, and forms, in respect of learning and research, an Encyclopædia unequalled in extent by any other work of the kind, either English or foreign.—*Dixon on Diseases of the Eye.*

Few modern books on any department of medicine or surgery have met with such extended circulation, or have procured for their authors a like amount of European celebrity. The immense research which it displayed, the thorough acquaintance with the subject, practically as well as theoretically, and the able manner in which [illegible] and experience [illegible] use, at once procured [illegible] the continent as [illegible] as a standard work [illegible] has there firmly [illegible] duty of every [illegible] and the [illegible] self familiar with this [illegible] the English language upon the [illegible] —*Med. Times and Gazette.*

MILLER (JAMES), F. R. S. E.,
Professor of Surgery in the University of Edinburgh, &c.

PRINCIPLES OF SURGERY. Fourth American, from the third and revised Edinburgh edition. In one large and very beautiful volume, leather, of 700 pages, with two hundred and forty illustrations on wood. $3.75.

The work of Mr. Miller is too well and too favorably known among us, as one of our best text-books, to render any further notice of it necessary than the announcement of a new edition, the *fourth* in our country, a proof of its extensive circulation among us. As a concise and reliable exposition of the science of modern surgery, it stands deservedly high—we know not its superior.—*Boston Med. and Surg. Journal.*

The work takes rank with Watson's *Practice of Physic*; it certainly does not fall behind that great work in soundness of principle or depth of reasoning and research. No physician who values his reputation, or seeks the interests of his clients, can acquit himself before his God and the world without making himself familiar with the sound and philosophical views developed in the foregoing book.—*New Orleans Med. and Surg. Journal.*

BY THE SAME AUTHOR. (*Just Issued.*)

THE PRACTICE OF SURGERY. Fourth American from the last Edinburgh edition. Revised by the American editor. Illustrated by three hundred and sixty-four engravings on wood. In one large octavo volume, leather, of nearly 700 pages. $3 75.

No encomium of ours could add to the popularity of Miller's Surgery. Its reputation in this country is unsurpassed by that of any other work, and, when taken in connection with the author's *Principles of Surgery*, constitutes a whole, without reference to which no conscientious surgeon would be willing to practice his art.—*Southern Med. and Surg. Journal.*

It is seldom that two volumes have ever made so profound an impression in so short a time as the "Principles" and the "Practice" of Surgery by Mr. Miller—or so richly merited the reputation they have acquired. The author is an eminently sensible, practical, and well-informed man, who knows exactly what he is talking about and exactly how to talk it.—*Kentucky Medical Recorder.*

By the almost unanimous voice of the profession, his works, both on the principles and practice of surgery have been assigned the highest rank. If we were limited to but one work on surgery, that one should be Miller's, as we regard it as superior to all others.—*St. Louis Med. and Surg. Journal.*

The author has in this and his "Principles," presented to the profession one of the most complete and reliable systems of Surgery extant. His style of writing is original, impressive, and engaging, energetic, concise, and lucid. Few have the faculty of condensing so much in small space, and at the same time so persistently holding the attention. Whether as a text-book for students or a book of reference for practitioners, it cannot be too strongly recommended.—*Southern Journal of Med. and Physical Sciences.*

MORLAND (W. W.), M. D.,
Fellow of the Massachusetts Medical Society, &c.

DISEASES OF THE URINARY ORGANS; a Compendium of their Diagnosis, Pathology, and Treatment. With illustrations. In one large and handsome octavo volume, of about 600 pages, extra cloth. (*Just Issued.*) $3 50.

Taken as a whole, we can recommend Dr. Morland's compendium as a very desirable addition to the library of every medical or surgical practitioner.—*Brit and For. Med.-Chir. Rev.*, April, 1859.

Every medical practitioner whose attention has been to any extent attracted towards the class of diseases to which this treatise relates, must have often and sorely experienced the want of some full, yet concise recent compendium to which he could refer. This desideratum has been supplied by Dr. Morland, and it has been ably done. He has placed before us a full, judicious, and reliable digest. Each subject is treated with sufficient minuteness, yet in a succinct, satisfactory style, such as to render the work one of great interest, and one which will prove in the highest degree useful to the general practitioner. To the members of the profession in the country it will be peculiarly valuable, on account of the characteristics which we have mentioned, and the one broad aim of practical utility which is kept in view, and which shines out upon every page, together with the skill which is evinced in the combination of this grand requisite with the utmost brevity which a just treatment of the subjects would admit.—*N. Y. Journ. of Medicine*, Nov. 1858.

MONTGOMERY (W. F.), M. D., M. R. I. A., &c.,
Professor of Midwifery in the King and Queen's College of Physicians in Ireland, &c.

AN EXPOSITION OF THE SIGNS AND SYMPTOMS OF PREGNANCY. With some other Papers on Subjects connected with Midwifery. From the second and enlarged English edition. With two exquisite colored plates, and numerous wood-cuts. In one very handsome octavo volume, extra cloth, of nearly 600 pages. (*Lately Published.*) $3 75.

A book unusually rich in practical suggestions.—*Am Journal Med. Sciences*, Jan. 1857.

These several subjects so interesting in themselves, and so important, every one of them, to the most delicate and precious of social relations, controlling often the honor and domestic peace of a family, the legitimacy of offspring, or the life of its parent, are all treated with an elegance of diction, fulness of illustration, acuteness and justice of reasoning, unparalleled in obstetrics, and unsurpassed in medicine. The reader's interest can never flag, so fresh, and vigorous, and classical is our author's style; and one forgets, in the renewed charm of every page, that it, and every line, and every word has been weighed and reweighed through years of preparation; that this is of all others the book of Obstetric Law, on each of its several topics; on all points connected with pregnancy, to be everywhere received as a manual of special jurisprudence, at once announcing fact, affording argument, establishing precedent, and governing alike the juryman, advocate, and judge. It is not merely in its legal relations that we find this work so interesting. Hardly a page but that has its hints or facts important to the general practitioner; and not a chapter without especial matter for the anatomist, physiologist, or pathologist.—*N.-A. Med.-Chir. Review*, March, 1857.

MOHR (FRANCIS), PH. D., AND REDWOOD (THEOPHILUS),

PRACTICAL PHARMACY. Comprising the Arrangements, Apparatus, and Manipulations of the Pharmaceutical Shop and Laboratory. Edited, with extensive Additions, by Prof. WILLIAM PROCTER, of the Philadelphia College of Pharmacy. In one handsomely printed octavo volume, extra cloth, of 570 pages, with over 500 engravings on wood. $2 75

NEILL (JOHN), M.D., [illegible]
Surgeon to the Pennsylvania Hospital, [illegible]

FRANCIS GURNEY SMITH, M.D., [illegible]
Professor of Institutes of Medicine in the Pennsylvania Medical College [illegible]

AN ANALYTICAL COMPENDIUM OF THE VARIOUS [illegible] OF MEDICAL SCIENCE; for the Use and Examination of Students. [illegible] and improved. In one very large and handsomely printed royal 12mo. [illegible] thousand pages, with 374 wood-cuts. Strongly bound in leather, [illegible]

The very flattering reception which has been accorded to this work, [illegible] upon it by the profession, as evinced by the constant and increasing demand [illegible] hausted two large editions, have stimulated the authors to render the volume [illegible] more worthy of the success which has attended it. It has accordingly been thoroughly [illegible] and such errors as had on former occasions escaped observation have been corrected, [illegible] additions were necessary to maintain it on a level with the advance of science [illegible] The extended series of illustrations has been still further increased [illegible] a slight enlargement of the page, these various additions have been incorporated [illegible] the bulk of the volume.

The work is, therefore, again presented as eminently worthy of the favor [illegible] been received. As a book for daily reference by the student requiring a guide to [illegible] text-books, as a manual for preceptors desiring to stimulate their students by [illegible] examination, or as a source from which the practitioners of older date may [illegible] a knowledge of the changes and improvement in professional science, [illegible] established.

The best work of the kind with which we are acquainted.—*Med. Examiner.*

Having made free use of this volume in our examinations of pupils, we can speak from experience in recommending it as an admirable compend for students, and as especially useful to preceptors who examine their pupils. It will save the teacher much labor by enabling him readily to recall all of the points upon which his pupils should be examined. A work of this sort should be in the hands of every one who takes pupils into his office with a view of examining them; and this is unquestionably the best of its class.—*Transylvania Med. Journal.*

In the rapid course of lectures, where work for the students is heavy, and [illegible] examination, a compend [illegible] it is almost a sine qua non [illegible] in most of the divisions, [illegible] of all books of the kind [illegible] newest and soundest [illegible] provements and discoveries [illegible] concisely, laid before the [illegible] to whom we very sincerely [illegible] a work its weight in silver [illegible] ates in medicine of more than [illegible] who have not studied medicine [illegible] perhaps find out from it that the science [illegible] now what it was when they left it off [illegible] scope.

NELIGAN (J. MOORE), M.D., M.R.I.A., [illegible]
(A splendid work. Just issued.)

ATLAS OF CUTANEOUS DISEASES. In one beautiful [illegible] cloth, with splendid colored plates, presenting nearly one hundred elaborate [illegible] disease. $4 50.

This beautiful volume is intended as a complete and accurate representation [illegible] of Diseases of the Skin. While it can be consulted in conjunction with any work [illegible] especial reference to the author's "Treatise on Diseases of the Skin," [illegible] profession some years since. The publishers feel justified in saying that [illegible] cuted plates have ever been presented to the profession of this country.

Neligan's Atlas of Cutaneous Diseases supplies a long existent desideratum much felt by the largest class of our profession. It presents, in quarto size, 16 plates, each containing from 3 to 6 figures, and forming in all a total of 90 distinct representations of the different species of skin affections, grouped together in genera or families. The illustrations have been taken from nature, and have been copied with such fidelity that they present a striking picture of life; in which the reduced scale aptly serves to give, at a coup d'œil, the [illegible] of each individual variety. [illegible] case is rendered more [illegible] of proportion [illegible] tion. Each figure is [illegible] has the artist been that [illegible] could not justly take [illegible] the execution of the [illegible] *Montreal Med. Chronicle,* [illegible]

BY THE SAME AUTHOR.

A PRACTICAL TREATISE ON DISEASES OF THE [illegible] American edition. In one neat royal 12mo. volume, extra cloth, of [illegible]

☞ The two volumes will be sent by mail on receipt of [illegible]

OWEN ON THE DIFFERENT FORMS OF THE SKELETON, AND OF THE TEETH. | One vol. royal [illegible] illustrations. $1.25. [illegible]

PIRRIE (WILLIAM), F.R.S.E., [illegible]
Professor of Surgery in the University of Aberdeen [illegible]

THE PRINCIPLES AND PRACTICE OF SURGERY. [illegible] NEILL, M.D., Professor of Surgery in the Penna. Medical College [illegible] Hospital, &c. In one very handsome octavo volume, leather, of [illegible] $3 75.

We know of no other surgical work of a reasonable size, wherein there is so much theory and practice, or where subjects are more soundly or clearly taught.—*The Stethoscope.*

Prof. Pirrie, in the work before us, has elaborately discussed [illegible] safe and effectual [illegible] Perhaps no work upon [illegible] is so full upon the [illegible] *Nashville Journal of* [illegible]

PARRISH (EDWARD),

Lecturer on Practical Pharmacy and Materia Medica in the Pennsylvania Academy of Medicine, &c.

AN INTRODUCTION TO PRACTICAL PHARMACY.

Designed as a Text-Book for the Student, and as a Guide for the Physician and Pharmaceutist. With many Formulæ and Prescriptions. Second edition, greatly enlarged and improved. In one handsome octavo volume of 720 pages, with several hundred Illustrations, extra cloth. $3 50. (*Now Ready.*)

During the short time in which this work has been before the profession, it has been received with very great favor, and in assuming the position of a standard authority, it has filled a vacancy which had been severely felt. Stimulated by this encouragement, the author, in availing himself of the opportunity of revision, has spared no pains to render it more worthy of the confidence bestowed upon it, and his assiduous labors have made it rather a new book than a new edition, many portions having been rewritten, and much new and important matter added. These alterations and improvements have been rendered necessary by the rapid progress made by pharmaceutical science during the last few years, and by the additional experience obtained in the practical use of the volume as a text-book and work of reference. To accommodate these improvements, the size of the page has been materially enlarged, and the number of pages considerably increased, presenting in all nearly *one-half more* matter than the last edition. The work is therefore now presented as a complete exponent of the subject in its most advanced condition. From the most ordinary matters in the dispensing office, to the most complicated details of the vegetable alkaloids, it is hoped that everything requisite to the practising physician, and to the apothecary, will be found fully and clearly set forth, and that the new matter alone will be worth more than the very moderate cost of the work to those who have been consulting the previous edition.

That Edward Parrish, in writing a book upon *practical* Pharmacy some few years ago—one eminently original and unique—did the medical and pharmaceutical professions a great and valuable service, no one, we think, who has had access to its pages will deny; doubly welcome, then, is this new edition, containing the added results of his recent and rich experience as an observer, teacher, and practical operator in the pharmaceutical laboratory. The excellent plan of the first is more thoroughly, and in detail, carried out in this edition.—*Peninsular Med. Journal*, Jan. 1860.

We know of no work on the subject which would be more indispensable to the physician or student desiring information on the subject of which it treats. With Griffith's "Medical Formulary" and this, the practising physician would be supplied with nearly or quite all the most useful information on the subject.—*Charleston Med. Journal and Review*, Jan. 1860.

This edition, now much enlarged, is one of the most useful works of the past year.—*N. O. Med. and Surg. Journal*, Jan. 1860.

The whole treatise is eminently practical; and there is no production of the kind in the English language so well adapted to the wants of the pharmaceutist and druggist. To physicians, also, it cannot fail to be highly valuable, especially to those who are obliged to prepare and compound many of their own medicines.—*N. Am. Med. Chir. Review*, Jan. 1860.

Of course, all apothecaries who have not already a copy of the first edition will procure one of this; it is, therefore, to physicians residing in the country and in small towns, who cannot avail themselves of the skill of an educated pharmaceutist, that we would especially commend this work. In it they will find all that they desire to know, and should know, but very little of which they do really know in reference to this important collateral branch of their profession; for it is a well established fact, that, in the education of physicians, while the science of medicine is generally well taught, very little attention is paid to the art of preparing them for use, and we know not how this defect can be so well remedied as by procuring and consulting Dr. Parrish's excellent work.—*St. Louis Med. Journal*, Jan. 1860.

PEASLEE (E. R.), M. D.,

Professor of Physiology and General Pathology in the New York Medical College.

HUMAN HISTOLOGY, in its relations to Anatomy, Physiology, and Pathology;

for the use of Medical Students. With four hundred and thirty-four illustrations. In one handsome octavo volume, of over 600 pages. (*Lately Published.*) $3 75.

It embraces a library upon the topics discussed within itself, and is just what the teacher and learner need. Another advantage, by no means to be overlooked, everything of real value in the wide range which it embraces, is with great skill compressed into an octavo volume of but little more than six hundred pages. We have not only the whole subject of Histology, interesting in itself, ably and fully discussed, but what is of infinitely greater interest to the student, because of greater practical value, are its relations to Anatomy, Physiology, and Pathology, which are here fully and satisfactorily set forth.—*Nashville Journ. of Med. and Surgery*, Dec. 1857.

We would recommend it to the medical student and practitioner, as containing a summary of all that is known of the important subjects which it treats; of all that is contained in the great works of Simon and Lehmann, and the organic chemists in general. Master this one volume, we would say to the medical student and practitioner—master this book and you know all that is known of the great fundamental principles of medicine, and we have no hesitation in saying that it is an honor to the American medical profession that one of its members should have produced it.—*St. Louis Med. and Surg. Journal*, March, 1858.

PEREIRA (JONATHAN), M. D., F. R. S., AND L. S.

THE ELEMENTS OF MATERIA MEDICA AND THERAPEUTICS.

Third American edition, enlarged and improved by the author; including Notices of most of the Medicinal Substances in use in the civilized world, and forming an Encyclopædia of Materia Medica. Edited, with Additions, by Joseph Carson, M. D., Professor of Materia Medica and Pharmacy in the University of Pennsylvania. In two very large octavo volumes of 2109 pages, on small type, with about 500 illustrations on stone and wood, strongly bound in leather, with raised bands. $9 00.

*** Vol. II. will no longer be sold separate.

PARKER (LANGSTON),

Surgeon to the Queen's Hospital, Birmingham.

THE MODERN TREATMENT OF SYPHILITIC DISEASES, BOTH PRIMARY AND SECONDARY;

comprising the Treatment of Constitutional and Confirmed Syphilis, by a safe and successful method. With numerous Cases, Formulæ, and Clinical Observations. From the Third and entirely rewritten London edition. In one neat octavo volume, extra cloth, of 316 pages. $1 75.

RAMSBOTHAM (FRANCIS H.), M.D.

THE PRINCIPLES AND PRACTICE OF OBSTETRIC MEDICINE AND SURGERY, in reference to the Process of Parturition. A new and enlarged edition, thoroughly revised by the Author. With Additions by W. V. KEATING, M. D. In one large and handsome imperial octavo volume, of 650 pages, strongly bound in leather, with raised bands; with sixty-four beautiful Plates, and numerous Wood-cuts in the text, containing in all nearly two hundred large and beautiful figures. $5 00.

From Prof. Hodge, of the University of Pa.

To the American public, it is most valuable, from its intrinsic undoubted excellence, and as being the best authorized exponent of British Midwifery. Its circulation will, I trust, be extensive throughout our country.

It is unnecessary to say anything in regard to the utility of this work. It is already appreciated in our country for the value of the matter, the clearness of its style, and the fulness of its illustrations. To the physician's library it is indispensable, while to the student as a text-book, from which to extract the material for laying the foundation of an education on obstetrical science, it has no superior.—*Ohio Med. and Surg. Journal.*

The publishers have secured its success by the truly elegant style in which they have brought it out, excelling themselves in its production, especially in its plates. It is dedicated to Prof. Meigs, and has the emphatic endorsement of Prof. Hodge, as the best exponent of British Midwifery. We know of no text-book which deserves in all respects to be more highly recommended to students, and we could wish to see it in the hands of every practitioner, for they will find it invaluable for reference.—*Med. Gazette.*

RICORD (P.), M.D.

A TREATISE ON THE VENEREAL DISEASE. By JOHN HUNTER, F.R.S. With copious Additions, by PH. RICORD, M.D. Translated and Edited, with Notes, by FREEMAN J. BUMSTEAD, M.D., Lecturer on Venereal at the College of Physicians and Surgeons, New York. Second edition, revised, containing a *résumé* of RICORD'S RECENT LECTURES ON CHANCRE. In one handsome octavo volume, extra cloth, of 550 pages, with eight plates. $3 25. (*Just Issued.*)

In revising this work, the editor has endeavored to introduce whatever matter of interest the recent investigations of syphilographers have added to our knowledge of the subject. The principal source from which this has been derived is the volume of "*Lectures on Chancre,*" published a few months since by M. Ricord, which affords a large amount of new and instructive material on many controverted points. In the previous edition, M. Ricord's additions amounted to nearly one-third of the whole, and with the matter now introduced, the work may be considered to present his views and experience more thoroughly and completely than any other.

Every one will recognize the attractiveness and value which this work derives from thus presenting the opinions of these two masters side by side. But, it must be admitted, what has made the fortune of the book, is the fact that it contains the "most complete embodiment of the veritable doctrines of the Hôpital du Midi," which has ever been made public. The doctrinal ideas of M. Ricord, ideas which, if not universally adopted, are incontestably dominant, have heretofore only been interpreted by more or less skilful secretaries, sometimes accredited and sometimes not. In the notes to Hunter, the master substitutes himself for his interpreters, and gives his original thoughts to the world in a lucid and perfectly intelligible manner. In conclusion we can say that this is incontestably the best treatise on syphilis with which we are acquainted, and, as we do not often employ the phrase, we may be excused for expressing the hope that it may find a place in the library of every physician.—*Virginia Med. and Surg. Journal.*

BY THE SAME AUTHOR.

RICORD'S LETTERS ON SYPHILIS. Translated by W. P. LATTIMORE, M.D. In one neat octavo volume, of 270 pages, extra cloth. $2 00.

ROYLE'S MATERIA MEDICA AND THERAPEUTICS; including the Preparations of the Pharmacopœias of London, Edinburgh, Dublin, and of the United States. With many new medicines. Edited by JOSEPH CARSON, M. D. With ninety-eight illustrations. In one large octavo volume, extra cloth, of about 700 pages. $3 00.

ROKITANSKY (CARL), M.D.,

Curator of the Imperial Pathological Museum, and Professor at the University of Vienna, &c.

A MANUAL OF PATHOLOGICAL ANATOMY. Four volumes, octavo, bound in two, extra cloth, of about 1200 pages. Translated by W. E. SWAINE, EDWARD SIEVEKING, C. H. MOORE, and G. E. DAY. $5 50

The profession is too well acquainted with the reputation of Rokitansky's work to need our assurance that this is one of the most profound, thorough, and valuable books ever issued from the medical press. It is *sui generis*, and has no standard of comparison. It is only necessary to announce that it is issued in a form as cheap as is compatible with its size and preservation, and its sale follows as a matter of course. No library can be called complete without it.—*Buffalo Med. Journal.*

An attempt to give our readers any adequate idea of the vast amount of instruction accumulated in these volumes, would be feeble and hopeless. The effort of the distinguished author to concentrate in a small space his great fund of knowledge, has so charged his text with valuable truths, that any attempt of a reviewer to epitomize is at once paralyzed, and must end in a failure.—*Western Lancet.*

As this is the highest source of knowledge upon the important subject of which it treats, no real student can afford to be without it. The American publishers have entitled themselves to the thanks of the profession of their country, for this timeous and beautiful edition.—*Nashville Journal of Medicine.*

As a book of reference, therefore, this work must prove of inestimable value, and we cannot too highly recommend it to the profession.—*Charleston Med. Journal and Review.*

This book is a necessity to every practitioner.—*Am. Med. Monthly.*

RIGBY (EDWARD), M.D.,

Senior Physician to the General Lying-in Hospital, &c.

A SYSTEM OF MIDWIFERY. With Notes and Additional Illustrations. Second American Edition. One volume octavo, extra cloth, 422 pages. $2 50.

BY THE SAME AUTHOR. (*Lately Published.*)

ON THE CONSTITUTIONAL TREATMENT OF FEMALE DISEASES. In one neat royal 12mo. volume, extra cloth, of about 250 pages. $1 00.

STILLÉ (ALFRED), M.D.

THERAPEUTICS AND MATERIA MEDICA; a Systematic Treatise on the Action, and Uses of Medicinal Agents, including their Description and History. In two large and handsome octavo volumes, of 1789 pages. (*Now Ready*, 1860.) $5 00.

This work is designed especially for the student and practitioner of medicine, and treats the various articles of the Materia Medica from the point of view of the bedside, and not of the shop or of the lecture-room. While thus endeavoring to give all practical information likely to be useful with respect to the employment of special remedies in special affections, and the results to be anticipated from their administration, a copious Index of Diseases and their Remedies renders the work eminently fitted for reference by showing at a glance the different means which have been employed, and enabling the practitioner to extend his resources in difficult cases with all that the experience of the profession has suggested. At the same time particular care has been given to the subject of General Therapeutics, and at the commencement of each class of medicines there is a chapter devoted to the consideration of their common influence upon morbid conditions. The action of remedial agents upon the healthy economy and on animals has likewise received particular notice, from the conviction that their physiological effects will afford frequent explanations of their pathological influence, and in many cases lead to new and important suggestions as to their practical use in disease. Within the scope thus designed by the author, no labor has been spared to accumulate all the facts which have accrued from the experience of the profession in all ages and all countries; and the vast amount of recent researches recorded in the periodical literature of both hemispheres has been zealously laid under contribution, resulting in a mass of practical information scarcely attempted hitherto in any similar work in the language.

Our expectations of the value of this work were based on the well-known reputation and character of the author as a man of scholarly attainments, an elegant writer, a candid inquirer after truth, and a philosophical thinker; we knew that the task would be conscientiously performed, and that few, if any, among the distinguished medical teachers in this country are better qualified than he to prepare a systematic treatise on therapeutics in accordance with the present requirements of medical science. Our preliminary examination of the work has satisfied us that we were not mistaken in our anticipations. In congratulating the author on the completion of the great labor which such a work involves, we are happy in expressing the conviction that its merits will receive that reward which is above all price—the grateful appreciation of his medical brethren.—*New Orleans Medical News*, March, 1860.

We think this work will do much to obviate the reluctance to a thorough investigation of this branch of scientific study, for in the wide range of medical literature treasured in the English tongue, we shall hardly find a work written in a style more clear and simple, conveying forcibly the facts taught, and yet free from turgidity and redundancy. There is a fascination in its pages that will insure to it a wide popularity and attentive perusal, and a degree of usefulness not often attained through the influence of a single work. The author has much enhanced the practical utility of his book by passing briefly over the physical, botanical, and commercial history of medicines, and directing attention chiefly to their physiological action, and their application for the amelioration or cure of disease. He ignores hypothesis and theory which are so alluring to many medical writers, and so liable to lead them astray, and confines himself to such facts as have been tried in the crucible of experience.—*Chicago Medical Journal*, March, 1860.

The plan pursued by the author in these very elaborate volumes is not strictly one of scientific unity and precision; he has rather subordinated these to practical utility. Dr. Stillé has produced a work which will be valuable equally to the student of medicine and the busy practitioner.—*London Lancet*, March 10, 1860.

With Pereira, Dunglison, Mitchell, and Wood before us, we may well ask if there was a necessity for a new book on the subject. After examining this work with some care, we can answer affirmatively. Dr. Wood's book is well adapted for students, while Dr. Stillé's will be more satisfactory to the practitioner, who desires to study the action of medicines. The author needs no encomiums from us, for he is well known as a ripe scholar and a man of the most extensive reading in his profession. This work bears evidence of this fact on every page.—*Cincinnati Lancet*, April, 1860.

SMITH (HENRY H.), M.D.

MINOR SURGERY; or, Hints on the Every-day Duties of the Surgeon. With 247 illustrations. Third edition. 1 vol. royal 12mo., pp. 456. In leather, $2 25; cloth, $2 00.

BY THE SAME AUTHOR, AND

HORNER (WILLIAM E.), M.D.,

Late Professor of Anatomy in the University of Pennsylvania.

AN ANATOMICAL ATLAS, illustrative of the Structure of the Human Body. In one volume, large imperial octavo, extra cloth, with about six hundred and fifty beautiful figures. $3 00.

These figures are well selected, and present a complete and accurate representation of that wonderful fabric, the human body. The plan of this Atlas, which renders it so peculiarly convenient for the student, and its superb artistical execution, have been already pointed out. We must congratulate the student upon the completion of this Atlas, as it is the most convenient work of the kind that has yet appeared; and we must add, the very beautiful manner in which it is "got up" is so creditable to the country as to be flattering to our national pride.—*American Medical Journal*.

SHARPEY (WILLIAM), M.D., JONES QUAIN, M.D., AND RICHARD QUAIN, F.R.S., &c.

HUMAN ANATOMY. Revised, with Notes and Additions, by JOSEPH LEIDY, M.D., Professor of Anatomy in the University of Pennsylvania. Complete in two large octavo volumes, leather, of about thirteen hundred pages. Beautifully illustrated with over five hundred engravings on wood. $6 00.

SIMPSON (J. Y.), M.D.,

Professor of Midwifery, &c., in the University of Edinburgh, &c.

CLINICAL LECTURES ON THE DISEASES OF FEMALES. With numerous illustrations.

This valuable series of practical Lectures is now appearing in the "MEDICAL NEWS AND LIBRARY" for 1860, and can thus be had without cost by subscribers to the "AMERICAN JOURNAL OF THE MEDICAL SCIENCES." See p. 2.

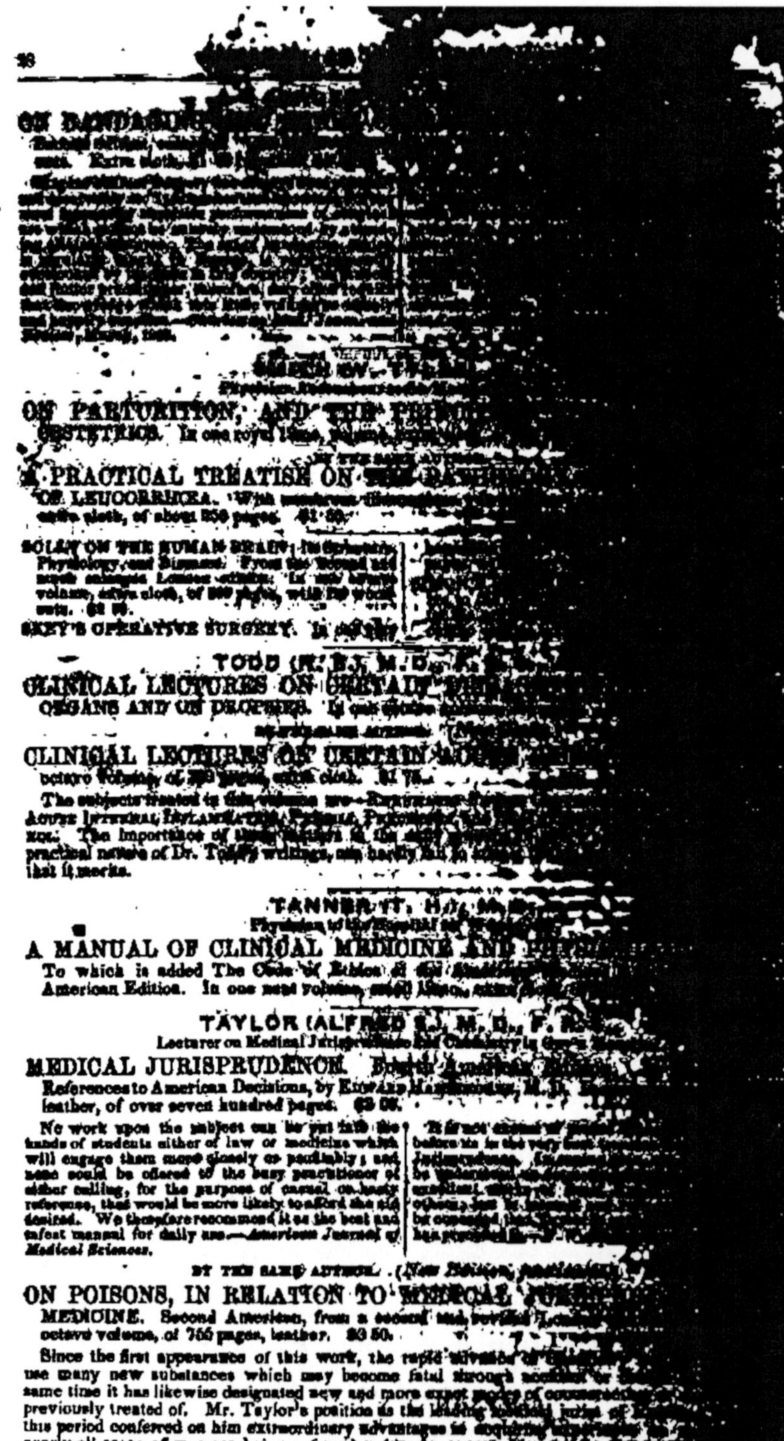

ON PARTURITION, AND [illegible]

OBSTETRICS. In one royal 12mo. [illegible]

A PRACTICAL TREATISE ON [illegible]

OF LEUCORRHŒA. [illegible] extra cloth, of about 250 pages. $1 50.

SKEY'S OPERATIVE SURGERY. In [illegible]

TODD (R. B.), M.D., [illegible]

CLINICAL LECTURES ON CERTAIN [illegible]

ORGANS AND ON DROPSIES. [illegible]

CLINICAL LECTURES ON CERTAIN [illegible]

The subjects treated in this volume are [illegible] practical nature of Dr. Todd's writings, can hardly fail to [illegible] that it merits.

TANNER (T. H.), M.D., [illegible]

A MANUAL OF CLINICAL MEDICINE AND [illegible]

To which is added The Code of Ethics of [illegible] American Edition. In one neat volume, small 12mo., [illegible]

TAYLOR (ALFRED S.), M.D., F.R.S., [illegible]

Lecturer on Medical Jurisprudence and Chemistry in [illegible]

MEDICAL JURISPRUDENCE. [illegible] References to American Decisions, by Edward Hartshorne, M.D. [illegible] leather, of over seven hundred pages. $3 00.

No work upon the subject can be put into the hands of students either of law or medicine which will engage them more closely or profitably; and none could be offered to the busy practitioner of either calling, for the purpose of casual or hasty reference, that would be more likely to afford the aid desired. We therefore recommend it as the best and safest manual for daily use.—*American Journal of Medical Sciences.*

BY THE SAME AUTHOR. (*New Edition*, [illegible])

ON POISONS, IN RELATION TO MEDICAL [illegible]

MEDICINE. Second American, from a second and revised London [illegible] octavo volume, of 755 pages, leather. $3 50.

Since the first appearance of this work, the rapid advance of [illegible] use many new substances which may become fatal through accident or [illegible] same time it has likewise designated new and more exact modes of [illegible] previously treated of. Mr. Taylor's position as the leading [illegible] this period conferred on him extraordinary advantages in acquiring [illegible] nearly all cases of moment being referred to him for [illegible] is generally accepted as final. The results of his labors, therefore, [illegible] volume, carefully weighed and sifted, and presented in the clear and [illegible] he is noted, may be received as an acknowledged authority, [illegible] implicit confidence.

TODD (ROBERT BENTLEY), M. D., F. R. S.,
Professor of Physiology in King's College, London, and
WILLIAM BOWMAN, F. R. S.,
Demonstrator of Anatomy in King's College, London.

THE PHYSIOLOGICAL ANATOMY AND PHYSIOLOGY OF MAN. With about three hundred large and beautiful illustrations on wood. Complete in one large octavo volume, of 950 pages, leather. Price $4 50.

☞ Gentlemen who have received portions of this work, as published in the "MEDICAL NEWS AND LIBRARY," can now complete their copies, if immediate application be made. It will be furnished as follows, free by mail, in paper covers, with cloth backs.

PARTS I., II., III. (pp. 25 to 552), $2 50.
PART IV. (pp. 553 to end, with Title, Preface, Contents, &c.), $2 00.
Or, PART IV., SECTION II. (pp. 725 to end, with Title, Preface, Contents, &c.), $1 25.

A magnificent contribution to British medicine, and the American physician who shall fail to peruse it, will have failed to read one of the most instructive books of the nineteenth century.—*N. O. Med and Surg. Journal*, Sept. 1867.

It is more concise than Carpenter's Principles, and more modern than the accessible edition of Müller's Elements; its details are brief, but sufficient; its descriptions vivid; its illustrations exact and copious; and its language terse and perspicuous.—*Charleston Med. Journal*, July, 1867.

We know of no work on the subject of physiology so well adapted to the wants of the medical student. Its completion has been thus long delayed, that the authors might secure accuracy by personal observation.—*St. Louis Med. and Surg. Journal*, Sept. '67.

Our notice, though it conveys but a very feeble and imperfect idea of the magnitude and importance of the work now under consideration, already transcends our limits; and, with the indulgence of our readers, and the hope that they will peruse the book for themselves, as we feel we can with confidence recommend it, we leave it in their hands.—*The Northwestern Med. and Surg. Journal*.

TOYNBEE (JOSEPH), F. R. S.,
Aural Surgeon to, and Lecturer on Surgery at, St. Mary's Hospital.

A PRACTICAL TREATISE ON DISEASES OF THE EAR; their Diagnosis, Pathology, and Treatment. Illustrated with one hundred engravings on wood. In one very handsome octavo volume, extra cloth, $3 00. (*Now Ready.*)

Mr Toynbee's name is too widely known as the highest authority on all matters connected with Aural Surgery and Medicine, to require special attention to be called to anything which he may communicate to the profession on the subject. Twenty years' labor devoted to the present work has embodied in it the results of an amount of experience and observation which perhaps no other living practitioner has enjoyed. It therefore cannot fail to prove a complete and trustworthy guide on all matters connected with this obscure and little known class of diseases, which so frequently embarrass the general practitioner.

The volume will be found thoroughly illustrated with a large number of original wood-engravings, elucidating the pathology of the organs of hearing, instruments, operations, &c., and in every respect it is one of the handsomest specimens of mechanical execution issued from the American press.

The following condensed synopsis of the contents will show the plan adopted by the author, and the completeness with which all departments of the subject are brought under consideration.

CHAPTER I. Introduction—Mode of Investigation—Dissection. II. The External Ear—Anatomy—Pathology—Malformations—Diseases. III. The External Meatus—Its Exploration. IV. The External Meatus—Foreign Bodies and Accumulations of Cerumen. V. The External Meatus—The Dermis and its Diseases. VI. The External Meatus—Polypi. VII. The External Meatus—Tumors. VIII. The Membrana Tympani—Structure and Functions. IX. The Membrana Tympani—Diseases. X. The Membrana Tympani—Diseases. XI. The Eustachian Tube—Obstructions. XII. The Cavity of the Tympanum—Anatomy—Pathology—Diseases. XIII. The Cavity of the Tympanum—Diseases. XIV. The Mastoid Cells—Diseases. XV. The Diseases of the Nervous Apparatus of the Ear, producing what is commonly called "Nervous Deafness." XVI. The Diseases of the Nervous Apparatus, continued. XVII. Malignant Disease of the Ear. XVIII. On the Deaf and Dumb. XIX. Ear-Trumpets and their uses. APPENDIX.

WILLIAMS (C. J. B.), M. D., F. R. S.,
Professor of Clinical Medicine in University College, London, &c.

PRINCIPLES OF MEDICINE. An Elementary View of the Causes, Nature, Treatment, Diagnosis, and Prognosis of Disease; with brief remarks on Hygienics, or the preservation of health. A new American, from the third and revised London edition. In one octavo volume, leather, of about 500 pages. $3 50. (*Just Issued.*)

We find that the deeply-interesting matter and style of this book have so far fascinated us, that we have unconsciously hung upon its pages, not too long, indeed, for our own profit, but longer than reviewers can be permitted to indulge. We leave the further analysis to the student and practitioner. Our judgment of the work has already been sufficiently expressed. It is a judgment of almost unqualified praise.—*London Lancet.*

A text-book to which no other in our language is comparable.—*Charleston Medical Journal.*

No work has ever achieved or maintained a more deserved reputation.—*Va. Med. and Surg. Journal.*

WHAT TO OBSERVE
AT THE BEDSIDE AND AFTER DEATH, IN MEDICAL CASES. Published under the authority of the London Society for Medical Observation. A new American, from the second and revised London edition. In one very handsome volume, royal 12mo., extra cloth. $1 00.

To the observer who prefers accuracy to blunders and precision to carelessness, this little book is invaluable.—*N. H. Journal of Medicine.*

One of the finest aids to a young practitioner we have ever seen.—*Peninsular Journal of Medicine.*

New and much enlarged edition—(Just Issued.)

WATSON (THOMAS), M. D., &c.,

Late Physician to the Middlesex Hospital, &c.

LECTURES ON THE PRINCIPLES AND PRACTICE OF PHYSIC.

Delivered at King's College, London. A new American, from the last revised and enlarged English edition, with Additions, by D. FRANCIS CONDIE, M. D., author of "A Practical Treatise on the Diseases of Children," &c. With one hundred and eighty-five illustrations on wood. In one very large and handsome volume, imperial octavo, of over 1200 closely printed pages in small type; the whole strongly bound in leather, with raised bands. Price $4 25.

That the high reputation of this work might be fully maintained, the author has subjected it to a thorough revision; every portion has been examined with the aid of the most recent researches in pathology, and the results of modern investigations in both theoretical and practical subjects have been carefully weighed and embodied throughout its pages. The watchful scrutiny of the editor has likewise introduced whatever possesses immediate importance to the American physician in relation to diseases incident to our climate which are little known in England, as well as those points in which experience here has led to different modes of practice; and he has also added largely to the series of illustrations, believing that in this manner valuable assistance may be conveyed to the student in elucidating the text. The work will, therefore, be found thoroughly on a level with the most advanced state of medical science on both sides of the Atlantic.

The additions which the work has received are shown by the fact that notwithstanding an enlargement in the size of the page, more than two hundred additional pages have been necessary to accommodate the two large volumes of the London edition (which sells at ten dollars), within the compass of a single volume, and in its present form it contains the matter of at least three ordinary octavos. Believing it to be a work which should lie on the table of every physician, and be in the hands of every student, the publishers have put it at a price within the reach of all, making it one of the cheapest books as yet presented to the American profession, while at the same time the beauty of its mechanical execution renders it an exceedingly attractive volume.

The fourth edition now appears, so carefully revised, as to add considerably to the value of a book already acknowledged, wherever the English language is read, to be beyond all comparison the best systematic work on the Principles and Practice of Physic in the whole range of medical literature. Every lecture contains proof of the extreme anxiety of the author to keep pace with the advancing knowledge of the day, and to bring the results of the labors, not only of physicians, but of chemists and histologists, before his readers, wherever they can be turned to useful account. And this is done with such a cordial appreciation of the merit due to the industrious observer, such a generous desire to encourage younger and rising men, and such a candid acknowledgment of his own obligations to them, that one scarcely knows whether to admire most the pure, simple, forcible English—the vast amount of useful practical information condensed into the Lectures—or the manly, kind-hearted, unassuming character of the lecturer shining through his work. —*London Med. Times and Gazette*, Oct. 31, 1857.

Thus these admirable volumes come before the profession in their fourth edition, abounding in those distinguished attributes of moderation, judgment, erudite cultivation, clearness, and eloquence, with which they were from the first invested, but yet richer than before in the results of more prolonged observation, and in the able appreciation of the latest advances in pathology and medicine by one of the most profound medical thinkers of the day.—*London Lancet*, Nov. 14, 1857.

The lecturer's skill, his wisdom, his learning, are equalled by the ease of his graceful diction, his eloquence, and the far higher qualities of candor, of courtesy, of modesty, and of generous appreciation of merit in others. May he long remain to instruct us, and to enjoy, in the glorious sunset of his declining years, the honors, the confidence and love gained during his useful life.—*N. A. Med.-Chir. Review*, July, 1858.

Watson's unrivalled, perhaps unapproachable work on Practice—the copious additions made to which (the fourth edition) have given it all the novelty and much of the interest of a new book.—*Charleston Med. Journal*, July, 1858.

Lecturers, practitioners, and students of medicine will equally hail the reappearance of the work of Dr. Watson in the form of a new—a fourth—edition. We merely do justice to our own feelings, and, we are sure, of the whole profession, if we thank him for having, in the trouble and turmoil of a large practice, made leisure to supply the hiatus caused by the exhaustion of the publisher's stock of the third edition, which has been severely felt for the last three years. For Dr. Watson has not merely caused the lectures to be reprinted, but scattered through the whole work we find additions or alterations which prove that the author has in every way sought to bring up his teaching to the level of the most recent acquisitions in science.—*Brit. and For. Medico-Chir. Review*, Jan. 1858.

WALSHE (W. H.), M. D.,

Professor of the Principles and Practice of Medicine in University College, London, &c.

A PRACTICAL TREATISE ON DISEASES OF THE LUNGS; including

the Principles of Physical Diagnosis. A new American, from the third revised and much enlarged London edition. In one vol. octavo, of 468 pages. (*Just Ready.*) $2 25.

The present edition has been carefully revised and much enlarged, and may be said in the main to be rewritten. Descriptions of several diseases, previously omitted, are now introduced; the causes and mode of production of the more important affections, so far as they possess direct practical significance, are succinctly inquired into; an effort has been made to bring the description of anatomical characters to the level of the wants of the practical physician; and the diagnosis and prognosis of each complaint are more completely considered. The sections on TREATMENT and the Appendix (concerning the influence of climate on pulmonary disorders), have, especially, been largely extended.—*Author's Preface.*

*** To be followed by a similar volume on Diseases of the Heart and Aorta.

WILSON (ERASMUS), F. R. S.,

Lecturer on Anatomy, London.

THE DISSECTOR'S MANUAL; or, Practical and Surgical Anatomy. Third

American, from the last revised and enlarged English edition. Modified and rearranged, by WILLIAM HUNT, M. D., Demonstrator of Anatomy in the University of Pennsylvania. In one large and handsome royal 12mo. volume, leather, of 582 pages, with 154 illustrations. $2 00.

WINSLOW (FORBES), M. D., D. C. L., &c.

ON OBSCURE DISEASES OF THE BRAIN AND DISORDERS OF THE MIND;

their incipient Symptoms, Pathology, Diagnosis, Treatment, and Prophylaxis. In one handsome octavo volume, of nearly 600 pages. (*Just Ready.*) $3 00.

The momentous questions discussed in this volume have perhaps not hitherto been so ably and elaborately treated. Dr. Winslow's distinguished reputation and long experience in everything relating to insanity invest his teachings with the highest authority, and in this carefully considered volume he has drawn upon the accumulated resources of a life of observation. His deductions are founded on a vast number of cases, the peculiarities of which are related in detail, rendering the work not only one of sound instruction, but of lively interest; the author's main object being to point out the connection between organic disease and insanity, tracing the latter through all its stages from mere eccentricity to mania, and urging the necessity of early measures of prophylaxis and appropriate treatment. A subject of greater importance to society at large could scarcely be named; while to the physician who may at any moment be called upon for interference in the most delicate relations of life, or for an opinion in a court of justice, a work like the present may be considered indispensable.

The treatment of the subject may be gathered from the following summary of the contents:—

CHAPTER I. Introduction.—II. Morbid Phenomena of Intelligence. III. Premonitory Symptoms of Insanity.—IV. Confessions of Patients after Recovery.—V. State of the Mind during Recovery.—VI. Anomalous and Masked Affections of the Mind.—VII. The Stage of Consciousness.—VIII. Stage of Exaltation.—IX. Stage of Mental Depression.—X. Stage of Aberration.—XI. Impairment of Mind.—XII. Morbid Phenomena of Attention.—XIII. Morbid Phenomena of Memory.—XIV. Acute Disorders of Memory.—XV. Chronic Affections of Memory.—XVI. Perversion and Exaltation of Memory.—XVII. Psychology and Pathology of Memory.—XVIII. Morbid Phenomena of Motion.—XIX. Morbid Phenomena of Speech.—XX. Morbid Phenomena of Sensation.—XXI. Morbid Phenomena of the Special Senses.—XXII. Morbid Phenomena of Vision, Hearing, Taste, Touch, and Smell.—XXIII. Morbid Phenomena of Sleep and Dreaming.—XXIV. Morbid Phenomena of Organic and Nutritive Life.—XXV. General Principles of Pathology, Diagnosis, Treatment, and Prophylaxis.

WEST (CHARLES), M. D.,

Accoucheur to and Lecturer on Midwifery at St. Bartholomew's Hospital, Physician to the Hospital for Sick Children, &c.

LECTURES ON THE DISEASES OF WOMEN.

Now complete in one handsome octavo volume, extra cloth, of about 500 pages; price $2 50.

Also, for sale separate, PART II, being pp. 309 to end, with Index, Title matter, &c., 8vo., cloth, price $1.

We must now conclude this hastily written sketch with the confident assurance to our readers that the work will well repay perusal. The conscientious, painstaking, practical physician is apparent on every page.—*N. Y. Journal of Medicine*, March, 1858.

We know of no treatise of the kind so complete and yet so compact.—*Chicago Med. Journal*, January, 1858.

A fairer, more honest, more earnest, and more reliable investigator of the many diseases of women and children is not to be found in any country.—*Southern Med. and Surg. Journal*, January 1858.

We gladly recommend his Lectures as in the highest degree instructive to all who are interested in obstetric practice.—*London Lancet.*

We have to say of it, briefly and decidedly, that it is the best work on the subject in any language; and that it stamps Dr. West as the *facile princeps* of British obstetric authors.—*Edinb. Med. Journ.*

BY THE SAME AUTHOR. (*Now Ready.*)

LECTURES ON THE DISEASES OF INFANCY AND CHILDHOOD.

Third American, from the fourth enlarged and improved London edition. In one handsome octavo volume, extra cloth, of about six hundred and fifty pages. $1 75.

The continued favor with which this work has been received has stimulated the author to render it in every respect more complete and more worthy the confidence of the profession. Containing nearly two hundred pages more than the last American edition, with several additional Lectures and a careful revision and enlargement of those formerly comprised in it, it can hardly fail to maintain its reputation as a clear and judicious text-book for the student, and a safe and reliable guide for the practitioner. The fact stated by the author that these Lectures "now embody the results of 900 observations and 288 post-mortem examinations made among nearly 30,000 children, who, during the past twenty-years, have come under my care," is sufficient to show their high practical value as the result of an amount of experience which few physicians enjoy.

The three former editions of the work now before us have placed the author in the foremost rank of those physicians who have devoted special attention to the diseases of early life. We attempt no analysis of this edition, but may refer the reader to some of the chapters to which the largest additions have been made—those on Diphtheria, Disorders of the Mind, and Idiocy, for instance—as a proof that the work is really a new edition; not a mere reprint. In its present shape it will be found of the greatest possible service in the every-day practice of nine-tenths of the profession.—*Med. Times and Gazette*, London, Dec. 10, 1859.

All things considered, this book of Dr. West is by far the best treatise in our language upon such modifications of morbid action and disease as are witnessed when we have to deal with infancy and childhood. It is true that it confines itself to such disorders as come within the province of the *physician*, and even with respect to these it is unequal as regards minuteness of consideration, and some diseases it omits to notice altogether. But those who know anything of the present condition of pædiatrics will readily admit that it would be next to impossible to effect more, or effect it better, than the accoucheur of St. Bartholomew's has done in a single volume. The lecture (XVI.) upon Disorders of the Mind in children is an admirable specimen of the value of the later information conveyed in the Lectures of Dr. Charles West.—*London Lancet*, Oct. 22, 1859.

Since the appearance of the first edition, about eleven years ago, the experience of the author has doubled; so that, whereas the lectures at first were founded on six hundred observations, and one hundred and eighty dissections made among nearly fourteen thousand children, they now embody the results of nine hundred observations, and two hundred and eighty-eight post-mortem examinations made among nearly thirty thousand children, who, during the past twenty years, have been under his care.—*British Med. Journal*, Oct. 1, 1859.

BY THE SAME AUTHOR.

AN ENQUIRY INTO THE PATHOLOGICAL IMPORTANCE OF ULCERATION OF THE OS UTERI.

In one neat octavo volume, extra cloth. $1 00.

Breinigsville, PA USA
19 October 2010

247609BV00002B/18/P

9 781143 673658